Gerioperative Nursing Care

Raelene V. Shippee-Rice, PhD, RN, is Associate Professor Emerita, former chair, University of New Hampshire, Department of Nursing and Associate Dean for Research, School of Health and Human Services. From 2003 to 2006, she was a member of the Clinical Nurse Leader Implementation Task Force of the American Association of Colleges of Nursing. In 1999 and 2000, she served as Education Associate, John A. Hartford Institute for Geriatric Nursing, New York University. She is the recipient of 14 grants on caring for older adults and the elderly. One grant led to the concept of care receiver burden. A two-time Fulbright Scholar, she studied family caregiving in Russia and Bulgaria. She served as visiting scholar at the University of Leeds, England, studying family caregiving. She has presented nationally and internationally on family caregiving, care receiver burden, and gerontological care of older adults. Dr. Shippee-Rice is a reviewer for four major research journals, a member of Sigma Theta Tau Honor Society in Nursing, and served as a board member to the Eastern Nursing Research Society and Association for Gerontology in Higher Education.

Susan J. Fetzer, PhD, RN, MBA, CNL, is tenured Professor at the University of New Hampshire, Department of Nursing and the Director of Nursing Research, Southern New Hampshire Medical Center. With over 30 years of nursing practice focused on surgical patients and perianesthesia practice, she has published widely, including in the *Journal of Perianesthesia Nursing*, and served as President of the American Board of Post-Anesthesia Nursing Certification. Dr. Fetzer is the recipient of research grants related to perianesthesia nursing and been recognized by the American Society of PeriAnesthesia Nurses with the Outstanding Researcher and Outstanding Achievement Award. She is an alumna of the Hartford Institute for Summer Research Scholars, an active member of the Eastern Nursing Research Society, and is a member of Sigma Theta Tau International.

Jennifer V. Long, MS, ANP, CRNA, is a nurse anesthetist with an 18-year health care career focused on elder care. Ms. Long was a staff nurse at the Veterans Affairs Medical Center in West Virginia for 3 years, where she focused on the care of World War II and Vietnam veterans. After obtaining her ANP certification, she practiced in an internal medicine primary care center for 4 years, concentrating on geriatric care. She is a member of Sigma Theta Tau Honor Society in Nursing, the American Association of Nurse Anesthetists (AANA), and the Pennsylvania Association of Nurse Anesthetists. She served on the Practice Committee for the AANA. Ms. Long has lectured on anesthesia care of the older adult emphasizing geriatric anesthesia as a subspecialty of anesthesia.

Gerioperative Nursing Care

*Principles and Practices of Surgical Care
for the Older Adult*

Raelene V. Shippee-Rice, PhD, RN
Susan J. Fetzer, PhD, RN, MBA, CNL
Jennifer V. Long, MS, ANP, CRNA

SPRINGER PUBLISHING COMPANY
NEW YORK

Springer Publishing Company, LLC
11 West 42nd Street
New York, NY 10036
www.springerpub.com

Acquisitions Editor: Allan Graubard
Production Editor: Dana Bigelow
Composition: Absolute Service, Inc.

ISBN: 9780826104700
ebook ISBN: 9780826104717

11 12 13 14 / 5 4 3 2 1

The author and the publisher of this work have made every effort to use sources believed to be reliable to provide information that is accurate and compatible with the standards generally accepted at the time of publication. Because medical science is continually advancing, our knowledge base continues to expand. Therefore, as new information becomes available, changes in procedures become necessary. We recommend that the reader always consult current research and specific institutional policies before performing any clinical procedure. The author and publisher shall not be liable for any special, consequential, or exemplary damages resulting, in whole or in part, from the readers' use of, or reliance on, the information contained in this book. The publisher has no responsibility for the persistence or accuracy of URLs for external or third-party Internet Web sites referred to in this publication and does not guarantee that any content on such Web sites is, or will remain, accurate or appropriate.

Library of Congress Cataloging-in-Publication Data

Shippee-Rice, Raelene V.
  Gerioperative nursing care : principles and practices of surgical care for the older adult / Raelene V. Shippee-Rice, Susan J. Fetzer, Jennifer V. Long.
    p. ; cm.
  Includes bibliographical references and index.
  ISBN 978-0-8261-0470-0 — ISBN 978-0-8261-0471-7 (ebook)
  I. Fetzer, Susan J. II. Long, Jennifer V. III. Title.
  [DNLM: 1. Geriatric Nursing--methods. 2. Perioperative Nursing—methods. 3. Aging—physiology. WY 152]
  LC classification not assigned
  618.97'0231—dc23
                        2011042452

Printed in the United States of America by Bradford & Bigelow.

Contents

Contributing Authors

David E. Durant, MS, APN, CRNA, has been practicing cardiac anesthesia with the largest open heart program in Delaware for 20 years. He is currently at Anesthesia Services P.A., Newark, Delaware. This has included both adult and pediatric cases. He is a member of the American Association of Nurse Anesthetists.

Kathleen M. Gilkey, MSN, CRNA, has a 29-year health care career including flight nursing, emergency department nursing, and medical/surgical/neurological intensive care unit nursing, and is currently employed as a Certified Registered Nurse Anesthetist at the Cumberland Anesthesia Associates, Cumberland, Maryland. She has been involved with prehospital medicine since 1980 and is the operating room clinical coordinator for paramedics at Western Maryland Regional Medical Center. She is a member of Sigma Theta Tau International and the American Association of Nurse Anesthetists.

Donna Pelletier, DNP, APRN, is certified in health coaching and interested in lifestyle behavior change, health promotion, and chronic disease prevention and management. Her professional career has spanned over 30 years of nursing experience in clinical practice and nursing education. Currently, she is a Clinical Associate Professor at the University of New Hampshire Department of Nursing, Durham, and works as a family nurse practitioner in an urgent care clinic. Previously, she cared for residents in a long-term care setting. Ms. Pelletier has a strong background in elder health issues and has presented regionally and nationally on geriatric care best practices in long-term care nursing, observing and understanding the older adult, geriatric syndromes, and assessing and managing common health problems of elders.

Illustrators

Elisabeth Miningham-Monsour started her formal study of oil painting under the direction of her grandmother, Caroline Haas, a prominent artist in the Philadelphia area, and continued formal art classes into college. Ms. Miningham-Monsour graduated with an occupational therapy degree and worked with the elderly for over 10 years in various health care settings. She now teaches art in middle and high schools in Pennsylvania.

Kathleen M. Gilkey, MSN, CRNA, has a 29-year health care career including flight nursing, emergency department nursing, and medical/surgical/neurological intensive care unit nursing, and is currently employed as a Certified Registered Nurse Anesthetist at the Cumberland Anesthesia Associates, Cumberland, Maryland. She has been involved with prehospital medicine since 1980 and is the operating room clinical coordinator for paramedics at Western Maryland Regional Medical Center. She is a member of Sigma Theta Tau International and the American Association of Nurse Anesthetists.

Foreword

Gerioperative Nursing Care is a wonderful addition to the sources of knowledge related to best practices for older adults. Dr. Shippee-Rice, Dr. Fetzer, and Ms. Long have edited an accessible textbook that will guide readers to the important literature related to best practices for surgical care of older adults. Why is this so important? Our hospitals and medical centers are increasingly becoming surgical centers for older adults admitted briefly for surgical procedures and then almost immediately discharged. In their introductory section, the authors make the point that there is extraordinary functional diversity in older adults and appropriate care for older individuals undergoing surgery requires an extensive knowledge of chronic disease, co-morbidities, pharmacologic complexity, and the high risk for iatrogenic complications. I further commend the authors for clearly describing the goals of each chapter with bullets related to what the readers will know upon completion of each chapter. In this era of knowledge explosion leaving us all in a true quandary over what to read given the array of academic materials published, this book is essential for nurses and other healthcare professionals who are involved in this practice arena. It's quite extraordinary to note the fact that older adults have a rate of general surgery three times higher than younger individuals and that one can anticipate an increased proportion of surgical intervention with aging, particularly in the gastrointestinal and orthopedic specialty areas. The importance of this book is reflected by the example that the total volume of hip arthroplasties is expected to grow by 174% and the demand for knee arthroplasties by over 500% by 2030. There is little wonder that these editors have seized the opportunity to compile a textbook that is focused on perioperative care of older adults, cleverly entitled *Gerioperative Nursing Care*. The chapters on the body systems are extremely well written and important given the necessity of all aging systems to successfully negotiate surgery. Ventilation, metabolism, and excretion are obviously critical aspects of recovering from surgery, and the authors have done an excellent job in making this complex content clear to even the newly licensed nurse.

I would further highlight the chapter on informed consent that is a crucial element in any pre-anesthesia scenario. The issues related to informed consent are well described with important dimensions such as the voluntary nature of consent and literacy underscored for both culturally competent care and ethical care.

Nurses need to know and understand how aging and age related changes make the care of older adults across the perioperative continuum different from other populations. Further, they need to think about what they know and how to use that knowledge for primary and secondary intervention. Prevention must be the lynchpin to successful care of older adults. Gerioperative care can be used as a model for restructuring clinical practice to focus individual provider, interdisciplinary teams, and systems attention to the transitional care needs of the older adult across the perioperative continuum. This text will help providers in their individual practice. It will assist members of the care team and systems to plan care in advance for what the older adult will need in the next step, while looking behind to understand how what happened in the past informs what is needed in the present and beyond. This process is the essence of transitional care.

In summary, I'm honored to provide a foreword to this text and to follow the work of these leading experts in geriatric care of older adults. *Gerioperative Nursing Care* will be a major asset to both undergraduate and graduate nursing programs, now and in the future.

Terry Fulmer, PhD, RN, FAAN
Erline Perkins McGriff Chair & Dean,
New York University College of Nursing
Former President, GSA

Preface

Surgery and anesthesia are inherently fraught with risks and complications, especially for the elderly. The increasing number of older adults who require surgical interventions continues to challenge caregivers on a daily basis. The complications experienced by older adults exceed those of younger adults. Gerioperative care is focused on improving the outcomes of older adults by carefully considering the implications and consequences of age-related changes on surgical recovery.

This book represents the first step in acknowledging that care of the older adult during surgery demands a different paradigm of care. Part I provides background on the need for gerioperative care and the resources required to provide gerioperative care. The role of the gerioperative care facilitator is introduced in Chapter 2. The chapter on medication safety highlights the difficulty of gerioperative pharmacology. The chapter on coaching formalizes the role of the health coach in helping family and friends promote older adults recovery and long-term health goals.

Part II uses a systems approach to describe age-related changes and their impact on perioperative considerations. Examination of age-related changes in a single system quickly lead to recognition of the complex interaction that occurs across systems. No body system stands alone. Age-related changes increase the intensity and complexity of the interaction creating the potential for a biologic cascade. That is, as one system fails, others are not far behind.

Part III selects specific areas of gerioperative vulnerability. The chapter on frailty emphasizes the effect of diminished reserve on elders. The chapter on depression and dementia stresses the risk these findings generate for postoperative complications and thus, the critical need for preoperative screening. Delirium and postoperative cognitive dysfunction is an emerging problem that has significant implications for patient and family awareness. The chapter on pain underscores that undertreated pain remains a significant gerioperative issue. Finally, by promoting a discharge wellness orientation, the gerioperative patient returns to a preoperative state at a higher level of health.

Each chapter of *Gerioperative Nursing Care* begins with a review of anatomical and physiological principles helpful in understanding age-related changes. Physiological age-related changes serve as a foundation for onset of many comorbid diseases. Diseases derived from age-related changes are highlighted to emphasize the progression of aging. The impact of age-related changes on care of the gerioperative patient follows the perioperative process from the beginning to end. By incorporating each phase of the perioperative process within the specific age-related changes of each chapter, an emphasis is placed on how surgery and anesthesia impact elders' ability to maintain homeostasis. In each chapter, a patient report is introduced at the beginning and resolved at the end of the chapter. The aim of each patient report is the illustration of key points of gerioperative care.

Throughout the delivery of gerioperative care, the emphasis is on assessment, prevention, early detection, and rapid intervention across the perioperative care continuum. Preoperative care includes care assessment and interventions from weeks prior to surgery to the day of surgery. The focus of preoperative considerations is to identify risk factors with the aim to initiate interventions to reduce or minimize complications. Intraoperative considerations identify events that add to gerioperative risks and strategies to reduce iatrogenic injury. Postoperative considerations present the assessment of the gerioperative patient's response to surgery and anesthesia.

Gerioperative recovery depends on the impact surgery and anesthesia place on different systems and elders' reserve potential. The integration of the perioperative continuum in each chapter emphasizes that knowing the assessment, prevention, and interventions at each stage contributes to the design and implementation of assessment, prevention, early detection, and rapid intervention in subsequent stages. Improving care at each stage of the continuum requires looking ahead to prevent undue events while also looking behind at what is causing them.

Gerioperative Nursing Care is designed as a basic text for the novice nurse and a refresher reference for practicing nurses across the perioperative continuum who may have received scant geriatric education. Nurses are the first line of defense with direct responsibility and accountability for the care older adults receive in the perioperative setting. As a result, nurses are the first to notice any changes that must be addressed. The value and importance of nurses' contribution to optimum gerioperative outcomes is evidenced throughout this text.

Other health care providers also can benefit from this text. Primary care providers, surgeons, and anesthesia providers who may not be familiar with the inherent impact of age-related changes on surgical outcomes will find this text useful in developing collaborative care of the gerioperative patient.

Raelene V. Shippee-Rice
Susan J. Fetzer
Jennifer V. Long

Acknowledgments

Thank you to the many people who contributed to this effort. A special thanks to Christopher Mills and Ann Kelley for their many hours of reading. To our work study students, Balil Bashik and Amanda St. Jean, thank you. You did whatever was asked and not only did it well but with grace and good humor. We extend a special appreciation to the authors and illustrators who shared their expertise, time, and effort to improve gerioperative care.

To Dale, with love, for your enduring optimism. To Jennifer, for joining me on this journey as a colleague and as a daughter. To Mattie, and the many older adults who taught me what it means to be a nurse.

RSR

To Woody and Lil, who I could only imagine as elders. To John, my colleagues and students who never tired in their inquiry of progress.

SJF

To Charles for his unending devotion and many hours of work on the farm while I was "away." To Margie Gacki, librarian at the Western Maryland Health System, for her support, and coworkers at Western Maryland Health System for hearing my passion for surgical care of elderly patients.

JVL

A special thank you to Springer Publishing for giving us the opportunity to share our passion about gerioperative care. If this book makes a difference in the care of even one gerioperative patient, it will have been worth the many hours, months, and years spent.

.

PART I

Introduction to Gerioperative Care

ONE

Gerioperative Demographics

Raelene V. Shippee-Rice, Susan J. Fetzer, and Jennifer V. Long

"While people over the age of 65 account for only 12% of the U.S. population, they undergo almost 40% of surgical procedures. They are also more likely to suffer a wide range of post-operative complications. In the future, the provision of high quality, "gero-sensitive" care will become an even more critical issue in the surgical and related specialties" (American Geriatrics Society, n.d.).

PATIENT REPORT: Mr. Warren

Mr. Warren is 78 years old. He enjoys hiking and having his regular Wednesday morning "coffee clache" with his friends from the photography club. Several times a year, he and his wife travel, often on family vacations with their children and grandchildren. He has been diagnosed with stage I colon cancer. When he entered the hospital for a colon resection, everything changed. Surgery went well, but on his third postoperative day, the morning report indicated he was incontinent and seemed confused but quiet. When his wife saw him, she asked the care team what was wrong with her husband: "He wasn't like this before." "He is a little confused," the team said, "but that's not unusual after surgery. It happens quite often." When she asked the nurses what could be done about it, she was told there really wasn't a lot they could do. He should come out of it in a few days. They told her he was probably a little confused before surgery, and she just didn't realize it. They added "...but we'll do everything we can." His meperidine was stopped; Mr. Warren recovered physically and returned home. After discharge, he continued to complain about feeling "fuzzy" in his head. He resumed hiking and the coffee claches but not with the same attention and vigor. His wife said, "he just isn't himself anymore. He's doing okay, but he isn't the same. They cured his cancer but...I don't know what happened. Why didn't they tell us about this?"

The observation that "People are never more alike than they are at birth, nor more different and unique than when they enter the geriatric era" (Silverstein, Rooks, Reves, & McLeskey, 2008, p. 35) attests to the wide variation in functional ability and health status among people aged 65 and older. This variation makes it challenging to recognize that, though age may impact physiological, physical, cognitive, and mental function, at least 20% of the elderly have no disabilities or medical problems; they remain healthy and active for many years. However, although chronologic age is not a sole, reliable indicator of health status, a significant percentage of the elderly is at risk for disease, iatrogenic complications, and adverse outcomes. Each year, over 16 million older adults (National Center for Health Statistics, 2011) seek the intentional trauma of surgery to alleviate complaints from adverse medical conditions. Surgical trauma can bring great benefit or great harm to the older patient. For the majority, surgery will improve the quality of life and extend lifespan; for others, surgery will lead to unnecessary complications, extended hospital stays, prolonged recovery periods, decreased quality of life, and even death.

In addition to taking into account the fundamental diversity among older adults, we need to consider that the need for surgical care of the elderly will only increase, especially over the next 30 years as the baby boom generation enters old age. Professional providers and the current health care delivery system are ill-prepared to meet the demands of this ever-growing older population. For example, less than 2% of health care professionals who provide care to the older surgical patient have adequate education or training in geriatrics or gerontology. Currently, there are only 9000 certified geriatricians in the United States, and the number of physicians sitting for geriatric certification is decreasing; a mere 1% of registered nurses are certified in the field of geriatrics (Kovner, Mezey, & Harrington, 2002). Few textbooks on geriatric anesthesiology or geriatric surgery have been published since 2000, and no nursing or allied health care textbooks specific to the surgical care of the older adult was found in current databases. Although the number of published articles on care of older adults in medical, nursing, and health care journals increases every year and information is becoming increasingly available through geriatric and health care websites, education and training in geriatrics and gerontology remains thin at all levels of education and practice. In fact, according to the Institute of Medicine (IOM) ". . .the education and training of the entire health care workforce with respect to the range of needs of older adults remains woefully inadequate" (2008, p.1).

> *Although old age is not the sole or most reliable indicator of health status, older adults are at risk for chronic disease, iatrogenic complications, and adverse health outcomes.*

Inadequacies of geriatric health care are exacerbated by the fact that as the demand for surgical care is increasing, the health care workforce is decreasing: not only is the general population aging, so is the health care workforce. Not enough students are entering the health professions to reverse the decrease; the number of students interested in the field of geriatrics as a clinical specialty is diminishing; and finally, nursing schools have closed or consolidated gerontology and geriatric advanced practice due to low enrollments. More troubling is that research shows that those entering the nursing profession often hold negative attitudes toward care of older adults or have inadequate education and training (Fox & Wold, 1996; Mezey & Fulmer, 2002; Shue, McNeley, & Arnold, 2005).

> *". . .The education and training of the health care workforce. . . in meeting the needs of elderly is woefully inadequate."*

In this chapter, we examine the profound changes occurring in the demographics of aging and explore the impact these changes are having and will continue to have on the demand for surgical care of the older patient. Having already indicated that current surgical care is inadequate, and is likely to become more so, we will lay the groundwork for the implementation of gerioperative care, a care management approach aimed at improving the surgical care of the older adult.

Demography of Aging

At a time of a shrinking health care workforce and a decrease in financial resources, the number of older adults is increasing worldwide at a pace unheard of in previous generations. Although geriatricians and gerontologists long predicted this trend, as well as the accompanying need for a workforce to care for this particular population, there is little evidence of a response from the health care disciplines. Over the last century, adults over 65 years of age increased from 4% of the population to 12.6%; that is, from 3.1 million in 1900 to 37.7 million in 2007, more than a 10-fold increase. By 2030, the current number of the elderly is estimated to double to 72 million. This figure would constitute 20% of the total population of the United States (Federal Interagency Forum on Aging Related Statistics, 2008). Figure 1.1 shows three population pyramids demonstrating the shift in numbers of age groups by sex between 1950, 2010, and 2050. A wider base is weighted toward younger ages whereas a wide top represents an aging population. Examination of the top rows of 1950, 2010, and 2050 pyramids show an aging population with the largest growth in those over age 85.

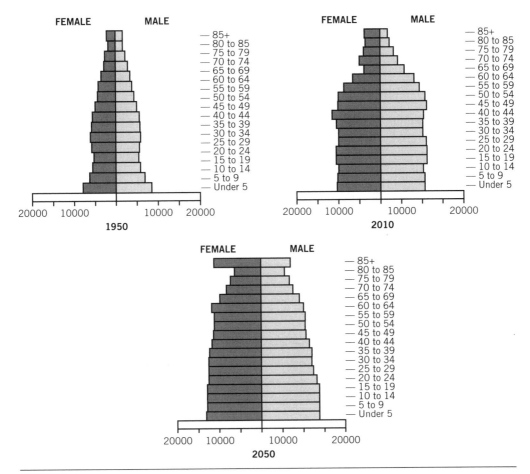

FIGURE 1.1

Population Pyramids 1950, 2010, and 2050

Data derived from National Center for Health Statistics, 2003 (1950) and U.S. Census Statistical Abstracts, 2011 (2010, 2050).

Longevity, the number of live births, and immigration all contribute to changes in demography. Lifespan increased in the 20th century as a result of multiple public health measures such as improved sanitary conditions, massive immunization programs, improvements in maternal and newborn care, and the advent of antibiotics, which greatly decreased the number of deaths from water- and airborne diseases and infections. In addition, advances in health care technology led to better diagnosis and thereby earlier and more effective treatment of disease. At the same time, a decrease in the birth rate increased the proportion of older adults in relation to other age groups. Figure 1.2 shows the percent changes in age group distribution in 1970, 2000, and 2030. The 25 and under population at 46% in 1970 is expected to decrease to 32.5% in 2030. The over 65 population is predicted to increase from 9.9% in 1970 to almost 20% in the same time period (U.S. Census Bureau, 2011). The use of the generic term "aging population" in reference to individuals age 65 and over might imply a homogeneity in this group. In fact, Whitbourne (2002) responds to the question "Who are the aged?" by noting "...there is no one single answer to this question" (p. 22). The aging population is comprised of groups with different demographic characteristics such as age, gender, race, and ethnicity. Examining these demographic subgroups provides a broader context for understanding the aging population as a whole.

AGING OF THE OLDEST OLD

The aging population can be subdivided into three subgroups: the young old, aged 64 to 74; the middle old, aged 75 to 84; and the oldest old, aged 85 and over. This last group is the fastest growing segment of the U.S. population. In 2000, this group was 4 million people; population projections from the U.S. Census Bureau suggest that this number will increase to

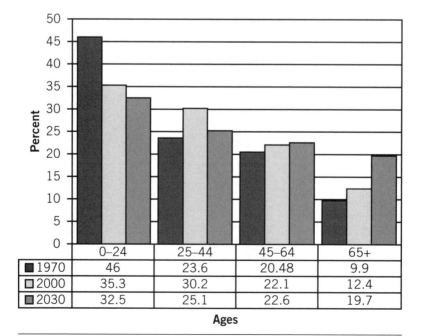

	0–24	25–44	45–64	65+
■ 1970	46	23.6	20.48	9.9
□ 2000	35.3	30.2	22.1	12.4
▣ 2030	32.5	25.1	22.6	19.7

Ages

FIGURE 1.2

Percent Change in Population Age Groups, 1970, 2000, 2030

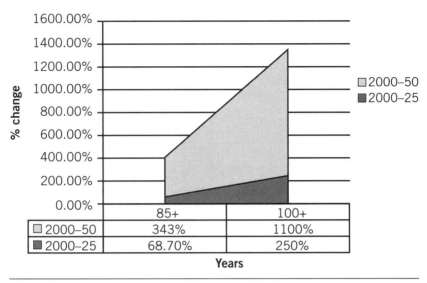

FIGURE 1.3
Percent Change in Ages 85+ and 100+, 2000–2025 and 2000–2050

more than 7 million by 2010 and to as much as 9 million by 2030. These figures represent an astonishing 50% increase in a 30-year period (U.S. Census Bureau, 2011).

Projections also indicate that many of the oldest old will be centenarians. Before she died in November 2008, Edna Parker had celebrated her 115th birthday the previous August, making her the oldest person in the United States at that time. In fact, the centenarian age group of the oldest old is growing. In 1990, the U.S. Census Bureau reported 37,000 people to be centenarians. By 2000, that number was 50,000. The 2008 National Population Projections states that there will be 600,000 by 2050, a 1100% increase since 2000 (Figure 1.3). These projections are only estimates (www.census.gov/popest/) and are subject to the multiple factors influencing population aging, including changes in disease processes, health care system access, and advances in knowledge and health care technology. Though the actual number may prove to be higher or lower, the evidence remains that there will be a dramatic increase in the number of the oldest old in the next 20 years, particularly among those who achieve 100 years and above.

AGING IN MEN AND WOMEN

In 1900, life expectancy was 47 years for men and only 2 years higher for women. Throughout the 20th century, life expectancy has increased steadily and continues to increase in the 21st century (Figure 1.4). By 1970, life expectancy was almost 71 years, with women outliving men by 7.5 years. In 2004, the median life expectancy was 77.8 years. The gender gap narrowed to 5.2 years with women, at birth, having a life expectancy of 80.4 years while men could expect 75.2 years. At age 65, a woman could expect to live another 20 years; a man can expect to live only another 17 years (Arias, National Vital Statistics Report, 2007). Women outnumber men in every age group from the youngest to the oldest old. Because women generally marry men who are older and who die earlier, it is easy to see why women across all older age groups are up to three times more likely than men

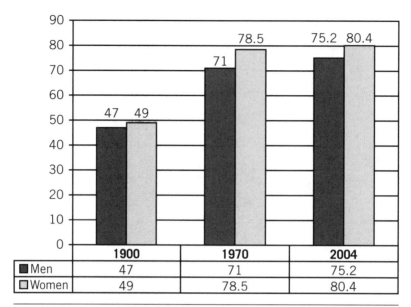

FIGURE 1.4
Life Expectancy, Men and Women, Years 1900, 1970, 2004

to be widowed. Men continue to have higher rates of being married even into the oldest old age group. Sixty percent of men over age 85 are married, compared with only 15% of women (Federal Interagency Forum on Aging Related Statistics, 2008). In the over 65 age group, there were 70 men for every 100 women. This ratio decreases with increasing age. By age 85 and over, there were only 41 men for every 100 women, a further indication of women's longevity. However, although women have lower mortality rates than men in every age group, they have higher rates of hypertension, asthma, arthritis, clinically relevant depressive symptoms, and lower functional status. They also have higher rates of frailty.

AGING IN RACIAL AND ETHNIC POPULATIONS

Race and ethnicity are additional factors that influence the gender differences in the aging population. Women live longer than men across every racial and ethnic minority in the United States. Figure 1.5 compares the life expectancy at birth and at age 65 of men and women for white and black older adults as reported by the Centers for Disease Control and Prevention. White women have the longest projected life expectancy at both birth and age 65. White women can expect to live an additional 19.9 years after age 65, compared to black or African American women's 18.7 years. Life expectancy for white men at age 65 is an additional 17.3 more years at age 65, compared to black or African American men at 15.2 more years, the lowest life expectancy of the group. Similar patterns exist regarding life expectancy at birth. White females live 4 years longer than black females (80.8 versus 76.8 years), longer than white males at 75.9 years, and longer than black males at 70 years (Centers for Disease Control and Prevention, 2011). Black or African American women have a slightly longer life expectancy at birth than white males. The gap in life expectancy in white women and men has narrowed to 5.0 years in 2004 from 7 years in the 1970s.

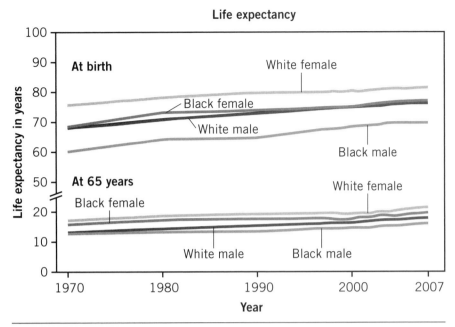

FIGURE 1.5
Life Expectancy by Gender and Race

Apart from gender issues, the U.S. Census Bureau findings for 2006 and projections for 2050 suggest there will be a profound shift in the racial composition of the aging population in the next 40 years (Federal Interagency Forum on Aging Related Statistics, 2008). Non-Hispanic whites comprised 81% of older Americans and 90% of the oldest old. White older adults report better health status across all older age groups than either non-Hispanic black or Hispanic of any race (Figure 1.6). The percent of older adults reporting to be in good health decreases with increasing age regardless of race.

In the same year (2006), 8.4% of older Americans were black, 3.2% Asian, and 6.5% Hispanic or Latino of any race. Projections for 2050, however, indicate that non-Hispanic whites will decrease to less than 61% of the over 65 age group, while Hispanic older adults of any race will increase to 17.5%. Black alone or Asian alone elders will increase to 12% and almost 8%, respectively.

Older adults who self identify as Hispanic or black are an ethnically diverse group that differs in relation to country of origin, number of generations in the United States, and predominant language spoken in the home. Most persons of Hispanic or Latino origin are from Mexico, South or Central America, Cuba, or Puerto Rico. Elders identifying themselves as Asian come from equally diverse countries, including China, Japan, the Philippines, Korea, Thailand, or India. It is easy to see that providing culturally sensitive care to racially and ethnically diverse older adults will remain a major concern for health care providers.

AGING AND CHRONIC DISEASE

Aging carries the risk of chronic disease with 80% of older adults reporting at least one chronic disease condition. The most common chronic diseases in older adults are arthritis, hypertension, heart disease, cancer, and diabetes. Heart disease, cancer, and stroke are the major causes of mortality. These chronic conditions decrease quality of life, impair functioning, and

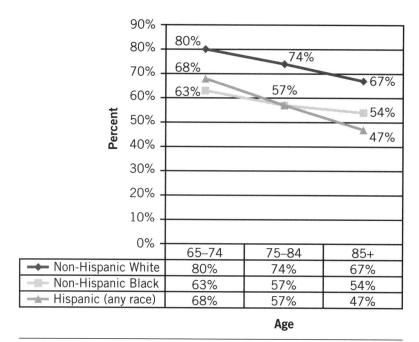

FIGURE 1.6
Self-Reported Good to Excellent Health Status by Age and Race

place older adults at higher risk for complications and adverse outcomes during hospitalization or surgery. Older adults from minority populations have disproportionately higher rates of chronic disease and earlier death from chronic disease. They also report lower rates of good to excellent health. Figure 1.6 shows the percent of older adults reporting good to excellent health by age group and race. Sixty-three percent of non-Hispanic black older adults and sixty-eight percent of Hispanic older adults between the ages of 65 and 74 report good to excellent health, compared with 80% of non-Hispanic white older adults. At age 85 and over, non-Hispanic white older adults continue to hold an advantage with 67% reporting good to excellent health, compared with 54% non-Hispanic black older adults and 47% Hispanic older adults. It is important to note that the rate of elders reporting good to excellent health declines with increasing age, regardless of race.

Heart disease accounted for almost 26% of all deaths in 2006 (Centers for Disease Control and Prevention, 2010) and is the leading cause of mortality. African American men are 30% more likely to die from heart disease than non-Hispanic white men, despite the fact that 10% of African Americans have heart disease as compared to 12% of whites. The Office of Minority Health reports that in 2006, 31.6% of African Americans had hypertension as compared to 22.4% of whites (Pleis, Ward, & Lucas, 2010). In addition, African American men are less likely than white men to have their blood pressure well controlled.

Cancer is the second leading cause of death in most aging populations in the United States. Adjusting for age, African Americans are 33% more likely to die from all types of cancer than white Americans. African American men are over twice as likely to die from prostate cancer. And though breast cancer is diagnosed less frequently in African American women than in white women, African American women are 34% more likely to die from the disease.

According to the Centers for Disease Control and Prevention, more than 20.8 million people in the United States have diabetes (Centers for Disease Control and Prevention, 2011).

Of this number, the elderly members of most racial and ethnic minority groups are disproportionately affected by both diabetes and pre-diabetes. For example, African Americans are 2.2 times more likely to not only have diabetes but to experience complications from the disease than members of the white population. The highest incidence of diabetes in African Americans occurs in the 65 to 75 range of years of age (Office of Minority Health, n.d.). When adjusted for age, African American women are more likely to be diagnosed with diabetes than African American men or members of other racial groups (Office of Minority Health Resource Center, 2006).

AGING AND HEALTH CARE

The proportion of elders using the health care system is higher than in the general U.S. population. Older adults make 20% more visits to the doctor's office than do young and middle-aged adults. They have longer hospital stays, take more medications, and require more home care visits. In addition, they spend more time in nursing homes and rehabilitation facilities than any other age group (Cherry, Burt, & Woodwell, 2001; IOM, 2008). Of the 2.2 trillion dollars of the 2007 U.S. health care budget, approximately 31% was spent on hospital costs. Older adults use 38% of all emergency medical services, constitute 40% of the total inpatient hospital population, and make up 60% of adult medical surgical patients (Amador & Loera, 2007). As the population ages further and as rates of heart disease, cancer, diabetes, arthritis, and cardiovascular disease increase, management of chronic illness will become the primary health care challenge in the United States. The management of chronic illness will also be a key factor in managing the surgical care of older adults and in the prevention of surgically related complications.

The number of older adults relying on the health care system creates a false assumption that aging is synonymous with frailty, disability, illness, disease, and dysfunction. Although age and associated physical and physiologic changes are risk factors for the onset of chronic disease and illness, chronologic age is not the sole indicator for determining health status and care needs. Social environment, health habits, lifestyle, level of social engagement, education, poverty, and access to health care are major contributing factors to the overall health of the older adult. For example, recent studies by Kuzawa and Sweet (2008) and Thorpe, Brandon, and Laveist (2008) argued that social and environmental factors are major elements in the consistent disparity in cardiovascular and hypertension rates between non-Hispanic white and African American populations.

Based on recent evidence supporting the relationship between social environment and chronic disease, it is arguable whether age alone or the accumulation of other risk factors over time could be the major determinant(s) of the decreased health and function that occur with increasing age. What is not arguable, however, is that there is a significant correlation between increasing age and morbidity (McCleskey, 1997). Findings documenting the interaction of age and disease challenge health care professionals to be vigilant regarding the effect of physical, physiologic, and psychological changes on aging body systems and functions while remaining sensitive to the wide variation among older adults and the diversity of the aging experience.

Aging and the Demand for Surgical Care

In addition to the disproportionate utilization of the health care system and health care dollars spent caring for the older population, an enormous growth in the demand for surgical procedures is expected. The demand varies depending on the surgical specialty and the

TABLE 1.1

Estimated Increase in Demand for Selected Surgeries

	2000–2020	2005–2030
General surgery	31.5%	
Cancer-related	46%	
General orthopedic		23%
Hip arthroplasty		101%–174%
Knee arthroplasty		565%–643%
Hip revisions		137%–175%
Knee revisions		600%

timeframe of the analysis. However, the evidence remains consistent that the demand for geriatric surgical procedures will increase at a faster rate than the increase in the number of elders in the population. Table 1.1 shows the predicted increases in demand for selected types of surgeries.

The elderly currently have a rate of general surgery 3 times higher than persons aged 15 to 44 and 1.6 times higher than those aged 45 to 64 (Liu, Etzioni, O'Connell, Maggard, & Ko, 2004). The most frequent surgery involves the gastrointestinal tract, followed by surgery of the breast and surgery for soft-tissue repair. Liu, Etzioni, O'Connell, Maggard, and Ko (2004) predicted an increase of 19% to 40% with an overall increase of 31.5%. The variation is due to the type of general surgery considered with gastrointestinal having the highest rate of growth.

Using an epidemiological model, Etzioni and colleagues (2003) studied the future demand for six surgical oncology procedures of the breast, colon, stomach, rectum, pancreas, and esophagus. Peak incidence of general cancer surgery was in the 70- to 90-year-old age group. Specifically, mastectomy, rectal resection, and stomach resection were highest in the 75 to 84 age group. Colon resection had the highest incidence in the over 85 age group. The study concluded that cancer-related surgery could be expected to increase approximately 46% by 2020 with the bulk of the increase in the over 65 age group. The largest increases, 45% to 51%, are resections due to gastrointestinal cancers and vary depending on specific disease site.

Between 2000 and 2020, the demand for orthopedic surgery will increase dramatically (Iorio et al., 2008). The most common orthopedic procedures are hip and knee joint replacements due to osteoarthritis, posttraumatic arthritis, hip fracture, and obesity. The volume of total hip arthroplasties is expected to grow 101% to 174% with demand for knee arthroplasties growing as much as 565% to 643% by 2030 (Iorio et al., 2008; Kurtz, Ong, Lau, Mowat, & Halpern, 2007). Although aging adults are not the only ones needing joint repair, the dramatic increase in the number of older adults strongly correlates with the anticipated increase in demand. For example, the incidence of arthritis and associated conditions increases as the population ages, and as the number of hip and joint replacement surgeries increase, there will be a concomitant increase in the need to revise joints previously replaced (Kurtz, Ong, Lau, Mowat, & Halpern, 2007). Kurtz and colleagues report that between 2005 and 2030, demand for knee revision surgery is expected to increase approximately 600%; for hip revisions, approximately 175%. Fractured hips occur most often in older adults, particularly among the oldest old, and can be expected to increase as the population ages. Although the increasing demand for surgery previously noted is not limited solely to older adults, this population will continue to be a major user of surgical services.

AGING AND SURGICAL CARE

Old age, no matter what medical or surgical interventions are sought, heralds a waning of vigor. And no matter how long the expected lifespan might become, old people will eventually die. Perhaps it is the fear and grieving associated with our own aging and the inevitable losses that it will bring, or the observation of the aging of those around us, that can lead to negative attitudes about the process of aging and about the elderly (Martens, Goldenberg, & Greenberg, 2005). These negative attitudes can lead to discrimination, unconscious or conscious, against an entire segment of our population: the elderly.

Ageism is an ingrained prejudice or discrimination against a particular age group, especially against the elderly. Butler first coined the term ageism in 1969. In 1975, he explicated the concept in great detail in *Why survive? Being Old in America*. Ageism is stereotyping the elderly and using "old" as a pejorative word when referring to the elderly.

In American society, the stereotype has long been negative, but ageism is by no means limited to the United States. It is pervasive across nations, societies, and cultures (Kite, Stockdale, Whitley, & Johnson, 2005). Negative stereotyping includes the characterization of the elderly as ugly, wrinkled, doddering, opinionated, and inflexible; in a social setting, the older adult is often viewed as an "old geezer." An equally damaging stereotype can be the image of an older adult as healthy and wealthy, who plays golf, travels, and enjoys life while younger counterparts struggle to make a living and have no leisure time. Even positive stereotypes of the elderly person can be seen as "evaluatively mixed": often the positive image of the older adult as someone warm and compassionate is perceived at the same time in a negative light, as someone who is incompetent and needs help (Cuddy, Norton, & Fiske, 2005). The image of older adults in America has changed in recent years due to the work of Butler and other leading experts in gerontology and geriatrics. Old age has an aura of new beginnings with time to devote to self-care and leisure. This is true for healthy young old age. The issue is as much a stereotype of illness and chronic disease as it is of age.

Healthism is another form of negative stereotyping directed at older adults. It is generally directed at elderly people who are in poor physical health. The assumption is that the older individual has a moral and personal responsibility for maintaining health and well-being. Elders who have chronic disease are often perceived as not meeting this responsibility and are therefore culpable (Clarke & Griffin, 2008). This attitude is reflected in provider comments when older adults have exacerbations of illness: "He just didn't do what he should have. Why couldn't he just do what I explained to him?"

The danger of stereotyping is the unconscious discrimination that accompanies it. Health professionals who succumb to ageism and healthism attitudes pose a risk for the elderly patient. However, stereotyping of the aged is by no means restricted to the medical community. Friends and family are prone to such discrimination as well. Older adults are equally subject to holding ageist attitudes.

> *Healthism is a serious barrier to care of older adults with chronic illness.*

Nurses, physicians, psychologists, social workers and other health care providers are not immune to the negative stereotypes directed at the aged. They often reflect the attitudes, beliefs, and norms of the larger society. In many ways, clinical practice caring for older adults with complex health needs reinforces negative stereotypes of "too old, too sick, too bad" (Moss & Halmandaris, 1977). Ageist discrimination is harmful to the physical and cognitive functioning of older adults (Ory, Hoffman, Hawdins, Sanner, & Mockenhaupt, 2003). Harmful effects result when health care providers dismiss elders' complaints, misdiagnose based on assumptions, provide inadequate treatment or overtreatment, or do not attend to care needs. Older adults are not always told that surgery is a treatment option even when it is reasonable. In a study by Hamel, Toth, Legezda, and Rosen (2008), older adults reported they were not informed that joint replacement was an option, or, if informed, they themselves refused treatment. A study on the effectiveness of surgery for pancreatic cancer (Billimoria et al., 2007) found that patients with selected sociodemographic characteristics such as increasing age, race, lower education, and Medicare/Medicaid insured, were less likely to receive surgical intervention for their condition. This was true even in situations where there were no identifiable contraindications. Both Hamel and colleagues and Billimoria and colleagues are careful to note there is no evidence to suggest discriminatory attitudes such as ageism and ageist attitudes as a reason for the lower rates of surgery.

Other investigators argue that there are situations where surgery can cause "greater harm" or will not improve the quality of life enough to consider doing a procedure. They cite preoperative comorbidities and risk ratio as justifiable reasons to defer surgical intervention with older adults (Velanovich et al., 2002).

Families are key players in shaping an older adult's treatment decisions. If family members harbor stereotypical and ageist attitudes toward their aging relative, they can become overprotective without actually considering the benefits of surgery. By communicating too much care and concern about the hazards or difficulty of a medical procedure, the family undermines the confidence and competence of the aging individual to make a decision (Nussbaum, Pitts, Huber, Krieger, & Ohs, 2005). As a consequence, the older adult may turn the decision-making over to the family or refuse surgery altogether, fearing that he or she is not capable enough to make a decision or strong enough to withstand the stress of a surgical procedure.

The aged themselves are not immune to ageist attitudes (Nelson, 2005; Nussbaum, Pitts, Huber, Krieger, & Ohs, 2005), which can influence how they make decisions about their own medical care. Meiner and Lueckenotte (2006) argued that even when given treatment options, older adults may refuse because they think they are "too old." Rothman, van Ness, O'Leary, and Fried (2007) found that 36 older adults in their sample of 226 community elders refused a medical or surgical treatment. Cardiac catheterization and surgery were the most common treatments refused. Two common reasons for elders' refusal were that (1) they would not be able to tolerate the feared side effects or (2) the treatment would not be effective. Other reasons included that they would not be able to return home, or that they were simply too old. Ms. A. used this type of decision-making regarding her treatment options. An 82-year-old woman, Ms. A. was admitted to the intensive care unit with a myocardial infarction. She lived alone, was independent in all the activities of daily living, and was very functional. At the time of her admission, she was alert and oriented to person, place, and time. She considered herself reasonably healthy but had a history of hypertension, hypercholesterolemia, and hypothyroidism, which were controlled with medication and lifestyle. The physicians explained to her that she had had a heart attack, and they outlined her treatment options: medical management, cardiac catheterization with possible stenting, or just watching and waiting for developments. The treatment recommended was cardiac catheterization with possible stenting as the treatment of choice based on her lifestyle and level of function. Though she was a good surgical candidate for cardiac catheterization, she chose not to proceed with surgery, preferring to "wait and see what happens." When asked about her decision, she replied, "I am too old to go through all that. I will just live out whatever time I have left."

Patients with attitudes similar to Ms. A.'s put themselves at risk. Kojodjojo et al. (2008) found that patient refusal of treatment was the primary cause of mortality in a group of patients aged 80 and over with severe aortic stenosis who were otherwise fit for surgery. Findings indicated that refusal of aortic valve replacement was associated with a greater than "12-fold increase in mortality risk" (p. 567). The authors conclude that the study's findings raise significant implications to ensure informed decision-making in fit, older adults with aortic stenosis.

Somewhat different than bias against the elderly is the reluctance to perform surgery at a time when it seems too dangerous a procedure. For example, Dr. Alton Oschsner, founder of the Oschsner Clinic in New Orleans, is quoted as stating, "In 1927, as a young professor of surgery at Tulane Medical School, I taught and practiced that an elective operation of inguinal hernia in a patient older than 50 years was not justified" (Lubin, Smith, Dodson, Spell, & Walker, 2006, p. 448) Thirty years later, P.D. Bedford, a well-known British surgeon and researcher, expressed a similar caution in a paper on cerebral effects of anesthesia in older adults: "Operations on elderly people should be confined to unequivocally necessary cases" (1955, p. 263). Thinking has changed, and surgery in the old, and even the very old, is common. Advances in anesthesia and medical technology, combined with a better understanding of the physiology of aging have made surgery a safer option for older adults. In 2006, one-third of all elective surgeries and half of all emergency surgeries involved adults over 65 years of age (Silverstein et al., 2007, cited in Amador & Loera, 2007).

Despite all the medical advances, however, the fact remains that surgery is a risk for older adults. Although the rates of surgical morbidity are higher in those aged 65 and older than in younger patients, chronologic age is not the sole predictor of risk. Other factors highly correlated with the number and severity of surgical complications are severity of comorbidities, overall health, level of cognitive function, type of surgery, intraoperative events, anxiety levels before and after surgery, and early detection of impending complications (Glover, Edwards, & Hitchcock, 2007). Table 1.2 presents an extensive list of commonly occurring surgical complications in older adults (Geriatric Interdisciplinary Advisory Group, 2006).

TABLE 1.2
Common Surgical Complications in Older Adults

- Myocardial infarction
- Pneumonia
- Infection
- Malnutrition
- Dehydration or fluid overload
- Functional decline
- Adverse drug events
- Pain and discomfort
- Delirium and postoperative cognitive dysfunction
- Incontinence
- Deconditioning and immobility
- Falls
- Pressure ulcers
- Thromboembolism
- Isolation
- Depression
- Readmission

In a study of 98 older adults undergoing posterior lumbar decompression and fusion for degenerative spine problems, 79, or almost 80%, experienced a surgical complication (Carreon, Puno, Dimar, Glassman, & Johnson, 2003). At least 21 patients (21%) had a major complication, most commonly a wound infection; 69% experienced a minor complication; and 50% had more than one complication. Confusion was a problem in 27% of the patients. The number of complications and their severity in this study population were associated with increased patient age, amount of surgical blood loss, length of the operation, and the number of fused spinal levels.

Clancy (2008) reported that up to 40% of surgeries result in a complication. Surgical site infections (SSIs) and venous thromboembolism (VTE) are two of the most common and often preventable complications with an annual rate of 780,000 SSIs each year and up to 25% of major surgeries resulting in a VTE when there is no prophylaxis. Clancy reported on a study indicating that postoperative complications were associated with a 22% rate of preventable deaths. The figures cited by Clancy are not limited to older adults, but, as noted, increased age is a contributing factor in postoperative complications. Clancy further noted that 27,000 postoperative myocardial events occur annually in Medicare patients.

Respiratory, wound, and urinary tract infections are among the most common surgical complications. Surgical sepsis is a major cause of mortality in older adults. In a study of surgical sepsis in Veterans Administration hospitals, Quartin, Schein, Kett, and Perduzzi (1997) reported that the onset of a postoperative infection decreased the mean lifespan of older adults from an expected 8 years to 5 years after surgery. Findings further showed that the severity of sepsis was linked with an increased mortality within 1 year after surgery, regardless of preoperative health status.

Finally, several postoperative complications such as cognitive dysfunction, delirium, malnutrition, pressure ulcers, and falls occur more often in older adults (Clancy, 2008; Wadlund, 2006) than in younger age groups.

Adding to the complexity of dealing with the postsurgical complications of an older population is the fact that significant racial disparities exist in rates of such complications. A retrospective record review by Fiscella, Franks, Meldrum, and Barnett (2005) examines the relationship between race and surgical complications. Study results indicate that non-white older adults have higher mortality rates and a 65% higher chance for surgical complications. Differences in comorbidity, length of stay, and hospital characteristics were significant in explaining these higher rates. Penrod and colleagues (2008) noted non-white patients with hip fracture have a higher mortality rate and a lower mobility rate than white patients. The authors of the study argued that more research is needed to determine the factors influencing racial and ethnic disparity in hip fracture complications and outcomes.

It also might be argued that future research should extend to factors that prevent complications and improve quality of outcomes for all surgical procedures involving older adults. Taking a preventative, wellness-oriented approach to surgical care of older adults could have the potential to decrease significantly the risk of postoperative complications across all racial and ethnic populations.

PATIENT REPORT: Mr. Warren

Gerioperative patients are at high risk for postoperative complications. Even though Mr. Warren is a healthy older adult, age-related changes increase his risk of surgical complications. Awareness of the unique needs and responses of the gerioperative patient to surgical stress enables health care providers to more effectively manage gerioperative care across the surgical continuum. Recognition of risk factors, prevention, early detection, and rapid therapeutic response are critical factors in decreasing onset and severity of surgically related complications and improving patient outcomes.

SUMMARY

Though many people live well into old age with few disabilities or medical problems, close to 80% of the elderly experience conditions for which surgical intervention is recommended or necessary. Though surgery will often improve the quality of life, there are times when it will prove to be a burden and a danger. To ensure the best outcomes of surgical intervention, and to prevent minor and major complications, the medical community needs to recognize the diversity of the ever-growing aging population. Demographic factors such as increasing longevity, differences and shifts in gender and ethnic groups, as well as persistent prejudices against the aged affect not only whether surgery is sought, but, once sought, also affect the outcome.

Decision-making related to care of older adults is a complex process involving knowledge, skills, beliefs, attitudes, health status, and options. Decisions are made in a time and situation context that is often complicated. The current workforce in the medical community is inadequate, ill-prepared, and disinterested in the special knowledge that is necessary to address the needs of the elderly. Care of the older surgical patient involves transferring the adult from one delivery care site to another or across surgical services. Each translocation means adapting to new surroundings and different health care practitioners or teams of providers. The process is uncoordinated and discontinuous, exacerbated by the fact that the aging population is diverse and often has complex health care needs. Miscommunication and lack of attention to patient-centered care is often the result, a result that leads to adverse events and poor outcomes. An integrated and specialized gerioperative care program is needed. It coordinates the care of older adults across the surgical continuum and forestall the complications and negative consequences often experienced in the current health care environment.

KEY POINTS

- The number of older adults is estimated to double to 72 million or 20% of the total population of the United States in the next 20 years.
- The 85 and over population is increasing faster than any other age group and expected to grow from 7 million to 9 million between 2010 and 2030.
- The over 65 population is heterogeneous, showing extensive variation in health status across individuals as well as population groups.
- Non-Hispanic white men and women report better health status, have lower rates of chronic disease, and experience fewer surgical complications than older adults who self-identify as non-Hispanic black or Hispanic of any race.
- The demand for surgical procedures is anticipated to increase between 45% and 600% by 2030, depending on type of surgery. Hip and knee arthroplasties will have the greatest increase in demand.
- Ageist and healthist attitudes in health care providers, families, and older adults can be harmful, resulting in adverse outcomes.
- Health care providers and the present health care system are ill prepared to meet the surgical care needs of older adults.
- Many of the surgical complications experienced by older adults are preventable or severity decreased through risk identification, prevention, early detection, and rapid therapeutic response.

TWO

Introduction to Gerioperative Care

Raelene V. Shippee-Rice, Susan J. Fetzer, and Jennifer V. Long

PATIENT REPORT: Mr. Tubman

Mr. Tubman was recently remarried after the death of his first wife, which occurred about 10 years ago. He and his wife enjoy traveling, dining out, and visiting with their many friends. At 78 years old, he describes his quality of life as outstanding. Recently diagnosed with colon cancer, Mr. Tubman agreed to surgery in hopes that he will have a few more years of "good times in him."

There was little time to prepare for surgery between the time of diagnosis and the time of surgery. He spent most of that time getting his affairs in order in case something should happen. His appetite had not been very good for several months, he had lost 17 pounds, and he "fell off" his exercise regimen. He admitted to not sleeping well due to his concerns about his wife if something should happen to him.

After surgery for a hemicolectomy, Mr. Tubman entered into a deconditioning, depleting reserve cascade. His pain was not well controlled, and he was not a candidate for epidural analgesia due to previous back surgery. As a result of intravenous narcotics, he developed a paralytic ileus, he was not allowed anything food or drink by mouth, and a nasogastric tube was inserted. He developed a urinary tract infection from the Foley catheter. Intravenous fluids were restarted after he began to show evidence of diminished urinary output via the catheter. He developed hypoactive delirium that remained undetected by nursing and physician providers.

His wife took care of him by changing his bed, bathing him, and providing ice chips. Providers remained distant as he had someone in his room all the time. He had a minimum of six physicians and multiple nurses caring for him but no other members of the health care team were involved. Each provider had a piece of the puzzle regarding his care needs and made treatment decisions accordingly.

On postoperative day five, a percutaneous central catheter was inserted, and he was started on total parenteral nutrition. Poor pain relief made it difficult for him to move, and staff argued he was "too sick to move." On postoperative day six, his oxygen saturation dropped, and his temperature and heart rate increased; the nurse assessed crackles in both lung bases. He was placed on a ventimask at FiO2 of 36%.

The complex care needs of older adults undergoing surgery can be approached in two ways. The gerioperative care (GOC) approach to surgical care of the older adult can be applied by any nurse at any stage of the surgical continuum. GOC is an evidence-based, humanistic model of care based on principles of gerontology and geriatrics. The second approach proposes a transitional care model: gerioperative facilitated care (GOFC). In this approach, a nurse care facilitator and a companion-coach work with the older adult and the interdisciplinary care team to facilitate the transition and care of the older adult across the surgical continuum.

Aging is a universal process that is multidimensional and complex. It occurs within a context of physiological and psychological changes, as well as personal, familial, and socio-cultural norms and expectations. There is tremendous diversity in the way people age and in how they respond to, adapt to, and manage these myriad changes. By the same token, there is tremendous diversity in the way the elderly respond to the trauma and stress of surgery. A major concern of older adults facing surgery, in addition to the uncertainty of the surgery itself, is what happens after surgery. Surgery is a pervasive assault on personal integrity and personhood that invades, modifies, and even mutilates the body, causing severe physical and emotional stress. One older woman described her feelings toward her anticipated surgery: "It is shocking. Some perfect stranger is going to see parts of my body that even I never see. Not only will he see those parts, but he will feel them and handle them, and all the time, I will be unconscious while he invades my body."

Though the patient is unconscious, patients under anesthesia experience the stress caused by surgery. Modern surgery is very different from that experienced by patients who did not have the benefit of anesthesia. During the Civil War, amputations were done routinely without anesthesia, causing unbearable pain and agony. In modern surgery, anesthesia relieves patients from the conscious experience of pain, but the body remains vulnerable to the trauma it experiences. This trauma triggers a physiologic stress response from the moment of incision, and though evidence suggests new techniques mitigate the intraoperative stress response, the problem remains (Goldmann et al., 2008). Clinicians caring for aging adults must remain acutely sensitive to the fact that the body and the psyche respond to surgical procedures as invasive, painful, and even agonizing. How the person responds to and tolerates the physiologic, physical, and emotional elements of surgical trauma depends on the health, situational context, and unique characteristics of the older adult.

Gerioperative Care

Less than 2% of nurses have education specific to the care of older adults. Nursing leaders have long advocated for the elderly as a vulnerable population, needing providers with specialized knowledge and skills. Knowledge of this vulnerable population is of particular importance when elders are undergoing the trauma of surgery. Yet, most surgical care for older adults is provided by generalists in medical-surgical nursing or clinicians with knowledge specialized to a disease process. Neither group attends to the effects of physiological, psychological, and sociological aging on a person's health, overall function, and quality of daily life before, during, and after surgery.

The term GOC is a framework that combines and applies knowledge and skills from geriatrics and gerontology to the care of the older adult throughout the perioperative continuum. Exhibit 2.1 identifies the core themes of the model. The goal is to improve geriatric

EXHIBIT 2.1 Concepts Integrated in Gerioperative Care

- The art, science, and ethics of gerontology and geriatrics
- Applying best evidence as a foundation for professional practice
- Developing, maintaining, and valuing collaborative relationships
- Navigating health care systems and cultures
- Effective therapeutic communication
- Coaching patients in wellness and self-care

surgical care by maximizing comfort, minimizing distress, preventing complications, and restoring the older adult to optimal functional health and well-being.

Three assumptions guide the provision of GOC:

- Quality care of older adults requires specialized knowledge and the application of evidence-based practice.
- Surgical trauma heightens vulnerability of older adults, increasing risk of complications.
- A wellness orientation based on preventative, holistic care is essential to minimize surgical complications and unexpected readmissions.

Key Elements of Gerioperative Care

McKinlay used the metaphor of "looking upstream" to describe the value of preventing a problem before it starts. In a meeting of the American Heart Association in 1974, he described his frustration at existing models of care that focused on intervention after a cardiac event occurred, rather than focusing on preventing the problem at the beginning:

> You know sometimes it feels like this. There I am standing by the shore of a swiftly flowing river and I hear the cry of a drowning man. So I jump into the river, put my arms around him, pull him to shore and apply artificial respiration. Just when he begins to breathe, there is another cry for help. So I jump into the river, reach him, pull him to shore and apply artificial respiration, and then just as he begins to breathe, there is another cry for help. So back in the river again, reaching, pulling, applying, breathing and then another yell. Again and again, without end, goes the sequence. You know, I am so busy jumping in, pulling them to shore, applying artificial respiration, that I have no time to see who the hell is upstream pushing them all in. (p. 9)

In applying McKinlay's analogy to surgical care, preventive measures "upstream" can decrease urgent and costly treatment "downstream." Preventive measures are of special importance when caring for older adults. GOC emphasizes the use of "upstream thinking" to improve patient care; prevent complications and adverse events; limit pain, discomfort, and suffering; and decrease costs. Key elements of upstream thinking in GOC are comprehensive collaborative assessment, risk identification, preventive care, and secondary prevention. Table 2.1 offers examples applying GOC key elements to practice.

TABLE 2.1

Identification of Key Elements and Selected Interventions of Gerioperative Care

Perioperative Phase	Elements	Selected Interventions
Decision-making/ informed consent	• Assessment • Risk identification • May not understand • Type of surgery • Preventive care • Early intervention	• Cognitive status and depression screening • Knowledge level and understanding re type of surgery, risks including potential for postoperative cognitive dysfunction, delirium, treatment options, benefit/risk balance, recovery needs and time line • Personal goals • Ageist beliefs, attitudes • Clear explanations of surgery, risk, treatment options and potential outcomes at appropriate level of comprehension • Use pictures, brochures, as well as verbal explanation • Have family or someone who has had similar surgery help with explaining surgery

Preoperative	• Assessment
	• Risk identification
	• Preventive care
	• Early intervention
		• Standard preoperative assessment and physical examination, preoperative tests
		• Conduct cognition and depression screening
		• Conduct additional assessments as indicated
		• Mobility problems post surgery due to diminished strength
		• Cognitive status
		• Medication
		• Prehabilitation
		  • Develop preoperative exercise and activity program
		  • Rest/activity schedule
		  • Nutrition and fluid program
		• Fall prevention protocol
		• In-bed strength exercises
		• Early ambulation

Intraoperative	• Assessment • Risk identification • Anticipated blood loss > 400 mL • Preventive care • Early intervention	• Anxiety level • Review data from preoperative assessment • Review risk potential • Review preventive actions and early intervention events • Fluid management • Blood availability • Provide reassurance during anesthesia • Decrease operative time • Control bleeding
Post anesthesia	• Assessment • Risk assessment • Potential for pain • Preventive care • Early intervention	• Cardiovascular and respiratory status • Initiate hypothermia protocol • Initiate pain management protocol • Initiate comfort measures • Provide reassurance • Revise pain protocol to needs of patient • Target comfort measures

(continued)

TABLE 2.1

Identification of Key Elements and Selected Interventions *(continued)*

Perioperative Phase	Elements	Selected Interventions
Postoperative	• Assessment • Risk identification • Blood loss • Medication • Pain • Wound healing • Dehydration • Preventive action • Early intervention	• Review intraoperative care with special attention to blood loss, surgical site • Assess side effects of positioning: neurological, skin, muscular • Associated with increased risk of delirium, cognitive dysfunction • Vigorous respiratory care • Vigilant pain relief • Assess wound healing addressing risk factors • Develop schedule for delirium and cognition assessment • Companion-coach, daily visitors to provide support, diminished sensory input • Rigorous pain management • Provide comfort measures • Distinguish delirium, depression, cognitive dysfunction • Implement preventive care to decrease infection, falls, medication error, skin changes, • Implement rest/activity plan • Medication review

Home-based care	• Assessment
	• Risk identification
	  • Bedroom upstairs
	  • Poor appetite
	  • Support systems
	  • Past medication adherence
	• Early intervention
	  • Medication adherence
		• Fall risk
		• Environmental hazards
		• Medication adherence
		• Support systems
		• Nutrition
		• Mobility
		• Skin
		• Environmental changes
		• Coaching medication adherence plan
		• Ensure access to pharmacy

ASSESSMENT

Assessment is the first critical step in decreasing surgical morbidity and preventing the functional loss associated with surgery and hospitalization in older adults. Assessment is essential in anticipating care needs, identifying strengths and risks, developing primary and secondary interventions, establishing realistic outcomes, and decreasing the potential for untoward events during hospitalization and after discharge. Comprehensive assessment, in addition to gathering data, serves as a medium for building relationships, conducting patient education, and reducing anxiety.

Older adults have lived long and complex lives that involve extensive psychosocial histories, multiple illnesses, and a myriad of therapeutic and alternative treatments. Sensory loss, decreased speed in cognitive processing, and diminished energy reserves can easily fatigue the older adult, especially when detailing a comprehensive history and undergoing physical examination. Fatigue is a concern when assessing older adults with preexisting disease, illness, or those with functional limitations. Pacing the interview and providing time for understanding the questions and reflecting on answers are important in obtaining accurate data.

A collaborative, relationship-centered interaction engaging the older adult and support persons facilitates information sharing and ensures that the older person's values, preferences, and concerns will be identified and discussed. Chapter 7 provides an extensive discussion on preoperative assessment.

In emergencies, the patient may not be able to provide information. A family member or close friend may be the primary informant. In situations involving a proxy informant, the collaborative, relationship-centered approach can help improve the quality of the information. Using valid and reliable standardized assessment tools are efficient and effective ways of gathering initial and continuing data. Specific tools that assess functional ability, social functioning, as well as physical, cognitive, psychological, and spiritual needs are discussed in Chapter 7. However, the application of standardized tools does not substitute for clinical judgment, using data gathered through interpersonal communication, observation, and physical assessment.

RISK IDENTIFICATION

Identifying elders' risk for surgical complications is critical to instituting effective primary care interventions that will prevent unnecessary discomfort, pain, dysfunction, and surgical morbidity. Analysis of risk involves evaluating the likelihood of a potential hazard, suffering, or any adverse effects that might occur. Based on risk identification, providers can develop strategies to mitigate or avoid the adverse event.

In surgery, risk identification is most commonly associated with anesthesia and patient safety in the operating room. The Surgical Care Improvement Project (SCIP), spear-headed by the Centers for Medicare & Medicaid Services and other leading health care organizations, is an effort to reduce postoperative complications: surgical site infection, adverse cardiac events, and venous thromboembolism. More needs to be done in the preoperative period to identify potential risks and institute measures that will prevent postoperative complications. It is important to recognize that adverse events are not limited to physiologic morbidities but include mental status, mood changes, functional loss, and changes in quality of life. Furthermore, risk needs to be predicted and monitored across the surgical continuum and not considered only in relationship to the immediate surgical intervention.

The standardized tools currently in use to detect risk are most effective in detecting the presence of a condition rather than identifying the level of risk that the condition could occur. Standardized risk assessment tools are available for pressure ulcers, falls, and incontinence. However, risk assessment is not available for many of the other surgical complications experienced by the gerioperative patient.

Knowledge of age-related changes, heterogeneity of individual patient response, level of functional health, impact of comorbidities, and factors associated with specific adverse events is needed to determine risk. As the patient transfers from one phase of the surgical process to another, documenting factors and specifying the risks are essential to establishing a database and information trail for the changing members of the health care team.

PRIMARY AND SECONDARY PREVENTION

Preventive care can be divided into primary and secondary prevention. In GOC, primary prevention refers to actions designed to preclude the development of a disease or unwanted surgical-related event. Primary prevention seeks to eliminate or modify risk factors. Preventive actions can be wide ranging, but they are generally targeted either to the specific risk or its associated factors in order to maximize the overall health, well-being, or functional status and minimize risk. SCIP identified a series of actions for preventing surgical site infections), venous thromboembolic events, and cardiac adverse events. However, these protocols are not specific to the elderly and must be adapted to the older adult's individual care needs and situation.

Anticipating risk or taking preventive actions is not always effective. Patients can respond in unexpected ways to the demands of surgery. Similarly, what appears to be a small risk can develop into something much bigger. If preventive action does not avert the problem, secondary prevention or early intervention is essential. In most care situations, early intervention can minimize the extent and severity of the problem. Consider the primary preventions that could be used to decrease the risks for Ms. Hall:

Mrs. Hall, a 79-year-old widow, is scheduled for a cardiac catheterization for evaluation of a mitral prolapse. She has a history of systolic hypertension and controlled atrial fibrillation. Current medications include digoxin, furosemide, and potassium chloride. Her health history includes frequent episodes of digoxin toxicity secondary to low potassium and increasing frequency of acute episodes of congestive heart failure with varying degrees of pulmonary edema. She lives alone, drives herself to her part-time job, and considers herself "doing pretty good."

She received large amounts of fluid during her cardiac catheterization and recovery in the post anesthesia care unit. Shortly after returning to the medical-surgical unit, she reported, "something isn't right." Within 15 minutes, she was dyspneic and panicked. She was rushed to the intensive care unit (ICU), where a central line was started and intravenous furosemide administered. She returned to her room after 24 hours in the ICU. She was weakened by the stress of the incident and upset that no one prevented it. Her hospital discharge was delayed 48 hours. After returning home, she developed a urinary tract infection and was in bed an additional 3 days. While in the hospital, she was prescribed prednisone 5 mg per day for fibromyalgia onset. The prescription did not follow her when she was discharged. She suffered severe pain and was unable to continue her cardiac rehabilitation program due to fatigue. This caused great distress as she was highly motivated to improve her health status. It was 6 weeks before her local cardiologist finally found the order in her medical record. By that time, she was so discouraged she did not return to her rehabilitation program.

GOC is a systematic, evidence-based approach to surgical care of the older adult. The goal is to improve geriatric surgical practice of individual practitioners, providing care in each stage of the surgical care continuum. Changing practice patterns of individual providers is necessary, but not sufficient, in the struggle to manage the discomforts and risks of surgery in the gerioperative patient more effectively. It is critical to providing effective and safe care to older adults as they move across different health care systems and units throughout the surgical process.

CARE TRANSITIONS

A single surgical procedure involves multiple care transitions. Care transition is the movement of patients from one health care setting to another or from one unit or department to another within the same institution (Coleman, 2003). In the course of elective surgery, older adults experience a minimum of 10 care transitions: home to primary care; primary care to surgeon; surgeon to preoperative outpatient assessment; home to hospital admission; during hospital admission: preadmission, operating room, post anesthesia care, post surgery, or medical-surgical care unit; hospital to post hospital setting. Older adults may be discharged to a rehabilitation unit before returning home. During each of these transitions, the older adult encounters an undocumented number of different care providers from different disciplines; some of them are professional providers, while others are support staff. Depending on preexisting illness, the complexity of the surgical procedure, the patient's response to surgery, and the presence of complications, the number of care transitions and providers increases rapidly and dramatically.

The potential for negative effects arising from frequent transitions and multiple care providers increases concerns about patients' well-being and safety. Patients who have multiple transfers are at risk for "medical errors, service duplication, inappropriate care, and critical elements of the care plan 'falling through the cracks' leading to 'poor clinical outcomes'" (Coleman, 2003, p. 549). Research reports on patient safety "demonstrates that the cumulative effect of mistakes . . . during care transitions can result in significant patient harm or even death." (Hughes & Clancy, 2007, p 289). The Institute of Medicine (IOM), in its 2008 report, *Retooling for an Aging America*, notes that older adults are "especially vulnerable" to harmful effects as they transition within and across care systems.

New models of care delivery are needed to improve health and well-being of older adults throughout the perioperative continuum and to prevent negative outcomes. The GOFC approach is introduced in response to these concerns as a way to improve safety, quality of care, and the well-being of older adults as they journey across the surgical continuum.

Gerioperative Facilitated Care

GOFC combines concepts from transitional care models and GOC as frameworks for a care delivery model that makes the surgical journey seamless, comfortable, and safe for older adults. Transitional care is "a set of actions designed to ensure the coordination and continuity of health care as patients transfer between different locations or different levels of care within the same location" (Coleman, 2003, p. 549). The approach is based on research establishing that:

- Surgical care involves multiple health care systems and subsystems that are related but often disconnected.
- Continuity of care is cost-effective.
- Transitional care improves patient outcomes.

The goals of GOFC are to enhance patient safety, well-being, and satisfaction; improve quality of surgical care; maximize patient outcomes; and minimize transition-related adverse events. Goals and outcomes of care are listed in Exhibit 2.2.

EXHIBIT 2.2 Goals and Expected Outcomes of Gerioperative Facilitated Care

Know and attend to current and emerging quality of daily life goals
- Goals are mutually determined
- Goals are reviewed regularly and revised as needed
- Older adult care and treatment preferences are respected

Facilitate transitions and translocations with minimal stress, risk, and discomfort for the older adult
- Receives anticipatory guidance prior to each transition
- Information shared with all members of health care team
- Translocations planned in advance attending to risk identification and preventive action

(continued)

EXHIBIT 2.2 **Goals and Expected Outcomes of Gerioperative Care** *(continued)*

Maximize health, safety, security, and comfort
- Health
  - Receives care to prevent secondary complications and surgical morbidity
  - Maintains or attains functional status
  - Reports health improved
  - Indicators satisfactory
- Safety
  - Has no adverse events
  - Preventive protocols implemented
- Security
  - Reports feeling comfortable
  - Engages in self-care
  - Demonstrates self-advocacy
  - Reports a supportive care-companion
- Comfort
  - Reports feeling part of planning and care processes
  - Reports pain well managed
  - Communicates needs to interdisciplinary team, staff, facilitator
  - Has accurate and timely information
  - Environmental design promotes comfort
  - Reports congruence between care providers, older adult, and family expectations regarding surgical goals and outcomes

Enhance self-care, independence, and function
- Has information and education for self-care
- Has needed equipment that supports self-care, independence, and maximum function available
- Has medication checklist for monitoring medication administration and changes in medication

Facilitate optimum care
- Receives assessment, care planning, and intervention activities that are evidence-based and reflect best practice
- Hospital length of stay decreased
- Evidence-based protocols are implemented
- Professional provider satisfaction is increased
- Relationship-centered care is evident between facilitator, patient, patient proxy, staff, and interdisciplinary team
- Care reflects mutually determined patient and provider goals

Prevent unexpected readmission
- Mutually developed transitional care plans reviewed periodically, revised as needed and implemented
- Referrals to health and social support services and resources
- Information on health and support services and resources is available
- System established for patient, proxy to report care concerns, questions

UNIQUENESS OF GERIOPERATIVE FACILITATED CARE

GOFC is innovative from two perspectives. First, GOFC focuses on older adults undergoing a surgical procedure while at the same time being an intentional, systematic coordination and integration of care throughout the surgical continuum, beginning with the decision to consider surgery and following through to stable recovery. Currently, no nursing care delivery models target older adults throughout the complete spectrum of surgical care.

The care situation at the beginning of this chapter highlights the need for the focus of care proposed by GOFC. In this situation, the patient's care needs could have been addressed more consistently and congruently if there was a single person coordinating care and someone had been assisting providers to remain aware of the patient's changing functional status and cognition. The interruption in continuity of care and the lack of coordination across systems contributed to his decline in health status. Knowledge of geriatrics and gerontology, in addition to surgical nursing knowledge, could have informed the care team about the patient's urgent needs for nutritional and cognitive support in the form of preventive actions.

In the current acute care system, the lack of continuity of care providers within and across care systems combines with inadequate time provided for "getting to know" the patient. Such constraints contribute to fragmentation of care, poor information sharing, and inconsistency in care. Further, these limitations impede the ability to provide adequate discharge planning and patient education, both of which can prevent unexpected readmissions of older adults. Unexpected readmissions occur as a result of poor care coordination and transfer of information. Focusing on *knowing* the older individual and the potential effects of aging and preexisting illness, coordinating care across the entire surgical continuum, and instituting preventive actions could have mitigated many of the factors that interfered with Mr. Tubman's quality of care.

GERIOPERATIVE FACILITATED CARE TEAM

GOFC relies on a team composed of the older adult, a GOC facilitator (GCF), and a companion-coach (CC) to support, monitor, and facilitate care across the surgical continuum. Exhibits 2.3 and 2.4 outline the role and responsibilities of the GCF and the CC.

EXHIBIT 2.3 Gerioperative Care Facilitator Responsibilities

- Support and advocate for the older adult and family or others designated by the patient
- Advocate for a patient-centered paradigm in the care of older adult
- Integrate plans of care across perioperative continuum
- Collaborate with members of the health care team using a patient-centered, relationship-oriented framework
- Serve as a resource to the health care team for information and clarification related to needs and goals of the older adult
- Promote implementation of gerioperative care
- Promote decisional support related to the older adult's care and outcome preferences on request
- Ensure the older adult has access to and understands care and treatment information as a basis for informed decision-making

EXHIBIT 2.4 **Companion-Coach Responsibilities**

- Be a friendly visitor
- Offer an attentive ear
- Respect the older adult as the decision maker
- Be a coach and encourage patient to notify staff about needs and concerns
- Report differences or changes in the older adults demeanor, needs, or condition
- Ask questions to clarify patient care information
- Collaborate with staff to ensure key elements of care are implemented
- Become a credible and active member of the team
- Be a cheerleader, coach, and support in helping the older adult perform recovery, self-care, and wellness activities

The GCF is a professional nurse who coordinates care decisions with the older adult, the family, individual care providers, and interdisciplinary care teams. The CC is a friend or family member who provides informal advice and encouragement as a coach and companion and acts as advocate or interpreter for the patient. The GCF and CC work together, following the older adult from care setting to care setting and unit-to-unit throughout the entire surgical journey. Figure 2.1 presents the GOFC model, showing the GCF supporting the efforts of the health care team and individual members across all stages of the surgical care continuum. The GCF and CC roles are discussed in greater detail later in this chapter.

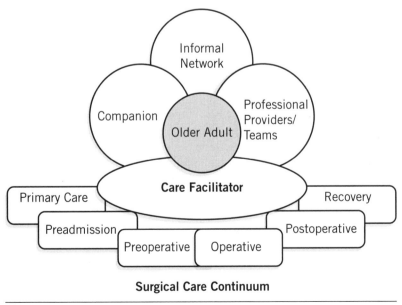

FIGURE 2.1
Gerioperative Facilitated Care Model

CORE PRINCIPLES

Guiding values noted in Exhibit 2.5 support the development of GOFC. The assumptions, key elements, and guiding principles are congruent with and reflect principles identified by the IOM for creating improved care delivery systems for older adults, and are shown in Table 2.2. The IOM principles include comprehensive care that is patient-centered, interdisciplinary, and seamless across delivery sites, and active partnership of patients and informal caregivers with the interdisciplinary care team. In line with these principles, a priority of GOFC is to honor the health and life hopes of the older adult. The older adult remains the center of the decision-making process; care activities are directed to maintaining the older adult's functional well-being, safety, and security. In the event the gerioperative patient becomes incapacitated during the gerioperative continuum or unable to participate in decision-making, the CC will already be aware of the elder patient's wishes and be an advocate for the patient's treatment and care until the patient recuperates or can make decisions once again.

An ounce of prevention is worth a pound of cure.

IMPACT

The GOFC approach changes the care delivery model, within and across care systems, as well as changes the focus of care transitions. The focus of all planning, activities, and actions is on the care needs of the individual older adult. The GCF promotes continuity of information between and among members of the care team leading to better and more informed decision-making. GOFC improves the internal consistency of care decisions and the congruency of care decisions with the elder adult's previously identified health and life goals.

EXHIBIT 2.5 Gerioperative Care Values

- An ounce of prevention is worth a pound of cure, or focusing surgical care on prevention yields better results at less cost.
- Care integrated within and across settings throughout the surgical continuum improves care and achieves better patient outcomes.
- Multiple care transitions involving multiple players and providers can be facilitated by a professional who "knits" the perioperative multiple transitions and players into an integrated whole.
- Comprehensive, collaborative assessment, effective risk identification, and effective primary and secondary interventions decrease patient suffering, surgical morbidity, and cost.
- Networks of health, social service, and community are critical resources.
- Best practice and evidence-based care increase care effectiveness.
- Collaboration among and between professional care providers and care teams improves communication and care outcomes.
- Relationship-centered care leads to better decisions, actions, and outcomes.
- Coaching older adults, caregivers, and families results in better elder self-care, health, and well-being.

TABLE 2.2

Comparison of GOC and IOM Care Principles

GOC Principles	IOM Principles (2008)*
• Facilitating comprehensive care across all phases of the surgical continuum • Referral to health care services and community resources and supports	"The health needs of the older population need to be addressed comprehensively."
• Instituting comprehensive assessment and taking appropriate preventive action and early intervention based on best practice guidelines • Using protocols to promote best practice and minimize adverse events • Using professional, nonprofessional, and informal providers as needed to provide treatment and care for the older adult	"Services need to be provided efficiently."
• Using relationship-centered care principles integrating all members of the care team • Respecting elder care and treatment preferences • Providing education, training, and support to older adult, family, patient companion, professional care providers, and support staff to support self-care and maximum independence of older adult	"Older persons need to be active partners in their own care."

*Institute of Medicine (IOM). (2008). Retooling for an aging America. Washington, D.C.: National Academies Press, p.76.

Care transitions are the most vulnerable periods of the surgical continuum. During care transitions, critical information can be lost. A significant change proposed by the GOFC is the level of support provided to the older adult during the most vulnerable periods of the surgical continuum and care transitions. The GOFC model provides support to health care providers and team members as they provide care at different times in different settings. The support is evident in the collaboration and coordination of information sharing. The GOFC decreases the effort needed in planning, implementing, and evaluating care consistent with the unique context of the individual older adult. Furthermore, by having the GCF following the patient across systems and units, duplication of effort, danger of care plans falling through the cracks, and delays in discharge planning are eliminated. The entire care process is more accessible and transparent to providers caring for the older adult as well as to the older adult and informal caregivers. Much of the work of the Institute for Health Improvement addresses the benefits of a more transparent care system and information sharing among team members. The GOFC role is consistent with these goals and provides an approach that moves these goals forward.

STRUCTURE

The structure of GOFC incorporates the functions and roles of the GCF in relation to other key players: older adult, health care providers, CC, and informal and formal support systems. This circle of support is depicted in Figure 2.1. The team circles rest on the care facilitator, suggesting that the level of support the facilitator provides to the older adult and the interdisciplinary health care team integrates and coordinates care throughout the surgical continuum. The surgical care continuum is depicted as stages. It is important to note that the continuum is progressive but not unidirectional. Older adults are apt to traverse the continuum with multiple moves back and forth across the different stages.

GERIOPERATIVE CARE FACILITATOR

The term *care facilitator* is rarely used in the United States to describe the role of support for patients within or across systems of care. The more common term is that of care manager or care coordinator. Distinguishing among these roles can be challenging due to the considerable overlap in roles and responsibilities. A facilitator makes progress easier; helps to maintain an open communication process among patients, families, and providers; and serves as a linking mechanism across the perioperative continuum.

A facilitator, the GCF, is the key to implementing the GOFC model of care. The GCF assesses and develops an understanding of the older adult's history, health status, needs, beliefs, and goals within the context of care. With this knowledge, the GCF engages with professional providers and direct caregivers to design and monitor treatment and plans of care that support the identified goals. GCFs are masters—prepared health care providers with education, training, and experience in the comprehensive care of older adults and in systems coordination. They are familiar with the surgical process and possess the necessary skills to be effective. Typically, GCFs are nurses, but they may be social workers, occupational therapists, or other professional clinicians. Clinical nurse leaders have the educational background in evidence-based practice, systems coordination, and clinical focus to be highly successful in the role. The GCF is a direct care provider, with knowledge of the type of care needed and the ability to work with patient, family, and provider teams. Important to the success of the model is the ability of the facilitator to establish positive relationships with older adults, their families, professionals, and support staff. Effective GCFs have a broad skill set as clinicians, scholars, educators, and interpreters.

GCFs must be adept at navigating the cultures of diverse care environments and care delivery systems. As a consultant to the patient, the facilitator will need to explain the GOFC model role and establish collaborative relationships with providers, support staff, and informal caregivers. The success of the GCFs as patient consultants and advocates rests on their ability to establish credibility and develop rapport with the heath care team.

The GCF supports the older adult by engaging as a clinician, scholar, interpreter, and educator (see Figure 2.2). When working to meet patient goals and the goals of GOC, the facilitator uses a set of processes and skills to implement the different roles. As clinician, the GCF uses clinical skills to ensure the integration of quality care. Having clinical knowledge and expertise is critical to understanding the care needs of the older adult and ensuring that the plan of care is directed toward achieving the individual's care goals and needs. As clinician, the GCF regularly conducts a risk assessment, identifies preventive interventions to minimize the identified risks, and collaborates with other providers to implement interventions. An expert clinician gains credibility with members of the interdisciplinary care team in order to effectively develop collaborative relationships. The GCF's expertise in geriatrics and gerontology can be a value to nurses who find the care of older adults challenging.

As educator, the GCF provides information to all members of the health care team. Promoting the older adult's self-care abilities and helping those in the informal support system be effective caregivers are instrumental in achieving the quality surgical outcomes of restoring optimal levels of function and well-being. Many older adults find it difficult to explain their concerns and care needs or to negotiate their plans of care when in primary care settings. Under the stress of surgery, being a self-advocate is an even greater challenge.

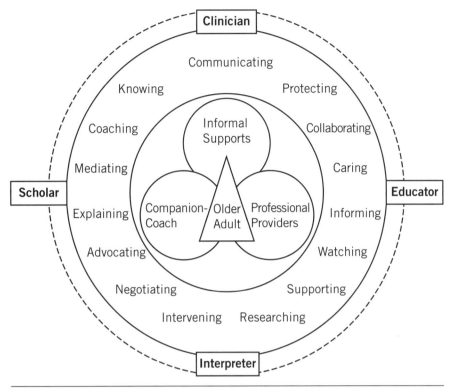

FIGURE 2.2
Gerioperative Care Facilitator Functions

Family members find it difficult to interpret the needs of an aging family member, communicate needs to providers, and negotiate with providers in a fast-paced acute care environment. Prior to surgery, the GCF coaches older adults and their support systems to communicate effectively regarding care needs and to navigate the acute care system. When the situation limits patients' ability to self-advocate, the facilitator serves as liaison to improve communication among and between the older adult, family members, CC, and professional providers.

As scholar, the GCF remains current regarding surgical care and practice in relation to the treatment of the older adult. Awareness of national patient care and safety guidelines to improve outcomes and prevent harm is essential. It is in the role of scholar that the facilitator ensures the older adult's care is based on best practice, incorporating evidence-based interventions grounded in the patient's specific health situation, preferences, and needs. The facilitator can share research findings with other care providers, who may not have the time or the knowledge to conduct literature searches and pursue emerging research. As innovator, the facilitator works with the health care team to use evidence-based care and to adapt interventions when needed to meet the specific care situation of the older adult.

In the interpreter role, the GCF is mindful of the differences in subcultures between patients and health care providers. The difference is present, even when members of both groups are from the same culture, and widens if members are from different minority, ethnic, or socioeconomic cultures. In addition, there are differences between older adults and care providers from younger generations regardless of other cultural beliefs. This mixture of cultures can affect the understanding of care needs and the care provided. The care facilitator in the interpreter role strives to promote cultural sensitivity and clarify understanding among members of these different cultures. The focus is to help the older adult make informed decisions based on the patient's values and preferences and an understanding of health-related information. Provider awareness and sensitivity to the multiple perspectives that influence and shape how information is presented and received is fundamental to patient-centered care.

GERIOPERATIVE COMPANION-COACH

The second key person in the GOFC model is a patient companion-coach (CC). The CC is a friend or family member who accompanies the older adult throughout the perioperative continuum. Key elements of the role of the CC role include support and encouragement during prehabilitation, surgery, and postoperative recovery, until after the follow-up visit with the surgeon or primary care provider. The CC encourages and works with the older adult to carry out prehabilitation as well as postoperative recovery and rehabilitation activities, including those required after discharge. The agreed on commitment by the CC ends after attending the post discharge surgeon and primary care follow-up visit with the older adult. As soon as the older adult identifies a person and throughout the perioperative continuum, the GCF coaches the older patient and CC as a team. Exhibit 2.4 outlines elements of the CC. Coaching the CC and older adult is described in Chapter 6.

Gerioperative Facilitated Care Practice Model

The GOFC model illustrated in Figure 2.3 is nested, indicating that concepts are interdependent. The increasing size of the segments suggests that the concepts in lower segments both rely on and support the concepts in the upper segments. The approach begins with comfort as a foundation for surgical care of the older adult. Comfort can be achieved with greater effectiveness and satisfaction when based on best practice and evidence. Relationship-centered care improves communication and collaboration required for best practice.

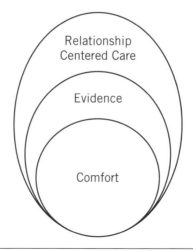

FIGURE 2.3
Concepts of the Gerioperative Facilitated Care Model

COMFORT THEORY

Comfort (verb) is action that leads to comfort (noun) as an outcome. The verb, to comfort, means to give strength and hope; to soothe, console, or reassure, to make physically comfortable; to relieve or alleviate as in to lessen pain or discomfort (Webster's New World Dictionary, 1970). Comfort, when used as a noun, means a feeling at ease; a sense of well-being, contentment, and satisfaction; a relief from affliction (Webster's New World Dictionary, 1970). The definitions identify comfort as both a care intervention and an outcome of care. Comfort incorporates physical, psychological, emotional, and spiritual dimensions. Surgical trauma challenges the older adult's comfort in each of these dimensions.

Kolcaba's (2001; Kolcaba, Tilton, & Drouin, 2006) theory of comfort originated from the behavior and responses of older adults with Alzheimer's disease. Kolcaba defines comfort as an immediate state of "being strengthened" by having the needs for relief, ease, and transcendence met physiologically, psychospiritually, socioculturally, and environmentally. Enhancing comfort leads to an individual's ability to be active in self-care. Comfort theory extends beyond the care of patients and families. Kolcaba, Tilton, and Drouin (2006) noted that meeting the comfort needs of professional caregivers improves clinical practice and, subsequently, better patient care outcomes.

Several authors have applied comfort theory to improving surgical care and practice. Wilson and Kolcaba (2004) used comfort theory to improve perianesthesia nursing practice. Comfort theory served as the framework for an acute care of elderly (ACE) unit for older adults having orthopedic surgery (Panno, Kolcaba, & Holder, 2000). A study by Wagner, Byrne, and Kolcaba (2006) on patient warming in the operating room used comfort as the study's theoretical framework.

In GOC, comfort is used as an action: the acts of providing comfort, a care outcome, and a maximum state of comfort and well-being. In addition to the patient's comfort, the GCF considers the application of comfort theory when interacting with family members, providers, and caregivers based on the knowledge that when family members, providers, and caregivers are comfortable, they can be more effective in meeting the comfort needs of the older adult.

BEST PRACTICE

There is no universal definition for best practice. Best practice and evidence-based practice are often used interchangeably, but there are notable differences. Evidence-based practice incorporates clinical judgment acquired through clinical experience combined with knowledge obtained from reputable research journals. Thus, evidence-based practice requires the clinician to apply published data in the context of clinical judgment and patient choice.

Best practice implies the use of standardized procedures and models found to be successful in meeting a desired outcome, usually based on empirical evidence. A second element in the definition of best practice is adaptation of the evidence to a current situation. Best practice integrates systematic research, expert opinion, and clinical judgment when making care and treatment decisions in the context of a specific care and patient situation (Sackett, Rosenberg, Gray, Haynes, & Richardson, 1996; Tanner, 2006).

Evidence-based practice and best practice both speak to the art and science of a discipline. GOFC is based on GOC—the integration of the art, science, and best practice from gerontology, geriatrics, and surgery.

RELATIONSHIP-CENTERED CARE

Relationship-centered care is "a philosophy that stresses partnership, careful attention to relational process, shared decision-making, and self-awareness" (Suchman, 2006, p. S40).

In relationship-centered care, the provider values relationships with patients, members of the health care teams, communities, and self as central elements in professional practice and the vehicle for achieving quality health care and optimal outcomes (Pew-Fetzer Task Force, 1994). Relationship-centered care calls for providers to be aware of their own beliefs, attitudes, values, and biases. Providers must respect and appreciate the experience and knowledge of patients, families, and colleagues; actively engage and communicate effectively; use reflection in action and reflection on action to improve practice; and remain open to alternative perspectives and paradigms.

The philosophy of relationship-centered care is akin to the ethics of personalism (dePender & Ikeda-Chandler, 1990), an ethic that argues "our most positive and lasting meaning comes from the quality of our relationships with ourselves and with other people" (p. 76) based on a "deep respect for the importance and worth of each person" (p. 77). Personalism extends traditional ethical principles of advocacy, beneficence, nonmalfeasance, and justice from a focus on the principle of recognizing the relationship as a medium for interpreting the problem and resolving the conflict. The IOM (2000, 2004) argues that improving patient-provider and provider-provider relationships and communication are significant contributions to minimizing medical errors and preventing harm. Nonsupportive or noncaring relationships between providers and patients or among providers can result in poor decision-making, due to incorrect information or inadequate understanding of the care situation.

Effective care and treatment decisions are dependent on the interactions between and among the key players and their awareness of how their perspectives, beliefs, attitudes, and paradigms influence the decision-making process and outcomes (Tanner, 2006).

Relationship-centered care paves the way for successful collaboration with and among members of the health care team (Gittel et al., 2000). Best practice and comfort care can be more effective in an environment when positive collegial relationships support open debate and discussion.

Evaluating Gerioperative Facilitated Care

The GOFC model is a proposed approach to care. While it has not been tested in practice, the tenets, principles, goals, key elements, and selected interventions are supported by the science of gerontology and geriatrics. GOFC is based on an ethic of care that is relationship-centered and committed to respecting the dignity, autonomy, and personhood of the older adult.

Process and outcome evaluation occurs with the older adult or designated members of the family. Criteria for evaluation reflect the GOFC's goals, aims, and outcomes: quality of care; number and severity of surgical complications; number and severity of adverse events; hospital readmission rate; elder and family satisfaction and goals; provider follow-up visits; and quality of relationships among and between members of the health care team and staff.

Access to the Gerioperative Care Facilitator

GCFs reflect goals outlined in the current arguments for improving transitional care. GOFC can be offered as a patient-centered service in hospitals, ambulatory surgical care centers, or outpatient surgical departments. It also can be offered through private enterprises, such as a surgeon practice group or independent contractors. Health care, nursing, and medical schools and colleges can offer GOFC as a clinical service that benefits students and older adults.

In an established health care system, GOFC may be implemented as an adjunct service through the surgical service or health care provider group available to any older adult undergoing a surgical procedure. Funding the service can be through fee-for-service, as a benefit of a health maintenance organization or insurance plan, or, when sufficient evidence demonstrates cost effectiveness, through Medicare reimbursement. The major direct cost is the GCF. Savings from decreased complication rates and non-readmission to hospital is expected to offset the cost.

A second implementation strategy for GOFC is through a private contractor or consultant model. In this strategy, an older adult or family contacts an agency offering the service directly in a contract for services.

All older adults facing the trauma of a surgical procedure and the care transitions associated with surgery can benefit from GOFC. Elders classified as II or above by the American Society of Anesthesiologists classification system may derive the greatest benefit and cost-effectiveness. A second group of elders who may find GOFC an important source of security and comfort are those with family living at a distance and not available to help the older adult manage care.

Regardless of the system providing GOFC, the older adult should provide written notification indicating that both the GCF and CC are part of the patient's health care team and should have access to health care information. Such documentation provides credibility to both the GCF and CC when sharing information about the older adult and when participating in decision-making and care coordination processes.

Related Transitional Care Models

Transitional care models to improve the health and well-being of older adults have been an ongoing enterprise for over 20 years. The IOM (2008) commissioned a review of care models offering comprehensive care services for older adults. Table 2.3 reviews selected interdisciplinary models described by the IOM and care transition models reviewed by Ryan (2011). Acute care delivery models include the Hospital Elder Life Program (Inouye, Bogardus, Baker, Leo-Summers, & Cooney, 2000), the Geriatric Evaluation and Management program (Rubenstein, Josephson, Wieland, English, Sayre, & Kane, 1984), and ACE (Landefeld, Palmer, Kresevic, Fortinsky & Kowal, 1995).

The purpose is to use geriatric specialty care units or consulting services to improve care and prevent iatrogenesis through interdisciplinary care teams, comprehensive geriatric assessment, and staff education and training.

Transitional care models generally focus on discharge planning and the transition of the older adult from hospital to home or nursing home to promote health and function after discharge and prevent hospital readmission. Common themes across transitional models are targeted discharge plans, improving patient self-care and management, and post discharge follow-up through home visits or telephone calls. The Care Transitions Intervention (Coleman, Parry, Chalmers, & Min, 2006), Transitional Care Model (Naylor, Brooten, Campbell, Maislin, McCauley, & Schwartz, 2004), and Guided Care (Boult, Gidens, Frey, Reider, & Novak, 2009) involve a specially trained nurse to implement the transitions intervention. The Guided Care nurse provides transitional care at time of hospital admission and discharge but does not follow the patient's during the hospital stay.

Mezey, Boltz, Esterson, and Mitty (2005) reviewed models that expanded or changed nurses' roles or responsibilities in caring for older adults in assisted living, home care, hospitals, and nursing homes. Nurses in acute care hospitals across the United States and Canada have created a number of nurse-led interventions under the auspices of the Nurses Improving Care

TABLE 2.3
Overview of Selected Transition Care Models

	Transition Focus	Patient Focus	Patient/Family contact	Length Intervention
Care Transitions Intervention (Coleman, Parry, Chalmers, & Min, 2006)	Hospital discharge	• Patient self-activation, empowerment • Medication management • Patient-centered record • Primary care/specialist follow-up • Identifying "red flags"	• Predischarge hospital visit • Post discharge home visit • Telephone follow-up	4 weeks
Transitional Care Model (Naylor et al., 1999)	Hospital discharge	• Patient self-management • Care coordination • Individualized plan of care • Medication reconciliation, management	• Predischarge hospital visit • Home visit • Telephone follow-up • Initial primary care visit	Up to 8 weeks
Guided Care (Boult, Gidens, Frey, Reider, & Novak, 2009)	Primary care	• Preventing hospital admission • Patient self-management • Smoothing hospital admission and discharge	• Throughout program	Long-term
Promoting a Geriatric-friendly Environment through Nursing Evaluation and Specific Interventions for Successful Healing (Baumhover & McNicoll, 2007)	Within hospital	• Improving quality care • Preventing iatrogenesis	• In hospital care	Hospital stay

to Health System Elders, initiated by the John A. Hartford Foundation Institute for Geriatric Nursing. Several models of nursing care rely on a geriatric resource nurse or clinical specialist.

Geriatric-friendly Environment through Nursing Evaluation and Specific Interventions for Successful Healing (GENESIS) is a nursing care delivery model described by Baumhover and McNicoll (2007). Program goals are to decrease complications and maintain functional capacity of hospitalized older adults. The key program elements were unit-based including staff education, environmental changes, and the use of nursing protocols. Nurses and certified nursing assistants received education on geriatric nursing care. The primary practice intervention involved implementing evidence-based mobility, sleep, pain, delirium, and nutrition nursing protocols. A planned expansion of the GENESIS project was to incorporate the GENESIS principles to care of geriatric patients across the perioperative continuum, including discharge planning.

An analysis of programs identifies common key elements and goals, suggesting there is a shared expectation among geriatric and gerontological advocates about changes that are needed to improve transitional care of older adults.

Implementing a GOC program expands current models of care. Each of the approaches described previously target a specific care setting or process. None address the unique transitional care needs of the older adult undergoing surgery. The GOC approach is unique in its scope and target population.

PATIENT REPORT: Mr. Tubman

Mr. Tubman died 2 weeks postoperatively. His condition was compounded by multiple providers who cared for parts of him, but no one integrated the care or facilitated care and communication processes among and between providers. His wife was told little about his condition and was left alone to care for him.

Although Mr. Tubman's case is extreme, it is not unusual. Mr. Tubman was ill-prepared physically, physiologically, or psychologically for surgery. Although he was active, he was bordering on frailty due to his weight loss, inadequate nutrition, poor sleep patterns, and lack of exercise. He had no preoperative coaching or plan of care to prevent complications based on his identified risk factors. His preoperative teaching focused exclusively on what to expect during and after surgery.

A GCF could have made the surgical journey easier for Mr. Tubman and for his wife. Mr. Tubman had a number of risk factors that needed to be identified during the preoperative period with plans for rehabilitation, post admission preoperative hospital care, and postoperative care. Coordinating the efforts of multiple providers, maintaining communication flow, and collaborating on plans for preventive actions especially around fluid management, nutrition needs, and potential for deconditioning is central to the care of patients with complex preexisting or emerging health problems. Identifying problems based on preoperative knowledge and working with the staff to identify nutrition needs, cognitive changes, sensitivity to antibiotics, and fluid management may have changed Mr. Tubman's outcome.

SUMMARY

GOC is an approach to the care of the geriatric surgical patient that can be implemented by a single practitioner, a unit, or an interdisciplinary team regardless of setting. The model emphasizes application of evidence-based gerontology and geriatrics in the care of the gerioperative patient.

The GOFC approach is a theoretical comprehensive practice approach that crosses the perioperative continuum. While not yet tested, evidence abounds that integrating care among multiple practitioners and practice settings *with attention to the patient's goals, preferences, and values* can improve care quality and patient outcomes, patient satisfaction, decrease length of hospital stays, and cut health care costs. This approach has not been addressed across the full continuum of care. Pieces of the continuum have and are being done within and across hospital units, and between single levels of care such as transitional or discharge planning from institution to home. It is time to knit the pieces into a complete fabric of care. Extending a transitional care model across the complete perioperative care continuum will improve care quality, achieve better patient outcomes, and be cost-effective.

KEY POINTS

- Preventing "falling through the cracks" and maintaining continuity of care for gerioperative patients continues to be a major health care issue decried by health policymakers, geriatricians, gerontologists, and geriatric nurse leaders for over 40 years.
- The perioperative continuum is a fragmented care system involving multiple transitions with multiple providers, increasing the risk of adverse events and poor patient outcomes.
- GOC can restructure clinical practice by focusing individual provider, interdisciplinary teams, and systems attention to the transitional care needs of the older adult across the perioperative continuum.
- A GCF who follows the gerioperative patient throughout the perioperative continuum can improve patient outcomes and decrease costs.

THREE

Gerioperative Practice Standards and Quality Care

Raelene V. Shippee-Rice, Jennifer V. Long, and Susan J. Fetzer

PATIENT REPORT: Ms. Mills

Ms. Mills underwent a hemicolectomy for colon cancer. She was 82 years old, an active crafter, and a volunteer at the local hospital. In the postanesthesia care unit (PACU), her vital signs remained stable and within her preoperative values. She was not a candidate for epidural analgesia, and after 40 minutes in the PACU she was awake and alert, rating her abdominal pain at a level of 5 on a scale of 0–10. The surgeon wrote an order for meperidine 50 mg intramuscularly (IM). As the PACU nurse reviewed the order, he recognized that Ms. Mills was 82 years old and that at 82 she would have decreased muscle mass. As the nurse considered his next steps, an echo from the past is the pharmacology professor sharing the rhyme about medications with anticholinergic properties: "can't see, can't pee, can't poop, can't spit." The nurse recalls that meperidine has anticholinergic properties and calls the provider suggesting a change in medication based on the following concerns: meperidine is contraindicated in older adults due to its anticholinergic properties, and risk of delirium. A final concern is the IM administration route. Older adults should not be given IM medications. The nurse presented the current order, analysis of the contraindications, and recommended a change in the medication order to hydromorphone 0.25 mg intravenously. The provider agreed and changed the order. On reassessment, Ms. Mills's indicated her pain was decreased to 2/10 and she was comfortable. She was discharged to the medical-surgical unit.

Gerioperative care is evidence-based and grounded in professional practice standards, best practice guidelines, research, and clinical judgment to ensure the safety, well-being, and care quality for the older adult. Surgical care of the older adult involves more than the response to the trauma and stress from the physiologic invasion caused by the surgical procedure. Many older adults have comorbid diseases affecting health status and functional capacity unrelated to the etiology of surgery. The quality of gerioperative care and standards for determining excellence in gerioperative practice must rest on more than the standards and guidelines of any one discipline. The measure of quality must be based on an integration of standards, guidelines, and protocols from multiple nursing and interdisciplinary clinical specialties. Currently, there are no standards identifying and mandating a broad, holistic perspective for ensuring the quality of surgical care of older adults in any discipline, and there is no interdisciplinary care standard. The primary focus of this chapter is to describe the potential contributions current nursing practice standards, position statements, and guidelines along with standards and guidelines used by other disciplines can make to quality surgical care of older adults. The chapter concludes with an argument that an interdisciplinary standard for gerioperative care is needed.

Professional Practice Standards

Gerontologic and geriatric nursing, primary care advanced nursing, perioperative nursing, anesthesia nursing, medical-surgical nursing, critical care, and community health nursing all guide the standard of care for gerioperative nursing practice standards and determine quality of care. Internal medicine, surgery, anesthesiology, medical clinical specialties, and allied health disciplines have professional practice standards or guidelines that guide the care of older adults' gerioperative care and provide additional sources of evidence. The need to incorporate and consider practice standards from nursing, clinical specialties, and allied health disciplines highlights the complex and challenging nature associated with providing safe, quality perioperative care to older adults.

Standards of practice, also known as standards of care, are criteria established by professional organizations and institutions for defining what is meant by professional practice. Standards determine what a professional practitioner should do and how professional practice should be enacted. Standards of practice that guide professional practice and the quality of patient care vary across disciplines. In some disciplines and health care contexts, standards describe minimum levels of performance or competence, whereas standards applied in other situations are used to measure the degree of excellence. *Minimum* standards establish what members of a profession or group consider an acceptable level of practice, what should be done, and how it should be done. When used as a measure of excellence, practice standards define what is meant by quality and measure performance against the established standards. Practice standards are authoritative rules and requirements and can be used to legally determine the actions and behaviors of professional practitioners.

Practitioner knowledge, skills, judgment, and attitudes needed to practice safely are based on identified practice standards. A basic premise of practice standards is that the practitioner holds the responsibility and accountability for professional practice behaviors and performance, either through direct action or through the actions of those to whom they delegate. In nursing, standards promote quality of nursing practice ". . .by delineating the professional scope and standards of practice and responsibilities of all professional registered nurses engaged in nursing practice, regardless of setting" (American Nurses Association, 2010, p. 29). Nursing standards are often used to create job descriptions, develop performance appraisal documents, and establish quality assurance or peer-review systems.

Standards of practice and standards of care are not fixed entities. They evolve as knowledge and evidence evolve, undergoing periodic review to ensure that new levels of expected practice behaviors and outcomes are developed in response to emerging evidence and expectations. Recognized experts or members of professional organizations write practice standards for their own professions that are then reviewed, edited, adapted, approved, and accepted by members of the profession.

NURSING SCOPE AND STANDARDS OF PRACTICE

Professional standards for nursing practice are developed by nurse leaders, clinicians, and educators who worked with American Nurses Association (ANA) members to create the *Nursing: Scope and Standards of Practice* document (2010). Members of the ANA and clinical nursing specialty professional organizations endorsed the scope and standards of the practice document, approving the application of the standards to all professional registered nurses regardless of specialty practice. The purpose of the standards is to describe the responsibilities for which the professional nurse is accountable and provide a framework for the evaluation of this accountability.

The *Nursing Scope and Standards Of Practice* (2010) document incorporates 6 standards of practice and 10 standards for professional nursing performance. The 2010 standards of practice and standards for professional nursing practice expand the responsibility of nurses for evidence-based practice and research, quality of practice, coordination and collaboration, and responsibility for evaluating personal practice. Exhibits 3.1 and 3.2 list care standards and nursing performance standards. The ANA standards serve as the foundation for all clinical nursing specialty practice standards.

Nursing is a complex, creative, and relational art juxtaposed with a science. As a profession, nursing is highly dependent on the continued acquisition of evolving knowledge, skills, and abilities. Performance standards describe the roles and behaviors expected of professional nurses based on practice standards. Integrating performance and practice standards creates a framework to support development of criteria for nursing excellence. The ANA nursing standards establish outcome expectations for meeting the criterion for quality nursing care. An element missing in earlier nursing standards was an explicit reference to the collaborative nature

---

EXHIBIT 3.1 Nursing Standards of Practice

Standard 1. Assessment
   The registered nurse collects comprehensive data pertinent to the health care consumer's health and/or the situation.

Standard 2. Diagnosis
   The registered nurse analyzes the assessment data to determine the diagnosis or the issues.

Standard 3. Outcomes Identification
   The registered nurse identifies expected outcomes for a plan individualized to the health care consumer or situation.

Standard 4. Planning
   The registered nurse develops a plan that prescribes strategies and alternatives to attain expected outcomes.

Standard 5. Implementation
   The registered nurse implements the identified plan.

Standard 5A. Coordination of Care
   The registered nurse coordinates care delivery.

Standard 5B. Health Teaching and Health Promotion
   The registered nurse employs strategies to promote health and a safe environment.

Standard 6. Evaluation
   The registered nurse evaluates progress toward attainment of outcomes.

EXHIBIT 3.2 Nursing Standards of Professional Performance

Standard 7. Ethics
The registered nurse practices ethically.

Standard 8. Education
The registered nurse attains knowledge and competence that reflects current nursing practice.

Standard 9. Evidence-Based Practice and Research
The registered nurse integrates evidence and research findings into practice.

Standard 10. Quality of Practice
The registered nurse contributes to quality nursing practice.

Standard 11. Communication
The registered nurse communicates effectively in a variety of formats in all areas of practice.

Standard 12. Leadership
The registered nurse demonstrates leadership in the professional practice setting and the profession.

Standard 13. Collaboration
The registered nurse collaborates with health care consumers, families, and others in the conduct of nursing practice.

Standard 14. Professional Practice Evaluation
The registered nurse evaluates her or his own nursing practice in relation to professional practice standards and guidelines, relevant statues, rules, and regulations.

Standard 15. Resource Utilization
The registered nurse utilizes appropriate resources to plan and provide nursing services that are safe, effective, and financially responsible.

Standard 16. Environmental Health
The registered nurse practices in an environmentally safe and healthy manner.

of the nurse-patient relationship. Although defined as a process, patient participation in making treatment decisions is also important to a professional practice outcome. In an environment of patient-centered care, professional standards must clearly state the collaborative nature of the nurse-patient relationship. The 2010 professional nursing practice standards clearly state the nature of the responsibility to collaborate with health care consumers and families.

Nursing practice and performance standards reflect a number of core themes. Selected themes can be adapted to guide a gerioperative model of nursing care. Examples of themes derived from ANA standards of particular relevance to gerioperative care include:

- Attending to the need for culturally, ethnically, and cohort-sensitive care.
- Maintaining an environment that is physically, emotionally, spiritually, physiologically, and ethically safe.

- Educating and assisting older adults and their families when making decisions about health care goals; treatment outcomes, options, and interventions; self-care and health promotion activities; and quality of life issues.
- Ensuring continuity of care throughout the perioperative continuum by:
  - Managing and sharing information.
  - Coordinating care among professional and informal caregivers across care settings.

NURSING CLINICAL SPECIALTY STANDARDS OF PRACTICE

Specialty nursing practice organizations have developed standards of practice or standards of care that reflect the uniqueness of the specialty practice. Specialty nursing standards must be consistent with the practice standards established by the ANA while reflecting the unique outcomes, expectations, and parameters of the clinical specialty. Gerioperative care engages nurses across diverse health care settings: primary care, hospital care, ambulatory care, rehabilitation, and home care. Therefore, the practice standards must reflect the unique care provided across these multiple settings and the type of care provided in each setting. The following nursing specialty practice standards can guide gerioperative care and development of standards for gerioperative practice:

- *Scope and Standards of Gerontological Nursing Practice*
- *Home Health Nursing: Scope and Standards of Practice*
- *Pain Management Nursing: Scope and Standards of Practice*
- *PeriAnesthesia Nursing Standards and Practices*
- *Perioperative Standards and Recommended Practices*
- *Scope and Standards of Medical-Surgical Nursing*
- *Scope and Standards of Nurse Anesthesia Practice*
- *Standards of Care for Acute and Critical Care Nursing*
- *Scope and Standards of Practice for Professional Ambulatory Care Nursing*

Although clinical specialty standards must reflect and be consistent with ANA standards, specialty organization standards are often more comprehensive in determining behaviors and expectations for nursing practice targeted to the unique needs and characteristics of the specialty clinical population. For example, the Association of periOperative Registered Nurses (AORN) nursing standards incorporate structure, process, and outcomes of perioperative care; practice guidelines and protocols specific to the perioperative setting; and position and policy statements.

ALLIED HEALTH PROFESSIONAL STANDARDS

Professional practice standards established by other disciplines direct the expected norms and activities of other health care providers on the gerioperative interdisciplinary team. Similar to the ANA nursing standards, the standards developed by each of the allied health professional organizations are not specific to care of the older adult but address the quality of care given to all persons. Recognizing and respecting professional standards that guide the practice of each member of the interdisciplinary team creates a core and norm of practice excellence that can be applied to care of the older adult. By working together, the health care team can tailor the practice standards of each profession to the needs of older adults, thereby providing a framework and expectation for quality care.

Position Statements

Position statements, broadly defined, are statements of intent or advocacy written by members of a professional society or group of experts representing an organization. The statements reflect expert opinions or an organization's philosophy or values about a specific topic or concern. The position statement often outlines specific goals or recommendations for a course of action by the group writing the statement or as a general policy for other organizations or groups to follow. Position statements are not binding; they serve as calls to action and mandates for change.

NURSING POSITION STATEMENTS

A number of nursing organizations have created position statements on nursing care of older adults. Position statements of particular relevance to gerioperative care are the statements on perioperative care of the older adults from AORN, the American Society of PeriAnesthesia Nurses (ASPAN), the Academy of Medical-Surgical Nurses, and the Association of Medical-Surgical Nurses, and the Hartford Institute *Specialty Nursing Association Global Vision Statement on Care of Older Adults* (2011). These vision statements can be found in Exhibit 3.3.

The AORN position statement addresses issues that are of direct and immediate importance to gerioperative care. The statements point to nurse competence in applying knowledge of physiologic, psychological, and social changes presented by older adults and the effect of these changes on the care needs of the older adult responding to the trauma and stresses of surgery.

ASPAN's position statement advocates promoting education, research, and clinical practice to improve nurses' knowledge about aging and care of older adults in the perianesthesia setting. The position statement also advocates that perianesthesia nurses inform other members of the health care team how education and research on age-related changes can promote positive outcomes in the perianesthesia setting.

The *Global Vision Statement* (2011) advocates eight principles of nursing education and practice that must be incorporated to ensure nurses have the knowledge, skills, and attitudes necessary for providing quality nursing care to older adults. Although the statements do not specifically address the needs of the older adult having surgery, the application of the principles will improve geriatric care, regardless of setting or health condition. The weight of the many professional nursing organizations formally approving the *Global Vision Statement* generates a call for action in changing nursing education and practice related to care of older adults.

Practice Guidelines

Practice guidelines are recommendations based on research, systematic investigations, systematic literature reviews, case control studies, or expert opinion. The purpose of a guideline is to assist health providers in making and implementing care and treatment decisions in specific clinical circumstances and to promote best practice. Practice guidelines are not rigid rules. They must be adapted to the care needs of the individual patient, clinical situation, health care setting, and available resources. Guidelines are reviewed and revised on a regular basis to ensure they remain consistent with emerging evidence from research and professional practice.

Health care organizations, professional provider organizations, government agencies, and expert panels composed of researchers, educators, or practitioners develop practice guidelines based on published data and best evidence. The National Guideline Clearinghouse (NGC) is an

EXHIBIT 3.3 Themes: Nursing Vision and Position Statements

Themes	Global Vision	AORN	ASPAN	AMSN
Age-related changes contributing to unique care needs of older adults	Older adults receive care sensitive to the physiological, functional, and psychological needs that set them apart from younger adults.	Perioperative registered nurses should recognize the physiological, cognitive/psychological, and sociological changes associated with aging and understand that age alone puts older adults at risk for complications.	Perianesthesia nurses seek knowledge of and develop skills in the care of geriatric patient to promote positive outcomes in perianesthesia settings.	The medical-surgical nurse should support the older adult and his or her support system in efforts to maintain a healthy and safe lifestyle, live independently, and manage the older adult's health care problems based on the individual's physical, mental, and financial limitations.
Respectful, patient-centered, elder-sensitive care	All nurses appreciate the wide spectrum of health of people aged 65 and over, and are responsive to the needs of "healthy" and "frail" older adults, taking into account cultural diversity.	Perioperative registered nurses should provide patient-centered care that takes into consideration the unique needs of older adults.	Perianesthesia registered nurses will be respectful, knowledgeable, and insightful of special considerations related to aging when caring for geriatric patients.	The medical-surgical nurse advocates for maintaining the dignity and rights of the older adult and the incorporation of the older adult's values and belief systems into health maintenance and health care decisions.

(continued)

EXHIBIT 3.3 Themes: Nursing Vision and Position Statements (*continued*)

Themes	Global Vision	AORN	ASPAN	AMSN
Evidence-based practice	All nurses are familiar with the evidence-based body of knowledge about care of older adults.		Encourage research activities related to perianesthesia geriatric considerations.	The medical-surgical nurse should be knowledgeable regarding issues affecting the health and well-being of the older adult.
Education and practice	All prelicensure and postlicensure nursing education programs incorporate competencies related to care of older adults.	Staff education competencies should be developed, initiated, and evaluated to assure perioperative registered nurses are proficient in addressing the needs of older adults.	Integrate issues related to geriatric considerations into perianesthesia education, research, and clinical practice.	The medical-surgical nurse pursues continuing education and/or certification in gerontology. The medical-surgical nurse can utilize tools available from the Hartford Institute for Geriatric Nursing in providing a safe environment for the hospitalized older adult.
Policy development	Care of older adults should be an essential element of hospital staff development education.		All perianesthesia registered nurses will familiarize themselves with and inform other members of the health care team of this position statement. Externalize information by sharing this position with regulatory agencies and professional organizations that interface with the perianesthesia nursing specialty.	The medical-surgical nurse supports health care reform that includes affordable and appropriate health care for the older adult.

Resource availability	Hospitals, home care, and institutional long-term care settings establish systems that support best practices in care of older adults.	Human and physical resources should be available to address the unique needs of older adults.	Develop guidelines to support and enhance knowledge and skills in the care of the geriatric patient.
	Care of older adults be seen as a responsibility of all nurses crossing all specialties.		
	Practicing nurses look to specialty nursing associations as resources for evidence-based clinical care information related to care of older adults.		

AORN, Association of periOperative Registered Nurses; AMSN, Academy of Medical-Surgical Nurses; ASPAN, American Society of PeriAnesthesia Nurses.

initiative of the Agency for Healthcare Research and Quality (AHRQ) in the U.S. Department of Health and Human Services. The purpose of the NGC is to collect, review, and disseminate practice guidelines for use by professional health care providers, organizations, and agencies to improve practice and patient care quality. A panel of experts reviews and approves all guidelines before they are listed with the NCG and released for dissemination. Each guideline includes:

- Structured, standardized abstracts (summaries) about each guideline and its development.
- A utility for comparing attributes of two or more guidelines in a side-by-side comparison.
- Syntheses of guidelines covering similar topics, highlighting areas of similarity and difference.
- Links to full-text guidelines, where available, and ordering information for print copies.
- Annotated bibliographies on guideline development methodology, structure, implementation, and evaluation.

Exhibit 3.4 lists selected websites that have practice guidelines for (1) perioperative care of adults, (2) care of older adults, and (3) perioperative care of older adults. Most guidelines are available to the general public as well as to professional care providers. Several of the websites describe protocols; they are included here for convenience. Protocols are described in the next section. Guidelines and protocols can be used by:

- Individual nurses and other providers to guide professional practices.
- Organizations and agencies as a basis for developing evidence-based practice protocols.
- Family members caring for an older adult before and after surgery.

Protocols

Protocols are more specific than guidelines, though the terms are sometimes used interchangeably. Protocols specify the steps to be followed in conducting an examination, carrying

---

EXHIBIT 3.4 Selected Clinical Guideline Websites for Gerioperative Care

Agency for Healthcare Research and Quality: http://text.nlm.nih.gov
American Pain Society: www.ampainsoc.org
American Society of Anesthesiologists: www.asahq.org
American Geriatrics Society: www.americangeriatrics.org
American Society of PeriAnesthesia Nursing: www.aspan.org
Association of periOperative Registered Nurses: www.aorn.org
American Association of Nurse Anesthetists: www.aana.com
The British Pain Society: www.britishpainsociety.org
Hartford Institute for Geriatric Nursing: http://consultgerirn.org
International Association for the Study of Pain: www.iasp-pain.org
National Guideline Clearinghouse: www.guideline.gov
University of Iowa Evidence-Based Practice Guidelines:
  http://www.nursing.uiowa.edu/hartford/nurse/ebp.htm
University of Iowa/Gerontological Nursing Interventions Research Center:
  http://www.nursing.uiowa.edu/excellence/nursing_interventions

out a procedure, or providing care for a particular condition or population. Using protocols allows for a standardized, evidence-based, identified level of care for each patient to assure an intended outcome. Major outcomes expected from the use of protocols are improved patient safety and error minimization. Clinical protocols can be an essential element for reducing variability in patient care. Based on national guidelines and practice recommendations or mandates, protocols are adapted to local practice environments and situations. For example, the Joint Commission universal protocol for preventing wrong site, wrong procedure, and wrong person surgeries in hospitals and outpatient settings consists of three steps:

1. Conduct a preprocedure verification process.
2. Mark the procedure site.
3. Perform a time-out.

The details for implementing these steps through communication methods, checklists, verification processes, marking procedures, and management of the time-out must be developed at the local hospital or outpatient surgical setting. The steps of the universal protocol are mandated, but the implementation procedures are determined in the local institution based on situation, context, resources, and patient population. Similarly, institutional protocols must be adapted to the needs of the individual patient. Expert clinicians, guided by published data and clinical judgment, are the foundation for adapting guidelines to protocols and for adapting protocols to individual patients. Neuman and colleagues (2010) conducted a survey of Pennsylvania hospitals to assess the prevalence of protocol or guidelines for selected patient care processes. Results indicated that over 85% of the 103 respondents had written protocols for general hospital practices recommended in the Surgical Care Improvement Project (SCIP) core measures. Almost 75% had written care documents or pathways for hip fracture. Protocols for inpatient geriatric consultation were in place in 39% of sampled hospitals. Less than 25% reported having standard protocols or guidelines for assessing delirium, a major geriatric syndrome and patient care concern. The authors recommended better dissemination and implementation of guidelines and protocols directed to clinical care of older adults.

A major resource for evidence-based geriatric protocols pertinent to gerioperative care is ConsultGeriRN.org. This geriatric nursing website is sponsored by the Hartford Institute for Geriatric Nursing at New York University's College of Nursing. The protocols listed on the ConsultGeriRN website describe nursing care of older adults experiencing common geriatric syndromes or care needs. Although the protocols are not targeted specifically to surgical care of older adults, many of the geriatric syndromes covered in the protocols are related to perioperative care issues. Exhibit 3.5 lists the protocols with particular relevance to surgical care of older adults. The protocols, when maintained in accordance to current evidence, should be required practice standards for gerioperative care. A sample of a delirium protocol adapted from Tullman, Mion, Fletcher, and Forman (2008) is available in Appendix I (Delirium Protocol I-1).

Order Sets

Order sets (previously known as standing orders) are pre-established, prescribed orders designed to expedite patient care. Order sets may reflect the orders of an individual care provider, a team of providers, or a clinical department. Order sets can also serve as protocols.

Postoperative orders sets direct interventions for specific patient care issues such as pain, mobility, and nutrition. Order sets can be more comprehensive, addressing multiple care issues for total patient care or for comprehensive care before, during, and after procedures.

EXHIBIT 3.5 Evidence-Based Geriatric Nursing Protocols*

Advance directives	Iatrogenesis
Age-related changes	Medication
Assessing cognition	Nutrition in the elderly
Atypical presentation	Oral health in aging
Critical care	Pain
Delirium	Palliative care
Dementia	Physical restraints
Depression	Pressure ulcers and skin tears
Ethnogeriatrics and cultural	Sensory changes
competence	Sleep
Falls	Substance abuse
Family care giving	Urinary incontinence
Hydration management	

*Available on ConsultGeriRN.org

Surgical order sets are generic, applying to a broad range of patients usually having a specific type of surgery. The sets often indicate specific medication(s), dose, frequency, or route of administration for treatment of a specific condition such as postoperative pain or as preparation for a procedure. It is not unusual for an order set to include a medication, dose, frequency, or route that is inappropriate for an older adult or that should only be used with a cautionary note.

When developing or using medication-related order sets, the orders need to be monitored and reviewed regularly to ensure they are consistent with geriatric care guidelines and practice standards. Exhibit 3.6 is an example of a generic order set for postoperative care of patients following orthopedic surgery. The order set sections that raise concerns for the gerioperative patient pertain to medications for pain management and the section labeled "misc." The sections are in bold italics in Exhibit 3.6 with explanatory notes. Order sets must be adapted to the clinical status and needs of the individual patient. Nurses are accountable for reviewing each order set before implementing the orders with a gerioperative patient and ensuring needed revisions are made.

Quality Care

"The purpose of the health care system is to reduce continually the burden of illness, injury, and disability, and to improve the health status and function of the people of the United States" (President's Advisory Commission as quoted by Berwick, 2002, p. 83). The question is, how can this purpose best be achieved? One answer is by continually seeking to improve the quality of care on the assumption that improving care quality improves health status and function.

As professional practitioners, providers have a professional obligation to actively participate in care and practice improvement efforts. For example, ANA standards of professional performance specifically state that, "the registered nurse enhances the quality and effectiveness of nursing practice" (American Nurses Association, 2004, p. 33) The question remains how to improve the quality of care. To answer, one must first define quality care.

EXHIBIT 3.6 Sample Orthopedic Postoperative Order Set

PT. WEIGHT: _____   PT. HEIGHT: _____

ALLERGIES/REACTIONS:

_____

DIAGNOSIS/PROCEDURE:

_____

┌─────────────────────┐
│   │
│ (Patient Information)│
│   │
└─────────────────────┘

MEDICATIONS

Pain Management

☐ ☐   Patient-controlled analgesia—See patient-controlled analgesia order form

☐ ☐ *   *Morphine 5–10 mg IM Q3H PRN pain. Give 5 mg for pain score 4 to 6 and 10 mg for pain score greater than 6. (If patient able to tolerate PO, see Oxycodone 5 mgm plus acetaminophen 325 mgm (Percocet) order.)*

☐ ☐   Oxycodone 5 mgm plus acetaminophen 325 mgm (Percocet): One to two tablet(s) PO Q4H PRN pain. Give one tablet for pain score 4 to 6 and two tablets for pain score greater than 6. [Each tablet contains 325 mg of acetaminophen.]

☐ ☐   Acetaminophen 650mg PO/PR (route per patient preference) Q4H PRN mild pain (pain scale 1–3), headache, or temperature over 101°F.

┌──┐
│ *Daily acetaminophen (APAP) dose not to exceed 4000 mg.*   │
│ *Caution when multiple APAP-containing products are given.*   │
└──┘

Misc.

☐ ☐   **IV Fluid**: _____ @ _____ mL/hr.

☐ ☐   *Lorazepam (Ativan) 0.5–1 mg PO/IV (PO preferred if tolerated) Q8H PRN anxiety.*

☐ ☐ **   *Diazepam (Valium) 5–10 mg IM Q3H PRN muscle spasm (when ordered, PO preferred if tolerated).*

☐ ☐ **   *Diazepam (Valium) 5–10mg PO Q6H PRN muscle spasm.*

☐ ☐ +   *Zolpidem (Ambiem) 5–10g PO QHS PRN insomnia. In patients less than 65 years old, may repeat dose once if still awake in 90 minutes.*

☐ ☐   *Multivitamin w/minerals: one PO Q24H.*

☐ ☐   *Sennosides (Senokot) 1 tablet PO BID, hold for loose stools.*

☐ ☐   *Liquid antacid (Maalox or equivalent) 15–30 mL PO Q6H PRN dyspepsia.*

☐ ☐   *Laxative:* _____

☐ ☐ **   *Promethazine (Phenergan) 25 mg PO/IM (PO if able to tolerate) Q4–6H PRN N/V.*

☐ ☐   **Ondansetron** (Zofran) 1 mg IV Q8H × 72 hours PRN refractory N/V. (When IV and ODT are ordered simultaneously, ODT route of administration preferred if tolerated.)

☐ ☐   **Ondansetron** (Zofran) 4 mg ODT on tongue Q8H × 72 hours PRN refractory N/V. [Moisten tongue first with ice chips, etc., for best effect]

Physician's Signature _____ Date _____ Time _____

Noted by _____ Date _____ Time _____

_____

*Intramuscular medications should not be administered to older adults. Loss of muscle mass and replacement with fat deposits alter absorption rates that can result in under or overdosing.

**Lorazepam, diazepam, and promethezine are considered inappropriate for use with older adults. If used, a cautionary note should be attached to the order.

+Zolpidem has been linked with impaired balance and increase fall risk.

Quality health care is an abstract concept that is not well defined. Mitchell (2008) argues, "quality does not exist as a discrete entity" (p. 1–1). Rather, quality is constructed, created by the interaction and agreement among health care providers, health care organizations, governmental and regulatory agencies, patients, and families about what norms and values should guide decisions related to what can be achieved to improve the health and well-being of patients. Webster's *New World Dictionary* (1970) defines quality as "a degree of excellence." Although there is a general agreement on this definition, how excellence is applied to health care is less clear. Is it based on what health care is delivered, how health care is delivered, or what health care (once delivered) achieves, and for whom? Several definitions of quality of care are in current use.

The Institute of Medicine (IOM) uses the following definition for health care quality: "the degree to which health services for individuals and populations increase the likelihood of desired health outcomes and are consistent with current professional knowledge" (IOM, 2001, p. 3). The AHRQ defines quality health care as the right care, at the right time, and in the right way, to achieve the best possible results (Clancy, 2009).

To meet the challenges created by the definitions of quality care stated by the AHRQ and the IOM, three basic dimensions (structure, process, and outcome) need to be considered (Mainz, 2003). Structure refers to the resources available in the health care system to meet the needs of the patient population: number and educational background of health care providers, availability of equipment and technologies, access to specialty care units, availability of clinical guidelines and evidence for practice, and communication resources. Process refers to what is done for and with the patient. Preoperative assessment, patient teaching, diagnosis, and therapeutic intervention are examples of process dimensions. Process is not limited to what is done; process also examines how something is done, such as patient-provider communication, interdisciplinary team communication, or transitional care planning and implementation. Outcomes are the results of care processes within a given structure. Outcomes look at the effect of care processes on the patient or group of patients. Examples of outcomes include number of complications, length of stay, health and functional status, well-being, quality of life, and satisfaction with care. Efforts to bring about changes in structure, process, and outcome dimensions are needed to establish a consistently safe, efficient, timely, effective, equitable, and patient-centered health care system (IOM, 2001). Achieving these changes can be done through monitoring clinical indicators as measures of quality care.

MEASURING QUALITY CARE: CLINICAL INDICATORS

Once quality of care is defined, it is necessary to know if care given meets the standard of quality care. One of the ways quality is measured is through the use of quality or clinical indicators. A clinical indicator is a measure used to monitor, evaluate, and subsequently improve the structure, process, or outcome of patient care. The goal is improving patient health and well-being (Birkmeyer, Dimick, & Birkmeyer, 2004; McGory, Kao, Shekelle, Rubenstien, Leondari, & Parikh, 2009). Indicators are used to identify problem areas, initiate quality improvement, establish benchmarks, compare data between institutions or before and after quality improvement initiatives, and support accreditation. Exhibit 3.7 lists examples of structure, process, and outcome surgical clinical indicators.

Professional, health care, and regulatory organizations and agencies, and experts in the field formulate quality indicators based on literature reviews, expert opinion, and standards of care.

SCIP is one of the first nationally targeted projects to attempt improving patient outcomes by mandating and monitoring discrete evidence-based practice items. SCIP identified a set of process and outcome core measures designed to decrease common postoperative

EXHIBIT 3.7 Definition and Selected Examples of Structure, Process, and Outcome Clinical Indicators for Gerioperative Care

Clinical Measures	Definition	Clinical Indicator
Structure	Health care system characteristics resource availability	Proportion of surgical procedures done with time-outs
		Number of certified geriatric or gerontological professional staff
		Availability of geriatric units or geriatric surgical units
		Nurse–patient ratios
Process	Care patients actually receive	Proportion of older adults receiving opioids also prescribed a bowel regimen
		Proportion of older patients at risk for delirium receiving systematic postoperative delirium assessment
		Proportion of older adults who receive medication reconciliation at time of hospital discharge
Outcome	State of health following care received; end results of surgical-related care	Proportion of older adults with postoperative deconditioning
		Proportion of older adults with unrelieved postoperative pain
		Proportion of older adults readmitted to the hospital

complications: surgical infections, venous thrombophlebitis, and cardiovascular complications. Exhibit 3.8 lists the SCIP process core measures and the recommended preventive interventions for each measure. Each of the core measures is based on published evidence of effectiveness for decreasing adverse events and improving patient outcomes.

Studies investigating the effectiveness of surgical infection core measures have not consistently demonstrated an association between adherence to the core process measures and postoperative infection rates (Stulberg, Delaney, Neuhauser, Aron, Fu, & Koroukian, 2010). The question raised by the work of Stulberg and colleagues is, how do we know if the measures used are the measures that should be used? Ongoing research that tests the relationship between process and outcome is needed.

The Patient Safety Indicators (PSI) developed by the AHRQ is an example of outcome indicators. The PSI differs from SCIP in that SCIP establishes clinical activities for preventing specific adverse events, while PSI identifies occurrence of potentially avoidable complications and iatrogenic events following surgeries and procedures in acute care settings. Knowing the incidence of potentially adverse events provides a basis for initiating a quality improvement process to address a specific problem.

EXHIBIT 3.8 Surgical Care Improvement Project Clinical Indicators

Variable	Indicator
Infection	Percent of surgery patients who received preventative antibiotic(s) 1 hour before surgical incision.
	Percent of surgery patients who received the appropriate preventative antibiotic(s) for their surgery.
	Percent of surgery patients whose preventative antibiotic(s) were stopped within 24 hours after surgery end time.
	Percent of cardiac surgery patients with controlled 6 a.m. serum glucose (less than200 mg/dL) on postoperative day 1 and postoperative day 2.
	Percent of surgery patients with appropriate surgical site hair removal. No hair removal or hair removal with clippers or depilatory is considered appropriate. Shaving is considered inappropriate.
	Percent of colorectal surgery patients with immediate normothermia (greater than or equal to 96.8°F) within 15 minutes after leaving the operating room.
Cardiac	Percent of surgery patients on beta-blocker therapy prior to admission who received a beta-blocker during the perioperative period.
Venous thromboemolism	Percent of surgery patients with recommended venous thromboembolism prophylaxis ordered.
	Percent of surgery patients who received appropriate venous thromboembolism prophylaxis within 24 hours prior to surgery to 24 hours after surgery.

From Clancy (2008).

GERIOPERATIVE CARE CLINICAL INDICATORS

The Assessing Care of Vulnerable Elder (ACOVE) project developed three sets of quality indicators aimed at improving quality care of older adults. Investigators used results from literature reviews and interviews with experts to establish and draft quality indicators. A panel of experts reviewed iterative drafts until a set of indicators met the criteria for face, construct, and predictive validity (McGory, Kao, Shekelle, Rubenstien, Leondari, & Parikh, 2009) for improving best practice and care quality. The results are process clinical indicators specifically directed to hospital and surgical care of older adults (Arora, McGory, & Fung 2007), elderly surgical patients undergoing abdominal surgery (McGory, Shekelle, Rubinstein, Fink, & Ko, 2005), and care of elderly surgical patients (McGory, Kao, Shekelle, Rubenstien, Leondari, & Parikh, 2009).

McGory and colleagues (2009) describe 91 clinical indicators categorized into a set of domains specific to surgical care of older adults. Those domains include comorbidity assessment, evaluation of elderly issues, medication use, patient-provider discussions, intraoperative care, postoperative management, discharge planning, and ambulatory surgery. The domains provide a holistic model for evaluating care of the gerioperative patient. Exhibit 3.9

EXHIBIT 3.9 Quality Indicator Domains With Sample Gerioperative Care Indicators

Domain	Sample Indicators
Comorbidity assessment	Prior to surgery, older adults should be evaluated for tobacco use and alcohol use.
	Older adults who smoke should be encouraged to stop smoking when the decision is made to perform surgery or 8 weeks prior to surgery.
Evaluation of elderly issues	Preoperative assessment results of nutritional status, cognition, depression, delirium risk, fall risk, functional status, mobility, and preferred decision-making process should be documented.
	Older adults should have a daily screening examination for postoperative delirium.
Medication use	Older adults should have an inpatient documentation of most recent outpatient medications with dosages.
	Standing orders should not include any potentially inappropriate medications according to the Beers criteria. If such medications are needed, cautionary notes and reason for medication should be provided.
Patient-provider discussions	Decision-making capacity of older adults should be assessed prior to signing an informed consent.
	Older adults who have specific treatment preferences should have those preferences documented on medical record.
Intraoperative care	Measures to maintain normothermia greater than 36°C should be instituted.
	Measurements to ensure proper positioning should be documented.
Postoperative care	Older adults who do not speak English should have an interpreter assist with communication between patient and providers.
	Pain assessments should be performed with each set of vital signs or whenever patient behaviors or communication suggests presence of pain.
Postdischarge function and well-being	Predischarge assessment should be conducted in the following areas and compared to preoperative levels: nutrition, cognition, depression, ambulation, and functional status.
	Discharge planning should ensure the gerioperative patient and caregivers can explain postdischarge care activities, how to perform them, and who to call if more information or assistance is needed.

Adapted from McGory, Kao, Shekelle, Rubenstien, Leondari, & Parikh (2009).

lists seven of the domains identified by McGory and colleagues (2009) with examples of indicators for each domain based on literature reviews.

Several clinical indicators identified by McGory and colleagues (2009) reflect previously identified clinical indicators for measuring quality in all adults having surgery, regardless of age. Establishing quality indicators for improving surgical care of older adults assumes a special urgency. The urgency for improving care stems from the heightened vulnerability of older adults to adverse events; the increasing number of vulnerable older adults undergoing minor, major, and complex surgeries; and the documented lack of knowledge, skills, and awareness among health care professionals about the unique care needs of vulnerable elders. The lack of knowledge, skills, and awareness of elder-sensitive gerioperative care limits the ability of health care providers' ability to prevent, evaluate, and intervene effectively to decrease risk and improve care outcomes.

Nursing protocols that address specific care needs of older adults were described previously in this chapter. The protocols have been published by Capezuti, Zwicker, Mezey, and Fulmer (2008) and are widely disseminated through the NGC and ConsultGeriRN websites. Several protocols, consistent with the surgical quality indicators identified by McGory and colleagues (2009), can be quickly implemented to improve clinical practice.

NURSING QUALITY INDICATORS

Nursing has a longstanding history of commitment to quality care, beginning with Florence Nightingale. As the "round the clock" care providers, nurses contribute assessment, analysis, and care decisions essential to meeting the standard of the right care at the right time in the right way. The ANA has long advocated the role of nurses in assessing, evaluating, and promoting quality patient care, and the value of nursing's contribution to monitoring the processes of care. A nursing workforce that is clinically savvy and well prepared in geriatric cares is key to achieving effective process and positive outcomes.

In 2004, the National Quality Forum, a nonprofit organization targeted to improving patient care, endorsed a set of outcome measures that directly reflected nursing care and nursing effectiveness. The measures came to be called "nursing-sensitive core measures." The concept of nursing sensitivity was important to the goal to measure the effectiveness and impact of nursing care on patient safety, quality of care, and outcomes. The nursing-sensitive measures address structure, process, and outcome domains.

Examples of structural domain measures are available supply of nurses, nursing education level, number of nurses certified in a clinical specialty, and nurse-to-patient ratio. Process measures are those that address the process of nurse-patient interaction and relationship such as nursing assessment, intervention, and evaluation. Examples include pain relief, patient teaching, nurse-patient communication, interdisciplinary team collaboration, discharge planning, and medication administration. Outcome measures are patient outcomes that occur in response to either a greater quantity or quality of nursing care. Examples are functional status, patient satisfaction, and patient falls.

GERIOPERATIVE CARE QUALITY INDICATORS

The IOM identified a set of health professional core competencies that establish a foundation for achieving quality gerioperative care. Core competencies include:

- Providing patient-centered care
- Collaborating with interdisciplinary health care team

- Implementing evidence-based practice
- Actively participating and instituting quality improvement
- Using informatics for communicating and documenting patient care

Quality gerioperative care depends on structures and processes that can lead to the best possible outcomes based on the most current knowledge and evidence. Implementing the IOM core competencies is a major step in providing a structure for gerioperative care. Structure depends on the availability of an adequate number of nurses, physicians, surgeons, anesthetists, and other health care providers with specialized gerioperative knowledge and skills who are able to work collaboratively on interdisciplinary teams to meet the care needs of older adults across the gerioperative continuum.

The hospital and surgical quality indicators developed through the ACOVE project serve as starting points for determining quality of gerioperative care. Geriatric nursing care protocols must be incorporated into quality care processes. Adapting guidelines, protocols, and order sets to the needs and clinical condition of the older adult and to the context of care should be a clearly stated indicator in measuring quality gerioperative care.

Nurses, physicians, anesthesia providers, and other members of the gerioperative interdisciplinary team across care settings must assume the accountability and responsibility for ensuring the quality of gerioperative care provided. Therefore, interdisciplinary collaboration is needed to develop, disseminate, and implement the structure and process measures needed to ensure best practice and achieve the best outcomes for gerioperative patients.

Implementing Quality Care

Having textbooks, documents, and statements outlining standards of practice, guidelines, protocols, and quality indicators will not produce quality care. Evidence-based practice can be applied to implementing standards, guidelines, and protocols as well as to the standards themselves. Translational research argues that guidelines, practice standards, and quality indicators are implemented most effectively when there is collaboration, cooperation, and collegial relationships among care providers, between providers and patients, and between providers and organizational leaders. Quality care is best achieved through a process of evidence-based practice derived from clinical judgment, experience, and published data. Quality exists not only in what is done but also in how it is done. Much of what constitutes quality care is intrinsic to the professional persona of the care provider. Standards and guidelines, like standing orders, attempt to ensure consistency of practice behaviors, attitudes, knowledge, and skills. The guidelines and protocols indicate what is to be done. It is the professional practitioner who determines the interpersonal and patient-centered process of how it is to be done. Structure must support the process if best outcomes are to be achieved. Quality requires attention to the individual practitioner-patient interaction and must be supported by the organization. Implementing quality indicators depends on the knowledge, attitudes, and skill of the care providers with the support of the organization and supportive health care policies.

PATIENT REPORT: Ms. Mills

After discussing the problem with the clinical nurse leader, the PACU nurse attended a meeting of the quality improvement committee (QIC) to discuss the use of meperidine in older adults. In preparation for the meeting, the nurse conducted a literature review. Guidelines from the American Geriatrics Society, the NGC guideline on managing acute postoperative pain, and a nursing pain management protocol documented that meperidine is contraindicated in older adults except to control shivering. The guidelines also stated IM administration routes are contraindicated. When the nurse met with the QIC chairperson, the nurse presented the results of the literature review and requested the committee remove meperidine as a pain relief intervention and all references to IM as a route for medication administration in older adults. Several months later, a list of potentially inappropriate medications for use with older adults was posted in the PACU. The nurse presented the list and the literature on meperidine at the next staff meeting.

SUMMARY

An integration of gerontological, medical-surgical, perioperative, perianesthesia, and pain management nursing practice standards and position and vision statements is needed to create a systematic, comprehensive approach to gerioperative nursing care. A gerioperative model of care must integrate standards and guidelines consistent with the health professions represented on the gerioperative interdisciplinary team. It is through such integration that a holistic, comprehensive, and best practice approach for the perioperative care of the older adult can be achieved.

KEY POINTS

- Gerioperative care is related to a wide array of nursing, clinical specialty, and interdisciplinary professional standards of practice.
- Practice guidelines and protocols are evidence-based tools that can be used to improve perioperative care of older adults.
- Standing orders directed at postoperative care of adults must be reviewed and adapted to the care needs of older adults.
- Quality indicators for measuring perioperative and hospital-based care of older adults have been published and should be used to guide gerioperative practice.
- Quality indicators, protocols, and order sets are tools to measure the care older adults receive. The quality of the care rests not in the tools but in the commitment, knowledge, skills, attitudes, and abilities of those providing the care.

FOUR

Gerioperative Informed Consent

Jennifer V. Long, Raelene V. Shippee-Rice, and Susan J. Fetzer

PATIENT REPORT: Mr. Barnard

Mr. Barnard is a 73-year-old patient. He is in preanesthesia awaiting abdominal surgery for colon cancer. He has been given morphine 4 mg intravenously for pain control. He is alert and oriented but drowsy. The surgeon arrives to obtain Mr. Barnard's consent for surgery. Is Mr. Barnard competent at this time to sign a surgical consent?

"Disclosure in medicine has served the function of getting patients to 'consent' to what clinicians wanted them to agree to in the first place" (Katz, 1984, p. 1). Written in 1984, much of this statement still holds true in clinical practice today. An older adult has the right and even the responsibility to consider options and make a personal decision to accept or refuse treatment. Many articles, research investigations, and white papers have addressed patient autonomy and informed consent. This chapter provides an overview of the doctrine of informed consent for treatment. The overview is followed by the application of informed consent to the care of the gerioperative patient. The chapter concludes with a review of informed consent for gerioperative research. Figure 4.1 depicts the pathway to informed consent.

Definition

Surgical informed consent is a patient's voluntary agreement to allow a health care provider to administer a medical treatment, procedure, or intervention only after the patient has been given complete information on the reason for the treatment, knowledge of all relevant facts including available treatment alternatives, and the risks and benefits associated with each available treatment. A patient's informed consent must be obtained before patients can receive health care treatment, procedures, or interventions, or are enrolled as participants in a research investigation. In addition to informed consent for surgery, some anesthesia providers conduct a separate informed consent process for anesthesia. The anesthesia consent process may or may not involve a signature.

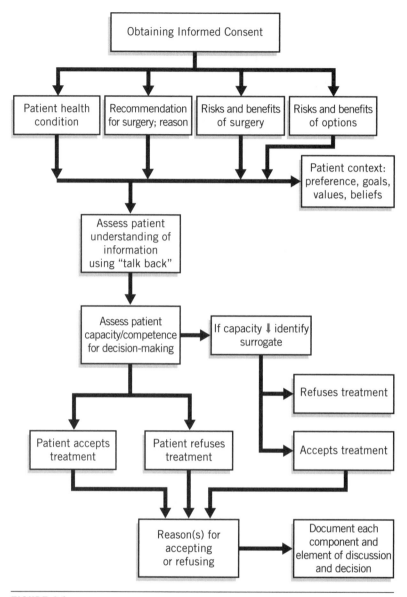

FIGURE 4.1
Informed Consent Pathway

Exceptions to the mandate for informed consent can be observed when the patient's health situation is critical and emergency surgery is needed, the patient is unconscious and unable to give informed consent, the patient is adjudicated incompetent by a court of law, the patient waives his or her right to information and to make a decision, or the physician determines that providing information will cause the patient greater harm than good. None of these exceptions is absolute. Making exceptions to the informed consent process must be done with caution and only after thoughtful assessment and sound clinical judgment, keeping in mind the best interests of the patient and the need to work collaboratively with family members and the interdisciplinary care team.

Legal Perspective

Informed consent results in a legal document, stemming from the right of a person to decide what is done to his or her body by another person or persons. The intent of informed consent is to protect the patient from unwanted treatment or personal invasion against his or her will. Providers are protected by the doctrine of informed consent resulting from permission by the patient to administer a treatment, procedure, or other action for therapeutic purposes, or as part of a research investigation. The principle of consent changes an action from battery, a physical contact "against" a person (without consent), to a physical action "with" the person (consent).

The legal application of surgical informed consent started in the early 1900s when a court determined that a physician should have informed a patient about the risks and benefits associated with surgery before the surgery occurred. In the 1950s, a series of court cases led to legal decisions stating a patient's consent must be based on having complete information and *full understanding* of the risks associated with the procedure. Legal consensus argues that it is the physician who has the responsibility to both inform the patient and to obtain the patient's consent before initiating treatment.

All American states have legislation identifying the need for a patient's informed consent prior to a medical or surgical procedure. The details of the informed consent process vary from state to state, but all states cite obtaining the patient's informed consent for treatment is the legal responsibility of the physician or surgeon who will be conducting the intervention, procedure, or surgery. Nurse practitioners have a legal responsibility for obtaining consent for procedures they perform.

Physicians cannot delegate any part of the informed consent process in some states, while in others they can delegate obtaining the patient's signature to nurses or other providers. However, all states affirm that the responsibility and accountability for the accuracy and validity of the informed consent process and full disclosure of risk and benefits for the surgery under consideration remain with the physician and cannot be delegated.

In informed consent, nurses have a professional, and in some states legal, responsibility to act as a patient advocate and as a witness to ensure the patient has received sufficient information to make an informed decision and that the patient is giving voluntary consent. Nurses caring for patients preoperatively should assess the patient's knowledge and understanding about the procedure and the associated risks and benefits. Assessing the patient's understanding can reveal concerns or questions that should be addressed prior to surgery. It is also the nurse's responsibility to ensure that the patient has, in fact, received sufficient information to be able to make an informed decision. If the patient indicates concerns, questions, misunderstandings, hesitancy, or lack of information about the surgery, the nurse must inform the physician and advocate for further discussion with the patient and physician. The nurse monitors the patient's response and decision-making in response to physician remediation of identified issues.

Ethical Perspective

Ethics is the foundation for the doctrine of informed consent and for the legal application of the right of a person to decide what is done to his or her body. It is the ethical perspective that establishes informed consent as a process of communication with respect for the personhood of the patient rather than a signature on a formal document. The ethical principles serving as the cornerstones for informed consent are autonomy, beneficence, non-malfeasance (also referred to as non-maleficence), and justice. These principles also provide the foundation for both advance directives and do not resuscitate orders, issues associated with informed consent for a surgical procedure.

Autonomy states that patients have the right and the responsibility to make, choose, or refuse recommended treatments. This principle, as used in informed consent, is to protect the rights of the individual from any undue influence or coercion to accept treatments that are unwanted or inconsistent with the patient's values, beliefs, or goals.

The principle of non-malfeasance is to prevent harm, a concept important in maintaining patient safety and well-being. Surgery does harm. It causes physical and physiologic trauma, increases stress, decreases immune function, and places the older adult in harm's way for postoperative complications. The harm associated with the surgery is mitigated by the ethical principle of beneficence, to "do good." The good, in the context of treatment alternatives and informed consent, is the best interest of the patient as determined in collaboration with the patient. In surgery, the "good" or benefit is the anticipated outcome: improvement in the patient's condition. The outcome may be palliative, as in removing a tumor causing pressure and pain, curative, as in removing a diseased gallbladder, or rehabilitative, as with joint replacement. It is the patient who must weigh the benefit to be derived from surgery with the harm caused by surgery. The decision must be consistent with the patient's preferences, values, and expected life goals. Surgery with frail older adults often raises concerns about "doing harm." Supporting older adults who make a decision to refuse surgery can be important in supporting the principle to do no harm.

Justice relates to fairness, a consistent conformity to rules or standards. Health care providers have a greater share of knowledge about treatment than the patients from whom they are obtaining consent. Yet it is the patients who have the responsibility, as well as the right, to accept or reject treatment. Justice requires those who have the necessary knowledge must share that knowledge with the person responsible for making the decision, the patient. Patients must not only receive the knowledge; they must be able to use it as a basis for decision-making. Therefore, providers have a duty to assist the patient in interpreting and understanding the information with respect to the patient's own needs and preferences. Exhibit 4.1 summarizes the definitions and applies the major ethical principles relevant to surgical informed consent.

Professional Standards

Informed consent is addressed in professional standards or principles and codes of ethics of physicians and nurses. The American Nurses Association's code of ethics and practice standards specifically address nurses' responsibility in informed consent. The American Medical Association has similar statements for physician practice. Anesthesia providers are responsible for meeting discipline-specific professional standards as well as the ethical standards of the anesthesia provider professional community. Ethical standards for informed consent emphasize patient's right to self-determination, participate in decision-making, receive understandable information, receive decisional support from providers and significant others, and be protected from undue influence. Professional providers are accountable for compliance with the informed consent process and ensuring the ethical rights of the gerioperative patient.

PROVIDER-PATIENT COMMUNICATION

Providing decision support is at the heart of informed consent. Informed consent is based on providing the information needed for the patient to make an informed decision and ensuring

EXHIBIT 4.1 Informed Consent Principles, Definitions, and Application

Principle	Definition	Application
Autonomy	Patient self-determination to choose or refuse surgical procedure	Respect patient's right to choose or refuse
		Protect patient's right to share decision-making with others (assisted autonomy)
Non-malfeasance	To do no harm; take action to prevent or minimize harm	Explain risk of treatment
		Recognize effects of ageism
		Ensure decision is informed and consistent with patient beliefs, values, and preferences
Beneficence	To do good; act in the best interest of the patient	Provide decisional support
		Act in accordance with patient strengths and limitations
		Recognize the patient's strengths and limitations
		Ensure decisional capacity
Justice	Giving to other what they are due; distribution of knowledge	Share knowledge with patient
		Use talk back to ensure the patient is able to interpret and understand information in context of own situation

the patient not only understands it, but can apply it to his or her own needs. Information exchange must be a shared process based on trust between patient and provider. The patient must be able to trust that the provider is interested in helping to arrive at the best decision for the individual. The provider must trust the patient will be engaged in the decision-making process and share patient-related information that will help the provider tailor the information to the individual patient.

Patient-centered, relationship-oriented communication involves more than information giving. It is a process in helping the patient interpret and apply the information in the context of his or her individual needs and goals. The communication process must be responsive to the patient's needs and questions, demonstrate respect, and maintain a consistent focus on the best interests of the patient. The provider must take time to listen to the patient, attending to what the patient says, while also listening for what may not be said that indicates unspoken concerns. Information must be offered slowly, clearly, and concisely, and be consistent with the patient's education, previous knowledge, functional ability, and level of comprehension.

Elements of Informed Consent

Three criteria must be met before informed consent can be considered valid. The patient must:

1. Be given sufficient information to make an educated decision.
2. Be able to comprehend and use the information to make a decision.
3. Provide voluntary consent.

INFORMATION SUFFICIENCY

A longstanding issue in informed consent is defining what constitutes sufficient information. The level of information needed to meet the criteria of an informed medical decision is an important one and is not easy to answer. The challenges to knowledge transfer from provider to patient are numerous. The transfer of information from patient to provider is equally challenging, but although it is an important element, it is not required.

The information listed as follows must be included when discussing the surgical procedure with the patient. The information that was discussed and the patient's subsequent decision must be documented in the medical record. Documentation should include:

- The nature of the health care problem including a diagnosis, if available.
- The nature of the surgical procedure under consideration with reason for recommendation.
- Treatment alternatives.
- Relevant risks, benefits, and uncertainties related to recommended procedure and each alternative.
- Evaluation of patient understanding.
- Patient decision to accept or refuse the procedure.

A common standard for determining information sufficiency consistent with a patient-centered framework is the "reasonable patient standard." This standard requires physicians to disclose information a patient would need or want to know. The reasonable patient standard sets a minimum level of information patients must receive as a basis for giving consent to surgery. Many patients may want or require more information; some may want less. The physician has a duty to provide the available level of information needed for the patient to make a decision; the patient can choose how much of the information to use in making a decision.

Health care providers face constraints that interfere with information transfer to patients. Constraints include provider and patient attitudes, beliefs, knowledge, and communication style. Provider attitudes and beliefs affect the language and interaction patterns they use and the points of information they emphasize. Providers also identify time as a major constraint that hinders their ability to have full and complete discussions with patients. Patient knowledge, attitudes, and beliefs influence the way they receive and interpret the provider's information and how they respond to provider power. Provider and patient characteristics interact in unique ways and take on a particular relevance when obtaining informed consent with patients from different cultures and cohorts, or who have poor health literacy.

CULTURE AND LANGUAGE

The concept of informed consent rests on the principle of individual autonomy. This principle is grounded in Western sociocultural norms and beliefs, and may not be consistent with the beliefs and values of patients from other cultures or age cohorts. In these cases, informed consent still applies, consent for treatment remains valid, and patients continue to need education and information about their health condition, treatment options, and decisions. The determination of informed consent is clear when cultural norms turn decision-making over to an authority other than the patient. The authority may be the health care provider, member(s) of the patient's family, or cultural community leader. The question of when the patient has the autonomy to turn decisions over to another person is a source of contention between health providers, organizations, and patients. Remaining true to respect for autonomy, patients who make a decision in the context of their values, beliefs, and preferences to delegate treatment decisions to another person must be allowed to do so (Berg, Appelbaum, Lidz, & Parker, 2001; del Carmen & Joffe, 2005).

Patients with limited English proficiency or who are non-English speaking must have a professional interpreter available for informed consent discussions. Family members face a number of challenges that inhibit their effectiveness in interpreting medical information between provider and patient. Those challenges include:

- Difficulty asking the patient questions the family member does not understand or when the family member is embarrassed.
- Lack of ability to translate information between English and the family member's own language.
- Family members' fear or concerns about care provider questions embarrassing or upsetting the patient.
- Disagreement with what the provider is saying.
- Miscommunication of the patient's message to the provider, preferring that the provider hear the family member's version of the situation.
- Emotional involvement with the patient and clinical situation, resulting in a tendency to protect the patient from bad news; therefore, the family member may edit or change information.
- Not giving the provider or patient "all this extra information."
- Patient hesitancy to disclose upsetting private information or secret issues in front of a relative.

LITERACY

Patients unfamiliar with medical terminology or who have learning disabilities, visual impairments, language barriers, or low reading levels cannot give informed consent if they do not understand the information or are unable to read the informed consent form that they sign. The informed consent must be written at a reading level consistent with the patient's literacy level with the information in short, clear sentences. A reading level in the range of sixth to eighth grade is most likely the maximum level for the general population. Patients unable to read the informed consent form or read it with comprehension should have the form read to them. The form should be read while the patient has the form in hand, allowing the patient to follow along as much as possible.

VOLUNTARY ACTION

Voluntary action refers to a lack of coercion, deceit, or duress in making a decision. Information must be provided in a way that does not unduly influence the patient to accede to or refuse treatment. Too much or too little information, overemphasis on either surgical risk or benefit, using medical terminology or value-laden words, and provider attitude and behaviors are all elements that can unduly influence a patient's decision.

When patients do not have time they need to review the information or consider its implications, patients can experience a level of duress that can negate an informed consent. There is a moral duty for patients to take time to consider options, risks, and benefits to ensure the choice is voluntary, informed, and not one of passive agreement. Providers have a moral duty to provide patients sufficient time to make decisions.

Urging or expectations by other persons, whether professional providers or family members, can lead to undue pressure that interferes with the element of voluntary action. For example, if a patient consents to a treatment or procedure because of concerns the physician will "no longer treat me if I refuse the procedure," the consent is not legitimate, even if the patient does not verbalize the concern to the provider.

MEDICATION ADMINISTRATION

Administration of preoperative analgesic or anxiolytic medication prior to obtaining informed consent is a longstanding concern among providers. A common dictum is that no pain or sedating medication should be administered before the patient has signed an informed consent. The reason for this dictum is the belief that patients who are medicated do not have the cognitive lucidity needed to make an informed choice. An absolute adherence to this dictum can be paternalistic and compromise informed consent.

Patients in severe pain or who are highly anxious may not meet the voluntary action element to give informed consent. When pain or antianxiety medications are withheld, patients can feel pressured to give consent in order to obtain medication and relieve their suffering. Providers must apply sound clinical judgment in making decisions about preoperative medications and completion of informed consent documents. Assessing the patient's level of emotional distress or pain to determine if the discomfort creates an undue influence is as much a negation of the informed consent process as is administering a medication. Assessing the patient may indicate there is a period when the patient is more alert and attentive to the informed consent process after medication administration but before onset of sedative effects. ". . .Pain medication should never be withheld from a suffering patient under the guise of obtaining informed consent" (Van Norman, 2008).

Nurses who administer medication prior to obtaining informed consent need to accurately document the situation. Documentation must include patient assessment data, identification of the problem, medication administered, demonstration of patient decisional capacity, and time delay between medication administration and informed consent signature.

COMPETENCE AND CAPACITY

Understanding of the information provided depends on the patient's decisional competence or capacity to make an informed consent. Decisional capacity is based on the ability to understand information, appreciate its relevance to one's own situation, and choose a course of action (choosing or rejecting surgery) based on awareness of possible consequences.

The terms competence and capacity are often used interchangeably to refer to the ability of patients to make a decision based on an understanding of the information presented and the consequences of a decision. Competence is a term that often carries legal implications. Courts are needed to determine that a patient is incompetent. Capacity is the preferred term when applying clinical judgment about an older person's ability to understand information and make an informed consent.

Decisional ability is evaluated as part of the informed consent discussion with the patient. Observations of the patient's verbal and nonverbal behavior in relation to attention, eye contact, listening behaviors, interaction, and asking questions indicate ability to make decisions. A more direct method for determining patient understanding is asking the patient to "repeat back" the information by (1) explaining the procedure, (2) identifying consequences (risks and benefits) of the intended procedure, (3) communicating verbally, nonverbally, or in writing his or her choice, and (4) presenting reasons for the choice.

In situations where clinicians are uncertain of a patient's ability to make informed decisions, a more extensive evaluation is needed. If the patient is unable to make independent decisions or if there is clinical uncertainty, formal court proceedings to determine legal competency may be required. If the patient is found incompetent, a formally appointed surrogate must be utilized when making treatment decisions. Although there may be differences in the formal definitions of competence, capacity, and comprehension, the issue of concern is whether the patient can understand and retain information, understand the implications, and has the functional ability to use information and implications to make decisions that are consistent with his or her own values, preferences, and beliefs.

Informed Consent and Aging

Older adults can benefit from decisional support when considering treatment decisions. Decision support is an interactive process whereby older patients are provided information and are supported when making choices regarding treatment options in the context of the person's needs, preferences, values, and individual circumstances. Age-related changes, illness, disease, and in social support make the process of decision-making more difficult for older adults.

Studies indicate that informed consent with older adults is compromised by poor comprehension, increased patient anxiety, and inadequate time for discussion. Increasing age is associated with inconsistent preferences and decreased comprehension. This holds true regardless of the level of education or income, gender, self-perceived skill and health, or decision-making style (Finucane, Slovic, Hibbard, Peters, Mertz, & McGregor, 2002). Up to 48% of older adults with acute conditions cannot adequately comprehend written informed consent documents (Appelbaum, 2007).

Care providers obtaining informed consent from gerioperative patients must remain true to the principles of autonomy, beneficence, non-malfeasance, and justice. The process also must adhere to the elements of informed consent: understanding, decisional capacity, and voluntariness. Health care providers must provide information in ways that will support the patient's ability to understand it. Using patient-centered, relationship-oriented communication and allowing sufficient time to answer questions, address concerns, and provide decisional support are integral parts of the process for maximizing informed consent.

DECISIONAL SUPPORT

Older adults have fears and concerns about the success of surgery, pain, and discomfort similar to that of many patients regardless of age. Older adults also fear loss of self-care ability and the associated increased dependency. A particular concern is becoming a burden to family members.

Older adults have values and goals that may differ from those of younger patients. Aging and age-related changes, alterations in health, clinical status, and availability of social support are important decision points for elders. Older adults with long-term chronic illness or who anticipate a potentially debilitating surgery with a long recovery period often balance the benefits and risks using different criteria from health care providers or other age groups. Risks and benefits may center on the question: "Does the use of resources (physical, physiologic, time for 'getting back to normal,' financial resources, time in a rehabilitation center, depending on family members) balance the 'number of days I have left?'" Ageism is common in older adults, often leading them to make decisions based on their beliefs about aging, rather than their beliefs about potential health or improved clinical condition.

Decisional support is helping the older person organize and interpret information related to the desired outcomes of surgery and the potential risks and benefits based on the individual's health condition, age, physical, and physiologic resources. An important aspect of decision support is helping the older person consider the context of the patient's own beliefs, values, health care information, and preferences. Surgery has different meanings for different patients. McKneally and Martin (2000) describe the surgical consent process as patients moving from a state of fear, vulnerability, and distress to a position of trust in the surgeon's ability to "care for them with vigilance" (p. 267). Patients describe similar trust in nurses' interest and ability to care for them.

Decision-making based on trust does not center on autonomous decision-making, but on a shared process of building trust that facilitates the patient's comfort in consenting to surgery. Older adults may not want to know or may be unable to absorb the details about the surgical procedure or balance the risks of surgical or anesthesia complications against the potential for benefit. They may make the decision based on trusting that those who care for them have their best interests at heart. The trust extends to family members who may be the decision-makers. Mitty and Post (2008) describe this as a process of assisted, supported, or delegated autonomy. When family members or friends have permission from the older adult to be active participants in the decision-making process, health care providers must provide them with the same decisional support they extend to the older adult.

GERIOPERATIVE COMMUNICATION AND INFORMED CONSENT

Communication

Age-related changes include decreased vision and hearing ability that affects reading consent forms and hearing explanations. Environmental stress further interferes with hearing and vision. Neurological age-related changes can result in decreased attention span and slowed response time, making it more difficult to sustain attention. Medication effects, fatigue, pain, and disease create further interference. Taking time to ensure the older adult is rested, has adequate pain relief, and decreasing environmental distractions improves the informed consent process. Considering the individual needs, strengths, and constraints of the older adult, adapting communication by allowing sufficient time for the older adult to absorb, process, and reflect on the information as the discussion progresses are key to best practice in informed consent communication. Awareness of the effects of age- and disease-related changes helps providers modify or adapt communication to the needs of the older adult.

Attention to emotional tone and creating a calm, unhurried manner helps the older adult focus on the interaction and consideration of treatment options and weighing risks and benefits. Care providers are often concerned that reviewing surgical risks can heighten patient anxiety, interfering with the ability of the person to attend to what is being said or to make an informed decision. Asking older adults about their discomfort when discussing surgical or anesthesia risks allows providers to provide additional support and adapt the discussion to patient's needs and comfort. Including family members or friends as a support system during discussions with the consent of the older adult can facilitate the informed consent process. It is important to remember the older adult, who is the patient, must have the information and must remain the focus of the provider's attention even when other persons are present. Keeping the older adult at the center of attention reminds all players, including the older patient, that it is the patient's preferences, values, beliefs, and health condition that must guide a decision, not the beliefs and values of family members. Exhibit 4.2 offers a checklist to facilitate communication with older adults.

A clear and concise presentation without medical jargon is helpful when discussing the patient's clinical condition, surgical procedures, and associated risks and benefits. Using a combination of verbal, visual, and written communication methods supports information sharing and can improve comprehension. Visual communication includes charts, diagrams, figures, and pictures. Written information can be especially useful for those with hearing impairment. Written information must be adapted to older adults who have impaired vision.

Having the informed consent document available and reviewing it with the patient contributes to helping older adults understand the document they are being asked to sign. Up to 70% of patients do not read, cannot read, or do not understand what is written in informed consent forms. Many times, patients are given the consent form, asked to sign it, and bring it

---

EXHIBIT 4.2 **Communication Checklist for Gerioperative Informed Consent**

- Evaluate patient's communication needs and preferred process of information before initiating discussion of informed consent.
- Have assistive devices clean, working effectively, and in place.
- Ensure patient is within a physical, psychological, and emotional comfort zone.
- Schedule when others important to the patient's decision-making are present.
- Face patient within cultural norms when speaking .
- Speak clearly at a pace and language level validated by the patient as comfortable.
- Allow time for patient to "take in" what is said, process it, and ask questions or respond.
- Stop frequently to invite patient to "reflect back" what is said in patient's own words and in context of personal preferences, values, and beliefs.
- Monitor patient's response to issues raised in informed consent and the level of physical, psychological, and emotional comfort.
- Ask patient to verbally clarify head nods, uh-huh, and yes responses or use cultural equivalent.
- Use written informed consent document as a talking point.
- Ensure informed consent document is written at fifth-grade level and is in large print on nongloss paper with key points highlighted or bulleted.
- Use pictures, graphics, white boards, nonverbal communication strategies, or other approaches that facilitates patient understanding.
- Provide interpreters with patient permission. Provide written materials to interpreter in advance to allow time for understanding and translation.

to the hospital the day of the procedure. Patients who forget the form are asked to sign prior to the procedure. Older adults sign the consent form with little to no understanding of what the consent form says or what it means. Older patients are unwilling to admit to their providers that they have difficulty reading or understanding the consent form for fear of being stereotyped or considered ignorant. An operating assumption in the basic informed consent process is that most patients can read the consent document. Older adults assume, "There must be something wrong with me if I can't read it, other people do." Few would consider that maybe something is wrong with the system and not them.

Reviewing the consent document with the patient allows providers to assess the patient's understanding, evaluate reading and health literacy, and respond to questions or concerns. Providers can explain (1) medical jargon if it is used, (2) clarify information that is unclear, and (3) interpret the document in light of the patient's own values, preferences, and clinical situation.

Computer-based programs are being developed to improve the process of informed consent. Benefits of computer programs for informed consent include giving patients time to read or listen to information, process what they read and hear, replay or read sections that are unclear, and make notes about what to review with the physician or surgeon. A major concern is the older adult's level of familiarity with computers. Asking an older adult who is apprehensive about surgery and unfamiliar with computers to review a computer program can quickly result in heightened stress and anxiety.

The effectiveness of computers in facilitating patient decision-making is not well established. Two studies examining the effect of computer-based programs on patient understanding and information retention show mixed results. Gyomber, Lawrentschuck, Wong, Parker, and Bolton (2010) compared the knowledge of radical prostatectomy in 40 patients, with a mean age of 61 years, after they had viewed either an interactive media presentation (IMP) or had a standard consent interaction with a provider. Patients were given a 26-item test to evaluate knowledge and retention of information. Patients who viewed the IMP had higher knowledge test scores. Patients who had a standard consent interaction improved their initial test scores after subsequent exposure to the IMP. A study comparing the use of a CD-ROM to the use of written instructions in explaining chemotherapy to 101 cancer patients found no differences in patients' recall of information (Olver, Whitford, Denson, Peterson, & Olver, 2009). Both studies focused on informed consent for treatment by examining the level of patient knowledge and information recall. The amount of information patients remember may not be the best test for determining if a patient's consent is informed. The relevance of the information to the patient's goals and preferences when making a decision may be more significant. The presence of a provider helps patients interpret information in light of their unique preferences, needs, and clinical situation and for providing decisional support. Exhibit 4.3 presents strategies for assessing elements of informed consent.

ELEMENTS OF INFORMED CONSENT AND THE GERIOPERATIVE PATIENT

Understanding

Overwhelming older adults with facts and statistics about surgical risks, benefits, and outcomes does not contribute to an understanding of their relevance to the patient. Placing information in the context of the older adult's goals, preferences, and clinical situation makes the information more meaningful and provides a more relevant context for making decisions. Discussion of risks and benefits should focus on information that is the most relevant to the patient's situation.

How well the older adult and his or her support systems understand the information can be assessed by asking the patient to do a talk back or explaining the information back to the provider (Fink et al., 2010; National Quality Forum, 2005). The National Quality Forum recommends health

EXHIBIT 4.3 **Assessing Elements of Informed Consent**

Element	Topics	Assessment: *Have patient explain the following information as if it was to another person (family member, friend, nurse).*
Patient understanding	The nature of the health care problem, including a diagnosis if available	The health care problem that needs surgery
	Nature of the surgical procedure under consideration and reason for recommendation	The type of surgical procedure the surgeon recommended
		What the surgeon will do in the surgery
		How long the surgical procedure will take?
		The reason for the surgery
	Treatment options	Other treatments available instead of surgery
		The possible problems and benefits of the surgery; of other treatments instead of surgery
		Why the surgeon considers surgery to be a better choice
Applying information to patient's own situation	Relevant risks, benefits, and uncertainties for surgery and alternative treatments	How the patient thinks surgery will help with the health problem
		Risks of having surgery
		The benefits of other treatments
		The risks of other treatments
		How surgery will help with what the patient wants to do in the future
		How surgery will interfere or make it difficult with what the patient wants to do in the future
Patient decision	Making the decision	How others can help the patient make a decision about surgery
	Factors influencing decision	What is important to the patient in making a decision?
		What worries the patient about making a decision?
		Other information the patient wish he or she had to help make the decision
Voluntariness		How the surgeon, nurse, family members, friends, or others have helped the patient's decision to have or not have surgery
		How others have made it harder for the patient to make a decision

care providers ask patients to restate (talk back) what patients heard the provider say. The talk back allows the provider to assess that what patients think they are agreeing to for surgery is consistent with the situation, to confirm patient understanding, and to ensure consent is informed.

The talk back process can be done after discussion of each component of the informed consent (description of the procedure and presentation of risks and benefits) and again at the completion of the informed consent discussion. The talk back can be used to identify areas of misunderstanding, allow for provider clarification as needed, and to assess elements of the older adult's capacity for making decisions.

Capacity

The majority of older adults are presumed to have the capacity to make decisions. Unless there is clear indication that an older adult is at risk for making an uninformed decision, the patient's decision prevails. When the decision capacity is uncertain, providers must intervene to ensure the older adult is protected (1) by allowing and advocating for the older adult to make decisions that are within the person's capacity to make, and (2) preventing harm due to provider abdication of responsibility to ensure decisional capacity.

Older adults and their providers must work together to ensure that the rights and responsibilities of each are met during the process of informed consent for surgery. Older adults are vulnerable not only due to patient characteristics, but also due to provider characteristics. Older adults may have capacity and make decisions to accept or refuse surgery consistent with preferences, may not have capacity and make decisions to accept or refuse surgery consistent with their preferences; may have capacity but not be allowed to make decisions consistent with identified preferences; or may not have capacity and are not allowed to make decisions or consideration given for preferences. Decisional capacity is decision-specific and not a global application. Assessing the older adult's preferences regardless of decisional capacity demonstrates respect for the personhood of the individual. Decisional capacity of the older adult should only be negated when there is overwhelming evidence that the older adult is cognitively or spiritually unable to make a choice or state a preference. The burden of proof for decisional incapacity rests with the provider to ensure that decisions not reflecting patient's best interests are not made by the patient or by the provider.

The process for determining decisional capacity is "neither complex nor overly burdensome" (Artnak, 1997, p. 59). Decisional capacity requires the ability to perform four functions:

1. Communicate a choice.
2. Understand the relevant information.
3. Appreciate a situation and its consequences.
4. Reason rationally.

Assess decisional capacity:

- *Abrupt change in mental status*
- *Refusal of treatment without explanation or negates attempts to correct misinformation*
- *Consents hastily without evident consideration of risks and benefits*
- *Risk factors present for misunderstanding information (psychiatric diagnosis, poor literacy, cultural barriers)*

Tunzi (2001) describes four situations that should lead providers to a more careful evaluation of the older adult's decision-making capacity. Situations include an abrupt change in the patient's mental status, refusal of a recommended treatment without explanation, a hasty response to consent without apparent consideration of information, or presence of known risk factors for interference with decisional capacity. The presence of any of these situations does not mean the patient cannot make a decision, only that the patient's clinical condition should be evaluated and the decision reviewed after the evaluation.

Transient Capacity

Transient capacity is capacity that fluctuates over time or changes with circumstances (i.e., a patient who experiences a "sundown syndrome" or increasing levels of fatigue throughout the day may be able to make decisions in the morning but not at night). Other conditions that can result in transient capacity are delirium, pain, anxiety, medication effects, or sensory disabilities. Older adults with transient capacity are often able to make reasoned decisions if approached at a time when capacity is intact. Care providers have a duty to ensure that judgments of decisional incapacity are not based on transient capacity. Older adults with transient capacity should be carefully evaluated to determine when the patient is best able to attend to information. Providers have an ethical responsibility to accommodate the patient to ensure the best possible process and decision outcomes.

Depression, Executive Function, and Decisional Capacity

There are few published studies data on the relationship between depression and informed consent to surgery. Lapid, Rummans, Pankratz, and Appelbaum (2004) investigated the ability of older adults with depression to consent to electroconvulsive therapy (ECT). The authors concluded that depressed elderly had adequate decisional capacities to consent to ECT. An important aspect of the study was the inclusion of education about the treatment and what to expect as it increased participants' decisional capacity. The authors concluded that providing education is important in maximizing older adults' ability to give informed consent.

Having the ability to make decisions is attributed to *executive functions*—the ability to plan, initiate, sequence, and monitor complex goal-directed behaviors. Executive function can be diminished in patients with depression, diabetes, hypertension, chronic obstructive pulmonary disease, or other chronic medical illnesses. Age-related cognitive changes affect executive function and decisional capacity. Loss of executive function is exacerbated in patients with age-related functional changes and comorbid disease.

A more detailed assessment is needed whenever care providers have reason to question the older adult's decisional capacity. However, assessing decision capacity depends to a large extent on clinical judgment. There is no "gold standard" assessment tool for determining the older adult's capacity to make a treatment decision.

The Mini-Mental Status Examination (Folstein, Folstein, & McHugh, 1975) is a test used for screening cognitive function. The CLOX: Executive Clock-drawing Task (Royall, Cordes, & Polk, 1998) is a screening tool to assess executive function.

The CLOX test assesses specific aspects of planning, organization, and behavior. The test was designed to assess for the presence of executive impairment (Royall, Cordes, & Polk, 1998). The test is easy to use in the clinical setting as a screening tool and takes only a few minutes to complete. The patient is given a pencil and a piece of paper with the instructions to draw a clock that says 1:45. The patient is instructed to set the hands and numbers on the face so that a child can read them. The CLOX test can be used effectively with older adults with limited English literacy or reading literacy. It has been validated in ethnically diverse populations. There is no information available on how well older adults with physical disabilities such as impaired manual dexterity in the dominant hand, severe vision impairment, or hand tremor can complete the clock drawing task. The ability to conduct the executive function elements of the CLOX test does not rest on physical ability.

Anxiety disorders, depression, bipolar disorder, schizophrenia, and personality disorders may be exacerbated during the postoperative period, requiring a geropsychiatric consultation to ensure the patient's capacity to make an informed decision. Requesting a geropsychiatric evaluation can help to resolve questions of decisional incapacity with older adults for whom there is clinical uncertainty about their mental status and for older patients with a history of a psychiatric diagnosis. Patients with a history of or demonstrating signs and symptoms of dementia often require a geropsychiatric evaluation to determine the degree to which the disease interferes with decision-making.

Provider Attitudes, Ageism, and Decision Capacity

Ethical conflicts can arise when the patient's decision does not coincide with the decision the health care system or provider recommends. Beneficent paternalism is when a health care provider or system tells patients what is good for them without regard to the patient's own needs or interests. This is in direct conflict with patient autonomy leading to one of the major conflicts in medicine today: the conflict between respecting a patient's right to make his or her own health care decisions and the provider's belief about what is in the patient's best interest. This form of paternalism can lead health care providers to override or change patients' decisions, especially if the provider is concerned that the patient is old and making poor decisions.

Ageism and beneficent paternalism violate the ethical principles of autonomy, justice, beneficence, non-malfeasance, and advocacy as well as opening the door to behavior that is unethical or immoral. Nurses may experience conflict when they disagree with a patient's decision regarding health care. They may be torn between the obligation to provide "best care" to the older adult and respecting the older person's right to make choices, even those that seem counter to the patient's best interest (Artnak, 1997). It is not the disagreement with the decision that is the problem, but the actions the nurse may take that places judgments on the patient or unduly influences the patient's decisions. The nurse should not accept the patient's decision when there is evidence the patient is unduly influenced by others or is demonstrating behaviors that raise concerns about capacity or understanding. Under these conditions, the nurse has a moral and professional obligation to not accept the patient's decision or allow others to accept the decision until the concerns are resolved.

Ageism is defined as discrimination against people based on their age. In the elderly, it is a cultural attitude that involves the belief that old people, especially old people who make decisions contrary to recommended treatment, are incapable of making informed decisions. Such attitudes can lead health care professionals to modify, discount, or altogether ignore medical decisions made by the older patient because the person making the decision is old. Ageism can interfere with the ability of the older adult to make a decision based on voluntariness.

VOLUNTARINESS

Age and illness makes elderly patients vulnerable to coercion by health care teams and family members. The coercion may be a perceived coercion, an inadvertent coercion, or a deliberate coercion. A significant percentage of elderly patients are poor, lack education about technical medical matters, or are physically and/or mentally impaired. These conditions can contribute to feelings of helplessness, which can make elderly patients open to being unduly influenced by others. Thus, it is crucially important that health care teams and families listen to the reasons for the decision made by the older adult.

Elders use less objective information when making decisions and rely heavily on people who they perceive as experts, whether the person is a health care professional or a family member. Older adults intuitively understand that they have incomplete knowledge and are vulnerable to make errors at a time of critical illness. Age-related changes in cognition could lead the older adult to rely on experts for analyzing information and recommending decisions. In addition, the clinician-patient relationship is one of unequal power in the clinical setting. This inequality stems from six sources: coercive power that carries a potential source of punishment, reward power that is a potential source of approval, legitimate power with the right to prescribe behavior, authoritative power that is admired, derived power based on expertise, and charismatic power that flows from information given in a convincing manner. In a medical setting, such power can be used for benefit or for ill; enhanced or diminished, it cannot be disowned (Cassell, 2005).

> *Older adults are vulnerable to provider power.*

Patients are acutely aware of these power disparities. In response, they delegate a certain amount of their freedom and entrust their care to others (Tauber, 2005). Tauber (2005) urges care providers not to turn away when older adults want information about their clinical condition, the kind of treatments that are available, or what the information means for their daily lives. However, there are no hard and fast rules. Older adults are unique individuals with diverse backgrounds, experiences, preferences, and views of their world. They should receive the level of information they want in a way that makes the information meaningful. Treatment decisions should be made in accordance with the older patient's preferences for level of involvement, need for decisional support, and the right to defer decisions to a family member or friend.

ANESTHESIA, CAPACITY, AND INFORMED CONSENT

Marcucci and colleagues (2010) caution that a patient's capacity for consent to surgery may not be at a level required to meet anesthesia informed consent. Anesthesia informed consent is a separate process from surgical informed consent. "Anesthesia involves more abstract concepts requiring a higher cognitive state than surgery, thus requiring a higher state of cognitive capacity for understanding" (Marcucci, Seagull, Loreck, Bourke, & Sandson, 2010, p. 596).

Preoperative Considerations

Nurses have a professional and moral responsibility and accountability to advocate for the gerioperative patient (American Nurses Association, 2001). Gerioperative nurses can ensure the ethical rights of older adults for informed consent by taking the following steps:

- Assessing decisional capacity
- Monitoring for anxiety, comfort, and response to unfamiliar surroundings that may influence the older person's ability to use reasoning and executive functions
- Conducting a repeat or talk back
- Eliciting patient questions, concerns, and feelings about the decision-making process and the decisions
- Encouraging and supporting the presence of a family member, friend, or significant other during discussions of informed consent
- Ensuring availability of an interpreter when needed
- Advocating for the older person's right to (1) decisional support from providers, families, or friends in making a decision, and (2) assisted, supported, or delegated autonomy

Advance Directives

Advance directives are written documents that allow a patient to indirectly participate in health care decisions if he or she becomes unable to do so. The Patient Self-Determination Act passed in 1991 requires that patients be informed of their right to participate in and direct health care decisions, the right to accept or refuse medical or surgical treatment, and the right to have an advance directive. The advance directive guides the decisions and actions of providers based on the patient's own wishes or preferences.

Two categories of advance directives are instructive and proxy directives. A living will is an example of an instructive directive. It allows an individual to predetermine what types of treatment the patient considers acceptable and prevents unwanted and futile invasive procedures at the end of life. The durable power of attorney for health care (DPAHC) is an example of a proxy directive and allows for the appointment of a surrogate decision-maker chosen by the patient. The surrogate decision-maker only has the power to make medical decisions if the patient becomes unconscious or incapacitated (Van Norman, 1998). The DPAHC is considered the document of choice as it permits delegation of health care decisions to someone who is aware of the individuals' health care preferences. Advance directive forms are available in most health care agencies including provider offices, hospitals, nursing homes, clinics, home health agencies, and hospice programs. Older patients should be told that a lawyer is not necessary for either completing the document or for the document to be legal or binding.

Studies indicate that approximately 70% of older adults have an advance directive. However, older adults with advance directives are more likely to be white with middle to upper socioeconomic status (Alano et al., 2010; McCarthy et al., 2008; Teno, Gruneir, Schwartz, Nanda, & Wetle, 2007). McCarthy and colleagues (2008) found that 69% of community dwelling elders had, at some time, discussed their wishes for medical care at the end of life with another person. Approximately two-thirds had a health care proxy. However, only 17% had discussed their preferences with a physician or health care provider. Nurses in all health care environments have a responsibility to assess if patients have an advance directive, encourage patients to prepare or revise an advance directive, especially the DPAHC, and supply information on obtaining and completing advance directive documents.

Prior to surgery, all older adults should be asked if they have a living will or durable power of attorney, and where a copy of the document is located. If there is a durable power of attorney, the patient should be asked who holds the decision-making proxy and if there are any limitations to the proxy. Finally, the patient should be asked if the wishes expressed in the advance directive are still valid. This is best done at the time of the preoperative assessment. Patients may need to review the document prior to making decisions about whether any changes to the document as stated are needed. Information about the advance directive should be documented in the patient's health care record.

The legal standing of advance directives can vary state to state. It is important that nurses and other health care providers as well as older adults and their families be aware of the state's position on advance directives. This is particularly important in older adults who have family in other states, who travel from state to state, or who have legal residences in more than one state.

Even in states that do not support a legal definition of advance directive, health care practitioners are expected to honor and respect patient preferences identified in such a document. The nurse should ensure that all health care providers are informed about and respect the advance directive and that the DPAHC is consulted as necessary. In the event that a provider disagrees or ignores an advance directive, charges of battery or emotional trauma may be filed. If there are disagreements between health care providers and/or family about the best care for the patient, every effort should be made to reconcile the parties in the best interest of the patient. An ethics committee should be consulted whenever there is an unresolved conflict.

If a patient states on the directive that a specific treatment or procedure such as mechanical ventilation or artificial feeding should not be used, but subsequently has a change of mind when faced with postsurgical complications, the nurse serves as an advocate for the patient and ensures the change is honored. The reverse is also true. Older adults who make the decision that they want to terminate treatment often need the support of nurses. As long as the patient is capable of making a decision, the advance directive is revocable or changeable (Van Norman, 1998).

Do Not Resuscitate

Cardiopulmonary resuscitation (CPR) is a set of medical procedures implemented as a supportive measure in the event of cardiac or pulmonary failure. CPR is designed to maintain perfusion to vital organs until a normal cardiac rhythm is reestablished. Two situations allow CPR to be withheld: when CPR is designated as having no medical benefit and when the patient has made a decision to not have CPR. In general, more geriatric patients have a do not resuscitate (DNR) order than any other age group (Cherniack, 2002).

CPR has been found to have minimal benefit in older adults with septic shock, acute stroke, metastatic cancer, and severe pneumonia. Likelihood of survival in these instances is near 0%. Survival rates of less than 4% are documented for hypotension, renal failure, acquired immunodeficiency syndrome, homebound lifestyle, and age over 70 (Van Norman, 1998).

DNR orders become problematic in the operating room (OR). Many institutions require DNR orders be suspended while in the OR and for 24 hours postoperatively. Arguments to discontinue DNR orders while in the OR stem from the difficulty of discerning resuscitation attempts from routine surgical and anesthesia care. While performing general anesthesia, many of the interventions such as mechanical ventilation, intubation, and administration of medications to prevent arrhythmias and hypotension, as well as blood products, are similar to actions performed during CPR. Secondly, practitioners argue that resuscitative measures in the OR are often more successful because they are witnessed and immediate. Third, many practitioners do not want to feel responsible for a death or potentially be involved in a legal action for being negligent (Sieber, 2007).

Advocates for maintaining DNR orders in the OR acknowledge that surgery may lead to poor outcomes and complications. Such adverse events may diminish patient quality of life and should be taken into consideration if CPR is to be performed. In general, surgeons and anesthetists often ask for a temporary suspension of a DNR order during surgery with a carefully negotiated timeline for reinstituting the DNR postoperatively.

Addressing questions and concerns about honoring or suspending a DNR order during surgery require attention to the ethical principles of autonomy, beneficence, non-malfeasance, and justice associated with informed consent for surgery. The American Society of Anesthesiologists established ethical guidelines for anesthesia care of patients who have documented DNR orders or advance directives. The guidelines clearly state automatic suspension of DNR orders during surgery is inconsistent with a patient's right to self-determination. The American College of Surgeons recommends the patient and physicians involved in the patient's care conduct a "required reconsideration" with the patient.

Discussion elements include the purpose of the DNR, the meaning of the DNR to the patient, the reasons for surgery, and the risks, benefits, and consequences of maintaining or suspending the DNR during surgery and for a period of time after surgery. Discussions about the DNR request should involve the older person, proxy decision-maker, and any other person requested by the older adult, as well as providers responsible for the patient's care. The DNR order should be discussed in relation to the goals of the proposed surgery, patient condition, personal values of the patient and family, as well as beliefs of the health care team. The decision should be documented and made readily available to all members of the intra-operative health care team.

If DNR orders are suspended temporarily for surgery, a timetable and process for reinstituting the DNR after surgery must be established and clearly documented in the preoperative record. Regardless of the preoperative decision, DNR decisions should be reviewed with the patient or proxy decision-maker after surgery prior to reinstituting the DNR to confirm the patient's wishes. Nurses can advocate for DNR review and document the discussion and decision.

PATIENT REPORT: MR. BARNARD

The answer to the opening situation as to whether Mr. Barnard is competent to sign a surgical consent after receiving analgesia is more complex than it may first appear. Some health care providers would argue Mr. Barnard has a diminished capacity secondary to receiving a potentially sedating medication. Others might contend that patients who are in pain and anxious are not competent as they are distracted by their discomfort. Others might argue that causing Mr. Barnard to wait for pain medication until the consent is signed is a form of coercion. Each of these could serve as a basis for determining that Mr. Barnard is not taking voluntary action, a criterion for informed consent.

The nurse stayed with Mr. Barnard after giving him his medication to assess his response to the medication and potential effects on his capacity. Mr. Barnard continued to be alert and oriented. The nurse remained in the room while the surgeon reviewed the surgery, and the associated risks and benefits, and asked Mr. Barnard about his decision. After the surgeon completed the explanation and left, the nurse asked Mr. Barnard to share what he heard about the surgery, his decision to have the surgery, and the reasons for that decision. When Mr. Barnard was able to share basic information and explain his reasoning for the procedure (Mr. Barnard would like the surgery so that he can do the things that he wants to do, like take his dog for a walk), the nurse concluded that Mr. Barnard was making an informed consent to surgery.

Informed Consent for Research

Research in the geriatric population presents its own set of ethical considerations. Many elderly patients have multiple disease processes and functional impairments at somatic and psychosocial levels. Most research is focused on one disease process or outcome, thus frail, older people are excluded from these studies. The preferred research design, large randomized clinical trials, is difficult to conduct in this age group secondary to multiple physical, social, and psychological limitations. Lastly, obtaining informed consent in this age group may be difficult.

Concerns related to research with older adults center on two major issues: protection of vulnerable populations and underrepresentation of older adults in clinical trials and intervention studies. Including older adults as research participants generates concerns about protection of vulnerable elders and ensuring informed consent.

Researchers often avoid aging research with elderly populations who present the most difficulty and greatest challenges to inclusion: the frail, those who have multiple disease conditions, or those who have combined physical and psychological alterations in health. Yet, these are the very elders who have some of the greatest need for research that will improve their care and clinical outcomes. Herrera and colleagues (2010) argue that low rates of elderly participants, especially the most vulnerable elders in study populations, limit generalizability of study findings, provide insufficient data about positive or negative effects of treatment among aging ethnic populations, and hinder much-needed access to new treatments.

A major difference between consent for clinical treatment and consent for research rests in the principles of beneficence and non-malfeasance. Clinical treatment is directed to the immediate benefit of the older adult, while the research procedure may not bring direct benefit; it may even cause harm. For example, clinical drug trials can carry risks for unintended consequences and side effects. Medical treatment and interventions often carry unintended consequences, but the risks may be clearer and more readily identified.

A major concern regarding research with older adults during the perioperative period is the effect of presurgical anxiety, pain and discomfort, surgical stress, anesthesia effects, and postoperative complications on the decision-making capacity of older adults. Pain can be a major impediment to information processes, comprehension, and voluntarism. Postoperative complications such as delirium, infection, and deconditioning can further impede informed consent.

In research, the risks are not always as readily apparent. Therefore, informed consent assumes an even greater importance. The history of exploitation in research of vulnerable older adults suggests the level of proof for attaining informed consent must rest with the research community. The burden of responsibility for ensuring informed consent must not be an excuse for excluding older adults from clinical trials or treatment intervention studies because of the ethical difficulties and challenges they present.

A decreased ability to compare information places the older adult at a disadvantage for research-based informed consent. In order to better understand and to better serve the patient, it is of special importance for providers to compare the risks and benefits of research participation, as well as to compare and recognize the differences between the role of the patient and the role of the research participant.

When the older adult is a patient and is asked to participate in research, the issue of adequate information and effect on voluntarism is more pronounced. Elders may be concerned that the right to say no to research participation may mean saying no to treatment or receiving other services. Decreased energy and increased fatigue interferes with the ability to "take in" the information. Taking in is being able to interpret and understand information at a personal, meaningful level for decision-making. The right to refuse participation is much more complex when older adults from minority or ethnic cultures depend on health care directed by persons from what is perceived as the majority culture.

Intervention research and clinical trials raise issues about benefits and costs to the individual in conditions where the individual receives no direct benefit from the intervention or trial. There is often an argument whether anyone should be subjected to the "control" condition. Research involves testing an intervention based on the anticipation that the intervention will lead to a better outcome. Should elders bear the burden of testing for the benefit of others at a cost to the self? How is an intervention or clinical trial explained in ways that non-researchers can understand? What does it mean to be in a "control" group versus being in an "experimental" group, especially when determination of the group assignment does not occur until after the consent form is signed? Is it harder to say "no" to participation after one has said "yes" and the project is underway? This is of special concern for elders who may have had changes in cognition that are not "impaired," but certainly may be constraining. Having a researcher or other health care professional present the request for informed consent may be sufficient to sway an older adult who relies on "expert opinion."

Elders often agree to be research participants when asked because they want to be thought of as "nice" or "not a burden." Although both of these motives may rest in the concept of generativity, they may also rest under the umbrella of undue inducement or implicit persuasion. Older adults have a fear that refusing to participate means something will be taken away from them or they will not receive something they would receive if they agreed. Their fears often center on not receiving a service or benefit they should receive or having a service or benefit discontinued. In the hospital, older adults fear being ignored or not getting the care they need if they refuse to participate. Although informed consent forms explicitly state this will not happen, elders often retain an underlying concern that refusing will cause some negative consequences.

An ethical concern highly debated in the bioethics and research community is the potential for coercion when participants receive payment for research participation. This ethical concern centers on the following questions: Will participants, who otherwise would not do so, participate in a study and act against their general welfare in return for funds offered? Is payment for research a form of exploitation, especially for elders without adequate financial resources? (Wertheimer & Miller, 2008). These questions may be of special concern when elders live with family members who bear the cost of the elder's care. It is possible that elders, who would say no if there were no financial inducements, would agree to participate based on self-talk similar to: "I should do this because I (or my family) need the money no matter what."

Is offering money to older adults for research coercion or inducement?

Wertheimer and Miller (2008) offer the argument that the opportunity to participate in research with or without payment is never coercion. However, payment may constitute undue inducement wherein the older adult may agree to participate regardless of the actual or perceived risks to the individual's own belief system, health, or well-being. The question is whether "distortion of judgment" (p. 391) occurs when payment is offered. How can the informed consent process protect the older adult from undue inducement and protect the research study from charges of inducement?

Older adults who are under the direct care of others, who see themselves as having little power over what happens to them, or who have health care needs that interfere with their ability to exercise personal power should not be exploited. Inviting older adults to participate in research, under the principle of "doing good," can be articulated in a way that is coercive to older adults. Older adults, especially those from certain generations or ethnic populations, are subject to the "guilt" of not doing one's share or meeting one's responsibilities to others. Understanding aging as a cohort issue with a set of norms and values, while understanding aging as a loss of perceived power to say "no," is critical to the researcher's understanding of "informed" consent. Older adults in acute care settings under the care of health care providers are at particular risk for loss of self-perceived power.

SUMMARY

While informed consent is legally and ethically important for all persons undergoing surgery, it is important to consider capabilities and limitations of the older adult, as well as the effects of age- and disease-related changes. Gerioperative patients should also have written documents related to advanced directives and CPR.

KEY POINTS

- Informed consent is a process based on legal and ethical principles.
- Elements of informed consent are to ensure the patient has sufficient information, has decision-making capacity, and consent is voluntary.
- The process of informed consent in older adults must take into consideration physical and psychological age-related changes that affect vision, hearing, information processing, decisional capacity, and communication needs.
- Decisional support is an integral aspect of the informed consent process with older adults.
- Advance directives and DNR orders are ethical issues that require application of principles of informed consent and gerioperative decision-making.
- Informed consent for research was the initial support for mandating patient's self-determination.

FIVE

Gerioperative Medication Safety

Raelene V. Shippee–Rice, Jennifer V. Long, and Susan J. Fetzer

PATIENT REPORT: Mr. Roberts

Mr. Roberts is 82 years old and lives with his wife of 40 years. He is admitted to the medical-surgical unit after surgery for a hip fracture. Mr. Roberts fell after slipping on the ice while shoveling snow off his porch steps. He was alert and oriented on admission. He takes alprazolam for anxiety "several times a week." He has moderately severe osteoarthritis in his left knee with effusion. His history reveals mild hypertension treated long-term with hydrochlorothiazide 25 mg. He self-administers acetaminophen 2500 mg/day for osteoarthritis pain, vitamin D, glucosamine, salmon oil, and multivitamins. He takes prednisone 10 mg a day for severe and recurring inflammation in his knee and polymyalgia rheumatica. Postoperatively, Mr. Roberts is alert, follows directions, and responds appropriately to questions. He occasionally loses focus and demonstrates a loss of affect. He denies hip pain and refuses pain medication. His wife tells the nurse there is something wrong with him, that he isn't "quite right." The nurse assesses his orientation questions, and he responds correctly except, "How would I know what time it is. I don't have a watch." After reassuring Mrs. Roberts that Mr. Roberts is fine but that it will take time for him to recover from the trauma of surgery, the nurse leaves the room.

Comprising approximately 13% of the total population, older adults consume almost 34% of all prescription medications. Approximately 40% of older adults take five or more concurrent prescription medications. In addition, over 90% of older adults take one or more over-the-counter (OTC) medications with diet supplements, cold medications, and analgesics as the most commonly used OTCs. Slightly over 25% of older adults take vitamins regularly, and 16% take two or more herbal remedies. Unfortunately, many OTC drugs interact with prescription drugs or cause physiologic responses that are potentially harmful to older adults.

Medication is a standard intervention for most acute and chronic diseases and minor ailments. A significant number of patients also use herbal and naturopathic remedies. Polypharmacy, the concurrent use of multiple medications, is a leading cause of adverse drug events (ADEs), a harmful effect associated with medication use. Age-related physiologic changes affecting pharmacodynamics and pharmacokinetics increase older adults' sensitivity to medications making ADE more likely. The goals of medication administration in the gerioperative patient are to optimize pharmacotherapeutic effectiveness, ensure patient safety, prevent avoidable ADEs, and minimize unavoidable effects.

This chapter describes factors associated with medication use and ADEs in the gerioperative patient. Focal areas center on age-related physiologic changes and perioperative considerations. Interventions to support safety and optimize medication outcomes are discussed as they relate to care of the gerioperative patient. Understanding the medication administration and safety needs of the gerioperative patient allows providers to develop interventions that maximize gerioperative safety and positive patient outcomes.

Pharmacokinetics and Pharmacodynamics

Pharmacokinetics describes drug absorption, distribution, metabolism, and excretion. A drug's pharmacokinetics determines the most important elements influencing its action, how rapidly it will act, how long it will act, and how much of the drug is available to create a physiologic effect.

Pharmacodynamics refers to the action of the drug once the target or receptor site is reached. The pharmacologic response depends on how much of the drug is available due to pharmacokinetics. Pharmacodynamics depends on the adequacy of target receptor sites. Drugs can have target selectivity, meaning that although drugs may use multiple receptor sites, they cannot access all receptors. Drug-selective receptor sites must be available, and the drug must be able to bind to the receptor. The drug must remain attached to the receptor site long enough for an action to occur. The concentration and duration of the drug at the receptor site influences the drug's effect.

The interaction of pharmacokinetics and pharmacodynamics determines the overall drug effect. Health status, physiological function, gender, and race influence the pharmacokinetics and pharmacodynamics for any single individual. The chemical properties of drugs combined with patient factors determine drug effects. Age-related changes that alter the pharmacodynamics and pharmacokinetics of drugs increase the sensitivity of gerioperative patient to drug effects. Figure 5.1 depicts the interaction of patient- and drug-related factors on drug effectiveness.

Age-Related Changes

Age-related changes in pharmacokinetics and pharmacodynamics are not uniform across individuals. There is wide variation at the individual level in how drug absorption, distribution, metabolism, and excretion are affected by aging. Individual variation is magnified with the number and severity of comorbid conditions. Recognizing the potential effect of age-related changes increases provider sensitivity to geriatric vulnerability to ADEs and the need to closely monitor the older patient's response to medications.

Drugs enter the body through oral and parenteral routes or are absorbed topically. Aging affects oral drug absorption by increasing gastric emptying time, slowing intestinal motility, and decreasing the available number of intestinal cells to absorb medication. However, these changes have minimal effect on the amount of drug absorbed.

Distribution is the extent to which the medication is transmitted within the body and to the specific site of drug activity. The extent of distribution is influenced by body size and composition of fat and water. Age-related changes affecting drug distribution are a decrease in body mass, increase in body fat, and decrease in body water.

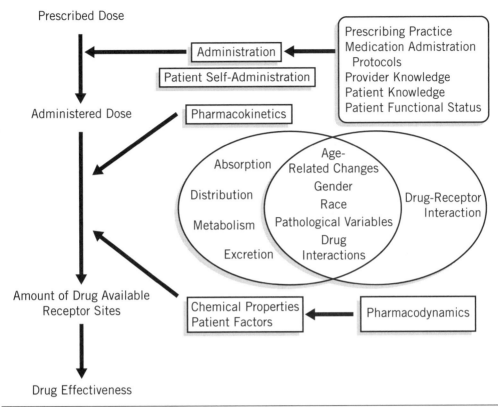

FIGURE 5.1

Factors Influencing Drug Effectiveness in the Gerioperative Patient

Physical size decreases with age, especially in the very old, primarily as a result of decrease in muscle mass. The change in physical size is one reason medication dosing must be decreased in older adults. The decrease in body mass and tissue volume allows drugs to become more concentrated in target tissues.

With increased age, body fat increases as much as 36% in men and 45% in women. The increased body fat means that fat-soluble drugs are distributed throughout the body for longer periods of time. Fat-soluble drugs hide in fat, thereby decreasing availability to the body. Fat-soluble drugs are also not available for degradation, leading to a longer half-life in the body. Cellular water content decreases up to 15% with age, forcing water-soluble drugs to become more concentrated. Use of diuretics or dehydration further decreases body water, adding to drug concentration in body tissues.

Once in the body, drugs are metabolized or broken down into an active form or inactive metabolites before being excreted. A decrease in liver function slows the rate of drug breakdown and elimination. The aging liver decreases as much as 40% in size, blood flow to the liver decreases, and hepatic enzymes are reduced. Heart failure, myocardial infarction, and liver disease compromise liver function even further. The effect on drug metabolism in the liver can vary depending on the extent of the change in liver size, blood flow, and enzyme activity.

Albumin, a protein made by the liver, binds drugs, reducing the serum concentration of "free" substance. Serum albumin levels tend to be lower in older adults. Low serum albumin levels caused by acute or sudden onset of malnutrition from surgery have an effect on protein binding capacity. When serum albumin is low, the drug remains unbound, causing elevated free drug levels. The combination of a low serum binding capacity and drugs with narrow therapeutic ranges results in a higher risk of adverse effects. Drugs such as warfarin, nonsterioidal anti-inflammatory drugs (NSAIDs), benzodiazepines, and antibiotics are problematic for elders. However, adequate kidney function can moderate some of the age-related changes in serum albumin. Even when serum albumin is low, adequate renal function eliminates the unbound drug.

Renal clearance is a major factor contributing to ADEs. Glomerular filtration rates can be significantly reduced by reduced renal blood flow. Dehydration and comorbid cardiovascular disease decrease renal blood flow, and glomerular filtration rates impair drug excretion even further. The kidney's ability to eliminate medications can be decreased as much as 50%, increasing risk for ADEs. Surgery places added stress on the kidneys over and above that caused by age-related or disease-related changes. Intraoperative fluid management must be adequate to ensure optimal kidney function (see Chapter 10).

Drug effectiveness is influenced by the amount of drug bound to target receptors and the response of the targeted receptor effects. Based on receptor site activity, drugs may have greater or lesser action in older people. Changes in action are due to the total number of receptors available or the degree of competition for receptors. Aging decreases receptor availability, thus increasing the amount of unbound drug and interfering or enhancing drug effectiveness. For example, warfarin binds to protein and albumin. With increasing age, albumin decreases, limiting the availability of receptor sites. The gerioperative patient typically requires a lower dose of warfarin to achieve the desired therapeutic effect while minimizing risk of excessive bleeding. Increased response to some cardiovascular drugs requires decreased dosage (i.e., diltiazem and enalapril).

Polypharmacy causes drugs to compete for the same receptor site, further interfering with drug availability. Changes in postreceptor age-related homeostatic mechanisms such as thermoregulation, visceral muscle function, and hemodynamic responses influence how the body responds to the drug after binding. Chronic illness also interferes with receptor availability and postreceptor response. The effects of age- and disease-related changes on the receptivity and expression of drug receptors is not well known.

Comorbidity

The intensity of a preexisting illness, onset of new disease, or interaction between preexisting and concurrent illnesses increases physiologic vulnerability to ADEs. Disease conditions have a dramatic effect on pharmacokinetics, while the effect on pharmacodynamics is less well documented. Changes in pharmacokinetics generate the potential for reduced therapeutic effect and increased adverse effects.

Aging predisposes the elderly to chronic medical conditions such as diabetes, heart disease, osteoporosis, and cancer. Most chronic health conditions are treated with medications. With the escalation in pharmaceutical technology, more intense medications are available for treating disease.

Multiple diseases requiring multiple medications lead to drug-disease interactions. Drug-disease interactions occur when a drug designed to improve one health condition makes another health condition worse. Up to 40% of hospitalized older adults experience drug-disease interactions. Most drug-disease interactions involve calcium-channel blockers in patients with heart failure or beta-blockers in patients with diabetes. Older adults undergoing surgery with multiple comorbidities and receiving five or more medications should be evaluated for drug-disease interactions.

Polypharmacy incorporates prescribed medications, OTC drugs, and naturopathic herbs, roots, and leaves. Multiple medications interfere with the therapeutic effects of some medications and create side effects by others. Drug-drug interactions are a major cause of ADEs in older adults. Warfarin is one of the most prescribed drugs in the elderly, and it reacts with many different OTC and prescription medications. Cimetidine, an OTC medication for indigestion, increases the effect of warfarin and can cause increased bleeding, which may result in hemorrhage.

Older adults are rarely included when new drugs are tested. Drug trials seek subjects without comorbid diseases. As a result, recommended drug doses do not consider age-related changes of elders or comorbid diseases and drugs. Given the lack of evidence supporting drug dosing, alterations in pharmacotherapeutic mechanisms in older adults requires attention to a basic principle of geriatric pharmacology" "Start low and go slow." Added to that principle is "with vigilant monitoring."

Adverse Drug Events

Many ADEs result in minimal harm to patients. However, more severe consequences include prolonged pain, extended hospitalization, delayed recovery, increased health care costs, and diminished functional status. Mortality from ADEs has been reported at 3.5%. The cost of ADEs has been estimated at nearly 4 billion dollars each year (Committee on Identifying and Preventing Medication Errors, 2006).

> *ADEs are one of the most common (AHRQ, 2010) complications of hospital mortality.*

EPIDEMIOLOGY

The risk of community-based ADEs increases to 50% with five or more prescriptions and is guaranteed with nine or more medications. Up to 35% of older adult hospital admissions are due to an ADE. Over two-thirds of ADEs are serious or life-threatening. Between 1997 and 2008, hospital admission rates for drug-related causes increased 96% in adults aged 65 to 84 and 87% in those 85 years of age and over (Agency for Health Care Quality and Research, 2010). Drug-induced delirium and overdoses of opiate-based pain medications were primarily responsible for the increase. In 2008, these two conditions accounted for 60% of drug-related stays for patients 65 to 84 years old and 78 percent of the drug-related stays in patients 85 years and older.

> *Motto of drug administration in gerioperative patients: "start low and go slow with vigilant monitoring"*

More than 50% of all drug-related adverse events in older adults are preventable depending on setting (community, hospital, or long-term care) and type of adverse event. Published studies underestimate the severity of ADEs in both community-based and hospitalized elders due to underreporting. In the community, many ADEs go unreported by older adults unless sufficiently severe to notify a care provider. The older adult often discontinues medications without notice. Alternatively, the older person may continue the medication and tolerate the adverse event, especially if the medication is ordered for a short period. Finally, the adverse event may never be known by anyone because there was no trigger to bring the event to attention.

ADEs are one of the most common complications in hospitalized older adults and one of the top five leading causes of in-hospital mortality. Most ADEs occur at time of admission, transfer to another unit, or at time of discharge.

Surgery is a high-risk center for ADEs. Multiple patient transfers involving multiple providers who prescribe and administer high-risk medications often under rapid-paced situations create adverse scenarios. ADEs occurring during perioperative care are reported to be around 7%. Intraoperative medication errors hover near 13% (Hicks, Becker, Krenzicheck, & Beyea, 2004; United States Pharmacopeia, 2007).

A major cause of surgical-related ADEs is the mix of high-alert medications and the complex medication regimens used to treat chronic and acute illness. High-alert medications have the potential to produce high therapeutic benefit with a high risk of injury (Institute for Healthcare Improvement, 2007; Institute for Safe Medication Practices, 2008). Table 5.1 lists common high-alert drugs administered during gerioperative care. Common high-alert drugs associated with ADEs in older adults are anticoagulants, narcotics, insulin, sodium chloride above 0.9%, and sedatives. In addition to surgery-related drugs, older adults are in contact with additional high-alert medications in the preoperative period such as cardiovascular and respiratory medications as well as glycemics.

Medications used to prevent or treat postoperative complications have a high degree of potency. Not only does the type of medication generate a risk, modes of administration such as intravenous or central routes make the drug available more rapidly. Patients undergoing surgery receive higher potency medications at higher doses and with more frequency. Potent medications in relatively high doses are often administered intra- and postoperatively, a time when elders' physiological vulnerability due to preexisting chronic and acute illness, surgery, pain, and postoperative complications is highest.

The fragmented nature of the surgical process with multiple transitions involving multiple providers is a second key factor in the escalation of ADE risk in the surgical care of older adults. Adverse events are more likely to occur when multiple providers, unfamiliar with the patient's health history and individual response to medications, prescribe and administer multiple medications to vulnerable older adults. Consistency of information and knowledge of the patient's individual situation are important variables to consider in improving medication safety.

TABLE 5.1

Examples of High-Alert Medications

Anticoagulants	Warfarin
	Heparin
	Aspirin
	Clopidogrel
	Enoxaparin
Hypoglycemic agents	Insulin
	Metformin
	Glyburide
Sedatives	Barbiturates
	Benzodiazepines
Anesthetic agents	Propofol
	Ketamine
Narcotic agents	Opioids
All intravenous solutions and medications	
All epidural and intrathecal medications	

MEDICATION ERRORS

Medication errors are the most common form of hospital-related ADEs. A medication error is any preventable event that may cause or lead to inappropriate medication prescription, administration, or utilization. Estimates suggest that medication administration constitutes approximately 38% of all medication errors, while prescribing errors constituting another 39% (Picone et al., 2008). Up to 95% of hospital-based medication errors are preventable.

Forty-six percent of medication errors occur with new orders written at the time of patient admission or discharge. Other sources of error result from poor communication, incomplete transfer of information, poor handoffs, inadequate gerioperative knowledge, lack of medication knowledge, errors in drug calculation, and lack of a "single point-person" to monitor progress of care. Transitions across hospital health care units account for up to 50% of all medication errors and 20% of ADEs in the hospital (Institute for Healthcare Improvement, n.d.).

Hospital ADEs remain underdetected. Symptoms caused by drug interactions or side effects are often overlooked due to provider and patient assumption that signs and symptoms are due to illness or "old age." Inadequate reporting practices by health care providers are a second cause of underestimation of hospital-based ADEs. Programs instituted by the Institute for Healthcare Improvement and the Institute for Safe Medication Practice have improved the reporting process through emphasis on quality improvement and shared responsibility.

Risk Factors

Surgically related medication errors in older adults result from patient characteristics and iatrogenic causes similar to those found in all hospitalized adults. Additional factors in older adults include age-related physiological changes and the sheer number of medications. Exhibit 5.1 lists predisposing risk factors to surgically related medication error.

A critical factor in the gerioperative patient is the increased vulnerability to the consequences of ADE. The increased vulnerability is due to decreased physiological reserve induced by surgical stress and anesthesia. Prescribing practices, medication administration, and system factors are the most significant causes of ADEs. System factors include environmental stress, number of providers, geriatric knowledge, nurse staffing ratios, communication systems, and number of transitions during the perioperative stay.

Promoting Medication Safety

Preventing medication errors is a major goal whenever a gerioperative patient requires one or more prescription medications. Sources of error include professional practice behaviors of medication prescribing and administration, provider knowledge, inadequate monitoring, and health care system barriers.

There is no universal definition for prescribing errors or administration errors. In general, prescribing errors include transcription errors, failure to communicate essential information, the use of drugs or doses inappropriate for the individual patient, or the over- or underutilization of medications to treat a disease or condition. Medication administration error is defined as "mistakes associated with drugs and intravenous solutions that are made during the prescription, transcription, dispensing, and administration phases of drug preparation and distribution" (Wolf, 1989, p.8).

EXHIBIT 5.1 **Factors Predisposing Older Adults to Surgically Related Adverse Drug Events**

- Patient factors
  - Age-related physiological changes
  - Number and severity of comorbidities
- Iatrogenic factors
  - Heightened physiological stress response from surgical trauma
  - Increased sensitivity to drug reactions and interactions
  - Effects of stress, pain, and analgesia on patient's ability to discriminate alterations in body function and sensation
- Provider factors
  - Polypharmacy
  - Drug-drug and drug-disease interactions
  - Use of high-alert medications
  - Use of potentially inappropriate medications
  - Prescribing cascade
  - Underprescribing medications
- System factors
  - Multiple transitions involving multiple providers
  - Inadequate communication
  - Discontinuity of care
  - Inadequate staffing
  - Environmental noise and distraction during medication administration

Lack of adequate nurse staffing, inattention to protocols, insufficient patient safety checks, rapid patient turnover, and rotating staff are common system-related factors contributing to adverse medication outcomes. Poor documentation and inadequate communication between and across providers during patient care and across unit transitions have been consistently cited as major sources of medication error.

A common prescribing error in older adults is the use of potentially inappropriate medications (PIM). Beers published inappropriate medications for nursing home residents in 1992. Five years later, the list was revised for elders in all settings (Beers, 1997). PIMs should be avoided or prescribed with extreme caution in patients 65 years of age or older. Reasons for not prescribing these medications for the elderly include lack of efficacy, harmful side effects, or treatment with other more suitable agents is available. The updated PIMs list (Beers criteria) is widely used for provider education and to assess and inform health care providers of altered medication prescribing practices for older adults across the health care continuum. Common drugs to be avoided in older adults are listed in Table 5.2.

In a retrospective review of 2004 data from 40 academic health centers, Bonk and colleagues (2006) reported up to 68% of hospitalized elders received at least one PIM; almost 20% received two or more. More recently, Hale and colleagues (2008) studied PIM use in 100 hospitalized older adults. Nearly 60% of the study sample received at least one PIM during hospitalization. Over half of the PIMs were new orders, while 43% were reorders of existing prescription home medications. In addition, PIMs were found on many preprinted standing orders and medication protocols.

TABLE 5.2

Examples of Drugs to Avoid or Use With Caution in Older Adults

Drug Category	Name
Gastrointestinal antispasmodic	Hyoscyamine Propantheline Belladonna/phenobarbital
Antihistamine	Chlorphenamine maleate Diphenhydramine Hydroxyzine Loratidine Cyproheptadine Promethazine
Muscle relaxant	Oxybutynin Methocarbamol Carisoprodol Chlorzoxazone Cyclobenzaprine
Antidepressant	Perphenazine/Amitriptyline Amitriptyline Doxepin
Antiarrhythmic	Lanoxin Disopyramide
Analgesic	Pentazocine/Naloxone Meperidine
Nonsteroidal	Indomethacin
Anxiolytics	Meprobamate Meprobamate
Long-acting benzodiazepines	Chlordiazepoxide Chlordiazepoxide/Clidinium Diazepam
Benzodiazepines	Alprazolam, Oxazepam Temazepam Triazolam Lorazepam
Antiemetic	Trimethobenzamide
Antacids	Cimetidine Ranitidine

Drugs with anticholinergic effects and benzodiazepines are well-documented high-risk medications in older adults. Anticholinergic medications cause adverse effects in the central and peripheral nervous system. Postoperative delirium, cognitive dysfunction, visual disturbances, memory changes, and respiratory depression are major central nervous effects. Other major side effects include constipation, urinary retention, dry mucous membranes, loss of coordination, blurred vision, and tachycardia.

Self-medication contributes to anticholinergic burden in older adults. Elders consume significant OTC drugs with significant anticholinergic effects such as antihistamines, sedatives, antacids, and antispasmodics used to treat incontinence and gastrointestinal complaints.

The Anticholinergic Risk Scale (ARS), developed by Rudolph and colleagues (2008), is a useful tool for detecting the level of anticholinergic drug burden in patient's medications. Selected common prescription and OTC medications are prescored from 0 to 3. Patient medications are scored based on the list. Patients with a total ARS score of 3 or higher are vulnerable to anticholinergic effects and should be closely evaluated for anticholinergic side effects.

Nurses need to be aware that standard orders may contain medications inappropriate for elders.

Long-acting benzodiazepines always should be avoided in older adults as they cause confusion, ataxia, psychomotor impairment, and pseudodementia in older adults. Older adults have increased sensitivity to certain benzodiazepines (such as diazepam) due to fat solubility. Drug effects last longer due to longer half-life in both fat-soluble and water-soluble benzodiazepines. The depressant effects of benzodiazepines are greater in the elderly, possibly due to age-related neurological changes.

Benzodiazepine use is common in older adults due to prescription practices of primary care providers. Primary care physicians report benzodiazepines are effective in treating anxiety in older adults, and patients are comfortable taking the medication. Many physicians consider the risk posed by benzodiazepine use in older adults to be overstated (Cook, Marshall, Masci, & Coyne, 2007). Older adults undergoing surgery need to be assessed for preoperative use of benzodiazepines.

The use of benzodiazepines preoperatively has been linked with emergence and postoperative delirium. Abrupt discontinuation of benzodiazepines after prolonged regular use causes withdrawal symptoms and, in severe cases, seizures. Routinely administered short-acting benzodiazepines should be withdrawn gradually over several weeks or longer.

PRESCRIBING CASCADE AND DRUG UNDERUTILIZATION

Prescribing cascades lead to overmedication. The prescribing cascade begins when a new medication is used to treat a new developing condition thought to be a new illness rather than a side effect of the newly prescribed medication. An example would be increased blood sugar after initiation of a beta blocker. The provider may consider adding another medication to treat the "diabetes" that is actually a side effect of the beta blocker. Onset of new symptoms after the initiation of a new medication should be considered side effects until otherwise determined.

Onset of new symptoms should be considered medication side effects until otherwise explained.

Medication underutilization occurs when a drug indicated for the treatment or prevention of a disease is not prescribed. Studies suggest that cardiovascular, respiratory, and hypoglycemic medications are the most underused medications. Underprescribing can occur regardless of the number of other medications a patient is receiving; underuse refers to appropriateness of medication and not the number of medications. A preoperative goal is to ensure that preexisting health conditions are well controlled. Ensuring the patient is receiving the right medication at the right dose is as important as not overmedicating with the wrong medication or the wrong dose.

Patients may omit or fabricate medication history.

Drug-drug interactions occur when two or more medications interact to cause a decrease in effectiveness of a drug, enhance effectiveness of a drug, or counteract the effectiveness of a drug. Causes of drug-drug interaction include competition for receptor sites, decreased protein for protein-bound drug binding, and altered absorption, distribution, metabolism, or elimination of medications. Polypharmacy increases the risk of drug-drug interactions. Older adults who take multiple OTC medications are more vulnerable to drug-drug interactions due to the multiple ingredients used in OTCs. Smoking may increase drug metabolism. Alcohol may enhance the effectiveness of medications such as benzodiazepines and valerian. An example of a deliberate drug-drug interaction is the use of naloxone to counteract the effects of narcotics. In the event of narcotic overdose, naloxone is administered to block the opiate receptors, making the narcotic ineffective. This deliberate drug-drug interaction can be lifesaving.

Gerioperative Care

PREOPERATIVE CONSIDERATIONS

The preoperative medication assessment establishes the individual's past and current medication history and identifies the potential effects on the surgical process and outcomes. Assessment involves asking the patient about past and current patterns of prescription and OTC medication use. Older patients can feel defensive about their medication use, particularly if they are not taking them as prescribed because of financial limitations or personal belief systems. Patients may omit important information about how they take their medications or forget to mention negative effects they may have experienced.

Nursing goals are to determine if medications are taken correctly, determine if the patient is taking only medications that are needed, identify any medications that may not be needed, monitor new medications ordered as part of preparation for surgery, and identify untoward effects from past, current, or new medications. All information should be documented in the patient's record. Exhibit 5.2 provides a sample list of questions to assess preoperative medication use. Ask the older adult to bring a "brown bag" with all prescriptions, OTC medications, and herbal remedies currently used or used in the recent past to the preoperative assessment interview. Many patients have their medications in an electronic medical record, making it easier to retrieve a medication history. However, the listing must be confirmed or updated.

Polyherbacy, the use of multiple herbals, and even single herbal use can lead to surgical complications. Gingko and ginseng are popular herbals that can cause bleeding complications. Ephedra can increase hypertension and tachycardia. Exhibit 5.3 lists common plants used for home remedies. Herbal information is important for nurses to document when reviewing patient's preoperative medications.

The gerioperative nurse can investigate potential factors that might affect absorption, distribution, or elimination of a medication. Surgery can add stress to body systems already stressed by diminished physiologic reserve, chronic disease, and polypharmacy. An important area to review is nutritional status to evaluate protein levels and body fat distribution that can alter pharmacokinetics.

Preoperative Testing
Renal and liver function should be evaluated in patients who have a history of hypertension, diabetes, or cardiac, liver, or renal disease, or of taking medications that have side effects related to kidney or liver function. Older patients with abnormal renal or liver function tests should be carefully monitored when patients are taking medications that impair function.

EXHIBIT 5.2 Conducting a Preoperative Medication Assessment

Coaching the patient on the medication assessment:

You will be receiving a lot of new medications during your surgery. Medications will be used to help you before surgery, during surgery, and after surgery. The after-surgery medications will be primarily for pain and sleep. Medications you take during surgery can interact with drugs you take at home. I need to ask you some detailed questions about all the medications and drugs you take. We want to avoid the possibility of having drugs interact with each other. You can help by sharing as much as you know about all the medications and drugs you have been taking before surgery.

- List current prescription drugs including:
  - Name of substance
  - Amount taken
  - Regular basis or as needed
  - Purpose of taking
- What concerns do you have about your medications?
- Have you ever had a reaction or side effect to any medication you are currently taking or have taken in the past?
- Do you take any medications to treat side effects caused by other medications?
- Please describe any allergies, sensitivities, or side effects you have been told about regarding your medication (e.g., to an antibiotic, pain medication, latex materials, local anesthetics).
- Have you or the doctor ever stopped a drug that was prescribed? If so, please describe what happened.
- How comfortable are you with taking your medications?
- How do you get your medications?
- How do you pay for your medications?
- Do you have any difficulty taking your medications (e.g., opening bottles, swallowing pills, counting out pills, organizing your schedule, whether you are taking them right)?
- Have you ever stopped taking a medication without telling your doctor or care provider? If so, please describe.
- What is important to you about taking prescription drugs, over-the-counter drugs, and/or home remedy medications?
- What medications do you purchase at the store that do not require a prescription (e.g., aspirin, ibuprofen or similar medication, acetaminophen, cold medications, sleeping pills, ointments, vitamins, minerals, herbal remedies, nutrition supplements, diet pills, etc.)?
- Do you purchase any herbal remedies, vitamins, sleeping pills, nutrition supplements, or diet foods at a health food or organic food store?
- What kinds of remedies do you buy?
- How often do you take them?
- Do you have a schedule for taking them?
- If so, what is the schedule?
- Have you ever had a reaction to any over-the-counter or home remedy treatment?

- Do you take any other drugs or medications that we have not yet discussed (e.g., eye drops, ear drops, analgesic heat rub, home remedies such as garlic, cinnamon, salmon oil, salves, poultices, or homemade teas)?
- What is important about taking your personal or nonprescription medications?
- How often do you drink coffee, tea, herbal teas, and/or sodas?
- How often do you drink beverages with alcohol such as wine, beer, mixed drinks, straight shots, or other beverage with alcohol?
- How many do you drink of each and when?
- Do you currently or have you ever used what are commonly called street drugs such as marijuana, cocaine, or other pills?
- Do you have any questions about taking your prescription or other pills?

Serum albumin is important for monitoring drug protein binding and can also be a guide to patient nutritional status.

Creatinine clearance is considered more reliable and valid than serum creatinine in determining kidney function. Reviewing creatinine clearance values during the preoperative and postoperative periods along with assessing hydration status is a standard of care in managing medications in older adults.

Preoperative Intervention

Engaging the patient as an active participant is one of the first steps in preventing ADEs. Conducting a medication review helps to identify current problems the elder may experience taking medications correctly. The medication review compares current medications with current health conditions, identifies medication underutilization either due to prescribing or patient decision to not take prescribed medication, and drug-drug, drug-disease, or prescription-nonprescription drug interactions. When questions arise about drug interactions or prescribing of medications, the nurse contacts the prescribing care provider or pharmacist for clarification or revision of existing orders. Interdisciplinary teams of pharmacists and nurses are effective in identifying medication-related issues that can affect preoperative prehabilitation, anesthesia administration, and postoperative outcomes.

EXHIBIT 5.3 **Common Plants With Anticholinergic Properties**

Angel's trumpet
Bittersweet
Burdock root
Deadly nightshade
Fly agaric
Jerusalem cherry
Jimson weed
Night blooming jessamine
Red sage
Wild tomato

Preoperative medication orders can involve complex directions and scheduling routines. Preoperative regimens include continuing current medications, revision of medication dose or scheduling, discontinuing current medications, and adding new medications. Patients can be easily confused about which medications to take the day of surgery and which should not be taken, and they require explicit information.

Herbals and OTC medications should be discontinued seven (7) days before elective surgery, as should medications with anticholinergic effect. The primary care physician, surgeon, and the anesthesia provider should be consulted about medications the patient should continue or discontinue prior to surgery. If discontinued, when and how the medication should be stopped must be clearly communicated to the patient and family. Different medications have different discontinuation schedules. Medication discontinuation schedules must be carefully written out and clearly explained for the patient and caregivers. This is particularly important for medications such as anticoagulants, anti-arrhythmic, antihypertensives, and glycemic medications.

Patients become easily confused about medications to take on the day of surgery.

Once the preoperative medication regimen is confirmed, the nurse coaches the patient and companion-coach on implementing it. The patient must agree with and accept the medication changes, especially for OTC and herbal medications. Having the patient demonstrate understanding of the preoperative medication regimen can be accomplished by having the patient conduct a talk back with the preoperative interviewer. The talk back asks the patient to explain the preoperative medication plan. Having the patient write out the directions using his or her words improves understanding. The nurse can review, clarify, and confirm direction until there is congruency between the patient's explanation and the medication plan.

The patient and a family member or significant other should receive a printout listing all prescriptions, OTC medications, and complementary drugs, herbs, and natural substances the patient reports. Any special needs of the patient such as swallowing difficulties or the need to take food with the drug to decrease side effects should also be on the printout. Drug allergies and sensitivities are highlighted. Inform the patient or family that it would be helpful to have multiple copies of the printout to take to the hospital or ambulatory surgical center at the time of admission. Copies should be given to the admitting nurse and later to the discharge nurse to assist with medication reconciliation and decrease discrepancies between preadmission and postadmission medication regimens. Encourage the patient to ask if the medication list was added to the patient's record and made available to staff. The patient should keep a copy of the preoperative medication list at the bedside for reference.

Preoperative coaching with the patient and family members includes review of the current medication regimen and plans for tracking medication changes throughout the surgical continuum. Patients and families can request a written list of hospital-ordered medications at time of admission and at any point throughout the surgical continuum. They can request to be informed when any changes are made in the patient's medication, the reasons for the change, and the purpose of the change.

Admission medications should be compared with the PIM list, paying special attention to any medications listed as high severity. Potential drug-drug and drug-disease interactions should be identified. The ARS lists common drugs exerting an anticholinergic type effect. Unnecessary prescription medications with anticholinergic effects should be discontinued unless there are overriding medical reasons. OTC and herbal drugs containing anticholinergic substances should be discontinued at least 7 days before surgery. New medication prescriptions must be evaluated for anticholinergic activity.

The surgeon and anesthesia provider should confirm all medications prior to administration in the preoperative holding area. Intravenous medications started in the holding area have high-risk or high-alert potential in older adults because of the speed of onset and effects of presurgical dehydration on pharmacokinetics. Older adults require close monitoring as environmental and physiological stressors along with medication effects can interfere with the patient's ability to recognize changes in his or her condition or to articulate changes clearly within a timeframe that will avert problems.

INTRAOPERATIVE CONSIDERATIONS

Nurses in the operating room are responsible for maintaining patient medication safety. Intraoperative medications are highly dependent on a patient's physiological status, comorbidities, medication history, and type of surgery. Having a medication history available that clearly documents the patient's medications prior to hospital admission as well as hospitalization medication regimens can determine intraoperative medication needs and potential for adverse anesthesia or medication effects. Assessment in the intraoperative period centers on monitoring the patient's response and reaction to preoperative and intraoperative medications including anesthesia. During the intraoperative period, the nurse should be available to double check high-risk medications such as insulin and heparin with the anesthesia care provider before administration.

POSTOPERATIVE CONSIDERATIONS

Nursing goals in the immediate postanesthesia period focus on avoiding prescribing and administration errors and maximizing therapeutic effectiveness. Postoperative care often involves the use of anticoagulants, analgesics, antibiotics, and cardiovascular drugs, all of which are high-alert medications. Many of the risk factors for ADEs are increased after surgery. Pharmacokinetics and pharmacodynamics can be altered due to changes in neurotransmitter and endocrine reactions, physiologic reserve, patient functional levels, and cognitive awareness.

Assessment involves monitoring patient progress, reviewing timing for restarting preoperative medication, determining level of therapeutic response, and avoiding adverse reactions. Assessment and intervention are critical to maintaining patient safety and recovery. A thorough and systematic assessment will identify changes in the patient's condition that require action for discontinuing, adding, or changing the dose or schedule of a medication. Reviewing standard protocols and medication prescriptions for PIMs and high-risk or high-alert medications should be part of the daily assessment of the patient.

INTERVENTION

Pain management is one of the most important and often most troublesome issues in the postoperative surgical care of the older adult. Prevention of acute and severe pain is important in avoiding pain and to achieving effective pain relief. Chapter 22 provides a detailed discussion of pain management. It is mentioned here because medication is the most often used intervention in alleviating acute surgical-related pain.

All high-risk medications should be double checked by the anesthesia provider and the circulating registered nurse.

The postanesthesia care unit (PACU) is a high-risk area for ADEs. Older patients are often not able to relay information that might indicate they are having side effects. Complex care, high patient turnover, and rapid changes in patient condition contribute to the potential for medication error and adverse effects along with therapeutic benefit. The fast pace of the environment limits availability of time to do a complete medication review. Discrepancies in allergies, medication orders, patient history, and prescriptions from multiple providers add to the confusion. Potential sources of error include prescribing, administering, monitoring patient's responses, and documenting the medication and the effects of the medication. Documentation is critical as adverse effects may not occur in the PACU but are delayed until transfer to the surgical unit.

> *Documentation is critical as adverse events may not occur until later.*

Medications associated with increased rate of errors are opiates, heparin, insulin, and intravenous solutions. Side effects and adverse outcomes of anticholinergic medications and benzodiazepines may not occur until after the operative period. Cognitive changes and postoperative delirium in response to preoperative or PACU medications may not develop until 24 hours or more after surgery. Anticholinergic and benzodiazepine medications need to be highlighted in the medical record and reported during patient handoff.

Postoperative care units continue to be the focus of medication safety. High patient-nurse ratios, multiple demands on nurses' time, daily staff turnover, multiple physician providers, and polypharmacy contribute to medication errors. Intensive care units with lower patient-nurse ratios but higher acuity patients are at higher risk for ADEs. Demands on time, prescribing by multiple providers, and rotation of nursing staff remain important risk factors affecting medication safety. Order sets that include the use of PIMs, over- or underprescribing, and dosing errors not adjusted to older adults increase the potential for negative effects.

MEDICATION RECONCILIATION

Vigilance begins with medication reconciliation. Medication reconciliation must be done every time a patient is admitted or transferred to a new unit or level of care. The list of medications the patient brought to the hospital can serve as a tool in the reconciliation process.

Effective communication is a second intervention in maintaining vigilance. Communication within and across team members must be based on the concept of relationship-centered care. Communication is critical in allowing caregivers to attend to one another, critically evaluate care practices, and identify near misses and actual errors. The patient and family can contribute to the vigilance by learning how to work with the team and reviewing medications as they are administered.

REDUCING POLYPHARMACY

Reducing polypharmacy and the use of PIMs decreases risk of drug-drug and drug-disease interactions. Having pharmacists review new medications can reduce duplicative drug effects. Comparing new drugs with disease conditions helps to ensure that each drug is targeted to a specific purpose. The gerioperative nurse should review standing orders and protocols to assess for medications that should not be prescribed to the elderly such as meperidine and NSAIDs. The medications should also be reviewed for dose, because many medications are effective in the elderly at lower doses. The use of best practice guidelines can promote safe management of anticoagulants and antibiotics.

Using nonpharmacologic interventions reduces polypharmacy and decreases risk for adverse effects. For example, sleep protocols rely on sleep rituals, soothing drinks, back rubs, and other comfort measures instead of medications to enhance sleep patterns. Back rubs, diversional activities, and music therapy have shown some promise in pain relief. Complementary pain measures can reduce reliance on pain medications, decreasing the risk of drug interactions and adverse events.

PATIENT-PROVIDER COMMUNICATION

Listening to the patient is important in maintaining medication safety. Patients often know what their care needs are and how they respond to medications. This is true even for older adults who may not adhere to medication regimens or who may not be able to verbalize their medication plan of care. When a patient tells a story about a medication, the nurse should listen carefully, question, and evaluate the information in context of the current situation. Whenever there seems to be a conflict between the professional perspective and the patient's story, it is essential the nurse take time to clarify the situation to avoid error or other adverse event.

REFLECTIVE PRACTICE

Self-reflection is a critical aspect of relationship-centered care. Self-reflection involves one's own patient care practices and interactions and relationships with other members of the professional interdisciplinary care team. Nurses who use self-reflection to assess and evaluate their actions and attitudes will be more effective in improving safe medication management, using evidence-based practice standards, and paying attention to the unique character and needs of older adults.

Any medication presents risks for side effects. Early detection is essential to minimize untoward effects. Monitoring the older adult's response to medication includes monitoring for onset of new signs and symptoms. Cognitive changes or changes in behavior are among the most common symptoms of adverse drug reactions in older adults. Older adults may describe a sensation of "feeling funny" that can indicate the onset of a drug side effect. Serum albumin levels, liver function, and renal function tests should be monitored whenever there is a change in the patient's condition that alters pharmacokinetics. Self-evaluation of practice patterns regarding attention to medication monitoring and listening to older adult's descriptions of their responses to medications is important in maintaining reflective practice.

DISCHARGE CONSIDERATIONS

Discharge to home, a rehabilitation center, or a long-term care facility poses potential and actual risk for medication errors in older adults. Errors result from inadequate medication reconciliation, discrepancies between providers and inattention to patient's knowledge, attitude, skill, and ability in managing medications. Discharge medication error rates including actual and potential errors have been reported as high as 70% (Wong et al., 2008; Pippins et al., 2008).

Early detection of side effects is essential to improve outcomes.

Foust and colleagues (2005) categorize posthospital medication errors as active or latent failures. Examples of active failures are discharge prescription errors and medication discrepancies. Latent failure is described as flawed discharge medication teaching, poor coordination and/or communication of changes in medication at time of hospital discharge, and inattention to medication-related risk factors.

A frequent discharge problem is that of omission. Omission includes not ordering preadmission and hospital-ordered medication that should be continued after discharge. Another example of omission is not prescribing a new medication that should be started after discharge. Incomplete prescriptions cause confusion in obtaining medication for the patient after discharge and are another source of error. The last form of active failure is prescribing inappropriate medications or underusing a medication to treat a patient's health condition.

Medication regimens get changed intentionally or unintentionally after hospitalization and surgery. Patients may be comfortable and knowledgeable about the medication regimen they had prior to admission. Changing to a new regimen requires time and adaptation. Obtaining the information needed to make the change is a challenge. Complex and complicated medication information delivered in the hospital environment by nurses who are harried and hurried can be beyond the capacity of the older adult or caregiver. Older adults need time to process new information and assimilate it into their daily lives. Patients and family members consistently report being unprepared to manage posthospital medications.

Medication errors occur when the patient is discharged home or transferred to long-term care and rehabilitation centers. Careful attention to the transfer of information during the handoff from the acute care setting to the postdischarge institution is needed if medication errors are to be prevented. Patients require the same type of discharge medication assessment regardless of discharge destination.

Discharge medication assessment begins with assessing the patient's ability to manage taking his or her own medications safely or the ability of caregivers to manage medication regimens. Building a relationship based on trust helps the patient ask questions and clarify information. Assessing the patient begins with determining the patient's functional abilities in cognition, vision, hearing, mobility, hand strength, and swallowing. Asking the patient about his or her attitude toward medications and intent to follow the medication regimen as prescribed is important in developing a self-care medication management plan. Determining the patient's level of knowledge and asking how the patient or responsible person will manage the medication regimen after discharge is an important first step in planning how much and what kind of information will be provided. One approach is to ask the patient or significant other to explain the medication regimen that was prescribed: name of the medication, dose and scheduling, expected benefit, and potential side effects.

Patients often do not know what they should do if they do not get the expected benefit or if side effects occur. The nurse needs to be clear about what needs to be reported and to whom. Patients need to be able to explain the routes of the medications and the kind and amount of food and fluid to take or avoid. Additional questions the nurse needs to ask are how and when the patient will be able to obtain prescriptions and when the person intends to begin taking medications. Asking about plans to resume herbal or OTC medications can identify potential problems and interactions that determine the need for further information.

Once assessment of the patient's knowledge, attitude, function, and skill is complete, the nurse can tailor information and coaching. Information on medication management, resources for obtaining medications, adaptive tools to assist in taking medications, and strategies to facilitate scheduling and retention of information are important areas to address.

Functional impairment can be a major contributor to ADEs at any stage of the surgical continuum. Cognitive impairment, changes in vision and hearing, decreased strength, and impaired mobility contribute to ADE risk in community elders. Changes in cognition and sensory abilities affect the older patient's understanding about his or her medication. Decreased strength and mobility interfere with obtaining medications and opening bottles or vials. Cognitive changes diminish awareness of medication side effects. Nonadherence to medication regimens results in poor therapeutic effect, which is important in older adults undergoing surgery. Poor or inadequate control of preexisting conditions increases surgical risk and contributes to subsequent perioperative and postoperative complications. Swallowing difficulties make taking medications more difficult. Older adults often drink insufficient quantities of liquid when taking oral medications to ensure pills clear the esophagus. Overall inadequate fluid volume interferes with effective drug distribution and renal clearance.

TRANSITIONAL CARE

Transitions to home or other health care setting are times of medication vulnerability for older adults. The process of transferring knowledge about medications across health care settings or the responsibility for taking and administering medications from the hospital to home or other institution is fraught with challenges. Errors in prescribing, transcribing, understanding, and administering drugs across the transition experience have been well documented. Prevention and early detection of actual and potential ADEs involves interdisciplinary teamwork, patient-centered care, and system-level actions.

Older adults at highest risk for discharge-related ADEs are those with multiple medications, new medications, or changes in medication. Drugs most commonly associated with ADEs are anticoagulants, antibiotics, and analgesic agents often prescribed after a surgical procedure. Anticoagulants are often stopped prior to surgery. Further, anticoagulants are often not restarted postoperatively even when indicated. Lack of follow-up and monitoring of patients with cognitive or mobility limitations are frequent causes of medication problems after discharge.

The gerioperative care facilitator (GCF) and companion-coach can be effective in improving quality and decreasing cost in older adults discharged after surgery. Transitional care provided by the gerioperative care nurse targets the individual needs of the older adult, allows for coordination of care from hospital to the posthospital care destination, and prevents what is commonly called "falling-through-the-cracks." In terms of medication management, the gerioperative care coordinator reviews the medication regimen with the patient or responsible care provider to ensure the patient is taking or receiving the medications appropriately, clarifies questions, identifies medication benefits, and assesses for side effects. The gerioperative nurse works with the interdisciplinary team throughout the transition period in preventing posthospital medication complications and resolving emerging problems.

Discharge medication reconciliation is essential in preventing errors and ADEs after hospitalization. Nurses are responsible for providing information that will empower and facilitate the patient, or those caring for the patient, to maintain effective medication management after discharge. Involving patients or family members in the medication reconciliation process by using the preadmission medication list is a good way to enlist family and patient involvement. While reviewing the preadmission medication list is an opportune time to review what preadmission medications need to be continued, assess how medications were being taken and clarify any safety issues or questions that may arise about previous medication management. Questions about herbal and OTC medications can be addressed. New medications can be put in the context of previous regimens, making it easier to incorporate change. The gerioperative care nurse and companion-coach can help the patient and family negotiate the medication reconciliation process with the interdisciplinary care team.

The review includes all preadmission, hospital-ordered, and discharge medications with the patient, family member(s), or other responsible person(s). The review should compare the name of the medication(s), dose(s), and schedule(s). Discrepancies should be noted and changes confirmed with the prescribing physician. The pharmacist is included to address any questions about medications. Drugs with anticholinergic effects should be evaluated and assessed for continuation. The medication list should be compared with Beers revised list of PIMs. If PIMs are required, doses should be reviewed to ensure the lowest possible dose.

Once the medication reconciliation process is completed and an accurate list of take-home medications is compiled, the nurse or gerioperative care coordinator should work with the patient and family to develop a medication management plan. A family member, friend, or the companion-coach selected by the patient should be involved in developing medication management strategies to help the patient as needed after discharge to put the medication management plan into effect.

Patient medication reconciliation lists help with medication management and changes.

A list of medications by name, dose, schedule, and expected benefits should be printed in large print and used as a reference source while explaining the medication plan to the patient and family. Patients and family members need to know what action should be taken if the expected benefits do not occur or if side effects occur. Reviewing minor and major side effects with information on what the patient should do if side effects occur is important in detecting early onset of adverse effects. Patients often ignore side effects or assume they are a normal part of taking medications until severe symptoms occur. Early intervention can help avoid rehospitalization. Comparing minor, major, and severe side effects along with actions the patient should take if side effects occur should be printed out, reviewed verbally, and then given to the patient to take home. Any potential drug-drug or drug-food interactions must be reviewed with strategies on how to avoid unwanted interactions.

Fluid intake with medications is often ignored in medication teaching. Older adults often do not take sufficient fluids with their medications. Adequate hydration is important in drug distribution and drug elimination. Fluid is also important in ensuring that oral medications pass into the stomach. This is of special importance for medications that can irritate the esophogeal mucosa. Patients are encouraged to drink adequate amounts of water with their medications. It is important to coach caregivers about fluid intake with medications as older adults who are given medications by another person are often given inadequate fluid for safe medication practice. Caregivers who assist the patient with medications also need to be informed about the importance of ensuring adequate fluid administration.

The patient should have copies of the medication reconciliation list for follow-up post-discharge visits to the surgeon and primary care provider. The medication list can be used to review patient adherence to the medication plan, review level of knowledge about safe medication practices, and identify potential problems. Revisions to the list can facilitate ongoing medication management as medications are discontinued or added, doses are changed, or administration schedules are revised. For patients transferred to another health care setting, the list can serve as the first step in a new medication reconciliation process.

Medication reconciliation and patient teaching for safe, effective postdischarge medication management is time-consuming. However, it is essential for patient safety and for avoiding hospital readmission due to ADEs. Including pharmacists as part of the patient's coaching team is particularly important for adults at high risk for experiencing an adverse drug event.

Follow-up telephone calls after discharge or visits to the patient's home are useful in monitoring medication understanding, adherence, therapeutic responses, and adverse side effects. Use of herbal remedies and OTC medications also can be assessed and monitored.

SYSTEM-LEVEL ACTIVITIES

Systems technology can be useful in facilitating medication reconciliation, improving patient teaching, and monitoring patient medication management. Linking medication records across systems of care facilitates medication review, prevents duplication, decreases drug-drug interactions, improves therapeutic effectiveness, reduces morbidity, and limits cost. These benefits can only accrue when all of the older patient's providers use the electronic system and systematically review, evaluate, and document medication management data.

PATIENT SITUATION: Mr. Roberts

Mrs. Roberts continued to worry about her husband's change in behavior. She told the nurses and physicians that he seemed "depressed" and not at all like himself. The staff continued to reassure her that depression is not uncommon after surgery, particularly hip fracture repair, and that she needn't be overly concerned. The gerioperative care facilitator met with Mr. and Mrs. Roberts as part of the daily patient visit and was told about the situation. The GCF knew that Mrs. Roberts is generally calm about her husband and would not be raising so much concern unnecessarily. Further, Mr. Roberts, although quiet, had a keen sense of humor that was noticeably absent. The GCF conducted a depression screening and reviewed the medication record along with the intraoperative and postoperative reports. Screening results showed that Mr. Roberts was experiencing a mild depression that could be surgery-related, as the providers noted. However, the history of benzodiazepine use in combination with prednisone use, traumatic injury, and surgical stress culminated in mood changes in response to alterations in central nervous system neurotransmitters. Mr. Roberts did not have the benzodiazepines or the prednisone reordered after surgery. His anxious behaviors went unnoted in the postoperative activities and lack of familiarity with his specific situation. He was started on a new medication to replace the aprazolam, and his prednisone was restarted. He completed his hospital stay a bit later than usual due to his loss of activity after surgery, but he was discharged to home, completed his physical therapy, and returned to his activities of daily living.

SUMMARY

Geriatric surgical patients are at high risk for ADEs due to surgical and anesthesia requirements for high-alert medications. Maintaining preoperative medication regimes, multiple transitions, and multiple providers involved in complex and complicated medication management contribute to increased risk of ADEs. Changes in renal function and albumin levels resulting from normal aging and secondary to surgical-related stress, changes in metabolism, dehydration, and malnutrition contribute to older adults' reactions to medications. Nursing care based on comprehensive risk assessment and preventative interventions ensures the safety and well-being of older adults. Preventing and minimizing ADEs across the surgical continuum is challenging. The gerioperative care nurse and companion-coach are integral in decreasing the risk, prevalence, and incidence of medication-related adverse events in older surgical patients.

KEY POINTS

- Age-related changes affecting drug distribution are a decrease in body mass, increase in body fat, and decrease in body water.

- Recommended drug doses do not consider age-related changes of elders, comorbid disease states, or polyphamacy.
- Surgery is a high-risk process for ADEs. Multiple patient transfers involving multiple providers who order high-risk medications under rapid-paced situations create optimum conditions for ADEs and errors in medication orders.
- Poor communication, incomplete transfer of information, inadequate gerioperative knowledge, incorrect drug calculations, and lack of systematic medication review contribute to medication error.
- Nurses in the operating room have a responsibility to double check all high-risk medication dosing such as insulin and heparin with anesthesia providers before administration.
- Accurate assessment and intervention are key to prevention of ADEs.
- Medication errors occur most frequently on transfer from one environment to another. The most frequent error is omission.
- Gerioperative nurses can facilitate medication changes across the surgical continuum and after discharge by reviewing medications with the patient, family, primary care provider, and pharmacist at each stage of transition.

SIX

Gerioperative Coaching

*Donna Pelletier, Raelene V. Shippee-Rice, Jennifer V. Long,
and Susan J. Fetzer*

PATIENT REPORT: Mrs. Dubois

Mrs. Dubois is a 77-year-old widow who is scheduled for an elective left total knee replacement in 4 weeks. She has suffered from osteoarthritis for almost 20 years, but her knee pain has become severe over the past year or so. Her severe left knee pain and moderate right knee pain makes it difficult getting out of bed in the morning, ambulating after sitting or standing for even a short period of time, and walking up or down stairs. She faithfully uses a cane since she fell while carrying her laundry 3 months ago. Mrs. Dubois recalls, "My left knee just gave out and I fell in my hallway, hitting my head on the floor." She incurred a broken left wrist and a mild concussion along with multiple contusions.

In hearing about her fall, her primary care provider referred her to an orthopedic surgeon for evaluation of her debilitating knee pain and decreased mobility and function. Radiographs of her left knee revealed marked narrowing of the joint space, osteophytes, and subchondral sclerosis. Home health services were ordered for a safety assessment and physical therapy. A bone densitometry scan revealed osteopenia with bone loss in both the hip and spine, and her vitamin D level was low.

Mrs. Dubois was visited weekly by a home care nurse, and a physical therapist visited twice a week to work on functional range of motion, balance, and strengthening her lower extremities. The therapist encouraged her to try using a walker now that her wrist has healed, but she "is comfortable using the cane" and prefers to keep one hand free to carry things if necessary.

Mrs. Dubois lives alone in a small farmhouse in a rural community. She was diagnosed with age-related macular degeneration about a year ago. Her blurred vision has worsened and she no longer drives. Her daughter and son live 1 and 4 hours away, respectively, and her daughter comes once a week to take her grocery shopping and help with housework. Her son rarely visits but does pay for someone to mow the grass and shovel snow. She has a long-time friend, Mrs. Martin, who lives nearby. Her neighbor calls every morning and frequently stops by to see if Mrs. Dubois needs any assistance.

Mrs. Dubois's medical history is significant for well-controlled essential hypertension, osteoarthritis of the hands and knees, mild obesity, macular degeneration, osteopenia, and invasive ductal carcinoma of the right breast, for which she had a lumpectomy 6 years earlier. Her current body mass index is 32, and she eats a diet high in salt and fat. She reports that she has smoked for over 40 years but now is an intermittent smoker, only smoking when she has cigarettes around. She does not drink alcohol. Her current medications include daily hydrochlorothiazide; vitamins A, C, D, and E; and zinc, copper, and calcium supplements. For pain medication she takes hydrocodone, acetaminophen, and ibuprofen on an as-needed basis. She has a strong family history of osteoarthritis, hypertension, and stroke, reporting that her mother and three of her four brothers had "bad knees" and died from a stroke. There is no history of diabetes.

Mrs. Dubois has an appointment at 2 p.m. today to meet with the gerioperative care facilitator (GCF) at the local hospital where she will receive her surgery. She has been asked to bring along her support team, her caregiver(s), and family member(s). Her daughter has arranged to drive her to the appointment and attend the meeting, but Mrs. Dubois did not ask her friend and neighbor Mrs. Martin, as she "didn't want to bother her."

Coaching is well known in sports, psychology, business, music, arts, and adventure for its success in motivating people and teams to reach personal and professional goals. More recently, nursing and other health care professions use health coaching to facilitate goal attainment for patients, caregivers and families. Coaching in gerioperative care is a framework for helping gerioperative patients attain optimal health status and function before surgery and maximum benefit in postoperative and postdischarge recovery activities. A surgical event is a "teachable moment." Preoperative preparation for surgery encompasses behaviors that are of equal value in improving overall health and well-being after surgery. Providing continuous coaching and decisional support aids older adults in making choices about their participation in preoperative prehabilitation and postoperative recovery actions. This chapter provides an overview of health coaching and motivational interviewing with application to perioperative care of older adults.

Definition

Health coaching has many definitions. Nursing defines health coaching as the practice of health education and health promotion within the coaching context to enhance the well-being of individuals and facilitate the achievement of their health-related goals (Palmer, Tubbs, & Whybrow, 2003). Health coaching in the gerioperative facilitated care (GOFC) model is considered *gerioperative coaching*. The GOFC approach assists older adults and their caregiver/family in navigating the health care system as it relates to surgery. Gerioperative coaching facilitates prehabilitation behavioral change, recovery adherence, and chronic illness self-management to improve health and prevent complications throughout the perioperative continuum.

Benefits

Gerioperative coaching provides opportunities to improve the overall health and well-being of the older adult. The GCF has the primary responsibility for guiding the patient/caregiver/family through the perioperative experience and minimizing the risk of adverse outcomes. The GCF coaches the patient, the caregiver/family, and the companion-coach (CC), who work as a team in partnership with health care providers to manage the patient's perioperative care.

As a facilitator, the GCF uses evidence-based health coaching techniques to assist the older adult prepare for surgery, engage in lifestyle behavior changes, improve chronic disease self-management, and manage the transition of care from hospital or ambulatory unit to home or other discharge destination. The GCF provides information and support as needed by the patient, the caregiver/family, and the CC, who serves as "cheerleader" for the patient throughout the perioperative experience.

Process of Gerioperative Coaching

Gerioperative coaching is a holistic approach to perioperative care targeted at health outcomes. With gerioperative coaching, the GCF initially meets with each older adult patient and his or her caregiver/family at the beginning of the perioperative process, develops rapport, and engagesthe patient and the patient's care team in a comprehensive geriatric assessment. An evidence-based perioperative plan of care evolves from the assessment in collaboration with the patient and the patient-designated participant in the care giving and support process. The plan of care centers on strategies to prevent perioperative complications and is shared with health care providers.

Gerioperative health coaching improves prehabilitation outcomes.

The initial meeting of the GCF with the gerioperative patient, caregiver/family, and CC centers on addressing the patient's questions, fears, or concerns and sharing information about the perioperative experience. Discussion emphasizes the value of patient choice, the intent to follow the patient's agenda, and to negotiate a process of shared decision-making in the event a situation arises. The GCF and CC roles and responsibilities are explained as they relate to the needs and concerns of the patient or caregiver/family member. The importance of a patient-centered relationship is emphasized. Ideally, the GCF and the interdisciplinary team involved in the patient's care commit to a decision support role that provides and clarifies information, and assists the patient and the patient's designated others to determine health and treatment goals and to make decisions. The entire health care team has the responsibility for ensuring that gerioperative coaching remains a patient-centered process driven by the patient's agenda.

With a comprehensive knowledge of the patient and caregiver/family, the GCF guides the patient and caregiver/family through the health care system, smoothing the transitions during the perioperative care continuum. In the preoperative period, the GCFcoordinates the patient's transitions between providers and care locations, providing continuing information on what the patient can expect as each phase of the perioperative process unfolds. Ongoing coaching assists the patient, caregiver/family, and the CC as they navigate the perioperative care system and begin to access community and health care resources. The CC receives coaching training from the GCF on ways to help the patient participate in self-care and conduct prehabilitation and postoperative behaviors while continuing to be a cheerleader for the patient. The CC encourages and supports the older adult in carrying out the identified action plan, acting as a personal coach focused on helping the patient get better by championing the patient's needs.

An important component of the pre- and postoperative action plan is the promotion of health for better patient outcomes. The GCF should be trained in motivational interviewing techniques to facilitate lifestyle behavior change, prehabilitation and recovery adherence, and chronic disease self-management. The motivational approach is well suited to a variety of clinical practice settings including gerioperative care. Gerioperative coaching enhances skills that support individuals in adopting new or modifying unhealthy behaviors, and managing chronic illness in the perioperative setting. Older adults living with chronic conditions require more than medical treatment from health care providers; they need support in mastering and sustaining the complex self-care behaviors that are necessary to enable them to live as healthy as possible. The GCF can assist perioperative patients with self-management behaviors such as following complicated medication regimens, adhering to diet and exercise instructions, monitoring and responding to symptoms, and coping effectively with stress.

> *The companion-coach is a key player in improving prehabilitation training in older adults.*

Based on information gained from the initial comprehensive health assessment, the GCF tailors motivational interviewing–based coaching interventions to the needs and goals of the individual. The CC supports the patient in health behavior change by being a cheerleader and may even engage in similar behaviors. For example, during prehabilitation, the CC takes walks with the older adult or participates in exercise activities. During postoperative recovery, the CC helps motivate the older adult to carry out pulmonary care, get out of bed, walk, eat, take fluids, and participate in self-care. The CC works with the older adult to make needs, questions, and concerns known to providers.

Throughout the perioperative experience, the GCF monitors the older patient and in doing so, gains detailed knowledge about the patient's preferred communication and learning styles. The GCF uses the knowledge to create action plans that target improvements in the patient's level of health knowledge and health behavior patterns. By understanding patient preferences and expectations, the GCF effectively collaborates with the interdisciplinary health care team who has briefer interactions with the patient and caregiver/family.

> *Telling people what to do does not work and is often perceived as confrontational.*

Evidence to Support Gerioperative Coaching

Health coaching has emerged as a fresh, new approach that guides health care professionals in using the patient's agenda to enhance compliance with healthy behaviors, prevent exacerbations of chronic illness, and support lifestyle change. The term *health coaching* emerged from motivational interviewing (Huffman, 2009).

Motivational interviewing is the only health coaching technique to be fully described and consistently demonstrated as causal and independently associated with positive behavioral outcomes (Butterworth, Linden, & McClay, 2007). Patients exposed to motivational interviewing–based health coaching versus "treatment as usual" are more likely to participate in follow-up visits, improve medication adherence, adhere to glucose monitoring, improve glycemic control, increase exercise, increase fruit and vegetable intake, reduce sodium intake, keep food diaries, and have less stress and fewer hospitalizations. The concepts of motivational interviewing–based health coaching are applicable to the goal of gerioperative care: improve gerioperative outcomes.

Health coaching interventions using a motivational interviewing approach require as little as 5 minutes. Extending the health coaching model throughout the perioperative continuum provides a new perspective on the use of health promotion and complication prevention to help older adults prepare for surgery, manage postoperative recovery, and maintain wellness after discharge from the surgical care setting. Health promotion and iatrogenesis prevention in older adults have been long standing goals of geriatric care providers and gerontologists. Health coaching that integrates the goals, preferences, strengths, and limitations of the older adult can be a cost- and time-effective innovation when done in collaboration with the

Health coaching begins with the patient's agenda.

health care team. It is a promising approach in prompting older adults to take new actions that will contribute to preoperative prehabilitation, postoperative recovery, and postdischarge wellness. However health coaching must be evaluated for use and adapted to meet the unique needs and preferences of the individual.

Stages of Change

Traditional strategies for motivating behavior change and self-management of chronic conditions, such as advice giving and patient education, are not effective. Traditionally, health care professionals have used their own agenda to determine what the patient needs to know and do to better manage their health conditions. Telling people what to do does not work and is often perceived as confrontational. Arguing for change while the patient argues against it is counterproductive. Suggesting that health care providers have all the answers for patients and families is misleading.

Health coaching, on the other hand, activates a patient's own motivation for change and adherence to treatment by focusing on the patient and the patient's goals. Health care providers can influence their patients' success in lifestyle management and treatment adherence efforts by embracing the fundamentals of behavior change science and using a patient-centered approach.

Health coaching is not "counseling." Health coaching offers specific conversations set within a tailored framework to guide the patient in discovering his or her own personal ambivalence toward health behavior change. Helping patients address ambivalence in making

Resolving ambivalence is a major focus of behavioral change.

changes in health behavior is a major focus of health coaching. Ambivalence indicates the patient is not ready to take action, stalling patient movement toward optimum health or preventing patient action all together.

Behavior change is rarely a discrete, single event. Some patients, when faced with a health care crisis and asked to change their health behavior, readily comply. But most patients are unable or unwilling to change, feeling discouraged or like a failure for not being able to change. Health care providers may feel discouraged that they are unable to assist patients in the change process. Ambivalence is the primary reason individuals do not change health behaviors. Health coaching is thoughtful guidance that engages the patient to discover why the ambivalence exists and guides them in developing new behaviors.

Health coaching helps the older adult resolve ambivalence, move through the stages of change, and achieve a desirable change that ideally results in improved health outcomes. For gerioperative patients, readiness for surgery or recovery from surgery is a key outcome. Identifying readiness for change allows the older adult, family, and provider to focus on behaviors of greatest importance to the patient, and therefore have a greater chance of success. As success is reached in one area, the process of change is translated into other areas. The transtheoretical Stages of Change model (Prochaska & Velicer, 1997) describes the behavioral change process.

The Stages of Change model describes how people modify a problem behavior or acquire a positive behavior. The model recognizes individual differences in motivation and readiness to adopt new health behaviors. Behavior change involves a progression though stages of motivational readiness, or stages of change, before adopting a health behavior. Prochaska's six stages of change are precontemplation, contemplation, preparation, action, maintenance, and relapse. Each stage of change is explained in Exhibit 6.1.

For most patients, a change in behavior occurs gradually, with the patient moving from being uninterested, unaware, or unwilling to make a change (precontemplation), to considering a change (contemplation), to deciding and preparing to make a change (preparation). Genuine, determined action is then taken and, over time, attempts to maintain the new

EXHIBIT 6.1 Six Stages of Change

Precontemplation	During the precontemplation stage, patients do not consider changing. Smokers who are "in denial" may not see that the advice applies to them personally. Patients with high cholesterol levels may feel "immune" to the health problems that strike others. Obese patients may have tried unsuccessfully so many times to lose weight that they have simply given up.
Contemplation	During the contemplation stage, patients are ambivalent about changing. Giving up an enjoyed behavior causes them to feel a sense of loss despite the perceived gain. During this stage, patients assess barriers (e.g., time, expense, hassle, fear, "I know I need to, but ...") as well as the benefits of change.
Preparation	During the preparation stage, patients prepare to make a specific change. They may experiment with small changes as their determination to change increases. For example, sampling low-fat foods may be experimented with or there may be a move toward greater dietary modification. Switching to a different brand of cigarettes or decreasing drinking signals that they have decided a change is needed.
Action	The action stage is the one that providers are eager to see their patients reach. Many failed New Year's resolutions provide evidence that if the prior stages have been glossed over, action itself is often not enough. However, any action taken by patients should be praised because it demonstrates the desire for lifestyle change.
Maintenance and relapse prevention	Maintenance and relapse prevention involve incorporating the new behavior "over the long haul." Discouragement over occasional "slips" may halt the change process and result in the patient giving up. However, most patients find themselves "recycling" through the stages of change several times before the change becomes established.

behavior occur. Relapses are almost inevitable and become part of the process of working toward continued lifelong change.

Implementing Gerioperative Health Coaching

Health coaching is a one-size-fits-all approach to behavior change that assumes the same behavior change strategies work for everyone, regardless of age or circumstances. Studies show that brief health coaching interventions using a motivational interviewing approach can be conducted in multiple health care settings and in the home to help older adults improve their health status. While the health coaching approach is the same for everyone, the application is tailored to the needs and circumstances of the gerioperative patient. Behaviors and interventions identified by the patient and health coach are individualized based on the patient's interests, abilities, and resources.

Older adults must make decisions about their participation in preoperative prehabilitation and postoperative recovery. The type of surgery and the patient's clinical status determine the time available to meet the goals of self-care and prehabilitation activities. Decisions to be involved in self-care behavior rest with the patient. Motivational interviewing and health coaching provide the patient with decisional support and encouragement.

> *The focus on prevention often gets lost in the harried environment of the acute care setting.*

Providers must keep in mind that older adults need clear communication. When providing health information or asking questions, it is important to use everyday language. Older adults are reluctant to ask health care providers to explain what they do not understand. This is an even greater concern when the provider is new and unfamiliar to the patient. The multiple transitions in perioperative care mean that most providers are unfamiliar to the patient, raising barriers to effective communication. Coaching the older adult about the critical importance of patient understanding of preoperative and postoperative instructions is essential for patient safety throughout the perioperative continuum. Informing the patient that providers expect patients to continue asking for explanations until the information is clear reassures the older adult that it is "okay" to ask as many times as needed until he or she fully understands. When and how to take medications, nutritional drinks, food, and fluid the day of surgery are some examples of where older adults must continue asking questions until there is a clear understanding. The provider has a responsibility to help the patient ask the questions.

Older adults may be embarrassed by questions posed in the health coaching approach, especially when asked about alcohol use, dietary intake, continence, or other personal behaviors. The gerioperative coach encourages patients to answer the personal questions as honestly as possible. Rephrasing the question in a way that is less personal decreases embarrassment. However, questions about personal behaviors need to be asked, and the patient should be supported in providing accurate, honest information. Prefacing questions using links to medical conditions makes the question seem less personal. For example, asking questions about smoking in relation to problems with breathing or about eating salty foods in relation to increasing edema can decrease a patient's uneasiness. The use of health screening instruments for alcohol use, nutrition, exercise, and smoking during the preoperative comprehensive assessment rather than direct questioning can make it easier for some patients to answer honestly. Avoiding the use of stigmatizing terms, such as alcoholic, obese, or overeating, preserves patient integrity.

In gerioperative coaching, the CC is a key figure. The CC participates in health behaviors with the older adult and serves as cheerleader, helping the older adult stay focused on the perioperative goals. The older adult identifies a person he or she can work with, have fun with, listen to when needed, and who can be supportive but assertive. Finding a person to carry out this role can be difficult for older adults living alone, who do not have family nearby, or who hesitate to burden family or friends. An alternative is matching a volunteer CC who has had similar health problems or surgery with the older adult. There are a number of disease-oriented nonprofit organizations that have volunteers willing to assume the role. Volunteers receive coaching on being a CC and health coaching from the GCF and patient.

DETERMINING READINESS FOR CHANGE

The perioperative prehabilitation or postoperative action plan is based on the patient's health coaching goal. Preoperative prehabilitation and postoperative rehabilitation require multiple behaviors that may be new to the patient. Behaviors associated with prehabilitation and recovery can be classified by priority or urgency. The GCF or provider explains the level of priority to the older adult based on the type and reason for surgery and the patient's health status. The older adult determines priorities based on what he or she is willing to change or feels able to accomplish. The gerioperative coach and patient develop a proposed perioperative action plan and goals based on priorities. The GCF explains the purpose of each action and goal as a prelude to helping the patient plan a perioperative action plan and goals. The goals should be specific, measurable, agreed on, realistic, and time-sensitive, and the roles and responsibilities for achieving the goal should be identified. Together, the gerioperative coach and the patient plan a process for meeting each of the stated goals. Although starting with a single goal is a preferred health coaching approach, the demands of preoperative and recovery timelines often require the older adult to attend to several behaviors at once.

With the priorities established and the patient's goals in view, the gerioperative coach asks a set of specific questions that elicit change talk and creative ideas. Change talk is the patient's use of language that suggests readiness for change. The GCF might ask the patient: "What prompts you to want to make this change?" "If you did decide to make this change, how would you do it?" "What are three benefits of making this change?" "How important is it for you to make this change?" "What do you think you will do?" "What are you already doing to keep yourself healthy?" The questions elicit the patient's thinking about engaging in perioperative-related health behaviors. Patients often say yes when told by providers to take their medication, start walking, or eat more fruits and vegetables in preparation for surgery. The degree of commitment to actually performing the behaviors is not usually discussed. The questions assess the older person's desire, ability, reasons, need, or commitment to doing the recommended activities. Following the initial set of questions, the GCF or interviewer uses three key strategies to promote behavior change: increasing importance, resolving ambivalence, and increasing confidence.

MEASURING CHANGE READINESS AND CONFIDENCE

Readiness for change and confidence for change are measured using simple, easy, and effective rulers or scales. The rulers can be used in the early stages of discussion or any time during the perioperative journey. The *Importance Level of Change* and *Confidence Level of Change* (Rollnick, Miller, & Butler, 2008) are tools used to determine the importance of the change to the patient and the patient's confidence in being successful in making the change. Readiness

0	1	2	3	4	5	6	7	8	9	10

Not at All
Important

Extremely
Important

FIGURE 6.1
Importance Level of Change Ruler

and confidence change rulers, or rating scales, are ranked from 0 to 10 (see Figures 6.1 and 6.2). Although many older patients are able to use rulers and scales in a purely verbal form, it is worthwhile to have the ruler drawn on a piece of paper or as a preprinted tool to ensure the patient's understanding and interviewer interpretation. Establishing a good rapport with the older adult and using a guiding style of communication improves the reliability of ruler results.

The *Importance Level of Change* ruler helps coaches evaluate how willing or "ready" the patient is for change. If the older adult does not see the change as important, it is unlikely the patient is ready to move forward and undertake the change. The *Importance Level of Change* ruler provides a quick assessment of a patient's motivational state relative to a specific behavior and serves as the basis for gerioperative coaching interventions to elicit behavior change. Readiness to change should be assessed regarding a very specific activity such as taking medications, improving nutritional intake, or exercising. Patients may differ in their readiness to change depending on the behavior.

Ask the patient, "On a scale from 0 to 10, where 0 is not important at all and 10 is extremely important, how important would you say it is to you to begin taking regular walks in preparation for surgery?" A "0" on the left side indicates "not at all important," which means the patient is not ready for change, and a "10" on the right side indicates "extremely important," which indicates the patient is ready to make a change. The gerioperative coach prompts the patient to consider reasons for not placing the mark further to the left, which elicits statements about the patient's motivational level. For example, "What is the reason you gave yourself a 6 and not 3?" The answer to this question indicates reasons the patient considers the change important (i.e., "change talk"). The gerioperative coach then asks the patient to indicate reasons for not placing the mark further to the right, which elicits perceived barriers. For example, "Why did you give yourself a 6 and not a 9?" The gerioperative coach asks what the patient suggests as ways to overcome

Change talk indicates the patient is moving toward change.

the identified barriers and to prompt actions that can be taken. To help prompt actions that might be taken, ask the patient, "If you were to make this change, what would it be like?" A score above 5 shows that a patient is willing to consider change and should be supported and encouraged in doing so by the GCF or provider and CC.

A similar tool, the *Confidence Level of Change* ruler, assesses patient self-efficacy. The same questions can be asked about the patient's confidence in the ability to change: "On a scale from 0 to 10, where 0 is not confident at all and 10 is extremely confident, how confident are you that if

0	1	2	3	4	5	6	7	8	9	10

Not at All
Confident

Extremely
Confident

FIGURE 6.2
Confidence Level of Change

you decided to begin walking in preparation for surgery, you could begin doing it? What number on the ruler would you give yourself right now?" A "0" on the left side indicates "not confident at all," which means the patient is certain that he or she is not able to change or to engage in change behaviors, and a "10" on the right side indicates "extremely confident," which means the patient is certain he or she is able to change the targeted behavior. After the rating, ask the older adult, "And why did you give yourself a 4 and not a 0?" This elicits the basis for the patient's confidence in his or her ability to change. Asking the patient, "What would help to get to a higher score?" or "How can I help you to move higher up on the scale?" can help boost the patient's confidence that with support he or she may be in a better position to enact the change.

The gerioperative coach's role is to help the patient increase the importance and confidence for change. If the importance or confidence level is low, the gerioperative coach determines if there is enough interest in or importance to the behavior to achieve change. If not, the patient is redirected to focus on a different health behavior. If the patient is somewhat interested or confident in the ability to change, the gerioperative coach supports and encourages the behavior change.

AMBIVALENCE

Ambivalence is a normal response when making a change. Older adults often do not consider the risks to keeping behaviors the same or do not recognize that maintaining current behaviors can be as harmful as taking on new ones. For example, a patient who experienced side effects from medications may see taking medication as harmful. The older adult may not recognize that not taking medication is also harmful as the disease will progress. Asking about the benefits and disadvantages of keeping things the same versus changing the behavior explores the patient's ambivalence. If the patient feels uncertain that he or she can change a health behavior, eliciting the patient's perspectives on benefits and disadvantages allows the patient to face that uncertainty in a supportive atmosphere. During the consideration of risks and benefits, the patient comes to realize his or her inner motivations that will support change. Asking the patient about the benefits of the status quo elicits arguments for not changing; asking about the disadvantages elicits change talk. By asking these questions, the patient becomes aware of both sides of his or her ambivalence. The essence of health coaching and motivational interviewing is to help patients resolve ambivalence and make conscious choices about behavior change.

Increasing exercise and activity are two priorities in gerioperative prehabilitation and postoperative recovery. Engaging the older adult in a discussion about initiating a more active exercise program, the gerioperative coach might ask with honest interest, "What do you like about not exercising?" Once the gerioperative coach has elicited the patient's perceptions of the positive aspects of not exercising, the coach follows up with a second question: "What's the downside for you about not exercising? What are the not-so-good things about being inactive?" After this conversation, the gerioperative coach briefly summarizes his or her understanding of the patient's account of the benefits and disadvantages of not exercising followed by a key question, "Where does this leave you now?" This question puts the patient in control of the next step, to either move toward change or remain static.

The GCF or provider incorporates health coaching strategies into gerioperative patient care and practice by asking key questions to facilitate health behavior change throughout the perioperative continuum. Health coaching is not limited to primary care settings. It is equally applicable to the ambulatory or in-hospital surgical setting. Engaging in health or wellness promoting behaviors promotes a positive surgical outcome. Attending to health behaviors begins with prehabilitation and continues through postoperative and postdischarge recovery. Nurses, GCFs, CCs, and other providers can apply health coaching in their practice to help patients work toward an optimal level of health and well-being. Using specific skills such as active listening, using open-ended questions,and summarizing the conversation facilitates conversations with older adults about changing health behavior.

Facilitating Change

The Stages of Change model suggests that interventions be matched to the individual's current stage of change. Most people go through the stages of change cycle several times before successfully achieving behavior change. Gerioperative coaching is most useful in the precontemplation or contemplation stages of change (Prochaska & DiClemente, 1983). To be successful, interventions are stage-matched and geared towars the needs of the patient. For example, it would be ineffective to try to increase walking speed or develop long-term exercise goals for someone in the contemplation stage who is still wrestling with the "why bother" question. Developing long-term strategies is better targeted toward older adults who are already active. Information sharing, counseling, and education targeted toward the patient's stage of change, assessing barriers to exercise, and determining the patient's confidence for change are more useful. For example, those in a contemplation state of mind can be offered walking options within their usual frame of reference such as taking the stairs, parking at the end of store parking lots for shopping, or walking to church. Goal setting involves asking the older adult to consider the following questions: How will I meet this goal? What are the potential obstacles that may interfere with my meeting this goal? What can I do or ask others to help me do to overcome these obstacles? A major barrier for older adults is asking for help in minimizing barriers or meeting goals. Many older adults are reluctant to ask for help because they do not want to be seen as incompetent, dependent, or a burden. Coaching older adults on ways to reach out to others can be integral to the success of health coaching. The presence of a designated CC may alleviate some of the older person's concerns about dependency and being a burden. Part of the responsibility of the CC is to reaffirm that the CC role is to help remove barriers and provide support. An evidence-based gerioperative coaching intervention to promote physical activity in an older adult matched to the stage of change is provided in Exhibit 6.2.

Feedback

Effective feedback is used throughout the perioperative continuum to assist in setting goals, to review progress, to help the patient discover ambivalence, to identify obstacles, and to determine caregiver/family support. Effective feedback consists of six components, which are shown in Exhibit 6.3.

The gerioperative coach provides both positive and corrective feedback. Positive feedback comes in the form of praise and rewards, and entails the coach saying what he or she liked about the patient's progress or behavior change, and explaining why. Corrective feedback is more complex. It involves the coach sharing concerns about the lack of progress or potential problems, and explaining the concerns. Describe the desired behavior in a manner that demonstrates concerns, reviews the goals, and helps the patient discover obstacles to the achievement of the desired outcome.

EXHIBIT 6.2 **Promoting Physical Activity Matched to Stage of Change**

Precontemplation	The gerioperative coach uses empathy and acceptance and "plants seeds" for change. Offering information on the benefits of exercise in meeting the challenge of surgery helps to make the activity more immediately relevant to the patient's current clinical condition and offers an opportunity for the patient to take actions that can promote a best outcome.
Contemplation	The gerioperative coach provides information on the reasons for the health benefits of exercise and discusses opportunities to exercise; emphasizes taking "baby steps" toward change; develops the coach-patient relationship; and reviews the perceived barriers and obstacles to change.
Preparation	The gerioperative coach investigates the motivation for change, works with the patient to set specific goal(s), devises a clear mutually agreed on plan, and schedules follow-up.
Action	The gerioperative coach uses inspiration and affirmation to encourage continued exercise, analyzes the challenges to exercising regularly, gives rewards, and offers support.
Maintenance and relapse prevention	The gerioperative coach recognizes the patient as a role model, gives rewards, is creative in helping the patient stay active, and discusses relapse prevention.

EXHIBIT 6.3 **Health Coaching Feedback**

Plan	Plan what you are going to say prior to the contact.
Use a behavior-focused approach	A gerioperative coach's focus is always on the behavior change that is desired—on the actions, not the individual.
Specific goal(s)	Identify specific goals that both the coach and patient agree to work toward.
Timeframe	Choose a realistic timeframe for next steps.
Balanced goal setting	Make certain that the patient does not address more than what is reasonable to be successful. The goal is to see progress toward the goal and build momentum with each achievement.
Privacy	When delivering positive feedback, it is acceptable to share this in the company of others. When the feedback is corrective, it should always be shared privately. The gerioperative coach must be careful not to discourage the patient or appear to be degrading. It is important to give a sense of motivation and a "Yes, you can!" attitude.

Implementing Health Coaching

Tomlin, Walker, and Grover (2005) published a trainer's guide to teach the basic concepts of motivational interviewing and the Stages of Change model, their relationship to each other, and their usefulness in clinical practice. The trainer's guide can be adapted to gerioperative coaching.

Important qualities of an effective gerioperative coach include being empathetic, empowering, supporting, respectful, understanding, nonjudgmental, patient, and accepting. These are particularly important when the older adult is in the precontemplation stage and not yet considering change or is unwilling or unable to change. The patient's inability to see that a problem exists may be considered denial, but this may not be a deliberate attempt to deceive the gerioperative coach, as the behavior may not be a problem within the patient's social context. The gerioperative coach's goal at this stage is to identify defenses and raise awareness of the problem behavior. The precontemplation stage is often the most frustrating stage of change, and the gerioperative coach's attitudes and beliefs about older adults affect outcomes. The gerioperative coach must establish rapport, ask permission, and build trust, and must elicit the patient's own doubts or concerns about the problem behavior. Strategies useful in precontemplation are provided in Exhibit 6.4.

In the contemplative stage of change, the patient acknowledges concerns and is considering the possibility of change. The gerioperative coach's goal is to assist the patient to make a decision for change. The coach normalizes ambivalence and helps the patient "tip the decisional balance scales" toward change. Suggested strategies are listed in Exhibit 6.5.

In the preparation stage of change, the patient is committed to and planning to make a change in the near future but is still considering what to do. Patients vacillate between the lure of comfort zones and the discomfort of needing to change. Affirmations and positive self-talk are important tools in assuring patients that in spite of their imbalance, they do have the power to make change. The knowledge that the gerioperative coach will be with a patient throughout the perioperative process appeals to a patient's sense of interconnectedness and diminishes feelings of anger, shame, and other negative emotions. The gerioperative coach's goal is to help patient get ready to make a change. It is important in this stage for the

---

EXHIBIT 6.4 **Strategies Used During Precontemplation Stage**

- Eliciting the patient's perceptions of the problem
- Offering factual information about the risks of the problem behavior
- Offering factual information about the reality of factors that may limit the patient's behavior while considering how patient strengths can be used to manage or adapt to the limitations
- Providing personalized feedback about assessment findings
- Exploring the pros and cons of the problem behavior
- Helping a significant other or companion-coach (CC) intervene
- Examining discrepancies between the patient's and others' perceptions of the problem behavior
- Expressing concern and empathy

EXHIBIT 6.5 Strategies Used in Contemplation Stage of Change

- Eliciting and weighing the pros and cons of the problem behavior and change
- Changing extrinsic to intrinsic motivation
- Examining the patient's personal values in relation to change
- Emphasizing the patient's free choice, responsibility, and self-efficacy for change
- Eliciting self-motivational statements of intent and commitment from the patient
- Eliciting ideas regarding the patient's perceived self-efficacy and expectations regarding treatment
- Summarizing self-motivational statements

gerioperative coach to take the time to clarify to patients about the coach's role in the change process. Strategies for the preparation stage are provided in Exhibit 6.6.

The action and maintenance stages of change are most comfortable for the patient and gerioperative coach, as typically the patient is changing and making progress toward improving the problem behavior. In the action stage, the patient is actively taking steps to change but has not yet reached a stable state. The gerioperative coach's goal is to support a realistic view of change through small steps, affirm patient successes, and assist with managing barriers encountered as change is negotiated. The gerioperative coach's goal is to affirm patient successes and assist with managing barriers encountered as change is negotiated, as well as reinforce active attempts to engage change with overt recognition of those efforts. Certificates, expressions of appreciation for follow-through, and supportive gestures are critical in preparing patients to cope with the reality of failure or relapse.

Health behavior changes unevenly until it becomes integrated into daily activities.

During the maintenance phase, the changes patients make are being integrated into their definition of who they are and what their lives are like with the problem behavior. At this stage of change, the support of others is important for the patient's ability to

EXHIBIT 6.6 Strategies for the Preparation Stage

- Clarifying the patient's own goals and strategies for change
- Offering a menu of options for change or treatment
- With permission, offering expertise and advise
- Negotiating a change or treatment plan and behavior contract
- Considering and lowering barriers to change
- Helping the patient enlist social support
- Exploring treatment expectancies and the patient's role
- Eliciting from the patient what has worked in the past either for him or her or others whom he or she knows
- Assisting the patient to negotiate finances, child care, work, transportation, or other potential barriers
- Having the patient publicly announce plans to change

EXHIBIT 6.7 **Strategies Useful in Maintenance Stage of Change**

- Provide hope for continued success
- Provide hope if setbacks occur; indicate that a setback does not mean failure
- Continue to acknowledge positive changes
- Identify and reinforce coping strategies
- Process any relapse experiences
- Monitor progress, remind patient of both short- and long-term goals

maintain changes. Strategies the gerioperative coach uses during this stage are outlined in Exhibit 6.7.

The gerioperative coach should help patients understand that change is a fluid and uneven process. Continuing a high level of trust enables patients to talk about failure, even after periods of success, without fear of recrimination and is critical to maintaining a sense of patient efficacy.

Brief Gerioperative Coaching Intervention

Prehabilitation and postoperative recovery are episodic interactions of information transfer critical to improving gerioperative patient outcomes. The effectiveness of information transfer is highly dependent on focused, caring, and effective communication. The FRAMES (*f*eedback, *r*esponsibility, *a*dvice, *m*enu of options, *e*mpathy, *s*elf-efficacy) model is a well-established model in substance abuse treatment in older adults. The model can be transferred to structuring brief intervention situations similar to those that occur in prehabilitation and postoperative recovery. The FRAMES model can be extended after discharge to a more comprehensive health coaching approach to help older adults maintain healthy behaviors and consider new behaviors for optimal health and wellness. Exhibit 6.8 explains each of the FRAMES components along with example provider statements.

Alternate Models

The OARS technique uses *o*pen-ended questions, *a*ffirmation, *r*eflective listening, and summarization to help patients identify and express their concerns about changing health behaviors. Miller (2010) suggests a three-step approach to facilitate the patient's change toward self-care and behavior change. Steps include educating and assessing willingness (step 1), setting goals and assessing readiness (step 2), and follow-up (step 3).

There are several other behavior change models that have been studied and found to be effective in assisting patients and families with change. One such model is the 5As Behavior Change Model, which is designed to facilitate an evidence-based, effective intervention in a short period of time with patients. The 5As—assess, advise, agree, assist, arrange—are used to assist clinicians and others in guiding patients and families that are coping with chronic conditions to develop goals and action plans for behavior change. An application of the 5As to helping a gerioperative patient stop smoking is described in Exhibit 6.9.

EXHIBIT 6.8 **Components of the FRAMES Model of Brief Intervention**

	Component	Example
Feedback	Give feedback on the risks and negative consequences of the problem behavior. See the patient's reaction and listen.	"Your tests show that you have an operable lung cancer, and this means you will need surgery."
Responsibility	Emphasize that the decision to change rests with the individual.	"You are responsible for the decision to make a change in your smoking."
Advice	Give straightforward advice on modifying the problem behavior.	"As your health coach, I strongly recommend that you quit smoking to lessen your risk of complications after your surgery."
Menu of options	Give menus of options to choose from, fostering the patient's involvement in the decision-making.	"There are a number of ways to help you quit. I'm happy to discuss them with you to figure out which one works for you."
Empathy	Be empathetic, respectful, and nonjudgmental.	"This isn't easy to hear. You've been smoking for a long time, and it's part of your life."
Self-efficacy	Express optimism that the individual can modify his or her problem behavior if they choose. Self-efficacy is one's ability to produce a desired result or effect.	"I'm confident that you'll be able to do this if you decide it's what you want to do."

Training for Health Coaching

The GCF can implement facets of health coaching using the skills developed during their professional education and through clinical practice. However, completing educational training specific to health coaching enables the GCF to more effectively support the patient, the caregiver/family, and the CC, and deliver coordinated and comprehensive perioperative care. Health coach training is required to become proficient in using motivational interviewing techniques for the promotion of perioperative behavior change and chronic disease self-management. Clinicians can become certified as a health coach by professional organizations. Certification programs vary widely in focus, intensity, cost, and time commitment.

Programs that utilize motivational interviewing–based health coaching and the Stages of Change model are more useful to someone in the GCF role than programs with life coaching–based health coaching approaches based on wellness models. Evidenced-based health coaching professional training, and certification programs for the health care provider, which can be used as training the trainer models, are available online through the National Society of Health Coaches at www.nshcoa.com, the HealthSciences Institute at www.healthsciences.org/, and the Motivational Interviewing Network of Trainers at www.motivationalinterview.org/.

EXHIBIT 6.9 5As Smoking Cessation Model

Component	Intervention
Ask	Ask for permission to discuss smoking and then proceed with further questions about the patient's smoking habits, interest in stopping smoking, and past experiences with quitting. Assessing the patient's smoking and related habits is the first step toward intervention.
Advise	Advise the patient to make permanent lifestyle changes by total smoking cessation. The gerioperative coach's advice to change a patient's behavior, shown to be effective in clinical trials, must be clear ("It is important for you to quit smoking now, and I will help you"), strong ("As your coach, I must tell you that quitting smoking is the single most important thing you can do for your health"), and personalized (provide specific information about the effects of smoking on their lifestyle and how these might improve of they stopped smoking).
Assess	Assess the patient's readiness to change, using the Stages of Change model. By "staging" a patient in this way, the gerioperative coach can better tailor the plan of action with the patient. If the patient is willing to quit at this time, continue with the 5As. If the patient clearly states that he or she is unwilling to make a quit attempt at this time, provide a motivational intervention and reassess readiness to change at the next visit.
Assist	Assist the patient in a plan of action. Smoking cessation guidelines and plans are available, and should be tailored for the patient's particular needs. It is at this stage that the gerioperative coach can give the patient specific materials and specific referral information for a smoking cessation program or self-help services (such as telephone quit-lines or websites). It is also at this stage that the gerioperative coach can assist the patient to set a quit date, give key advice on successful quitting, and encourage pharmacological therapy as appropriate.
Arrange	Arrange for some kind of clinical follow-up with the patient, ideally within 2 weeks after the patient's quit date. This is important for the patient to know that the health care system, as well as their gerioperative coach, will be following their progress. Minimally, the gerioperative coach should document with chart reminders to follow-up at each subsequent visit, but there are more intensive strategies including phone contact and follow-up visits.

PATIENT REPORT: Mrs. Dubois

The GCF greeted Mrs. Dubois and her daughter in the waiting area and brought them into her office. Seated in comfortable chairs, the GCF asked Mrs. Dubois to tell her story of the events that led up to her knee surgery being scheduled. Mrs. Dubois explains that, "it all started with my fall at home." She related that she was doing fine except for her constant knee pain until she fell. She further explains that, "my bone doctor said that I have nothing left in my knee joints" and that her problems "will not get better unless she has surgery." Mrs. Dubois as not exactly sure what "nothing left in my knee joints" really meant, although she understood that it is the cause of her pain. The GCF engaged Mrs. Dubois's daughter to share her thoughts on her mother's condition and the impending surgery. Her daughter shared worry that her mother will fall again and maybe break her hip the next time. Her daughter had met with resistance in trying to get her mother to sell the house and move closer to her. Mrs. Dubois was quiet but when asked to share her feelings on relocating, she said that she intended to live her life out in her home. She grew up in the farmhouse and does not want to live anywhere else.

The GCF performed a comprehensive preoperative assessment and discovered that Mrs. Dubois wants to regain mobility and function and believes that she needs to have surgery for this to happen, although she is not looking forward to it. Her surgical history included a total hysterectomy at 48 years old due to multiple fibroids and a lumpectomy for breast cancer 6 years ago. There were no postoperative complications with either of these surgeries. On physical examination, the GCF noted that Mrs. Dubois had a steady gait and good balance with a cane assist, decreased flexion and extension of both knees with the left more affected than the right, clear lung fields, and loss of central vision. Analysis of her preoperative history and physical exam indicated that Mrs. Dubois is at increased risk for intraoperative and postoperative complications due to a 40-pack-per-year smoking history, limited activity level, obesity, decreased muscle strength in hands and lower extremities, persistent and acute knee pain, occasional opioid use, porous bones, poor nutrition, central vision loss, and increased fall risk.

To facilitate health behavior change for better perioperative outcomes, the GCF asked Mrs. Dubois, "What is your greatest concern regarding your health?" "Well," Mrs. Dubois said, "Everyone has been telling me to stop smoking because it make my bones weaker and with my family's stroke history, it makes sense to stop." The GCF replied, "How has your smoking affected you?" Mrs. Dubois states, "I don't think it is a big deal 'cause my breathing is pretty good. . . but. . . if it weakens my bones then I might fall again." This statement indicated that Mrs. Dubois is in the contemplation stage of change and should be encouraged and supported. The GCF recognized the ambivalence in Mrs. Dubois's internal argument and recapped what Mrs. Dubois said, "So you feel that if you continue to smoke then you might have a stroke, which runs in your family, and it might also cause you to fall due to the fact that smoking makes your bones weaker." Mrs. Dubois nodded her head and said, "Yes, my doctor recently told me that I have weak bones on top of my arthritis and gave me two more medications to take everyday to help my bones stay strong. And to be honest, I am afraid that I will die from a stroke just like my mother and brothers. One of my brothers had a massive stroke and died a short time after his hip surgery. It was such a shock."

The GCF used gerioperative coaching to further explore Mrs. Dubois's commitment to stop smoking. She showed Mrs. Dubois an importance ruler and asked, "Mrs. Dubois, on a scale from 0 to 10, where 0 is not important at all and 10 is extremely important, how important would you say it is for you to stop smoking?" Mrs. Dubois responded, "I would say about 4." The GCF then tried to elicit change talk by asking, "Why did you give yourself a 4 and not a 1?" Mrs. Dubois explained, "Because I know it can give me lung cancer and make my bones weaker, and people who smoke have more heart attacks and strokes." Then the GCF attempted to elicit perceived barriers, "Why did you give yourself a 4 and not a 7?" Mrs. Dubois said, "Because my breathing is pretty good and I really like to smoke. I find it relaxing. And besides I have already gained weight since I have been unable to walk much or work in my garden. . .or even do housework like I used to. . .and if I quit I am worried that I will gain even more weight." The GCF asked Mrs. Dubois for suggestions to overcome these obstacles, and Mrs. Dubois responded, "I guess I could try something else to help me relax and maybe watch what I eat so I don't gain more weight." The GCF followed with another question to identify what actions might be taken, "If you were to stop smoking, what would it be like?" Mrs. Dubois thought for a few seconds, and then said, "I would not have to worry that I am weakening my bones or increasing my chance of having a stroke. . .and I would save money that I spend on cigarettes."

The GCF went through the same line of questioning using a confidence ruler. She asked, "On a scale from 0 to 10, where 0 is not confident at all and 10 is extremely confident, how confident are you that if you decided to stop smoking, you could do it?" Mrs. Dubois said, "Probably a 6." The GCF followed with, "And why did you give yourself a 6 and not a 0?" Mrs. Dubois said, "Well, I have run out of cigarettes a few times in the past few months and it wasn't so bad." The GCF then asked, "How can I help you to move higher up on the scale?"

Mrs. Dubois paused and then said, "If you could help me find another way to calm my nerves then I think I could give it a try."

The GCF, Mrs. Dubois, and Mrs. Dubois's daughter discussed stress management strategies including relaxation exercises and deep breathing for coping with stress and nicotine cravings. Mrs. Dubois decided she will stop smoking in 1 week, after she smokes her last pack of cigarettes. The GCF wrote the plan down, and both the GCF and Mrs. Dubois signed a health behavior change contract with the specific goal to stop smoking in 1 week by recognizing her stress triggers, practicing breathing relaxation techniques, and taking "breathing breaks" throughout the day. The GCF asked Mrs. Dubois to identify someone to be her CC. Mrs. Dubois immediately thought of Mrs. Martin, her friend and neighbor. The GCF asked Mrs. Dubois to decide which members of her support team will be responsible for holding her accountable. She chooses her daughter and Mrs. Martin, if she agrees to be her CC. They make another appointment for 2 weeks and set the agenda for the next meeting, which includes talking about what is working or not working with the relaxation strategies and ways to eat healthier. Mrs. Dubois agrees to ask Mrs. Martin if she would like to come to the next meeting.

The GCF prompted herself to call Mrs. Dubois after 5 days to see if Mrs. Dubois was able to identify what situations, people, or emotions cause her stress; how practicing the relaxation techniques is going; and to remind her of her smoking quit date. Mrs. Dubois was pleased to receive the call and admits that looking forward to quitting, as she has read that people who do not smoke have fewer problems after surgery. The GCF promised to call in 2 days to celebrate Mrs. Dubois's first day of commitment to stop smoking. At the follow-up meeting, the GCF applauds that Mrs. Dubois has not had a cigarette in 1 week and gives her a certificate of achievement. She reminded Mrs. Dubois that quitting smoking is not easy and shares some support numbers she can call if needed. The GCF reviewed what to expect in preparation for the surgery; coordinated where Mrs. Dubois needs to go, who she will see, and when she needs to be there for preoperative care; explained the roles and responsibilities of each member of the patient care team; and educated Mrs. Martin as the designated CC on how to be a cheerleader for Mrs. Dubois. The GCF then repeated the gerioperative coaching approach with Mrs. Dubois, who now desires to start eating healthier foods in preparation for surgery.

SUMMARY

Health coaching and motivational interviewing is a new approach for partnering with the older adult to improve health status before and after surgery. Older adults must make decisions about engaging in new behaviors. Health coaching is a patient-centered, relationship-oriented model that informs and supports behavior change processes. Health coaching and motivational interviewing can be tailored to the unique situations and focus of prehabilitation and postoperative recovery behaviors. The Stages of Change model explains the way patients change behavior and suggests ways to help older adults navigate the change process. Helping older adults prepare for surgery requires the active involvement of the older adult, CC, and GCF as well as other support persons identified by the patient and the interdisciplinary care team. The CC is integral in supporting the older adult through the change process. There are several well-researched approaches for delivering a brief health coaching intervention. The gerioperative coach can use the FRAMES model or the 5A's model to simplify change facilitation. Health coaching is useful in meeting immediate prehabilitation and postoperative patient outcomes as well as help the gerioperative patient move forward after surgery to achieve behavioral change that promote longer-term achievement of health and well-being.

KEY POINTS

- Coaching in gerioperative care is a framework for helping gerioperative patients attain optimal health status and function before surgery and maximum benefit in postoperative and postdischarge recovery activities.
- The GCF has the primary responsibility for guiding the patient/caregiver/family through the perioperative experience and minimizing the risk of adverse outcomes.
- The 5As—assess, advise, agree, assist, arrange—assists clinicians and others in guiding patients and families coping with chronic conditions to develop goals and action plans for behavior change.
- The health coaching approach is the same for everyone, but the application is tailored to the needs and circumstances of the gerioperative patient.
- The GCF explains the purpose of each action and goal as a prelude to helping the patient plan a perioperative action plan and goals. The goals should be specific, measurable, agreed on, realistic, and time-sensitive, and the roles and responsibilities for achieving the goals should be identified.
- The essence of health coaching and motivational interviewing is to help patients resolve ambivalence and make conscious choices about behavior change.
- The FRAMES (feedback, responsibility, advice, menus of options, empathy, and self-efficacy) model is effective for use in brief counseling interventions.

SEVEN

Gerioperative Assessment

Raelene V. Shippee-Rice, Jennifer V. Long, and Susan J. Fetzer

PATIENT REPORT: Mr. Morris

Mr. Morris is scheduled for a Whipple procedure for stage II pancreatic cancer in 4 weeks. A widower, Mr. Morris lives alone in a small apartment with his cocker spaniel, Daisy. He does not cook for himself, eating most of his meals out or doing what he calls "grazing." Although he has many friends and his daughter and family live nearby, Mr. Morris does not like to ask for much help. "I like doing my own thing," he tells his gerioperative nurse.

The comprehensive geriatric assessment (CGA) reveals an 80-year-old man who plays golf once a week during the summer, has an extensive social network, and travels around the country visiting friends and family. Mr. Morris has not been active during the winter months except to go to shopping.

Previous medical history in addition to his diagnosis of pancreatic cancer includes osteoarthritis of increasing severity over several years in his right knee. He has an open wound on the second metatarsal of his left foot that has not healed and was recently diagnosed with osteomyelitis. The osteoarthritis in his right knee limits his walking ability and makes it difficult to move from a sitting to standing position. He uses an electric cart to golf and has a handicap sticker for easier access when shopping.

Medications include acetaminophen 750 mg four times a day to manage his osteoarthritis pain and daily multivitamins, chondroitin/glucosamine pills, and a liquid he takes daily for this osteoarthritis. He has no information on the contents of the liquid. He has a history prior to his diagnosis of cancer of having two to three glasses of wine with meals and after dinner.

His preoperative testing includes a recent bone densitometry that revealed no osteopenia, serum albumin of 3.9 g/dL, hemoglobin of 12.8 g/dL, and hematocrit of 38.2%. He has lost 15 pounds over the past 2 months due to chemotherapy and loss of appetite. Although he was 30 pounds overweight before his diagnosis, the weight loss presents a concern about his general nutritional status and potential for deconditioning when combined with his inactivity.

Based on his weight loss, impaired mobility, lack of appetite, and preoperative testing results, Mr. Morris borders on frailty, placing him at high risk for postoperative complications.

Surgery is a highly effective intervention to improve the quality of life for even frail older adults. However, older adults are more vulnerable than younger patients to intraoperative and postoperative complications. The older adult's preoperative level of wellness is more important than age alone in influencing surgical outcomes. Preoperative wellness is influenced by comorbid disease, physical and physiological reserve, functional capacity, cognitive and emotional strength, availability of social support, and general preparedness for surgery.

Identifying risk factors supports prevention for promoting gerioperative patient outcomes.

Poor health status, polypharmacy, and lack of provider attention to prevention as an intervention increases risk of surgical complications. To achieve positive outcomes, predisposing and potential precipitating risk factors must be identified and treated before surgery. The preoperative assessment provides a gateway to risk identification as well as an evaluation of patient strengths. This chapter is an overview of the preoperative assessment in older adults with special attention to preoperative intervention. A more detailed description of perioperative considerations related to aging in different body systems is presented in subsequent chapters, as identified in Table 7.1.

Preoperative assessment collects and analyzes patient information. Patient strengths and limitations, health and disease, reserve capacity, functional ability, and physical and psychological readiness for surgery are assessed and evaluated. Assessment results are used to develop prevention and intervention action plans for use throughout the perioperative continuum. Goals are directed to helping the patient achieve an optimal state of psychological, emotional, and physical health prior to the surgical procedure and to inform the patient of actions needed after surgery to promote recovery and long-term health.

Preoperative assessment is a focused facilitative communication process that allows the provider to obtain information about the older patient's health status, functional capacity and psychosocial well-being before the surgical procedure. The preoperative assessment is an opportunity to identify current and potential health problems and initiate interventions that not only minimize surgical risk but also achieve long-term health benefits. Data from the preoperative assessment are used to design a prevention and intervention plan that will

TABLE 7.1
Chapters Related to Gerioperative Assessment

Gerioperative Assessment	Chapter
Gerioperative coaching	6
Informed consent, advance directives	4
Functional status	13, 19
Mobility	13
Cognition and depression	20
Pain	22
Nutrition	15
Hydration	9, 10, 15
Polypharmacy	5
Sleep	12

optimize preoperative wellness and minimize intraoperative and postoperative risk. The value of accurate comprehensive preoperative data collection and analysis as a basis for prevention of complications cannot be overestimated. The preoperative assessment is the foundation for safe, quality care across the perioperative continuum.

The major outcome of the preoperative assessment and health coaching is obtaining the information needed for providers to stay ahead of problems by initiating prevention programs and protocols. Staying "ahead of the curve" saves the patient from unnecessary suffering and promotes optimum outcomes.

Communication

Discovering the patient's physical and psychosocial readiness for surgery relies on a communication process that facilitates sharing and exchanging of information between patient and provider. Accurate information is needed about the patient's strengths, limitations, clinical status, and concerns. A facilitative communication model elicits information in the context of the patient's unique situation. Information obtained in context of the individual's strengths, needs, and concerns allows the nurse to provide support, educate, coaching, and comfort appropriate to the patient and the situation.

Communication during the preoperative assessment supports a process of discovery. Learning the patient's story helps the nurse to discover patient expectations and understanding about the surgical procedure and postoperative recovery. Eliciting the story can be a challenge for the care provider. The stress of a difficult illness, anxiety about the

Active listening means attending to what patients do not say as well as what is said.

impending surgery, and age-related changes in sensory abilities, cognition, and energy create barriers to effective communication. Eliciting information pertinent to the older person's physical, psychological, and social resources and limitations requires active listening skills and the ability to establish a patient-centered relationship.

Active listening is a process of simultaneously hearing, interpreting, evaluating, and responding. Active listening also involves hearing what the patient does not say as well as what the patient says. Older adults are reluctant to acknowledge incapacities, especially those they hide because of fears about being dependent or being forced to move to a different living situation. Establishing a patient-centered relationship demands that care providers demonstrate a respect and commitment to the patient's best interests. Motivational interviewing skills help the older adult prepare for surgery and identify the older adult's readiness for prehabilitation and postoperative recovery activities critical to achieving optimal surgical outcomes.

Obtaining a history from an older adult who is depressed or has cognitive impairment yields inaccurate or incomplete information. These inaccuracies involve information from patient to provider but also from provider to patient. Having a friend or family or companion-coach (CC) attend the preoperative visit facilitates data collection and information sharing. When family members or others attend the preoperative interview with the older adult, it is important for the interviewer to establish rapport with the older adult and keep the focus of the assessment on developing a relationship with the patient. However, including the CC and family members depends on the wishes of the older adult and should be assessed at the beginning of the interview. The CC can be a source of overall support and reassurance to the older adult as well as provide gentle reminders that help the patient present a coherent and comprehensive history. With the older adult's permission, the CC or family can actively participate during the interview providing direct answers, as long as the information remains within the knowledge of the patient. Alternatively, the patient may request that those attending the preoperative interview participate in the interview only when explicitly invited to do so.

Including the CC and patient-designated caregivers is important regardless of diagnosis of cognitive or mood status of the older adult. Even in cognitively intact older patients, anxiety, sensory impairment, energy level, or fatigue can interfere with information exchange. Older adults frequently have undetected cognitive impairment, depression, or anxiety that impairs understanding with resulting inadequate knowledge exchange. In early dementia, mild cognitive impairment, or early stage depression, the older adult may not be aware of cognitive changes and unknowingly skew or misrepresent information.

Assessment Environment

The assessment and information sharing process begins at the time surgery is recommended. Follow-up assessments and patient information sessions are conducted in ambulatory and outpatient surgical settings, physician's offices, preoperative assessment clinics, emergency departments, and inpatient hospital settings. The depth, breadth, and detail of assessment depend on the setting, type of surgery, patient characteristics, and preoperative timeframe. A preoperative assessment conducted several weeks in advance of the procedure allows time for patients to become better prepared physically and mentally. Often, the preoperative assessment for an outpatient procedure is conducted the day of surgery, leaving little time for establishing rapport, obtaining patient data, or to do patient coaching for preoperative preparation or postoperative recovery. Older adults should always undergo the preoperative assessment in a timeframe that allows for follow-up assessment, intervention, and evaluation as needed.

Outpatient surgery is increasingly recommended to older adults as anesthesia and surgical techniques continue to improve. A benefit of outpatient surgery is avoiding the hazards associated with hospitalization. However, management of postoperative recovery at home is a disadvantage for many older adults who do not have support systems on which they can rely. Environmental supports and assistance from friends or family are needed to ensure safety and security postoperatively. In addition to the stress, fears, and anxieties about surgery, older adults may have similar concerns about being a burden to others or not having adequate support at home. Attention to the patient's postoperative situation and detailed patient education about postoperative recovery during the preoperative assessment interview are important considerations for ensuring successful outpatient outcomes.

Inpatient surgery includes urgent, emergent, or elective conditions. Preoperative assessment is significantly influenced by the timeframe of surgery. Elective surgery allows time for more detailed assessments and attention to getting the patient ready for surgery. Urgent and emergent surgery assessment focuses on the most critical factors to determine surgical risk. There may be little time to prepare the patient for surgery. Establishing rapport and trust and building a patient-centered relationship is critical when older adults are undergoing urgent or emergent surgery. Uncertainty about surgical outcome and fears of death or dying create higher levels of anxiety and stress with little time for resolution before surgery. Attending to the older person's psychological, spiritual, and physical comfort becomes an urgent and integral aspect of the preoperative preparation.

Obtaining information from the patient and providing patients with information is accomplished through telephone interviews, paper- or computer-based patient self-administered or family-completed health and medication history, in-person interviews, home visits, or preoperative seminars. Each strategy has benefits and disadvantages (Table 7.2).

TABLE 7.2

Benefits and Disadvantages of Preoperative Assessment Strategies

	Benefits	Disadvantages
Self-administered assessment	• Patient self-paced • Saves provider time • Patient privacy • Low patient burden • Established due date	• Increased risk of misinterpretation • Literacy concerns • English fluency • Patient may have impaired vision • Skewed data • Incomplete data • Constrained data • Closed information • Lack of nonverbal cues • Lack of motivation • Forgetting to return data • Not all tools translated • Lack of knowledge on the part of family/caregiver • Unknown respondent
Telephone assessment	• Scheduled timeframe • Bidirectional questions to clarify information • Able to use interpreter • Open-ended questions • Increased motivation to share information • Familiar environment • Shared information • Limited caregiver/family member participation	• Difficulty managing attention • Environmental distraction • Lack of nonverbal cues • Hearing impairment • English language fluency • Fatiguing • Questionable data
Face-to-face assessment	• Observation • Access nonverbal cues • Open-ended questions • Scheduled timeframe • Bidirectional feedback • Clarification of questions • Scheduled timeframe • High motivation to share information • Shared information • Effective patient coaching • Involvement of family members	• Fatiguing • Stressful • Transportation expense • Transportation availability • Expensive for patient and provider: time, resources • Difficulty scheduling • Unfamiliar environment
In-home assessment	• Scheduled • Environmental context • Comprehensive data • Patient familiar with environment • High-value data • Observation of nonverbal data • Observation of family interaction • Able to use interpreter • Shared information	• Time-consuming • Scheduling • Expensive • Travel time

(continued)

TABLE 7.2

Benefits and Disadvantages of Preoperative Assessment Strategies *(continued)*

	Benefits	**Disadvantages**
Multimodal	• Able to clarify data from other sources • Incorporates best of other assessment methods • Cost-effective when targeted to key concerns • Family evaluation and observation	• Expensive • Time-consuming

Time constraints limit gerioperative assessment in ambulatory care settings.

Outpatient preoperative assessment at clinical sites or ambulatory surgical settings can be difficult for older adults as a result of transportation availability or mobility problems. Telephone interviews are difficult if the older person has a hearing impairment. Self-administered health and medication histories require familiarity with the English language, literacy, and health literacy. Knowledge of computers is needed for self-administered computer-based questionnaires. Family members or friends who assist older patients with self-administered forms may not have complete information. The older adult may be hesitant to share some of the information out of embarrassment or need for privacy. A health care provider should review data from self-administered health histories with plans for a follow-up telephone or in-person interview to ensure completeness and accuracy of information.

Telephone interviews require preplanning and advanced scheduling. Prior to the interview, sending copies of the health and medication assessment questionnaires, patient education materials, surgical preparation information, or other documents that will be reviewed during the telephone conversation can facilitate data gathering and information sharing. All information sent to older adults should be in large print with space for writing notes. Older adults who have a hearing impairment may want a family member or friend to participate in the telephone call to help ensure information clarity. Having another person who is fluent in English and is health literate is especially important for older adults with English as a second language or limited health literacy.

Extended and detailed telephone conversations can be difficult for older adults. Telephone listening and maintaining attention for long periods of time is fatiguing. Divide telephone assessments into sections to keep each conversation within a comfortable timeframe. Respect and concern for the provider's time and not wanting to admit to limitations inhibit older adults from admitting to discomfort or weariness during "business" health care calls. One way to assess for attention span is to ask the older adult to explain back a part of the conversation recently concluded. The "talk back" assesses the older person's understanding of the information under discussion as well as his or her attention ability.

Face-to-face interviews can be tiring for older adults with severe chronic illness. Dividing personal interviews into several shorter timeframes creates multiple problems involving scheduling, transportation, diminished energy, and mobility impairment. In-home visits are often less tiring than telephone or clinical interviews. The security of a familiar milieu, not needing to travel, and having a person physically present when asking questions or explaining information in a face-to-face encounter can lower stress and stress-related fatigue. Family members may find it easier to participate in a home interview. Home interviews allow the care provider to observe environmental barriers and facilitators and availability of local resources. This type of information is highly relevant in anticipating discharge plans.

When preoperative assessments occur on the day of surgery, nurses are faced with little time to establish rapport with the older patient. Time constraints interfere with the ability to fully assess risk of postoperative complications and provide patient and family teaching about postoperative care, prevention of complications, and observations of patient changes that require consultation with providers.

Assessment Elements

The basic elements to be included in a standard preoperative assessment remain the same in any surgical setting or type of surgery: health and medication history, physical examination, psychological and social assessment, and results of laboratory, imaging, and diagnostic work-ups. Analysis of patient information is used to identify actual and potential problems, risk factors for intraoperative and postoperative complications, and areas for patient education.

Critical patient findings requiring immediate follow-up evaluation include decreased cardiac function, presence of infection, bleeding, alterations in mental status, rash, or changes in medication. Patient education is directed at relieving patient fears and anxieties, explanations of the surgical procedure and process, preoperative instructions, presurgical procedures, postoperative recovery activities, and pain management.

COMPREHENSIVE GERIATRIC ASSESSMENT

Assessment of the older adult requires more extensive data gathering and analysis than the basic elements of a standard assessment. Older adults have complex health and medication histories that span many years. Age-related changes affect physiologic function and functional capacity even in the absence of disease, adding to the vulnerabilities caused by disease. Assessments that receive limited attention in younger populations assume a higher priority in older adults. A higher priority rests on the documented association of age with intraoperative and postoperative complications. The purpose of the gerioperative evaluation is to screen for potential or actual risk factors of special importance in older adults: comorbid disease, functional capacity, cognitive function, depression, nutrition and hydration status, polypharmacy, fall risk, continence, skin condition, and social support such as availability of caregivers and accessibility of support services. Findings from the preoperative screening provide an indication for initiating a more extensive CGA.

The CGA involves a "multidisciplinary evaluation in which the multiple problems of older persons are uncovered, described, and explained, if possible, and in which the resources and strengths of the person are catalogued, need for services assessed, and a coordinated care plan developed to focus interventions on the person's problems" (National Institutes of Health, 1987). The CGA covers the same elements as the gerioperative screening assessment. The difference is the depth of evaluation and the involvement of the multidisciplinary team in conducting the evaluation.

The CGA identifies older adults at risk for developing intraoperative and postoperative complications, length of hospital stay, delayed recovery, and prolonged debilitation. The CGA is reserved for older adults at greatest risk for poor surgical outcomes. The population most in need for a comprehensive assessments includes gerioperative patients with complex medical histories, poorly controlled comorbid disease, degree of age-related changes, diminished reserve capacity, poor nutritional status, or who are undergoing a major surgical procedure. Identifying older adults most vulnerable to postoperative complications and poor outcome allows for the development of individualized care plans and implementation of comprehensive interventions to reduce risks and improve outcomes.

A geriatric comprehensive screening is a shortened version of the interdisciplinary approach to CGA. CGA screening indicates a need for a more detailed evaluation by the interdisciplinary care team. Table 7.3 identifies elements with suggested questions to be included in a CGA preoperative screening.

SCREENING GERIOPERATIVE ASSESSMENT

Informed Consent

Informed consent reflects an older patient's understanding about the procedure to be performed, the expected outcome, and associated risks and benefits. Older adults who sign informed consent documents often do not have a clear understanding of what is to be done or to have forgotten the details of the informed consent discussion (see Chapter 4).

An important part of the preoperative assessment is to determine that the patient has a clear understanding of the planned surgery. Asking the patient to explain the reason and outcomes of the planned procedure and any concerns about possible risks and benefits allows the interviewer to answer questions, allay concerns, and clarify misunderstanding. Older adults who have a poor understanding of the planned surgery may need to be reevaluated to ensure consent is informed.

Advance Directives

Advance directives for perioperative patients are treated differently than for other populations. In some institutions advance directives are waived in the operating room. The patient undergoing surgery is assumed to want all measures taken to maintain life. It is important to ask the older adult if there is an advanced directive, if a surrogate decision-maker is designated, and if the older adult has discussed advanced directives with the surrogate decision-maker. It is also important to determine the patient's preferences in the event a treatment decision is needed during the perioperative continuum and the patient is unable to respond. Obtain a copy of the advance directive, living will, or other document prepared by the patient. Older adults who do not have an advance directive must be counseled about the process before surgery.

Comorbid Disease

Comorbidity or preexisting disease is the presence of disorders or diagnoses other than the disorder requiring surgery. Preexisting disease severity has a strong correlation with poor surgical outcomes, postoperative complications, and decreased quality of life after surgery, regardless of age or type of surgery. Comorbid disease may be well or poorly controlled. Preexisting diseases that are poorly controlled create higher risk for surgical complications.

The greater the number and severity of preexisting medical conditions, the greater the risk of intraoperative and postoperative complications. Medical conditions, unless poorly controlled, are often overlooked due to attention on the surgical management and recovery of the older adult. Many of the complications encountered during intraoperative and postoperative care occur due to preexisting age-related and disease-related changes combined with the trauma of surgery and anesthesia rather than the result of surgical trauma alone. Being aware of these changes before the patient experiences surgery allows providers to initiate preventative and therapeutic interventions before surgery that prevent later onset complications.

TABLE 7.3

Elements to Be Included in Preoperative Comprehensive Geriatric Assessment

Screening Element	Suggested Questions
Informed consent	What is the surgery or procedure you are having? What is the purpose of the surgery? How do you describe what is important to you about this surgery?
Advance directives	Do you have an advance directive or living will? Have you identified someone to make treatment decisions if you are not able to make them?
Preexisting/comorbid disease conditions	What health problems do you have? What medical diagnosis have you been told? What do you do to take care of your health problems?
Functional status	Do you have someone help you with everyday activities such as showering, dressing, or walking? Does anyone help you with paying bills, shopping, or taking your medications? What do you do for social activity?
Mobility/fall risk	How easy is it for you to stand up from a chair? How far do you walk outside the house? Have you fallen in the past 6 months? Are you afraid of falling?
Cognition	Have you had difficulty remembering things? Do you find that you have forgotten how to do things that used to be easy for you?
Sensory changes	Do you have difficulty reading even with glasses? Do you find that you have to turn up the television to hear? Do you have numbness, tingling, or loss of sensation in lower legs or feet?
Depression	Do you often feel sad or depressed? Have you lost pleasure in doing things over the past few months? (If yes, assess suicide risk.)
Pain	Do you have any current pain? Do you have any pain on a regular basis?
Nutrition and hydration	Have you lost more than 10 pounds in the last 6 months? Has your appetite changed in the past month?
Polypharmacy/medication safety	How many prescription medications do you take? How do you take your medications? What kind of nonprescription medications do you use?
Sleep	Do you fall asleep often during the day without intending to? How often do you wake up during the night? How many hours of sleep do you generally get at night?
Social support	Do you have a family member or friend who helps you? Is there someone who can be a companion-coach with you during your surgery? Who will be helping you after your surgery? Who will be your companion-coach during your surgery?

(continued)

TABLE 7.3

Elements to Be Included in Preoperative Comprehensive Geriatric Assessment *(continued)*

Screening Element	Suggested Questions
Spiritual support	What or who do you turn to when you are feeling distressed or overwhelmed? Do you have a minister, pastor, or other person you would like contacted to meet with you before or after surgery? What can the staff do to help provide you with spiritual support?
Patient strengths	What would you describe as your biggest strengths? How do you cope when faced with special challenges, like this surgery? What do you want the people who will be taking care of you to know that will be most helpful to you while you are going through this surgery?

Chronic disease screening relies on the older patient's self-report of diagnoses and a review of the patient's medical record. Older adults may not have complete recall of their diagnoses, particularly if the list is extensive. Using a self-administered checklist or reading the checklist to the older adult can help improve recall. Determining how well the disease is controlled during a screening assessment is based primarily on patient self-report of current symptoms, observation, physical examination, and laboratory results. Investigating the presence of comorbid disease extends beyond the presence or severity of disease. The effect of disease on functional, cognitive, and psychosocial capacity as well as physiologic capacity is important in the care of the gerioperative patient. The ability of the older adult to participate in and conduct postoperative recovery and rehabilitation activities is critical in achieving successful patient outcomes.

Evaluation of cardiovascular disease, pulmonary disease, and renal diseases are of special concern in older adults. Cardiovascular disease is the most common and serious perioperative event. Presence of heart failure, ischemic disease, valve disease, and dysrhythmias are the strongest predictors for postoperative complications. Preoperative pulmonary function accounts for 40% of all postoperative complications, while preoperative renal disease predicts risk of postoperative renal failure and adverse drug events. Musculoskeletal impairment is associated with rapid deconditioning after surgery. Gastrointestinal alterations are linked with nutritional intake.

Functional Status

Functional status or functional capacity is a measure of how well and to what extent the older adult is able to carry out basic, instrumental, and advanced activities of daily living. Basic activities of daily living (BADLs) include eating, dressing, ambulating/walking, toileting, bathing and hygiene, and transferring. Instrumental activities of daily living (IADLs) are more complex, requiring a higher level of cognition and integration of multiple tasks. IADLs involve shopping, making telephone calls, self-managing medication, managing household tasks, and monitoring finances. Advanced activities of daily living are defined as carrying out social roles, occupations including volunteer work or participation in a hobby, or leisure and recreational activities. Impairment in BADLs and IADLs is associated with postoperative immobility and associated complications: atelecta sis, delirium, multisystem deconditioning, falls, and early death. Conducting a screening evaluation of functional status is useful in predicting risk for postoperative complications and identifying interventions to decrease the risk.

Standardized tools or self-report is used to evaluate functional status. Commonly used tools for BADLs are the Katz Activities of Daily Living Scale and the Barthel Index (Mahoney & Barthel, 1965). IADLs can be readily evaluated using the Lawton-Brody IADL to evaluate an older person's ability to use the telephone, shop, do laundry, use transportation, manage personal medications, handle finances, prepare a meal, and do moderate to heavy housework (Katz, Down, Cash, & Grotz, 1970).

Self-report data provide insight into the patient's perspective of his or her functional status. Patient perception of functional ability is often inconsistent with observed functional ability. For example, Mr. Morris reported he was doing "pretty well" getting around. Provider observation revealed that Mr. Morris constantly held door handles, leaned against a wall, and had severe difficulty rising from a sitting position even when using both arms for leverage. When asked about the apparent inconsistency, Mr. Morris. revealed he was happy to be able to "get up and get around at all," leading to his statement he was not doing "too bad." Mr. Morris's description was not based on his lack of awareness of his limitation. The inconsistency between his description and the observed reality was the meaning of the limitations in light of his goals and expectations. Honoring the patient's perspective while recognizing limitations and their importance in planning postoperative care is crucial in helping the patient retain self-esteem and competence.

Mobility

Impaired mobility is a major cause of postoperative complications in older adults. Ambulation, mobility, balance, and gait are critical for postoperative recovery activities and for preventing falls. Conducting a fall assessment is an integral element of the gerioperative assessment. Determining functional mobility in the preoperative period suggests prehabilitative interventions to strengthen mobility prior to surgery. The Timed Get up and Go (see Chapter 13) is one of the most commonly used tools to assess mobility and ambulatory function in older adults. The test asks the older adult to stand from a seated position, walk, turn around, and return to seated position. The entire sequence is timed.

Cognition

Changes in cognition are associated with postoperative delirium, falls, postoperative cognitive dysfunction, and prolonged recovery. Cognitive changes are prevalent in older adults due to age-related neurological changes and pathologic conditions such as dementia or depression. Older adults with cognitive age-related changes are at greater risk for delayed identification of perioperative complications because the effect of cognitive changes on the patient's thinking and behavior are unnoticed or ignored (Lawton & Brody, 1969). Providers may interpret behaviors or missed cues as an expected consequence of aging without attending to the impact such changes have on the older person's ability to attend to information, hear instructions, or interpret environmental and verbal cues accurately. Any older adult demonstrating changes in cognition such as memory loss, decreased problem-solving ability, and diminished attention span, should be evaluated for early detection of changes in cognition. Early detection leads to early intervention that can slow progression of disease-related cognitive changes. Cognitive function should be systematically assessed in all older adults before surgery.

Standardized tests are used to assess the absence or presence of impairment. The Mini-Mental State Examination (MMSE; Folstein, Folstein, & McHugh, 1975) and the Mini-Cog (Borson, Scanlan, Chen, & Ganguli, 2003) are tests commonly used in clinical settings to screen for changes in cognitive function. The MMSE is easy to use and score. Results of the MMSE can be influenced by the patient's level of education, language facility, and verbal ability. The Mini-Cog is more efficient to administer and score than the MMSE and is not influenced by patient literacy or verbal ability (see Chapters 20 and 21). The Trail Making

Test, oral version (Ricker & Axelrod, 1994), evaluates problem solving and planning associated with executive function.

Older adults with age-related preexisting cognitive changes are highly vulnerable to postoperative delirium and postoperative cognitive dysfunction. Screening for cognitive changes can uncover unexpected deficits associated with undetected mild cognitive impairment.

Preexisting cognitive changes predict difficulty with attention span and concentration due to anxiety associated with surgery or hospitalization. Stress increases vulnerability to misinterpretation and missed information. Adapting communication methods includes providing time for the older adult to hear, attend, and respond. Further evaluation and follow-up may be required for determining the presence of dementia.

Sensory Changes

Sensory changes create patient safety issues related to difficulty reading or hearing instructions. Changes in sensory function also interfere with balance, gait, and coordination. Ask the patient about recent vision and hearing testing and use of assistive devices. A change in color discrimination is common with aging and important for patients who often think about their medication according to pill color rather than name. Often, older adults are not aware of changes due to the slow onset of many vision and hearing conditions. With the permission of the patient, ask a family member or CC if the patient has changed light sources, changes the volume on media devices, asked family members or friends to repeat verbal statements more often, or complained about difficulty reading or hearing.

Depression

Preoperative depression contributes to postoperative delirium, increased pain severity and analgesia use, wound infection, delayed recovery, and postoperative cognitive dysfunction. Symptoms of preoperative depression are often masked by symptoms of disease, loss of functional ability, changes in cognitive function, or medications. Preoperative depression is overlooked when care providers expect older adults to be depressed or exhibit depressed behavior in response to being old, sick, alone, and losing friends and family to death and disease. However, depression is not a normal part of the aging process; it is an altered health state that must be assessed, diagnosed, and treated before surgery. Depression is so common in older adults undergoing heart surgery that the American Heart Association recommends that all older adults be preoperatively screened for depression.

Recent grief or loss, appetite changes, changes in sleep patterns, longstanding chronic illness, or persistent pain are well-noted risk factors for depression. Patients with history of one or more of these risk factors should be screened for depression prior to surgery.

Older adults undergoing cardiac surgery or orthopedic surgery have higher rates of depression preoperatively and postoperatively. The correlation of poor postoperative rehabilitation and depression in older adults is sufficiently strong that older adults undergoing joint replacement should be screened for depression. The Geriatric Depression Scale–Short Form is a brief, 5-minute standardized tool that can be used to screen for depression in older adults (see Chapter 20).

Pain

Preoperative pain limits prehabilitation activity and increases postoperative pain severity. Pain is a common cause of depressed mood and changes in cognition. Assessing preoperative pain and pain relief methods provides information essential to management of postoperative pain and preventing postoperative complications. Chapter 22 presents an extensive discussion of gerioperative pain and pain relief.

Nutrition and Hydration

Older adults are highly vulnerable to nutritional deficits and dehydration. Malnutrition occurs in up to 15% of older adults, 65% of hospitalized older adults, and 26% of institutionalized elders (Williams, Jones, & Pofahl, 2008). Age and disease, environmental factors including inadequate social resources, and functional impairment all contribute to poor nutrition. Low serum albumin levels indicating poor nutritional status are common in older adults with chronic illness. Inadequate nutrition contributes to perioperative risk for complications. Chronic dehydration occurs in up to half of community dwelling older adults and up to 35% of older adults living in nursing homes. Chronic dehydration can be difficult to detect as it occurs slowly and older adults adapt to low fluid levels. Complications from chronic dehydration include loss of muscle tone, medication toxicity, impaired renal failure, and difficulty with temperature regulation. Older adults who have multiple chronic diseases or impaired ambulation need to be carefully evaluated for dehydration.

Nutritional status is assessed by evaluating body mass index and diet history. Asking the older adult about meals provides an overview of general nutritional intake. Many older adults have difficulty recalling specific foods for each meal. Asking for general categories followed by asking for specific foods makes recall easier. Preparing meals alone and eating alone can decrease nutritional intake. Often, older adults fall back on easy to prepare foods such as cereal, frozen meals, or canned soups. Asking for details about the specific kinds of cereal or frozen meals is important as there is a wide variation in nutritional quality. Fluid intake questions should consider type of fluid as well as amount.

Onset of sudden illness, vomiting, or diarrhea prior to surgery dramatically diminishes the older adult's dietary and fluid intake. An older person with chronic poor nutrition or dehydration becomes rapidly malnourished and at increasing risk of renal failure after surgery (see Chapter 10).

Polypharmacy

Older adults comprise approximately 12% of the population in the United States but account for 34% of all medication use. Age-related changes in pharmacokinetics and pharmacodynamics (see Chapter 5) increase the potential for adverse medication effects. Many medications used for preexisting conditions or as self-treatment interact with perianesthesia, anesthesia, and postoperative analgesic medications. Conduct a careful and detailed drug history including prescription and over-the-counter medications, as well as manufactured and homemade herbal remedies. Older adults frequently take medications with anticholinergic properties that can cause cognitive disruption and delirium, urinary retention, dry mucous membranes, and constipation. Anticholinergic medications interact with anesthesia medications during surgery. Sedative hypnotics, antianxiety agents, and psychotropic medications also cause adverse drug events in older adults. Table 7.4 lists common prescription and over-the-counter medications that are considered inappropriate for use or must be administered using a lower dose and scheduling for older adults.

Requesting that the older adult bring a "brown bag" of all the medications used in the past month to the preoperative interview allows providers to have a more comprehensive view of the patient's medication use. Older adults may not recall the details of their medication regimen. They are often hesitant to admit to nonadherence or abuse of prescription, over-the-counter, or other drugs such as alcohol or illegal substances. Developing trust and a patient-centered relationship promotes sharing of medication information. Reinforcing that questions about medications are important for the patient's safety during and after surgery can remove the potential stigma older adults may experience about the use, misuse, or abuse of prescription, over-the-counter, and herbal drugs.

TABLE 7.4

Commonly Used Medications of Concern in Older Adults

Prescription Drugs	Over-the-Counter Drugs	Herbal Remedies
Anticholesterol	Analgesic	Ginkgo balboa
Bone absorption inhibitor	Antihistamine	St. John's wort
Proton pump inhibitor	Sleep aids	Saw palmetto
Antidepressants	Cold medication	Senna
Beta blockers	Caffeine	Cascara
Diuretics	Alcohol	
Hypoglycemic		

Medication concerns, especially for potential of drug-drug interactions and number of medications, are reviewed with the interdisciplinary team in relation to preoperative discontinuation or changes in treatment regimens. Discussion of concerns and decisions about prevention and intervention strategies are documented in the patient's record for use by caregivers across the perioperative continuum.

A medication reconciliation is completed on admission to the surgical setting. Hospital or surgical setting medication orders are compared with prehospital medications to identify potential drug-drug interactions and ensure that drugs to be continued have a start date and drugs not needed are discontinued. The companion-coach and informal caregiver are given written documentation of medication changes and explanations for the changes.

Sleep Patterns

Sleep is an important consideration in the gerioperative patient. Sleep apnea has been linked with pulmonary complications with anesthesia significantly disrupting postoperative sleep. Over 50% of community dwelling older adults have inadequate sleep patterns (Foley, Monjan, & Brown, 1995). Older adults with high levels of fatigue due to poor sleep are less likely to complete prehabilitation activities. Inadequate sleep interferes with cognition, metabolism, muscle strength, and increases fall risk.

Smoking

Preoperative smoking cessation is a major focus area for prehabilitation and postoperative recovery. Smoking cessation is encouraged immediately upon the decision to have surgery. Surgery fears can act as a stimulus to discontinue smoking due to fear of complications.

Ask the patient about duration of smoking, number of cigarettes, or other smoking materials used per day, and patient physiological and psychological response to smoking. If the older adult indicates smoking was discontinued, assess when the patient ceased smoking and responses to the change.

Social Support

Assessing the availability of social support is an integral aspect of gerioperative assessment. Impending surgery increases psychological distress, feelings of vulnerability, and uncertainty about the future. Higher levels of emotional distress and anxiety are linked with increased response to surgical stress, higher complication rates including pain severity and analgesia use, and longer hospital stays. Availability of social support improves outcomes for gerioperative patients. Social support is the belief that one is care for and cared about. Older adults who perceive themselves as having high levels of social support demonstrate less preoperative anxiety, lower postoperative pain scores, lower rates of analgesia, shorter hospital stays, and reduced hospital readmissions.

Social supports include emotional and instrumental support systems. Emotional support is having friends or family who help the older adult feel cared about and valued. Emotional support relieves feelings of isolation, loneliness, stress, and hopelessness. Instrumental support is the most direct form of support including providing transportation, shopping assistance, meal preparation, personal care, and monitoring activities. Identify the availability of family members or friends who provide instrumental support during the assessment to plan postdischarge home care.

> *Surgery increases patient's feeling of distress, vulnerability, and uncertainty about the future.*

Asking the older person who they rely on for help provides a social support list. Follow-up questions distinguish the type of support available to the patient and the extent of the support network. Encouraging the older adult to identify a family member or friend to be a companion-coach facilitates transfer and interpretation of information between patient and provider and within the patient's support network while maintaining patient confidentiality.

The availability of instrumental support systems and resources contributes to developing an initial discharge planning process as part of the preoperative assessment. Plans for postdischarge care depend on the availability of a support system that is willing to monitor patient safety, well-being, and continuation of discharge medications and recovery activities. Having someone available who can identify the onset of complications is important for ensuring early intervention and the avoidance of hospital readmission. If the patient does not have a support system available, formal systems will be needed through community agencies. The Aging and Disability Resource Centers (ADRCs) offer options counseling to help older adults make decisions about the type of services and supports needed to remain at home after discharge from the hospital. Asking the older adult about a referral to the local ADRCs at the time of the preoperative assessment ensures sufficient time for an options counselor to meet with the older adult to determine hospital discharge needs.

Family members provide the majority of care giving for older adults living in the community. While family members may have provided care giving for a number of years, postsurgical care can involve specific skills such as dressings, colostomy care, intravenous or central access lines management, prevention of pressure ulcers, and encouraging mobility. Knowing what to do, how to do it, and how often to do it are common caregiver concerns. Assessing pain, decisions about pain relief medications, and decreasing analgesia create additional concerns. Interviewing the designated caregiver identifies needed areas for coaching and training. Document the availability of a caregiver and an analysis of caregiver needs throughout the care continuum in preparation for discharge.

Home Environment

Patient safety remains an important discharge concern. Ask the patient to describe the home environment to assess environmental barriers that can impact recovery. Assessment involves basic safety measures such as access to and within the home and availability of basic amenities such as a bathroom, bed, safe water supply, cooking, and refrigeration. Type of transportation and availability of transportation for grocery shopping and pharmaceutical supplies are important areas to assess. Conducting a home visit improves the older adult's confidence about being discharged to the home after surgery. During the preoperative home assessment, the need for assistive equipment after discharge can be evaluated and placed before the patient is discharged. Environmental hazards can be assessed more effectively through a home visit than through patient description. Older adults have less preoperative anxiety related to returning home when a preoperative assessment determines the type of adaptations needed and implemented before surgery.

Spiritual Support

The prospect of surgery is a frightening experience. Exploratory surgery, cancer care, or surgery involving general anesthesia creates feelings of vulnerability and dread. Disability, becoming a burden, or "being worse off than before I started" are of greatest concern for older adults, often more worrisome than death. Fear of the unknown, uncertainty about outcomes, and concerns about pain raise questions of "Is it (surgery) worth it" and "Why bother." Over their lifespan, older adults have developed ways of coping with life's adversities including illness, death of loved ones, and loss. Finding meaning in these struggles leads older adults to create a life full of meaning and spiritual resources. Surgery can raise doubts or reaffirm strengths in spiritual beliefs. Asking what the older adult "holds onto" in times of stress or life's difficulties gives nurses and providers insights into how the older adult is coping with the prospect of surgery. Identifying the older adult's spiritual strengths or needs for spiritual support guides patient care. Providers can help older adults use their spiritual resources within themselves or in a formal religious network or community. Older adults struggling to find spiritual comfort may need support and comfort from the nurse, spiritual counselor, or pastor. Asking the older adult to describe his or her spiritual or religious beliefs opens the door. Nurses provide spiritual support through their caring. Patients reported that when nurses listen, comfort, and show caring or presencing behaviors, they are providing spiritual care. Spiritual care is not an intervention that nurses do. Listening to patients' concerns and answering their questions during the preoperative assessment is the essence of spiritual care and comfort.

Patient Strengths

Patient health status, comorbid disease, and presence of risk factors become focal points for the preoperative assessment. As a result, preoperative assessment becomes biased, focusing only on patient problems and ignoring strengths and personal resources older adults bring to the surgical challenge.

Health care providers underestimate the strengths of older adults and their ability to navigate surgical adversity. Old people have extensive histories that involve overcoming challenging life situations. They have learned coping skills and have found ways to overcome many of the barriers adversity presents. The strengths older adults bring to the surgical experience should be identified, acknowledged, and used to manage risk factors and prevent potentially adverse events. "Old people are tough old birds. They don't get to live to be 80 or 90 without having survived a lot of crises through stamina, strength, and resilience" (Wells, personal communication, 1979).

The ethic of care carries a responsibility to support how older patients cope with the threat of surgery by helping the patient recognize how he or she can apply skills and strengths to the current challenge. Assessing personal resources, strengths, and coping ability is as important a part of the preoperative assessment as health history and physical examination. Personal resources provide a different perspective and insight into the older person's ability to withstand the rigors of surgery. Older adults have the ability to be an active partner and meet the surgical challenge if health care providers educate, coach, support, and use a collaborative team approach to care and decision making.

Conversely, health care providers underestimate the potential vulnerability of even healthy older adults to the adverse effects of surgery and surgical stress. Increasing age brings a decreasing physiologic reserve. Subclinical disease and diminished reserve can go unnoticed until surgery, anesthesia, or complications stress organ systems beyond their capacity to respond. Care providers must maintain vigilance while respecting the strengths of older adults, recognizing the limitations and being acutely aware of tipping points that push the older adult from clinical, psychological, or functional stability to instability (see Chapters 9–18).

Asking the older adult to describe what is most useful in helping him or her meet the challenge of surgery serves several purposes. It reinforces that providers and staff are interested in helping the older person be comfortable throughout the perioperative continuum. The question stimulates the older person's analysis of what will make the surgical process easier. The answer saves time eliciting concerns and support methods so that they are available and ready to use as needed across the perioperative continuum.

PHYSICAL EXAMINATION

The standard physical examination for any patient takes on special significance in older adults depending on the type of preexisting disease and functional capacity. The physical assessment relies on identifying and understanding age-related changes. The following provides a brief overview of elements to be included in gerioperative assessment. More detailed descriptions of assessment can be found in the chapters associated with physiological systems.

Preoperative Testing

McGory and colleagues (2009) developed a set of clinical indicators for surgical care of vulnerable older adults. Recommended preoperative screening includes the following tests: hemoglobin and hematocrit, electrolytes, serum albumin, urinalysis, blood urea nitrogen/creatinine, and electrocardiogram within 6 months of surgery, as well as height and weight. Additional screening depends on comorbidity, type of surgery, and anesthesia.

PREVENTION AND INTERVENTION: PREHABILITATION

Patient fitness and readiness for surgery are major priorities in achieving successful surgical outcomes. The goal of preoperative care is for the patient to be in an optimal state of physical and psychological readiness with social supports available to assist in care transitions.

Warner (2005), in reviewing smoking cessation programs, described surgery as an "opportunity to help smokers quit permanently with the potential for long term health benefit to the patient. . ." (p. 252). Using surgery as an agent for change can be extended beyond smoking to exercise, disease control, nutrition, and medication use. Poor physical conditioning, uncontrolled comorbid disease, inadequate nutrition, and incorrect use of medications are all associated with increased postoperative complications. Providing patient coaching and education on ways to improve their readiness for surgery through prehabilitation can decrease surgical risk and improve outcomes.

Prehabilitation optimizes the health status, functional capacity, and well-being of the older adult prior to surgery. Initially used to prevent sports injuries in children and young adults, prehabilitation is a multimodal, evidence-based program preparing older adults to meet the challenges imposed

Prehabilitation addresses health problems amenable to intervention.

by surgical stress. Prehabilitation rests on the theory that maximizing functional capacity before surgery improves the older adult's ability to withstand the stress of surgery, thereby decreasing postoperative complications and returning the patient to preoperative level of function more quickly. Prehabilitation has been shown to decrease surgical morbidity, hospital length of stay, and recovery time in older adults undergoing orthopedic surgery and colorectal surgery. While evidence suggests that prehabilitation can improve outcomes and decrease risks, more research is needed to determine the benefits and risks of using prehabilitation in gerioperative patients.

The prehabilitation plan is directed to optimize areas amenable to intervention identified during the patient history and physical examination as risk factors. Behaviors amenable to intervention are exercise and activity, nutrition, comorbid disease management, medication, mental health, smoking cessation, and alcohol use. Prehabilitation also involves practicing postoperative recovery skills such as deep breathing, use of an incentive spirometer, and non-pharmacologic pain relief methods. Table 7.5 lists most common prehabilitation and post-recovery interventions for older adults undergoing surgery. Type of surgery and functional status further influence type of activity.

Prehabilitation can be used for individual patients or a group of patients with similar risk factors or a similar type of surgery. For individuals, the prehabilitation program must be targeted to the needs, limitations, and strengths of the individual. Smoking cessation programs are an example of a program designed for a group of patients with a similar risk factor. Exercise programs are conducted with groups of older adults who are having total joint replacement surgery or abdominal surgery.

A prehabilitation program is most effective when it is offered as a comprehensive program through a center with access to an interdisciplinary team of providers such as physical and occupational therapists, dieticians or nutritionists, social workers, nurses, geriatricians, anesthesia providers, respiratory therapists, and surgeons. A gerioperative care facilitator can integrate a prehabilitation program, coordinating the recommendations of the interdisciplinary care team and organizing therapeutic activities. Comprehensive programs are generally offered through health clinics, ambulatory surgical centers, or hospital-based programs. When a comprehensive program is not available, a prehabilitation plan can be developed for the patient to carry out independently with support from family or friends.

It is imperative that the older adult actively participates in designing prehabilitation goals and plan of activities. Many older adults will have difficulty achieving goals that are not established in the context of the patient's clinical condition and situation. External barriers can limit the type and extent of activities patients can accomplish.

Health coaching and motivational interviewing are successful methods that can increase older adults commitment and participation in prehabilitation activities (see Chapter 6). Balancing the strengths of the older person with the limitations imposed by disease, illness, surgical-related fears and anxieties, and age-related changes require astute clinical judgment. Older patients are strong yet vulnerable. They speak their mind while remaining hesitant to risk being seen as incompetent or unable to meet expectations. They avoid talking about constraints they think will diminish them in the eyes of others. Clinicians must be skillful, able to develop the trust that supports freedom to discuss constraints and fears. The patient may not be cognizant of his or her feelings or the focus of fears and concerns. Excellent active listening skills help the older adult to become aware of unrealized expectations and concerns that can interfere with prehabilitation and with involvement in postoperative care. Knowing the patient's constraints and strengths helps to develop a prehabilitation plan that is realistic and achievable but that also challenges the patient to achieve his or her maximum potential. Helping patients find the motivation to initiate behaviors that will better prepare them for surgery is a fundamental component of prehabilitation.

Preferably, prehabilitation begins 6 to 8 weeks before the scheduled surgery to enable interventions to be effective. While older adults have higher rates of urgent surgery than younger patients short-term prehabilitation programs provide physiological and psychological benefit. Prehabilitation plans are directed to the needs of the individual older adult, clinical status, and type of surgery. A benefit of prehabilitation is that most action plans can be continued after surgery as part of an ongoing health behavior change program to improve the overall health and well-being of the older adult. Action plans are tailored to the functional capacity of the older adult so that even frail older adults are able to improve function and reserve prior to surgery. Prehabilitation focuses on smoking cessation, exercise and activity, nutrition and hydration, medication, chronic disease management, depression, and cognition.

Preparing the patient for surgery involves more than providing information. Mr. Samson

TABLE 7.5

Common Prehabilitation and Postrecovery Interventions for Older Adults

Assessment Element	Prehabilitation/Postoperative Strategies
Preexisting comorbid conditions	Related to disease condition Examples: glycemic control, pain relief, hypertension control, dysrhythmia stability, beta blockers, venous thrombosis prophylaxis, pulmonary hygiene
Functional status	Adaptive or assistive equipment as needed Physical therapy, occupational therapy referral Related to specific dysfunction Related to type of surgery and postoperative interruptions in function
Mobility, fall risk	Exercise to tolerance Range of motion Chair yoga Walking Balancing exercises Easy stretching Nutrition Moving, standing, and walking in relation to type of surgery
Cognition	Social interaction Board games Crossword puzzles Jigsaw puzzles Computer games Coaching on informing providers about postoperative changes in sensation, thinking, and feelings
Sensory changes	Encourage use of assistive devices Evaluate effectiveness of assistive devices
Depression	Exercise Nutrition Ensure social support Family coaching Cognitive behavioral counseling Interdisciplinary team consult
Pain	Medication review Coaching, nonpharmacologic pain relief Exercise to tolerance Range of motion Coaching on pain assessment methods Coaching on pain communication with care team
Nutrition	Increase or decrease caloric intake depending on clinical situation Small high-nutrition meals five to six times a day High nutrition snacks Nutrition consult
Hydration	Increase or maintain fluids at 1200–1400 mL/day unless medical restriction Decrease caffeine intake Restrict alcohol use Limit early evening fluids if nocturia interrupts sleep

(continued)

TABLE 7.5

Common Prehabilitation and Postrecovery Interventions for Older Adults *(continued)*

Assessment Element	Prehabilitation/Postoperative Strategies
Polypharmacy	Medication review related to: Is this drug necessary? Is this drug recommended for use with older adults? Is the drug dose at lowest effective dose? Is this drug interacting with other drugs? Does this drug have potential interactions with anesthesia? Pharmacy review if five or more drugs Coaching on over-the-counter drug use and herbal remedies
Sleep	Adequate pain relief Listen to quiet or preferred music Eliminate television at least 30 min before bedtime Meditation/relaxation activities Comfortable room/in bed temperature Apply warm blankets, heating/cooling devices as preferred Limiting fluids before bedtime Physical and mental exercise/activity during day Evaluate/treat sleep disorders, depression, incontinence Review medications to determine if any interfere with sleep
Smoking	Health coaching regarding smoking cessation Pulmonary hygiene Demonstration deep breathing, coughing Demonstration incentive spirometer Exercise regimen Increase fluid intake
Social support	Identify a companion-coach Identify a postoperative caregiver Provide coaching to postoperative coach and caregiver dependent on type of surgery Demonstrate, coach, and evaluate skills needed for postdischarge care
Spiritual support	Discuss spiritual needs and concerns with patient Respond to patient based on patient needs Referral to spiritual counselor, priest, or minister per patient's permission and request

was scheduled for a toe amputation for osteomyelitis as an outpatient. He was given a brochure with the date of his surgery and a postoperative follow-up appointment with the surgeon. He signed an informed consent form. He was told to call before surgery to get the time of surgery. When he got home, his family asked about the surgical plan, but Mr. Samson was unable to provide any details. When asked, he said no one went over the brochure with him or gave him any details. He later received a phone call telling him to contact his primary care provider for a "presurgical physical." Mr. Samson was inadequately prepared for surgery due to mild cognitive impairment that was not noticed or addressed by the surgeon or the staff responsible for giving him information.

Patient coaching and decisional support is targeted to the specific needs, questions, and concerns of the older adult. Coaching prompts the older adult to use information in making decisions about how he or she will participate in prehabilitation activities and prepare for postoperative and postdischarge recovery plans. Examination of barriers enables the preoperative interviewer to work with the older adult, companion-coach, and family on removing or reframing perceived barriers to action. Identifying the level of patient commitment to prehabilitation helps the patient make more conscious and less reactive decisions. However, when barriers cannot be reframed or removed, the interdisciplinary team must adapt prehabilitation and postoperative recovery plans.

Preparing the patient and caregivers for postdischarge begins during the preoperative interview. Discussion of any needed adaptations to the home environment is based on type of surgery, surgical setting, functional capacity, and clinical condition of the older adult. Family caregivers are instrumental in seeing that needed modifications are made for the patient transfer to home. Depending on the type of surgery and home environment, older adults may transition from hospital to a rehabilitation facility before being discharged home. Explaining the anticipated discharge plans allays concerns for the future. The older adult and family must be prepared that the preoperative plan for discharge may be altered depending on patient's hospital recovery, postoperative comfort, and postoperative complications.

PATIENT REPORT: Mr. Morris

Mr. Morris states he is willing to do whatever he needs to do to make sure his surgery is a success. The gerioperative facilitator suggests that he ask someone to be his companion-coach. Mr. Morris is reluctant as he does not want to bother anyone, and as he states, "I can take care of myself." The GCF suggests that may be true during his prehabilitation activity, but in the hospital he will have less energy and find it easier to not do something than to do it. Similarly, once he gets back to his home he will find continuing postdischarge recovery activities difficult without assistance. Mr. Morris agrees and finally identifies a friend, not a close friend, who will make sure he does what he needs to do.

The CC is not available during the initial preoperative interview. A follow-up meeting is scheduled for the next week with Mr. Morris, the gerioperative facilitator, and the CC.

Based on the geriatric assessment, the gerioperative facilitator explains to Mr. Morris that due to his inactivity over the winter, an exercise/activity program will help strengthen his upper arms and lower legs in preparation for ambulating after surgery. The upper strength will be important if he needs to use a walker during initial ambulation. Mr. Morris expresses concern about his knee and toe interfering with an exercise program. After discussing what he can do, the gerioperative facilitator suggests doing chair yoga and using a therapy band for upper body strengthening. The facilitator demonstrates several chair yoga exercises. Chair yoga helps to increase muscle strength but also increases range of motion and flexibility, equally important in ambulation and balance. The facilitator suggests the possibility of walking around his apartment several times a day or daily walks around the local grocery store or mall. Mr. Morris is confident he can do the chair yoga and the therapy band if he has diagrams or pictures to follow and written information about how many times to do them and when. The facilitator works with Mr. Morris on a schedule for his exercise routine and provides him with several chair yoga pictures, reviewing them with Mr. Morris. He is referred to physical therapy for additional conditioning due to the severe osteoarthritis.

A second major issue is nutritional and fluid intake. Mr. Morris states he has no appetite. He just does not feel like eating. He denies nausea or that the smell of food is bothersome, restating only that he does not have any appetite that prompts him to eat or drink. The interviewer reminds him about his statements that he is a "grazer," that is, eats snacks multiple times a day and asks if this would be easier than trying to eat regular meals. Mr. Morris is not sure but says he can try. The facilitator and Mr. Morris work out a small meal or grazing schedule. A nutrition consult is scheduled to detail the type of foods that will be easy for Mr. Morris to prepare or obtain. They discuss the benefits and disadvantages of eating alone or making sure he has the CC or other friends eat with him at home or out of home as this is his usual routine. The nutritionist reviews how to select high nutrition foods when eating out. The gerioperative facilitator suggests they stay in contact via telephone over the first week to see how he is progressing and make decisions about continued follow-up before surgery depending on his progress. Mr. Morris agrees.

SUMMARY

Surgery is an intervention to improve the health and function of well elders as well as frail elders. Gerioperative assessment is a preoperative analysis of the older adult's physical, physiological, and psychoemotional readiness for surgery. Analysis is based on information obtained through integration of a standard preoperative assessment with a screening CGA. The preoperative assessment can be carried out in many different ways. However, preoperative assessment conducted in the home is cost-effective, most comfortable for the patient, and provides the most comprehensive information. Preoperative assessment using a patient-centered, active listening approach is the foundation for developing patient-focused prevention and intervention strategies for use throughout the perioperative continuum to improve care quality and patient outcomes throughout the perioperative continuum.

KEY POINTS

- The purpose of the gerioperative assessment is to screen for potential or actual risk factors. Information attained during the preoperative assessment is used to develop prevention and intervention action plans for use throughout the perioperative continuum.
- Establishing rapport and trust, and building a patient-centered relationship is critical when gerioperative patients are undergoing the stress of impending surgery, especially urgent and emergency surgery.
- Home interviews are often the easiest for gerioperative patients and allow the gerioperative care provider to observe the environmental barriers, facilitators, and local resources highly relevant to planning and implementing the patient's transition to postdischarge care.
- Elements of preoperative assessment that require immediate health care provider notification include cardiovascular changes, presence of infection, bleeding, abnormal laboratory values, alterations in mental status, changes in skin integrity, changes in respiratory function, and medication changes.
- Assessing the availability of social support is an integral aspect of gerioperative assessment.
- While family members may provide many types of care giving, postsurgical care can be intimidating and requires personal coaching by the gerioperative nurse.
- Nurses provide spiritual support through their caring. Patients report that when nurses listen, comfort, and demonstrate presencing and caring behaviors, they are providing spiritual care.
- Nurses and care providers must maintain vigilance while respecting the strengths of older adults, recognizing their limitations and being acutely aware of tipping points that can push the older adult from clinical, psychological, or functional stability to instability.
- A prehabilitation program is most effective when offered as a comprehensive program through a center with access to an interdisciplinary team incorporating physical and occupational therapists, dieticians, nutritionists, social workers, anesthesia providers, nurses, respiratory therapists, surgeons, and geriatricians.

PART II

Aging and Gerioperative Care

EIGHT

Gerioperative Anesthesia

Jennifer V. Long, Susan J. Fetzer, and Raelene V. Shippee-Rice

---

PATIENT REPORT: Mr. Tung Ming Wang

Mr. Tung Ming Wang is a 92-year-old retired engineer who was born in China and has lived in the United States for the past 50 years. He lives at home with his 82-year-old wife. He is active, having returned from a recent trip to Portugal and Spain. He is in fairly good health except for a mild stroke 5 years ago, from which he has residual expressive aphasia, but only when speaking English when he is fatigued. He is on statins for elevated cholesterol and 81 mg aspirin per day. Recently, he has complained of frequent urination in small amounts. After treatment for a urinary tract infection, it was found that he had an enlarged prostate. For the past 3 weeks, he has used an indwelling catheter, and he is admitted for transurethral resection of the prostate. He has been taking an antibiotic for 1 week to treat his urinary tract infection.

"People are never more alike than they are at birth, nor more different and unique than when they enter the geriatric era" (Silverstein, Rooke, Reves, & McLeskey, 2008).

Providing anesthesia to patients at either end of the age continuum can be challenging. Pediatric patients are not "little adults," nor are geriatric patients "old adults." However, while the pediatric population responds similarly to anesthetic stress and medications, the geriatric population is a heterogeneous one. The anesthesia plan must consider the gerioperative state of the individual as no two older adults are the same. Elders have different age-related changes, disease processes, medications, reactions to stress, body compositions, and metabolisms. These differences create diverse reactions to anesthesia and the surgical process.

> *"Start low and go slow" with vigilant monitoring is critically important during surgery because of the powerful adverse side effects of anesthetic agents.*

This chapter presents anesthesia considerations that apply to the care of the gerioperative patient throughout the perioperative period. Common medications and techniques used for anesthesia are reviewed. Implications for gerioperative nurses to anticipate potential problems as well as implement appropriate interventions to minimize their impact on elders are presented.

Preoperative Assessment

The American Society of Anesthesiologists (ASA) developed a classification system in 1961 to assess the physical state or degree of illness of a patient prior to selecting an anesthesia technique for surgery. The ASA classification is universally used by the anesthesia community for documentation and communication purposes, as well as providing a basis for comparing anesthesia outcomes. While the ASA classification system was not intended to predict surgical risk, insurance companies often use ASA classifications to determine reimbursement policies.

The ASA classification ranks individuals from 1 to 6 depending on their functional ability and comorbid illness (Table 8.1). The addition of "E" refers to emergency. However, the ASA classification does not consider age or underlying physiological changes. For example, there is no classification for pregnancy, though many anesthesia providers will rate a healthy pregnant woman as an ASA 2 secondary to normal physiologic changes of pregnancy that affect anesthesia care. A patient with uncontrolled hypertension may be an ASA 2 to one provider but ranked as

> *The ASA classification does not consider age or underlying age-related changes.*

TABLE 8.1

The American Society of Anesthesiologists' Physical Status Classification System

Grade*	Status	Explanation
1	A normal healthy patient	Patient has no clinical evidence of disease beyond the surgery; excludes very young and very old.
2	Patients with mild systemic disease	Patient has a well-controlled disease of one body system with no functional impairment. Cigarette smoking without COPD; mild obesity. **
3	Patients with severe systemic disease	Patient has disease from any cause. Severity imposes a functional limitation on activity, with no immediate danger of death; stable disease (e.g., heart failure, angina, prior myocardial infarction, obesity, chronic renal failure).
4	Incapacitating systemic disease(which is a constant threat to life)	Patient has at least one severe disease that is poorly controlled or at end stage; presents a constant threat to life; unstable angina, symptomatic COPD, symptomatic heart, kidney, or renal failure.
5	A moribund patient (unlikely to survive 24 hours with or without surgery)	Patient is not expected to survive >24 hours without surgery; imminent risk of death; multiorgan failure, sepsis syndrome with hemodynamic instability, hypothermia, poorly controlled coagulopathy.

COPD, chronic obstructive pulmonary disease.
*"E" after the grade indicates emergency surgery.
**Patients aged 75 and older are classified category 2 even if there are no disease-associated health changes due to normal age-related changes or increased risk of postoperative complications.

an ASA 3 by a different provider. Ranking of elders is similarly subjective. A patient rated as ASA 2 that is 75 years old may be rated as an ASA 3 to account for age-related changes that affect anesthesia. In spite of these drawbacks, the system is widely used and is generally well understood in the anesthesia community. It is important for perioperative nurses to appreciate that the ASA classification is an indicator of health or illness. An ASA 5E is sicker preoperatively than an ASA 2. Elders, by virtue of age-related changes, are not in poorer health than their younger counterparts but have greater potential to have their health compromised as a result of age-related changes.

Anesthetic Medications

The elderly are more susceptible to the effects of anesthesia medications due to age- and disease-related changes in pharmacodynamics and pharmacokinetics. Elderly patients have a slower circulation time that results in a longer lag time between effective plasma concentration and actual onset of action. Also, the brain and central nervous system is the target of many anesthetic agents. The normal age-related changes to the nervous system account for the increase in sensitivity to anesthesia agents in the gerioperative patient. The general rule for medication administration in the elderly is that anesthetic medication doses should be decreased and the intervals between doses should be increased. "Start low and go slow" is the motto for elderly medication administration in general and is even more important in the operating room (OR) secondary to the powerful adverse side effects of anesthetic agents. The amount of decrease and the intervals between doses varies depending on drug class.

BENZODIAZEPINES

Benzodiazepines are anxiolytics and include midazolam, diazepam, and lorazepam. The intent of premedication with benzodiazepines is to minimize anxiety. Other reasons include perioperative amnesia, sedation, and as an adjunct to regional and local anesthesia. Midazolam is most often used in the perioperative arena due to its short half-life, fast recovery, and amnesic effects. In the elderly, benzodiazepines have a longer half-life, double that of younger individuals. Age-related changes in the brain make older adults' brains more sensitive to benzodiazepines. Midazolam has been identified as inducing postoperative delirium and postoperative cognitive dysfunction. Due to the longer half-life, increased brain sensitivity, and side effects, premedication with benzodiazepines is strongly discouraged in the elderly.

Interventions

Preoperative anxiety is normal. Elderly patients often have less preoperative anxiety than younger patients due to life experiences. Preoperative anxiety can be allayed during the preoperative interview after meeting with the perioperative team. In the event that the gerioperative patient is anxious and not assured during the preoperative interview, then premedication with benzodiazepines is indicated. The dose for patients over the age of 60 should be decreased by 20% and by as much as 75% in patients over 85. An alternative is lorazepam 1 mg by mouth. Oral lorazepam has been found to be well tolerated by geriatric patients. Lorazepam has a half life of 8 to 12 hours with no active metabolites. However, lorazepam, as well as other benzodiazepines, can cause hypoxemia, especially when combined with fentanyl.

Due to the longer half-life, increased brain sensitivity, and side effects, premedication with benzodiazepines is strongly discouraged in the elderly.

Premedicated patients must be monitored, including pulse oximetry, and provided with supplemental oxygen. When monitoring the oxygen saturation, the nurse must be aware of the heart rate and monitor the pulse oximeter wave form. Benzodiazepines can cause hypotension when administered with fentanyl, so blood pressure (BP) must be frequently monitored. Paradoxical reactions to benzodiazepines can occur in gerioperative patients. Instead of becoming less anxious and sedated, the patient becomes irritable and overactive. The mechanism of paradoxical reactions is not known but may be secondary to aging.

In the event the patient has a reaction or stops breathing, flumazenil reverses the effect of benzodiazepines. However, the duration of effect of flumazenil may not be as long as the duration of benzodiazepine. The patient must be carefully monitored for at least 2 hours after administration of flumazenil, and repeat reversal doses should be given if necessary. Flumazenil should not be given to patients who take benzodiazepines on a routine basis as reversal can lead to acute withdrawal and seizures.

Medications used by older adults can interact with benzodiazepines. Cimetidine reduces metabolism of diazepam, and erythromycin prolongs the action of midazolam. Heparin displaces diazepam from protein binding sites and increases the amount of free drug available. An increase in drug availability can result in diazepam overdose.

Gerioperative patients discharged the day of surgery should always be provided with verbal and written discharge instructions. The registered nurse should review instructions with the patient, caregiver, or family member. The side effects of benzodiazepines should be discussed with the responsible adult that will be caring for the elder in the next 24 hours. The caregiver should be coached to monitor the gerioperative patient for any sedation effects or respiratory depression.

The elderly patient should not climb stairs or attempt any activities that require concentration as benzodiazepines cause residual confusion. The caregiver should also be coached about the risk of delirium (see Chapter 21) over the next 24 to 48 hours.

NARCOTIC MEDICATIONS

Narcotic medications are used preoperatively for sedation and analgesia. Intraoperatively, narcotics are used synergistically with induction agents to initiate induction and block autonomic response to intubation and surgery. Narcotics are effective and administered in small doses throughout the perioperative period for analgesia.

Gerioperative patients are more sensitive to opioids, and clearance rates are slower than their younger counterparts. However, during surgery and in the immediate postsurgical area, gerioperative patients may require a dose of narcotic similar to younger patients in order to control postoperative pain. The interval between dosing of medications may be longer, due to longer clearance times.

Interventions

The perioperative and postoperative nursing considerations for care of patients receiving narcotics are similar regardless of the narcotic. Narcotics cause respiratory depression in the elderly, especially when combined with other medications. The risk of respiratory depression secondary to opioid administration is nearly three times greater in patients 61 to 70 years old than in patients 16 to 45 years old. More importantly, narcotics decrease the respiratory system response to hypercapnia, meaning the stimulus to breathe is decreased. Elders receiving opioids must receive supplemental oxygen therapy.

Intramuscular (IM) administration of narcotics is not recommended for older adults. Changes in muscle tone and erratic absorption in the gerioperative patient can result in an overdose or underdose of medication, making adequate pain control difficult. Intravenous (IV) administration is rapid and easily titrated. Onset is faster and duration is similar to IM injection. However, administration of IV pain medication produces a peak and valley syndrome, making steady state difficult to obtain. Patient-controlled analgesia or oral medications can produce a better steady state and can better pain control (see Chapter 22). IM injections are painful. There is no need to cause pain to treat pain when other administration routes are available.

Another risk of IM administration involves patients on anticoagulant medications. Many elders take medications such as clopidogrel or warfarin, increasing the risk of hematoma formation and nerve damage. The risk of nausea from narcotics decreases 13% with each decade, but constipation is an important postoperative side effect of narcotics in the elderly. Gerioperative patients often complain of bowel difficulties, and narcotic constipation in this population can be significant. The nurse should ensure that stool softeners are ordered at the same time that narcotic orders begin. Patients being discharged home on narcotics should be informed of the need to take stool softeners. If there is no bowel movement after 3 days, laxatives are recommended. Hydration is important in maintaining bowel function.

MORPHINE SULFATE

Morphine sulfate is the gold standard narcotic to which all other narcotics and analgesics are compared. Morphine is used postoperatively as a long-acting narcotic for pain control. Side effects of morphine in the elderly are secondary to age-related changes in hepatorenal function. Morphine must be administered with caution in patients with decreased renal clearance or liver disease due to build up of morphine metabolites. Morphine effects can be enhanced when administered to patients on ranitidine. Many patients take over-the-counter ranitidine and should be questioned about this medication preoperatively to avoid morphine overmedication and side effects.

FENTANYL

Fentanyl is the most common narcotic perioperative medication due to quick onset of action and relatively short duration. Fentanyl is 100 times more potent than morphine, requiring close monitoring of the dose and titration. Fentanyl is the recommended drug of choice for pain control in renal patients and has a favorable drug profile for use in the elderly. Due to potency, it must be used with caution. Fentanyl can also be given intrathecally for pain control in epidurals and spinals.

HYDROMORPHONE

Hydromorphone is a narcotic agent that is 8 to 10 times more potent than morphine. It is well tolerated by gerioperative patients when given in doses and intervals compatible with the individual patient's pharmacokinetic profile. Many medications taken by the elderly are metabolized by cytochrome P450. When elder patients take too many medications, cytochrome P450 may not be able to completely metabolize these medications, including narcotics, leading to the possibility of a narcotic overdose. Because hydromorphone is not metabolized by the cytochrome P450 system, it is safer to use in elderly patients on multiple medications and is safer than morphine in renal patients.

Elders receiving opioids must receive supplemental oxygen therapy.

MEPERIDINE

Meperidine is not indicated for pain control in the elderly due to increased build up of normeperidine metabolites secondary to age-related changes in renal function. Normeperidine can cause delirium and seizures. Meperidine can cause orthostatic hypotension and transient tachycardia, both of which are poorly tolerated by gerioperative patients. Meperidine has anticholinergic properties that can cause delirium in gerioperative patients. As a result, meperidine has been identified as a leading cause of delirium in surgical and hospitalized older patients. Meperidine is contraindicated in patients with renal failure or seizures. In the event that gerioperative patients exhibit postoperative shivering, a single dose of 12.5 mg IV can be administered. Physicians often prescribe oral meperidine for postoperative pain. Oral meperidine has many side effects and is virtually ineffective in the elderly. It is not recommended for use in older adults.

SUFENTANIL

Sufentanil is a very potent narcotic that is 1,000 times more potent than morphine. Due to its potency, sufentanil is only administered by anesthesia providers in the OR. After sufentanil is metabolized, the gerioperative patient will need another narcotic such as hydromorphone or morphine to maintain pain control.

ALFENTANIL

Alfentanil is a synthetic narcotic that is 25 times more potent than morphine. Alfentanil is administered only in the OR by an anesthesia provider. Due to a short half-life and extreme nausea and vomiting, it is usually administered as an IV infusion with propofol during monitored anesthesia care (MAC) or total IV anesthesia (TIVA). Erythromycin can significantly prolong the duration of alfentanil. When alfentanil is used, the postanesthesia care unit (PACU) nurse will need to administer another narcotic for pain control.

REMIFENTANIL

Remifentanil is similar to fentanyl in its potency, approximately 100 times more potent than morphine. Remifentanil has an extremely short onset and duration of action. Remifentanil is primarily used in the OR, usually as an IV infusion with propofol for MAC or TIVA. The advantage of remifentanil is safety for elders as it does not build up in tissues and does not need adjustment for hepatorenal changes. However, it is virtually ineffective 10 minutes after the infusion stops. The patient will need a longer acting narcotic agent to control pain in the PACU.

NALOXONE

Naloxone reverses narcotics by binding to the mu receptor site and blocking the ability of the narcotic to bind to that receptor. Naloxone is administered in very small doses of 0.1 to 0.4 mg IV in response to narcotic-induced respiratory depression or muscle rigidity. The smallest dose is administered first and then titrated upwards. Onset of action is usually 1 to 2 minutes. However, circulation time and response time to naloxone may be delayed in the elderly. The delay means that titration must be slower than in younger adults. Naloxone duration is typically 60 minutes but may be somewhat longer in the gerioperative patient. As the narcotic is reversed and the patient begins to feel pain, naloxone administration causes sympathetic stimulation with heart rate, BP, and respiratory rate increases. The nurse must monitor the patient for dysrhythmias, potential for congestive heart failure, and pulmonary edema. Most importantly, the naloxone may wear off before the narcotic. The nurse should monitor the patient closely for return of signs of opioid-induced respiratory depression.

NONOPIOID PAIN CONTROL

Acetaminophen

Acetaminophen is a well-tolerated nonopioid pain medicine for older adults. Acetaminophen is effective, has few side effects, and allows for narcotic dose reduction in the gerioperative population. It must be used with caution in older adults with hepatic disorders or decreased hepatic blood flow.

Nonsteroidal Anti-Inflammatory Drugs

Nonsteroidal anti-inflammatory drugs (NSAIDs), such as aspirin, ibuprofen, and naproxen, are metabolized by the kidneys and therefore used sparingly or not at all in the elderly, with the exception of low-dose aspirin for cardiovascular disease. NSAIDs can cause ulcers, especially in the elderly, and increase bleeding times.

Ketorolac

Ketorolac is an NSAID and not recommended for the gerioperative patient. If necessary to administer, the dose should not exceed 15 mg IV. It is important to remember that ketorolac is an NSAID and cannot be given to patients with a stated allergy to aspirin or ibuprofen. Care must also be taken when administering the drug to asthma patients, as many asthma patients cannot take aspirin.

Induction Agents

Onset of anesthesia, known as induction, is faster with IV agents than inhalation agents. All induction agents can be administered to the gerioperative and frail gerioperative patients. Gerioperative patients are more sensitive to induction agents secondary to age-related changes in physiology, lower volume of distribution, and increased sensitivity. Dosage should be carefully and patiently titrated to response. In general, while it is common knowledge that gerioperative patients require lower doses of all anesthetics than younger individuals, the mechanism is poorly understood. Unfortunately, in practice, many anesthesia providers continue to overanesthetize the gerioperative population.

During induction, older adults exhibit a slower time to unconsciousness, often prompting unnecessary doses of induction agents. Additional doses of induction agents, especially propofol, can cause significant hemodynamic depression and undesired prolonged recovery times. Recovery times from vasodilation are prolonged due to diastolic cardiac insufficiency often found in older adults. As a result of the hypotension, significant amounts of IV fluid and vasopressors are utilized to maintain mean arterial pressure with

In practice, many anesthesia providers continue to overanesthetize the gerioperative population.

resulting fluid overload and increased myocardial oxygen consumption. These complications could be avoided if lower doses of medication were administered. The recommended decrease in dose of propofol for gerioperative patients is 30% to 50%.

PROPOFOL

Propofol is used in MAC, TIVA, and general anesthesia (GA). Propofol has a rapid onset and is quickly redistributed, allowing for a short duration of action. There is no lingering sedation, so it is the anesthetic agent of choice for elderly surgical patients going home after surgery and for MAC procedures where the patient will be discharged home. Propofol has an antiemetic effect.

Propofol is often administered in the intensive care unit (ICU) as a continuous IV infusion for sedation of ventilated patients. Because the elderly brain is more sensitive to propofol and has hemodynamic side effects, IV infusions are started low and cautiously titrated in gerioperative patients. The nurse must check the BP frequently after beginning an IV infusion of propofol as it can cause significant hypotension.

Propofol keeps the patient unconscious but does not provide pain relief. The nurse must administer pain medications to patients on propofol drips when the nurse suspects the patient is having pain. The nurse may have to reduce the IV infusion rate of propofol after pain medication is administration. Outside of the ICU, propofol is administered only by anesthesia providers for acute procedures as it causes severe respiratory depression, respiratory arrest, and hypotension significant enough to lead to cardiac arrest.

ETOMIDATE

Etomidate is the induction agent of choice in emergency surgery or in elderly patients with dehydration, cardiac history, or other comorbidity that can lead to hypotension. Etomidate has been used in some emergency rooms by physicians for minor procedures. The safety of this practice is questionable as etomidate has unpleasant side effects as well as deadly adverse effects. Etomidate can cause burning on injection, myotonic contractions (uncontrolled muscle movements), nausea, vomiting, and hiccoughs. Adverse effects include hypotension, respiratory depression, and adrenal suppression. Adrenal suppression in the gerioperative patient can be significant and may require treatment with hydrocortisone (see Chapter 18). Antiemetic therapy is needed for patients receiving etomidate. While etomidate causes less hypotension than propofol, hypotension is still likely in frail elders. Even though respiratory depression is not as significant in etomidate as other induction agents, etomidate can still cause respiratory arrest. The dose of etomidate needs to be reduced by 15% for the gerioperative patient.

The PACU nurse must be alert to the nausea side effects of etomidate. During handoff, the report should include information regarding administration of antiemetic therapy. If antiemetic therapy was not given, the nurse should obtain an order for ondansetron for immediate administration to prevent nausea. Handoff to the surgical unit nurse should include the need for careful attention to BP effects of etomidate. While adrenal suppression may not be manifested for 24 hours, a symptom of adrenal suppression is refractory hypotension. In the event the patient becomes hypotensive and is not responsive to fluid boluses or medications, adrenal suppression should be considered. After notifying the physician of hypotension and administration of etomidate during surgery, the nurse should obtain an order for hydrocortisone 100 mg IV. Family members should be aware of signs of adrenal suppression that may only be described by the patient as dizziness or fatigue. Other signs and symptoms of adrenal crisis include muscle weakness; abdominal, back, and leg pain; and poor urine output secondary to decreased adrenal function. The family should be coached about the importance of notifying a health care provider if problems occur when the patient returns home.

KETAMINE

Ketamine, a structural analogue of phencyclidine, is a dissociative anesthetic. A dissociative anesthetic causes a depression of some areas of the brain and stimulation of others. Ketamine produces a catatonic state in which the eyes are open; at low doses, the recipient may be able to respond to external stimuli but does not remember the events after administration of the drug. At larger doses, ketamine produces unconsciousness. Respiratory depression is much lower with ketamine, and it is often used for moderate sedation in obese patients with suspected sleep apnea. Ketamine has pain-relieving properties that other induction agents do not possess, so it may not be necessary to administer narcotics, reducing the risk of respiratory depression during the procedure. Ketamine produces a dose-dependent increase in BP and heart rate. Due to its cardiac stimulation, ketamine is often used for induction of anesthesia in trauma patients experiencing hypotension secondary to blood loss. Ketamine must be used with caution in gerioperative patients due to tachycardia that can contribute to myocardial ischemia and intraoperative myocardial infarction.

One of the most undesirable adverse effects of ketamine is an effect on the psyche. Ketamine can produce vivid dreams and dysphoria that usually occur on emergence and recovery. Premedication with a benzodiazepine often mitigates these adverse effects.

Propofol and ketamine are often used together during MAC or TIVA, particularly in elderly patients with an unstable cardiac history. Ketamine reduces the hypotensive and respiratory depressive effects of the propofol and provides analgesia. The propofol decreases the psychogenic side effects of the ketamine. During the PACU handoff, information about ketamine administration is important to prepare the nurse for any psychological or cardiac adverse effects.

METHOHEXITAL, THIOPENTAL

Methohexital and thiopental are infrequently used since propofol and etomidate were introduced as induction agents. Significant side effects of methohexital and thiopental include hypotension and reflex tachycardia on induction of anesthesia. Adverse effects generally wear off prior to leaving the OR.

MUSCLE RELAXANTS

Muscle relaxants are administered during GA to provide for insertion of the endotracheal tube (ETT), paralysis for mechanical ventilation, and skeletal muscle relaxation for the surgical procedure. During abdominal surgery, muscle relaxation allows the surgeon better access into the abdomen. Muscle relaxants block transmission of nerve impulses from the nerve to the muscle at the neuromuscular junction (see Chapter 13). There are two types of muscle relaxants: depolarizers and nondepolarizers.

SUCCINYLCHOLINE

Succinylcholine is a depolarizing muscle relaxant that works by mimicking acetylcholine at the neuromuscular junction. The succinylcholine binds to the cholinergic receptor site on the muscle cell, causing depolarization. The muscles remain paralyzed as long as cholinergic receptor sites are blocked. Succinylcholine has a rapid onset and is metabolized by pseudocholinesterase, an enzyme produced by the liver to break down succinylcholine in 5 to 10 minutes. Once succinyl-choline is metabolized, it cannot be reversed. A deficiency of pseudocholinesterase will cause prolonged muscle paralysis and can prolong intubation up to 24 hours. Pseudocholinesterase deficiency is genetic and can be deadly if a patient is given succinylcholine and extubated too early when the muscles of respiration are still paralyzed and respirations are ineffective. Obtain-ing a preoperative history of previous difficulty with anesthesia or of family history of anesthesia complications can identify patients at risk for pseudocholinesterase deficiency.

Succinylcholine presents a risk for hyperkalemia. Knowledge of the patient's baseline serum potassium level is mandatory. Succinylcholine cannot be used for patients with stroke history or recent bed rest. Potassium released from unused and paralyzed muscles results in hyperkalemia. Due to the potential adverse effects of succinylcholine, its use is often reserved for rapid sequence intubation or for intubation of patients with difficult airways.

ROCURONIUM AND CISATRACURIUM

Recuronium and cisatracurium are nondepolarizing muscle relaxants that act by blocking acetylcholine from reaching the receptor site on the motor end plate. Neuromuscular trans-mission is blocked and results in paralysis. These agents act longer than succinylcholine at 20 to 45 minutes. While the paralyzing effects can wear off, gerioperative patients need to receive reversal agents. Reversal prevents silent aspiration caused by residual paralysis of small muscle groups in the pharynx. These small muscles require longer to recover from nondepolarizing agents.

Interventions

When the gerioperative patient receives GA, the PACU nurse should obtain information as to the type of muscle relaxant and if the patient was reversed. Residual muscle weakness postoperatively due to nonreversal of muscle relaxants or nonmetabolism of succinylcholine can cause ineffective respirations leading to hypoxia and hypercapnia. Additional signs are decreased muscle strength, inability to talk, and ineffective swallowing leading to aspiration.

In the event of recurarization, the nurse should secure the airway and provide oxygen, and the anesthesia provider must be notified immediately.

The PACU nurse should monitor GA patients closely for signs of muscle reparalysis, or recurarization. Recurarization is rare with the newer, shorter-acting muscle relaxants but can still be a serious postoperative complication. Recurariza-tion is the return of some degree of muscle relaxation after the administration of reversal agent. One cause of reparalysis is hypothermia. Hypothermia can prolong the duration of action of the muscle relaxant, and the reversal may wear off before the muscle relaxant. Patients may complain that they cannot breathe or that they may not be able to talk above a whisper. In the event of recurariza-tion, the nurse must first secure the airway and provide oxygen. The anesthesia provider should be notified immediately. Close observation of GA in gerioperative patients is essential.

REVERSAL AGENTS

Anticholinesterase inhibitors, such as neostigmine, pyridostigmine, and edrophonium, reverse the effects of nondepolarizing muscle relaxants, such rocuronium and cisatracurium. The reversal agents differ by onset, duration of action, and metabolism. Neostigmine is the most commonly used reversal agent, working by binding to the enzyme acetylcholinesterase. By binding acetyl-choinesterase, acetycholine is not broken down and can build up in the neuromuscular junction, displacing the muscle relaxant and restoring muscular function. Side effects of anticholinesterase inhibitors include bradycardia, hypotension, bronchoconstriction, and excessive salivation. In order to prevent these side effects, neostigmine is administered with the anticholinergic glycopy-rolate, which blocks the adverse effects of the anticholinesterase inhibitor.

ANTICHOLINERGIC MEDICATIONS

Glycopyrolate

Glycopyrolate is an anticholinergic agent that is relatively safe for the geriatric population. It does not cross the blood-brain barrier and does not cause the confusion and agitation often seen with anticholinergics. Glycopyrolate can cause tachycardia, dry mouth, urinary retention, and blurred vision. Rather than a 1:1 ratio of neostigmine to glycopyrolate, by administering one more milliliter of neostigmine than glycopyrolate, the side effects can be reduced. The ratio prevents the gerioperative patient from becoming tachycardic, which can be an unwelcomed side effect.

ATROPINE

Atropine is an anticholinergic administered in surgery to prevent bradycardia. IV atropine may cause confusion and agitation in the gerioperative patient. The nurse should closely monitor older adults who receive atropine for postoperative delirium and urinary retention.

INHALATION AGENTS

All inhalation agents have similar characteristics. They induce rapid unconsciousness, are absorbed into the alveoli for systemic absorption from the pulmonary circulation, alter the neuronal activity of the central nervous system, are eliminated with ventilation, and are independent of hepatorenal metabolism. While inhalation anesthesia is easily titrated in the gerioperative patient, the level of potency increases with patient age. Minimum alveolar concentration should be reduced by 30% by age 80 to prevent adverse effects of myocardial depression and hypotension.

SEVOFLURANE

Sevoflurane is the best inhalation anesthetic for the gerioperative patient. It is relatively safe, does not cause irritation to airways and coughing, protects the myocardium with coronary vasodila-tion effects, and is quickly eliminated with ventilation. Sevoflurane has replaced isoflurane, origi-nally the gold standard for anesthetic gases. Isoflurane takes longer to reach a therapeutic level and requires a longer elimination time after procedure, so wake up times are longer.

DESFLURANE

Desflurane is the fastest of the anesthetic gases, with a quick onset and offset. However, it is irritating to airways and can cause severe cough, especially in patients with chronic obstruc-tive pulmonary disease or who smoke. It also causes tachycardia, a side effect to be avoided in elderly patients. While research has found that patients are more alert after desflurane, patients have a more intense and faster onset of postsurgical pain. Due to the coughing, tachycardia, and earlier onset of pain, desflurane may not be the best anesthesia choice in the gerioperative patient.

NITROUS OXIDE

Nitrous oxide (N_2O), an odorless and nonirritating anesthetic gas, is always administered with oxygen to prevent hypoxia. N_2O has mild analgesic properties with minimal cardiac depression. N_2O may be mildly stimulating to the sympathetic nervous system. Nitrous oxide is often used as an adjunct to sevoflurane or isoflurane because it does not provide the same level of muscle relaxation as other inhalation agents. N_2O can be used alone for minimal procedures.

INTERVENTIONS

The PACU nurse should be aware of the inhalation agent administered to gauge the sedation and pain perception of the patient. Patients who received isoflurane will be less alert than patients who received sevoflurane and those that received desflurane. Patients who received desflurane will be more alert and need pain medication sooner than patients who receiving sevoflurane or isoflurane. Patients that were administered desflurane may have hyperreactive airways and continue to cough. In the event of a persistent cough, lung sounds should be assessed and a respiratory treatment considered.

Nitrous oxide can decrease the hypoxic drive to breathe. Patients who have had nitrous oxide must be carefully monitored for ventilatory effort in the PACU. Nitrous oxide may cause postoperative nausea and vomiting, although research supporting the association is contradictory.

Types of Anesthesia

The goal of anesthesia is to provide hypnosis, analgesia, amnesia, loss of autonomic reflexes, and skeletal muscle relaxation. With many ways to anesthetize a patient for surgery, the anesthesia provider determines the anesthesia method that is safest for the patient and allows the surgeon optimum surgical conditions to perform the procedure.

GENERAL ANESTHESIA

GA creates a deep level of unconsciousness and generally requires administration of anesthetic gases. GA requires protection of the airway with an ETT or laryngeal mask airway.

Intubation with an ETT is the safest way to protect the airway in patients receiving GA. An ETT is always used in acute abdominal surgery, laparoscopic surgery, obese patients, or patients with gastric reflux. Surgery requiring patients to be prone, side lying, or sitting also requires an ETT. Insertion of the ETT is extremely stimulating to the sympathetic nervous system, resulting in tachycardia and hypertension. When intubating the gerioperative patient, it is important to prevent this hemodynamic response to intubation, because tachycardia and hypertension leads to increased myocardial oxygen consumption. Therefore, fentanyl and occasionally esmolol are administered to blunt the response to ETT insertion. The patient is paralyzed with succinylcholine or a nondepolarizing muscle relaxant prior to intubation to provide the best visualization and open the vocal cords. Paralysis decreases the risk of injury while the ETT is inserted. While intubation is possible without muscle relaxation, a sufficient amount of other medication, such as etomidate, propofol, or fentanyl, must be administered in order to ensure an adequate depth of anesthesia, which would allow for intubation without tachycardia or hypertension. After inserting the ETT, it must be secured in place with an ETT holder rather than tape. Tape harms the gerioperative patient's skin.

Induction of anesthesia and extubation are the most critical periods for patient safety during anesthesia. The nurse can help with cricoid pressure, handing the ETT to the anesthesia provider, and helping to hold the face mask on the patient's face during preintubation. Face mask ventilation can be difficult in edentulous elderly patients. Large, edentulous older adults require two-handed mask holding in order to ventilate. In that case, the nurse may compress the bag valve mask while the anesthesia provider secures the mask. The nurse must be alert to circumstances involving patient safety and be ready to assist in the event of a difficult intubation or patient desaturation.

> *Elders often breathe shallower and at a faster rate.*

Once intubated, mechanical ventilation in the gerioperative patient differs from younger adults. Elders often breathe shallower and at a faster rate. The gerioperative patient is given smaller tidal volumes with more breaths per minute. Peak end-expiratory pressures are maintained, and oxygenation is kept at 50% to prevent atelectasis secondary to denitrogenation caused by 100% oxygenation. At the end of a general anesthetic case, re-expansion of atelectatic alveoli can be accomplished with a few assisted deep breaths that are let out slowly. This is known as recruitment and should be done to expand alveoli prior to extubation.

The laryngeal mask airway (LMA) can be substituted for the ETT when GA is required. The LMA allows the patient to breathe on their own with minimal assistance from the anesthesia provider after the initial period of apnea. The patient is not paralyzed, eliminating the need for anesthesia reversal and the associated side effects from the anticholinergic such as tachycardia, dry mouth, and urinary retention. The LMA is contraindicated in obese patients or those with a significant history of acid reflux. However, older adults often have comorbidities such as smoking and diabetes that can predispose them to gastric reflux. In these cases, even if the patient is asymptomatic, the anesthesia provider must weigh risks and benefits when choosing an LMA or ETT.

MONITORED ANESTHESIA CARE

MAC is a type of anesthesia provided for short uncomplicated procedures that create less sensory stimulation of pain receptors than more complicated surgeries. MAC can also be used in conjunction with a local or regional anesthetic such as a spinal or regional block. The local anesthetic blocks the pain sensation, and the MAC sedation provides amnesia and a light sleep. Fentanyl and midazolam can be administered by the nurses under the direction of a physician for minimal sedation during outpatient procedures. However, MAC allows the use of propofol, which provides moderate sedation. Midazolam is not recommended in older adults, as benzodiazepines create residual effects. MAC decreases physiologic stress with medications that are easier to metabolize. The goal of MAC is to speed recovery, avoid functional decline, and provide early home discharge. MAC promotes one of the most important aspects of gerioperative care: to maintain independence of older adults.

During MAC, IV agents are administered less frequently and in smaller doses due to elders' increased medication sensitivity. Infusion rates are one-third and boluses are half of doses given to younger patients. Even though propofol is rapidly redistributed and recovery is fast, the gerioperative patient may take longer to wake up after a propofol infusion due to slower redistribution rates.

MAC promotes one of the most important aspects of gerioperative care: to maintain independence of older adults.

Hypotension is a common occurrence of elders undergoing MAC. Close monitoring is essential with medications titrated to keep BP in the elder's usual range. If hypotension is not corrected with medication reduction, vasoconstrictors or fluid administration is needed. It is essential to maintain BP to perfuse the heart and brain of the gerioperative patient.

During MAC, elders must be closely monitored for airway obstruction. Age-related changes to the facial muscles and oropharynx increase the risk of impaired ventilation. Airway obstruction can occur at lower doses than younger counterparts.

Monitored Anesthesia Care Postoperative Considerations

MAC requires monitoring for recovery using the same criteria for other types of anesthesia. Preoperative and postoperative management of possible cardiac and respiratory complications is important to prevent morbidity and mortality. Patients breathing on their own can become drowsy and decrease ventilatory effort in the PACU. Vital signs (VSs) should be closely monitored. In the event the elder continually obstructs the airway, an oral or nasal airway is inserted to maintain patency.

MAC, similar to GA, predisposes the gerioperative patient to postoperative cognitive dysfunction and delirium (see Chapter 21). However, less sedation appears to decrease the risk of these complications.

TOTAL INTRAVENOUS ANESTHESIA

TIVA is similar to MAC but produces a deeper level of anesthesia. TIVA includes administration of IV infusions of propofol and another agent, such as ketamine, sufentanil, alfentanil, or remifentanil. TIVA provides GA without muscle relaxation, allowing the patient to maintain independent ventilatory efforts. The recovery process is similar to MAC.

REGIONAL, SPINAL, AND EPIDURAL ANESTHESIA

Regional anesthesia is the application of local anesthetics to the area surrounding a nerve or group of nerves in order to block nerve impulses to the brain. Local anesthetics inhibit nerve conduction by preventing cellular permeability to sodium ions. By blocking depolarization, the action potential is not generated, and the nerve impulse is not conducted. Regional anesthesia can be peripheral or central. Peripheral blocks affect the limbs, such as an interscalene block for shoulder surgery or femoral nerve block for knee surgery. Central regional anesthesia includes spinal and epidural anesthesia.

Spinal anesthesia involves placing a small amount of local anesthetic into the intrathecal space or spinal canal below the first lumbar vertebrae, which avoids trauma to the spinal cord. Epidural anesthesia involves larger amounts of local anesthetics injected into the epidural space. Alternatively, a catheter can be inserted into the epidural space, and a continuous infusion of local anesthetic administered. Placement of an epidural catheter provides pain relief for several hours or days. Epidurals can be placed in the thoracic or lumbar area depending on the area and spinal level of the pain to be treated. Spinal and epidural anesthesia can be used alone or with sedation.

Peripheral nerve blocks are often used with sedation, such as Bier blocks. Interscalene blocks for shoulder surgery are often used for postoperative pain control; during surgery, GA is utilized.

FLUID ADMINISTRATION

Many gerioperative patients are hypovolemic and require IV fluid for hydration (see Chapter 10). Elders with a history of heart failure may also be hypovolemic, as fluid available in the tissues is not in the vascular system. Hypovolemia causes hypotension and tachycardia. Patients with a history of hypertension, diabetes, or renal insufficiency may be hypovolemic preoperatively due to disease processes and medications. During surgery, the anesthesia provider administers fluids based on surgical events, length of surgery, and fluid requirements for body type. Intraoperatively, urine output is documented by the circulating nurse. Fluid balance calculations are an integral part of the postoperative handoff. Fluid volume deficits or excessive administration of fluids influences the postoperative course. The surgical unit nurse must consider the perioperative fluid input and output when evaluating postoperative renal function.

Fluids administered perioperatively are usually mobilized and shifted back into the vascular system by the third postoperative day. At this time, hormonal changes in antidiuretic hormone changes return to normal and diuresis occurs. Fluid overload in the elderly that is not mobilized may be the source of a potential cardiac problem and requires further follow-up.

AGE-RELATED ANESTHESIA CONSIDERATIONS

The type of anesthesia, GA, regional anesthesia, or TIVA, has little influence on gerioperative mortality, morbidity, or complications such as postoperative delirium. The quality of the anesthesia delivered is more important than the type of anesthesia.

There are many variables to be considered when determining the optimum anesthesia including the type, duration, urgency, and invasiveness of the surgery; patient medical comorbidities; mental status of the patient; as well as the skill and expertise of the anesthesia provider and surgeon. One of the most important considerations is to optimize the overall management of the gerioperative patient during the perioperative period and to maintain anesthetic techniques that are safe for the older adult. Regional anesthesia techniques appear to be healthier for the gerioperative patient because there is minimal sedation during the procedure, patients are breathing on their own, and excellent postoperative pain control decreases the amount of medications administered to the patient. Also, the risks of thromboembolic events, blood loss, and the incidence of deep vein thrombosis (DVT) are diminished following hip surgery under spinal anesthesia.

> *The quality of the anesthesia delivered is more important than the type of anesthesia.*

However, age-related changes in the nervous system cause an increased sensitivity to local anesthetics in older adults. Decline in the number of neurons, deterioration of the myelin sheath, slowed conduction velocity, and changes to the anatomy of the spinal column, along with slower clearance time of local anesthetics, require decreased doses of local anesthetic and decreased intervals between doses. While there are differences between local anesthetics, large doses of local anesthetic are to be avoided in the gerioperative population.

Interventions

The general rule of gerioperative medication administration ("start with a low dose") is also true for local anesthetics. Systemic toxicity from local anesthetics generally occurs due to accidental intravascular injection. However, toxicity in the elderly may be dose-related. There is no reversal of local anesthetic agents, so supportive care is provided until the medication is metabolized. Symptoms may begin as lightheadedness, dizziness, tinnitus, a funny or metallic taste in mouth, and disorientation, and may progress to muscle twitching and seizures. Cardiovascular symptoms include hypotension or increased PR and QRS interval noted on the cardiac monitor. Local anesthetic toxicity is a medical emergency. Once assessed, the perioperative nurse must be prepared to implement advanced cardiac life-saving interventions and supportive care.

Spinal anesthesia carries greater risk and technical difficulty for older adults than in younger adults. Patient positioning and needle insertion can be more difficult due to arthritic changes to the spine. Common side effects of spinal anesthesia in all patients include hypotension, bradycardia, urinary retention, nausea and vomiting, and extensive spread of the anesthetic agent to high spinal levels. In older adults, hypotension can be more pronounced due to preoperative dehydration secondary to nothing-by-mouth status, disease processes, and medications. Administration of additional IV fluids to elderly patients prior to the spinal can mitigate the hypotensive effect. A high spinal can be detrimental to the gerioperative patient by causing dramatic hypotension, respiratory compromise, and bradycardia that can result in poorer outcomes than for the younger surgical patient. The perioperative nurse must closely monitor older adults receiving spinal anesthesia for changes in respiratory and cardiovascular status. Early intervention is critical.

Epidural anesthesia is also technically more difficult to perform in the older adult than a younger adult. Arthritic changes to the back make needle insertion difficult, and there is an increased risk of nerve damage, especially in the thoracic area. Age-related changes increasing permeability of the dura, and increasing size of the arachnoid villi result in rapid onset of epidural anesthesia. It is necessary to reduce the dose of local anesthetic bolus and infusion in the elderly to avoid the increased risk of severe hypotension and respiratory depression. Perioperative nurses must closely monitor the older epidural anesthesia patient for any hemodynamic or respiratory adverse effects.

Urinary retention can be a problem following epidural anesthesia, especially in the elderly. Postoperatively, if there is no urine output for several hours, a bladder scan is done to assess the patient's need for a straight or Foley catheter. Check lower extremities frequently for neuromuscular function. Neurological checks should be performed to assess for changes in mental status related to local anesthetic toxicity. Assess the skin on the back for breakdown secondary to the epidural dressing or moisture from catheter leakage. The epidural tubing should be checked to ensure it has not become disconnected and that the catheter is not contaminated. The epidural catheter length needs to be documented because the epidural catheter can shift secondary to patient movement. The patient's pain control is carefully monitored as pain control will change in the event that the catheter shifts.

Intraoperatively, during regional anesthesia, patients may be mildly sedated on a continuous low-dose propofol infusion. Because the patient is essentially awake, positioning is important. Elders' arthritic changes make it difficult to position a patient to comfort. Proper positioning devices, padding, and head support are imperative. During the procedure, the nurse should keep in mind that the region of the body that is blocked does not feel pain, but other areas remain sensitive. Gerioperative patients become stiff and sore lying on a hard OR table. Administration of small doses of fentanyl along with the propofol drip improves patient comfort. Minor repositioning under the drape during surgery redistributes pressure off sore areas or changes alignment of uncomfortable limbs.

Patients on antiplatelet therapy are not candidates for spinal or epidural anesthesia due to the risk of hematoma formation and potential nerve injury. Communication with the anesthesia provider during the preoperative assessment, when information on use of warfarin, clopidogrel, aspirin, or heparin is identified, is crucial. Additional information on the time and date of the last dose is important. Elders who have not taken antiplatelet drugs for several days may be candidates depending on number of days and laboratory values. Coagulation studies can confirm risk of bleeding and abnormal results are reported immediately to the surgeon and anesthesia provider.

Positioning

The procedure and the surgeon's preference determine how the patient is to be positioned for the duration of the surgery. However, severe complications such as pressure ulcers and nerve damage can be attributed to improper positioning. The surgical team, nurse, anesthesia provider, and surgeon should collaborate to ensure the gerioperative patient is safely positioned for comfort and physiologic stability. Patient positioning is often a balancing act between the demands of the surgeon, the particular position necessary for the procedure, and the needs of the patient (Table 8.2). Positioning becomes complicated for older adults due to age-related disease processes and comorbid conditions (Table 8.3).

The preoperative interview of the older adult includes identifying any limitations to range of motion or movement. Knowledge of previous surgeries impacts surgical position. The nurse and anesthesia provider should determine if the elder has any neck, back, or leg pain preoperatively. Muscle weakness or numbness and tingling in the feet, legs, hands, or fingers must be documented. If the gerioperative patient has significant back or leg problems and the patient will be supine during surgery, it can be suggested to the patient that positioning can occur prior to induction of anesthesia. In these cases, the patient will be able to communicate any pressure areas or pain due to positioning prior to the induction of anesthesia.

> *Patient positioning is often a balancing act between the demands of the surgeon, the particular position necessary for the procedure, and the needs of the patient.*

Anesthesia impacts positioning by causing analgesia, amnesia, elimination of reflexes, and muscle relaxation. Anesthesia blocks the body's response to pain and pressure increasing the gerioperative patient's vulnerability to injury. Without pain, a patient's joints can be overextended or a

TABLE 8.2
Important Considerations for Operative Positioning

- Access to airway
- Access to surgical site
- Ability to monitor all vital signs
- Patient safety
- Patient comfort

TABLE 8.3
Individual Considerations for Operative Positioning

- Patient age, height, and weight
- Preexisting conditions
- Limited range of motion
- Previous surgeries
- Presence of joint prosthesis
- Present or past fractures

nerve compromised, injuring the nerve or muscle. Even if muscle relaxation permits, the patient's normal range of motion must never be exceeded. Anesthesia causes autonomic dysfunction and vasodilation that contributes to low BP. Positioning can often exacerbate the problems of vasodilation and poor perfusion. Hypovolemia contributes to hypotension and decreased tissue perfusion. The combination of muscle relaxation, poor positioning, and hypoperfusion leads to pressure ulcer formation (see Chapter 14).

Many sources of pressure exist during surgery, including the pressure of the patient's body on the OR table, equipment leaning or rubbing against the skin, personnel leaning on the patient during the procedure, and positioning devices such as leg and arm holders. The intraoperative team must work together to prevent any skin injuries, pressure ulcers, or nerve injuries while the patient is anesthetized and helpless. The nurse must become the patient's advocate and be vigilant while positioning to prevent injury. When there is a difference of opinion about a patient's positioning, the nurse must advocate for patient safety first and work to find a compromise.

The most common positions for anesthesia are supine, lithotomy, lateral, prone, and positioning on the fracture table. Each position has different pressure points and complications that can affect the gerioperative patient.

SUPINE

In the supine position, the gerioperative patient is at increased risk for backache secondary to laxity of vertebral ligaments that put additional pressure on vertebral joints. Alleviate the pressure by placing a pillow under the heels, relieving strain on the vertebral joints. Many elderly patients are kyphotic. The patient's neck and upper back must be supported to prevent injury. Piling up pillows and blankets often provides enough support. As the pillows and blankets are applied to support the neck and back, more blankets must be placed under the arms to prevent brachial plexus stress and strain. The arm must be supported at the level of the shoulder. After positioning, the nurse palpates over the anterior shoulder joint to assess for any sensation of stretch over the brachial plexus. Extra padded elevated arm support is needed for supine obese patients or when a sandbag is used for positioning.

Elderly patients may have conditions such as adhesive capsulitis (frozen shoulder) or other mobility issues that prevent them from stretching their arms out on the arm boards. Arms can be protected by tucking them to the sides to prevent injury. The elbows must be padded to prevent ulnar nerve injury from pressure against the edge of the mattress. Injuries to the radial nerve have been noted from arms falling off the arm board or by surgical personnel leaning on the arm. To prevent these complications, arms are secured with arm straps. The circulating nurse and anesthesia provider must monitor personnel during surgery and direct them to change position if leaning is noted.

Gerioperative patients often have contractures to the elbows and knees that may prevent them from placing the extremities flat against the OR table or on an arm board. Pillows placed under knees provide support, as do pillows and blankets under the hands when arms are not able to stretch and lay flat on the arm board. The supine position increases pressure over the sacrum, elbows, heels, and back of the head. These areas must be padded for protection. In the case of the back of the head, a donut pillow is used for long procedures to prevent pressure alopecia.

BEACH CHAIR

The beach chair position is a modified supine position that sits the patient, allowing for access to the shoulder. The position takes pressure off the vertebral ligaments but increases pressure to the sacrum. The biggest risk in this position is hypotension and decreased cardiac output as much as 20% to 40%, which occurs when blood is shifted downward away from the upper body. A known complication of this position is loss of eyesight, possibly related to hypotension and hypoperfusion to the eyes. In order to compensate for hypotension, fluids can be administered, and vasopressor drips such as neosynephrine can be initiated. The BP goal for older adults is to maintain the systolic BP within 20% of normal range to sustain organ perfusion. The use of vaso-constrictors increases the risk of pressure ulcers secondary to decreased peripheral tissue perfu-sion. If vasoconstrictors are required, the postoperative handoff report must include information about the hypotension and the need to assess for pressure ulcers during surgical recovery.

LITHOTOMY

The lithotomy position is used for surgeries requiring access to the perineal area. The litho-tomy position is a precarious position for elders and is used for urologic, gynecologic, and rectal procedures, as well as some abdominal and perineal surgeries. Nerves at risk for injury in this position include common peroneal, obturator, saphenous, and femoral. Placing geri-atrics' legs, with decreased range of motion, up in the air and abducted can be uncomfortable. There are several variations of lithotomy position based on the degree of elevation of the legs: low or less than 45 degrees, standard 45 to 90 degrees, and exaggerated 100 degrees or higher, with the pelvis lifted off the bed.

The lithotomy position results in postoperative hip, back, and inner thigh pain. To mini-mize the positioning effects, the sacrum and knees must be padded and the legs well sup-ported. The hips must not be flexed greater than 90 degrees to prevent postoperative hip pain. Abduction should be as narrow as possible to allow the surgical team to work without stress-ing the hips of the gerioperative patient. Patients with hip replacements are especially vul-nerable to abduction and external rotation. Special care must be taken to prevent dislocation of the prosthesis. Age-related changes to peripheral circulation require that the circulating nurse make frequent checks of pedal pulses and color of the feet throughout the procedure. Accurate assessment can identify if the leg position has occluded major blood vessels and compromised the circulation.

Legs placed in stirrups produce an autotransfusion of blood from the legs into the cen-tral circulation. The fluid shift increases cardiac output and venous return. At the end of the procedure, the legs must be removed slowly to prevent sudden fluid shifts. As the legs are placed down on the OR table, the blood is diverted from the central circulation back to the legs causing temporary hypotension. In the elderly, recovery from hypotension takes longer and may need to be supplemented with vasoconstrictor and fluids to minimize decreased perfusion to vital organs.

The lithotomy position imposes challenges to respiration and ventilation. Elderly patients in general, especially those with kyphosis, will find it more difficult to breath due to increased abdominal pressure and decreased diaghramatic movement. Even if patients are sedated or anesthetized, ventilation can become an issue secondary to stiff rib cages and increased pressure from abdominal contents. Changes may need to be made in ventilatory settings, and LMA breathing may need to be assisted to achieve larger tidal volumes.

In the lithotomy position, arms are placed abducted on padded arm boards. Elders with decreased shoulder range of motion and obese patients present a challenge. Taping the arms across the chest may be considered if abdominal exposure is not necessary.

LATERAL POSITION

The lateral position is used for orthopedic, kidney, and thoracic procedures. Nerves at increased risk for injury are the suprascapular nerve, peroneal nerve, and axillary nerve. The major concern for the gerioperative patient in this position is ventilation-perfusion mismatch (see Chapter 11), which can be best addressed with mechanical ventilation.

The arms should have no muscle tension, pressure, or nerve compression.

In the lateral position, body alignment in the elderly is essential. After the axillary roll is placed, the neck must be aligned with the body. Alignment often requires a pillow or blanket under the head and neck to maintain cervical thoracic support. The ears must be flat on the down side and the eyes without pressure. Legs must be aligned and padded with flexion at the knee. A pillow between the legs maintains leg alignment. Arms must be placed on arm boards and padded. In the elderly, it may be difficult to extend the arms due to normal age-related muscle contraction. Pillows are placed under the arms for support. When providing support to maintain the lateral position, many padded braces have plastic covers that can stick to elders' skin and cause abrasions when removed. The circulating nurse must ensure that tape used to stabilize the patient is not directly against the skin.

In the event the bed is flexed for additional exposure, the patient's position must be rechecked and additional support provided as necessary. Pooling of blood in the extremities predisposes the elderly to DVT. Surgical compression devices are put in place prior to entering the OR suite.

PRONE

The prone position is used for spinal procedures, craniotomies, orthopedic procedures, and some rectal procedures. Positioning the older adult patient in this position can be challenging. The patient must be log rolled from the stretcher to the OR table. Arms must be brought up by the head and flexed, padded, and placed on arm boards or secured at sides. This must be done carefully as elders have brittle bones and decreased range of motion. The arms must be protected from muscle tension, pressure, or nerve compression. Radial pulses need to be checked regularly to assess for circulation compromise.

The knees are flexed with padded knee pads, and feet are elevated slightly. In the prone position, fluid can accumulate in dependent areas of hands, feet, face, and eyes. The transient edema can exacerbate conditions such as intermittent carpal tunnel syndrome.

The head is placed in a special "prone" pillow that is designed to support the head and prevent pressure to the eyes and nose. The eyes and nose must be checked frequently. The neck must be in alignment with the body to prevent neck injuries.

The patient is placed on rolls or gel pads at the hips and shoulders to elevate the abdomen and keep it free of pressure. Elderly patients with large abdomens can have decreased venous return secondary to abdominal pressure in the prone position. Supporting the patient on a special bed frame, blankets, or gel rolls frees the abdomen and decreases the risk of epidural vein engorgement and decreased venous return. Elderly patients are often kyphotic, and special positioning must be used to accommodate the spine curvature. The penis and scrotum must be free of pressure or compression.

Vision loss is an uncommon but devastating complication of the prone position. Risks also include hypotension, diabetes, anemia, blood loss, fluid management, adverse drug effects, and extended prone position. Prevention includes ensuring that there is no pressure to the eyes, replacing blood loss, maintaining normotension, and monitoring fluid replacement.

FRACTURE BED

A fracture bed is necessary to position patients for femur and hip fracture repair. The bed applies traction to the operative leg to manipulate, realign, and fixate the fracture in a position for hardware insertion. The arm on the fracture side is taped over the chest. A padded vertical pole is placed in the perineal area to stabilize the pelvis. The pole puts pressure on the perineal area and may cause damage to the pudendal nerve and the genitalia. Positioning on this bed is difficult, and the nurse and anesthesia provider must work together to prevent further injury to the patient.

Positioning the elderly for surgical procedures can be time-consuming and labor-intensive. The circulating nurse, anesthesia provider, and surgeon must work together to ensure that the best possible positioning for patient safety is attained. Shifts during surgery can alter even the best positioning. Frequent checking of arms, legs, eyes, nose, neck, and head prevents pressure and nerve injuries.

Anesthesia Emergency

MALIGNANT HYPERTHERMIA

Malignant hyperthermia (MH) is a life-threatening reaction triggered by exposure to anesthetic gasses and succinylcholine. MH is hereditary. The risk of an unidentified case of MH among older adults is low. Many elderly have previously undergone anesthesia and would have experienced an MH episode. During the preoperative interview, the patient should be asked about a family history of anesthetic reactions or previous reactions to anesthesia.

Surgical Care Improvement Project

The Surgical Care Improvement Project (SCIP) is a national quality improvement project designed to improve the care of hospitalized surgical patients. A goal was to decrease surgical complications by 25% by the year 2010. SCIP is utilized in hospitals to promote patient care. The surgical complications targeted in SCIP include surgical site infections (SSIs), DVT, intraoperative myocardial infarction, hypothermia, and glucose monitoring during open heart surgery.

Postoperative SSIs are a primary cause of postoperative morbidity and mortality. The gerioperative patient is particularly susceptible to SSIs secondary to diminished immune function, skin changes, changes to wound healing, decreased nutrition, and changes to mobility and function that may directly impact wound care. SCIP methods to decrease wound infections include ensuring that antibiotic prophylaxis is administered within 1 hour of incision, that the right antibiotic is administered for the procedure being done, that prophylactic antibiotics are discontinued within 24 hours of surgery, and that correct surgical hair removal has been performed. All of these measures are critical for the gerioperative patient due to age-related changes (see Chapter 17).

The same day surgery nurse, surgical unit nurse, circulating nurse, and PACU nurse must all work together and communicate through handoff reports to enforce the SCIP guidelines. The nurses, anesthesia providers, and surgeons must all work together as a team to ensure compliance with the guidelines and patient safety. All involved must make sure that allergies are carefully annotated and that appropriate antibiotics are prescribed considering the patient's allergies. Surgical areas should be trimmed or clipped with an electric clipper rather than shaved with a handheld razor. Razors cause nicks in the skin and introduce sources of infection.

DVT is discussed in Chapter 16. The major complication of DVT, pulmonary embolism (PE), is reviewed in Chapter 11. The gerioperative patient is more susceptible to DVT and PE secondary to changes in vasculature, atherosclerosis, circulation, and mobility. Comorbid disease such as stroke, heart failure, chronic obstructive pulmonary disease, and lower leg injuries also increase the risk of DVT. The elderly often do not have signs and symptoms of DVT and often do not have chest pain with PE.

> *Prevention of hypothermia is less labor-intensive and cost-effective compared with efforts and equipment required to warm a hypothermic patient.*

Advanced age is an independent predictor of mortality from DVT and PE. Even though the risk of DVT is higher in older adults, studies have indicated that up to 50% of hospitalized patients do not receive DVT prophylaxis. Elderly patients are less likely to receive pneumatic compression devices and heparin prophylaxis than younger patients. SCIP recommendations include chemical and mechanical DVT prophylaxis, including subcutaneous heparin and pneumatic compression devices for all surgical patients. Again the surgeon, anesthesia provider, and nurse must work together to ensure DVT prophylaxis is ordered and correctly implemented.

The compression provided by the pneumatic stocking can disrupt skin integrity. The skin under the device must be assessed prior to placing the pneumatic stockings. Compression stockings are used with caution in elderly patients with peripheral vascular disease, as the compression may actually decrease circulation to the lower extremities. Knee-high compression stockings placed on the legs must be wrinkle free.

Hypothermia is defined as a core body temperature below 36° C (98.6° F). Hypothermia produces vasoconstriction, which can impair neutrophil phagocytosis and decrease function of the immune system. In the older adult, there is less vasoconstriction per degree fall in temperature. The decrease in vasoconstriction promotes greater heat loss to the environment. Hypothermia increases the risk for infection, myocardial infarction, arrhythmias, blood loss, prolonged mechanical ventilation, and mortality. Hypothermia can decrease the rate of drug metabolism, increasing the time to wake up after general anesthesia.

Older adults are more susceptible to hypothermia due to changes in body composition. Elders have less muscle mass, which decreases basal metabolic rate, and less subcutaneous fat. A lower rate decreases the amount of heat produced, while less fat decreases insulation ability.

Shivering increases heat energy; however, the shivering mechanism is delayed in the elderly secondary to changes in the hypothalamic-pituitary-adrenal axis. Elders may not shiver until the core temperature has fallen by 2° C. Anesthesia and surgery further contribute to cooling due to vasodilation and surgical exposure. Prevention of hypothermia is less labor-intensive and more cost-effective compared with efforts and equipment required to warm a hypothermic patient.

While the circulating nurse and the anesthesia provider work together to keep the gerioperative patient warm, elders are also susceptible to overheating due to atrophy of sweat glands. When using warm ambient OR temperatures, forced air warming devices, heated IV fluids, and humidivents to warm and moisturize anesthetic gases, patients must be closely monitored for overheating.

The gerioperative patient is susceptible to intraoperative myocardial infarction secondary to cardiac and vascular changes (see Chapter 9). The SCIP protocol calls for patients on beta blockers to receive them prior to surgery. During the preoperative interview, elderly patients taking beta blockers need to be carefully coached to take the beta blocker on schedule, either the morning of surgery or the night before surgery. The nurse, anesthesia provider, and surgeon must determine whether the beta blocker was taken. If the oral beta blocker was not taken, an order is obtained to administer the oral beta blockers in the preoperative holding area with water, as soon as possible.

Hyperglycemia is a common response to anesthesia, metabolic stress, and critical illness. Surgical stress and trauma cause release of cortisol, glucagon, epinephrine, and growth hormone (see Chapter 18). Perioperative hyperglycemia leads to impaired chemotaxis and phagocytosis, increased adhesion of cells, decreased complement function, and decreased vasodilation. The changes increase elders' vulnerability to infection, decrease wound healing, and multiorgan dysfunction. Intraoperative hyperglycemia is detrimental. However, less clear is the goal for glucose control in the OR, as hypoglycemia can be detrimental to brain function. Depending on the glucose control of the individual patient, what may be perceived as hypoglycemic to the brain may be relative to what the normal blood sugar is for that patient. As an example, if a patient's normal blood sugar is poorly controlled, with average readings of 275 mg/dL, decreasing the blood sugar to 100 mg/dL may be hypoglycemic to the patient's brain. It seems reasonable that until there is clear evidence about the best glucose control for surgical patient, the blood sugar should be maintained close to what is normal for that particular patient.

PATIENT REPORT: Mr. Tung Ming Wang

After consulting with the surgeon, the anesthesia provider determines that spinal anesthesia may be a good choice for Mr. Wang. The surgery is relatively short, and the lithotomy position is necessary for the procedure. The spinal anesthetic, positioning, and infusion of medication for light sleep (propofol) are discussed with Mr. Wang. The potential side effects of midazolam are also discussed. Mr. Wang decides he would like the spinal anesthetic but does not want to risk the side effects of midazolam. He is taken to the PACU for preoperative insertion of the spinal anesthetic. He is given 100 mcg of fentanyl IV, and placed on oxygen and monitors. The spinal is inserted without difficulty by the anesthesiologist. Mr. Wang tolerates the procedure well. The nurse anesthetist comes to the PACU to retrieve the patient for surgery, and a minimal transition report is given. The nurse anesthetist is not informed about the IV fluids given in PACU. The patient is taken to the OR suite and subsequently moved onto the OR table with a slide board. In the process of moving the patient, the IV is dislodged. As soon as the patient is secure on the OR table, VS monitors are attached, and VSs are checked. The BP is

80/40 and heart rate is 80. With no IV to administer fluids or medications, oxygen is placed on the patient and VSs monitored continually. The circulating nurse restarts the IV and phenylephrine is given by the anesthesia provider. The nurse reviews the chart and finds the patient did not receive a fluid bolus in the PACU prior to spinal administration. A 500-mL fluid bolus is administered along with the phenylephrine, and the BP climbs to 130/80. The phenylephrine drip is maintained while the patient is sedated to maintain a BP around 140 systolic. The propofol drip is started. The combination of propofol and fentanyl provides Mr. Wang with a light sleep during the procedure. When he wakes up after the procedure, he is alert and oriented. He does not remember anything after the propofol drip was started, and he states he has no pain. Mr. Wang is transported to the PACU without the phenylephrine drip.

In the PACU, his VSs are stable, and his BP is 130/80. Over the course of the next half hour, the BP drops steadily to 110/50. The PACU nurse checks the preanesthesia VSs and realizes the patient's normal BP is 160/65. The nurse realizes that although a BP of 110/50 is "normal," for Mr. Wang it is not high enough to maintain brain perfusion in a 92-year-old man who has had a previous stroke. The nurse notifies the anesthesia provider who orders a phenylephrine drip to maintain BP between 140 and 150 systolic until the spinal anesthesia wears off. As the anesthesia wears off, the BP increases and the phenylephrine drip is weaned. Mr. Wang is transferred to the floor without the vasoconstrictor, and his BP at time of transfer is 156/55.

SUMMARY

Each gerioperative patient requires an individualized anesthetic plan. Older adults are more susceptible to the effects of anesthesia medications. Anesthetic medication doses in the elderly should be decreased, and the intervals between doses should be increased. "Start low and go slow" with vigilant monitoring is critically important during surgery because of the powerful adverse side effects of anesthetic agents. Anesthesia impacts all body systems. Promoting patient safety in the OR should be the top priority of all team members.

KEY POINTS

- Geriatric patients are not just "old adults." Geriatric patients have a unique set of risks and complications.
- Anesthetic medication doses should be decreased for older adults and the intervals between doses should be increased.
- During surgery and in the immediate postsurgical area, gerioperative patients may require a dose of narcotic similar to younger patients in order to control postoperative pain.
- Induction of anesthesia and extubation are the most critical periods for patient safety during anesthesia.
- The nurse, anesthesia personnel, and the surgeon should make sure the gerioperative patient is safely positioned for the patient's safety, comfort, and physiologic stability during the surgical procedure.

NINE

Cardiovascular

David Durant, Susan J. Fetzer, and Jennifer V. Long

PATIENT REPORT: Mr. Brookshire

Mr. Brookshire, a 67-year-old widower, visits the surgical nurse practitioner (NP) for his preoperative evaluation. He is scheduled for a femoral-popliteal bypass in 4 weeks. He brings his brown bag of medications and his son as a companion-coach to the appointment. During the interview, he tells the NP that he has had trouble walking more than a block for the past month. He is a retired postal carrier and walked several miles a day without problems before he retired 2 years ago. He was forced to retire because of a heart attack. His past medical history includes an appendectomy and cholecystectomy. His medications include metoprolol, a baby aspirin, and cilostazol.

The NP completes her assessment and notes that Mr. Brookshire has a midsternal scar. Upon questioning, Mr. Brookshire says that he had a double bypass after his heart attack, but has not had any pain since then. The nurse assesses Mr. Brookshire's risk for cardiac complications. He has major clinical predictors and moderate functional ability and will undergo a high-risk procedure. According to his medical record, Mr. Brookshire has not had an electrocardiogram (EKG) for a year. The NP orders a preoperative EKG. As Mr. Brookshire has difficulty walking, the NP requests a preoperative dobutamine stress test. Mr. Brookshire and his companion-coach will return to the preoperative clinic after the stress test is performed.

The cardiovascular system exerts the most influence on anesthesia and perioperative outcomes. Cardiovascular changes occur at the structural, functional, and molecular level. Declining cardiac function is accelerated and exacerbated by chronic diseases. Age-related changes to the cardiovascular system combine with genetic predisposition and lifestyle, making elders vulnerable to the stress of surgery, anesthesia, and recovery. Though the heart generally functions well under resting conditions, age-related changes diminish cardiac reserve. This chapter reviews the anatomical and physiological changes in the cardiovascular system with aging. Gerioperative care to minimize and detect cardiac complications is presented.

Cardiac Considerations

The cardiovascular system includes the four-chambered heart and great vessels, arteries, and veins. Included in the anatomic structure of the heart is an electrical system that controls contractions of the four chambers to ensure the heart pumps in a controlled, regulated fashion in response to the physical demands of the body. The components of the electrical system include the sinoatrial (SA) node, the atrioventricular (AV) node, the bundle of His, and the left and right bundle ventricular branches, which conduct the electrical impulses to the myocardium of the ventricles. The heart is composed of three layers: the outside epicardium containing the coronary arteries and veins, the middle myocardial or muscle layer, and the inner endocardial layer. The muscle mass of the left ventricle exceeds that of the right ventricle, allowing it to generate more force under greater pressure. Surrounding the heart is a thin pericardial lining, with pericardial fluid excreted by the cells of the pericardium into the space between the epicardium and the pericardium. The pericardial fluid lubricates the membranes allowing them to slide over one another with each contraction.

Blood begins flowing into the heart as it returns through the venous system via the superior and inferior vena cava. Entering the right atrium passively, blood passes through the tricuspid valve, which is open during diastole or rest. A signal from the SA node causes the atria to contract and deliver the remaining blood in the atria into the ventricle. At the same time this process is occurring, the right ventricle is re-expanding, having just completed its own ejection of blood. Because it is relatively empty and re-expanding, the pressure within the right ventricle is lower than the pressure from the inflowing blood from the right atrium and so the blood flows freely into the ventricle. The added amount of blood forced into the ventricle during atrial contraction is the atrial "kick" and accounts for approximately one-third of the ventricular volume.

Atrial contraction or kick contributes one-third of diastolic volume.

Following the active filling of the ventricle, the impulse from the SA node has traversed to the gatekeeper or AV node. Passage of the impulse continues down the bundle of His to the left and right bundle branch of the ventricle ending at the Purkinje fibers of the myocardium. The electrical stimulation excites muscle contraction, resulting in ventricular contraction. Contraction increases ventricular pressure, closes the tricuspid valve, and opens the pulmonic valve, sending the blood forward into the pulmonary circulatory system. The process is repeated in the left side of the heart as the left atria passively receive oxygenated blood returning from the pulmonary system. After passively filling the left ventricle through an open mitral valve, the SA impulse from the SA node in the right atria conducts to the left atria, and the remaining blood is forced into the left ventricle. The electrical impulse continues through the AV node, bundle branches, and Purkinje fibers, and the powerful left ventricular myocardium contracts. The mitral value closes under pressure, the aortic value opens, and blood is ejected into the aorta and the systemic circulation. Ejection can be detected as the pulse wave travels to smaller vessels such as the brachial and radial arteries. As the pulse wave travels to smaller vessels, further from the heart, blood pressure increases. Thus, the blood pressure in the lower extremities is different than in the upper extremities.

Blood flows through the arterial system under pressure. Systolic pressure from myocardial ejection forces the blood forward. Peripheral resistance occurs as the arteries leading to arterioles become smaller. Diastolic or resting pressure is affected by the peripheral resistance. During vasoconstriction, peripheral resistance increases, forcing the heart to pump harder to eject blood.

Nitric oxide, produced by the endothelium, inhibits platelets.

The arteries are composed of three tissue layers: the internal intima or endothelial layer, the middle or media layer, and the outer or adventia layer. The intima, composed of endothelial cells, is in constant contact with blood cells and plasma. The endothelial cells produce and release nitric oxide (NO). The NO releases signals to the surrounding vessel to vasodilate, inhibits platelets from aggregating, and prevents white blood cells from adhering to the cell wall. Chemicals such as acetylcholine, histamine, and thrombin stimulate additional release of nitric oxide. The media layer is composed of smooth muscle and elastin fibers with innervation by the sympathetic nervous system. The media layer of the larger arteries can have five to seven layers of circular and longitudinal muscle cells. The outer adventitia layer includes collagen and more elastin fibers. The adventitia layer anchors the vessel to surrounding tissues. Elastin provides flexibility while collagen provides strength and support. The muscle layer allows arteries to contract or relax in response to nervous system stimulation. The muscle layer ranges from the diameter of the aorta at 3 cm to the capillary, which is one cell wide.

The venous system holds 60% of the body's blood volume.

After exchanging oxygen for carbon dioxide at the cellular level, blood returns to the venous system. Unlike arteries, veins have few organized muscle fibers in the media layer. The intima layer has folds within the vein that serve as one-way valves. The valves prevent the blood from pooling in the extremities due to the lack of muscle in the vein. The venous system has the capacity to hold 60% of the body's blood volume.

Blood is supplied to the heart by three coronary arteries. Two ostia, or openings, in the aorta just past the aortic valve lead to the right coronary artery and the left main coronary artery. The left main coronary artery is very short, dividing after 25 mm into the left circumflex and left anterior descending coronary arteries. During systole, the aortic valve cusps open and cover the coronary ostia. It is only during diastole that blood flows into the coronary arteries and supplies the heart with needed oxygen. When the heart rate increases, the period of diastole, or rest, decreases, reducing the amount of oxygenated blood delivered to the myocardium.

Heart filling and cardiac oxygenation during diastole is severely compromised when the heart rate increases.

AGE-RELATED CHANGES

Heart muscle cells, or myocytes, lack the ability to regenerate and are programmed at birth for apoptosis, or cell death. Approximately 25 million myocytes per year undergo apoptosis, and the remaining muscle cells compensate by increasing their cellular components. The hypertrophy of the remaining viable myocytes results in an increased ventricular mass. As myocytes die, they are replaced by fibroblasts (see Chapter 16). The fibroblasts continue to divide, producing collagen and stiffening the heart muscle. The ventricle of an older adult is less compliant. The increased stiffness and reduced compliance impairs passive ventricular filling during diastole.

With age, the heart valves degenerate. The valve opening, or annulus, dilates, and calcium deposits along the edges of the valve leaflets. Calcified leaflets are stiff and hard. By 80 years old, nearly 50% of aortic valves and 40% of mitral valves will be calcified. When valve calcification is severe, usually over age 70, symptoms of valvular stenosis will occur. Aortic stenosis requires that the left ventricle contract harder and longer to eject blood. If the ventricle is unable to compensate, cardiac output will drop. Classic symptoms of aortic stenosis include syncope, angina, and sudden death. Age-related changes accounts for over 50% of the prevalence of aortic stenosis. Mitral valve insufficiency results in a stretched mitral annulus. Blood regurgitates during systole, increasing left atrial pressure; over time, this results in left atrial dilation. As blood is ejected backward into the pulmonary system, the pulmonary vascular pressure increases. Gas exchange is impaired, and the elder complains of dyspnea on exertion.

Gender differences exist with aging as women appear to have more active myocytes than men of similar age, even though their hearts are smaller. Ventricular hypertrophy in women tends to be concentric, while men are more likely to develop hypertrophy eccentrically (see Figure 9.1).

Concentric hypertrophy is the result of pressure overload such as with chronic hypertension. The heart must compensate for higher systemic pressure by developing more sarcomeres parallel to existing sarcomeres to increase strength of contraction against pressure. This causes increased ventricular wall thickness with resulting smaller ventricular chambers. As the process continues, the ventricular walls become stiff and less compliant affecting ventricular filling; diastolic heart failure (HF) often results. When hypertension is diagnosed and controlled, the process can be interrupted.

Eccentric hypertrophy is often the result of volume overload. In order to maintain cardiac output and compensate for increased fluid return, the ventricular sarcomeres lengthen. Ventricular chamber dilation occurs, and ventricular wall thickness remains the same or becomes thinner with stretching. As this process continues over time, the heart becomes less able to compensate, and systolic HF is the result. Again, the pathophysiologic process can be interrupted with effective diagnosis and treatment.

Aging affects the conduction system of the atria and ventricles. Fibroblasts and fat invade the SA node. The number of pacemaker cells in the SA node declines from 50% in younger adults to less than 30% in older adults. Less than 10% of the SA node cells in a 75-year-old are capable of initiating a stimulus. The AV node and ventricular conduction branches become fibrotic and are affected by calcium deposits on nearby heart valves. The age-related changes in

SA node function declines 90% by age 75, resulting in atrial arrhythmias.

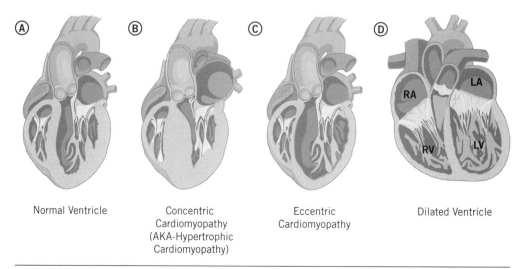

(A)	(B)	(C)	(D)
Normal Ventricle	Concentric Cardiomyopathy (AKA-Hypertrophic Cardiomyopathy)	Eccentric Cardiomyopathy	Dilated Ventricle

FIGURE 9.1

Changes in Ventricular Anatomy With Age and Heart Failure

the heart's conduction system produce common rhythm disturbances of old age including atrial fibrillation, sick sinus syndrome, and second and third degree heart block. Over 85% of the 100,000 pacemakers inserted each year are implanted in patients over 65 years old.

With age, the SA node is more resistant to autonomic nervous system regulation of heart rate. Heart rate variability declines and is less able to increase when the body requires additional cardiac output. Elders exhibit less heart rate variability. The maximal heart rate response to exercise is reduced by one-quarter.

Isolated ectopic beats originate in the atria and ventricles with increasing frequency. Atrial premature beats occur in 10% of healthy older adults. Up to 80% of healthy elders demonstrate ventricular premature beats with asymptomatic ventricular tachycardia occurring in 4 out of 100 elders. Atrial fibrillation occurs in up to 6% of healthy older adults without coronary artery disease (CAD). Atrial fibrillation may be asymptomatic and frequently alternates with sinus rhythm.

Age-related changes in the vascular system result in a decrease in elastin and an increase in collagen. As the aorta and larger arteries contain more elastin, they are more prone to collagen deposits. Flexibility and elasticity of the vessels decrease. The intimal layer thickens with lipid, collagen, and mineral deposits replacing elastin, even in the absence of atherosclerosis (see Figure 9-2). NO

> *Elastin decreases and collagen increases, making vessels stiff and less flexible.*

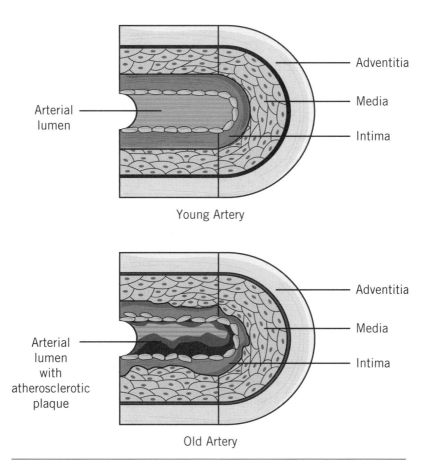

FIGURE 9.2

Young Arteries and Old Arteries With Atherosclerotic Plaques

production decreases with age, as does the ability of the endothelium to increase NO with stress. A decline in NO promotes arterial inflammation and localized platelet aggregration. The decline occurs earlier in men than women. The ability of the endothelium to vasodilate progressively declines with age. As a result, vessels are more reactive to vasoconstrictors. A disturbance in NO synthesis has been associated with diabetes, smoking, hypertension, and high cholesterol levels. Exercise appears to increase NO availability. The NO vessel wall changes help to explain the increased risk of myocardial infarction (MI), stroke, and thrombosis with age.

The calcium content of the arterial wall increases with age. A two- to threefold increase in thickness in the wall occurs between age 20 and 90 with an increased risk of cardiovascular disease. As the vessel wall thickens, the artery dilates and stiffens. The loss of elasticity decreases the aorta's ability to distend when the left ventricle ejects blood during systole. The stiff vessels transmit the pulse wave to the periphery with increased velocity. As arteries stiffen, the systolic pressure increases and diastolic pressure decreases, resulting in a wider pulse pressure. Pulse pressure is a useful indicator of arterial elasticity.

The ability of the cardiovascular system to supply tissue with oxygen depends on preload, afterload, and contractility. The sympathetic nervous system modulates heart and vessel hemodynamics. The parasympathetic system influences the heart via the vagus nerve.

Preload. Preload refers to the stretch of the myocytes, or individual myocardial fibers, at the end of diastole. Preload determines stroke volume, which is the amount of blood ejected by each cardiac contraction. Preload relies on the amount of blood in the venous system available to stretch the myocytes. Increased preload from increased venous return results in an increased stroke volume. When preload is decreased during blood loss or dehydration, stroke volume is reduced because the myocyte has not achieved an optimal stretch.

Afterload. Afterload refers to the resistance that the ventricular contraction must overcome to eject stroke volume. Resistance is produced by the weight of the blood, the flexibility of the aortic valve, and the diastolic pressure in the aorta. When there are more red blood cells in the plasma or the aortic valve is stiff or the opening narrow, afterload increases. The most common cause of increased afterload is increased peripheral vascular resistance responsible for diastolic hypertension.

Contractility. Optimum preload and afterload are necessary for contractility. However, when not provided with oxygen and sufficient nutrients, when products of cell metabolism are not removed, or when cells over stretched from invading organisms, myocytes cannot adequately function. Myocyte dysfunction results in a less forceful contraction, less blood ejecting from the heart, and less oxygenated blood supplying body tissues.

Heart volumes. The normal adult ventricle has the capacity to hold approximately 120 mL of blood when filled at the end of diastole (end diastolic volume [EDV]). The average stroke volume that leaves the heart during each contraction is 70 mL of blood. The remaining 50 mL of blood remains in the heart as the end systolic volume. The fraction of blood ejected each beat (ejection fraction [EF]) is 70 mL/120 mL, or 58%. The EF represents the efficiency of the heart's ability to pump. The amount of blood provided to the body in 1 minute of cardiac output is determined by multiplying the heart rate by the stroke volume. The cardiac output in a normal adult can range from 4 to 8 L/min.

> Optimum preload and afterload are necessary for contractility.

Nervous system influence. The heart ventricles contain a large number of beta-2 adrenergic receptors that are linked to muscle contraction. The sympathetic nervous system, through its neurotransmitters norepinephrine and epinephrine, stimulates the receptors to increase heart rate, increase contractility, and dilate and constrict peripheral vessels in response to the body's need. Working muscles, participating in the flight-or-flight response, require additional cardiac output. The muscle energy consumption produces heat, which is controlled by dilating the vessels of the skin.

The parasympathetic nervous system innervates the SA node via the vagus nerve. The vagus nerve releases acetylcholine, which acts by decreasing pacemaker cell firing. When the acetylcholine receptors are blocked, vagal tone is reduced, allowing the sympathetic nervous system to increase SA node firing. Atropine sulfate blocks acetycholine receptors.

Baroreceptors, pressure-sensitive receptors located in the aortic arch and carotid arteries, regulate blood pressure by changing heart rate (see Figure 9.3). When a healthy individual stands up, up to 1 L of vascular volume can pool in the legs. The decrease in preload results in a decreased cardiac output and a drop in blood pressure. The drop in blood pressure causes the baroreceptors to slow their rate of firing to the medulla of the brain. The brain responds by increasing

The loss of atrial kick can be life-threatening to an elder.

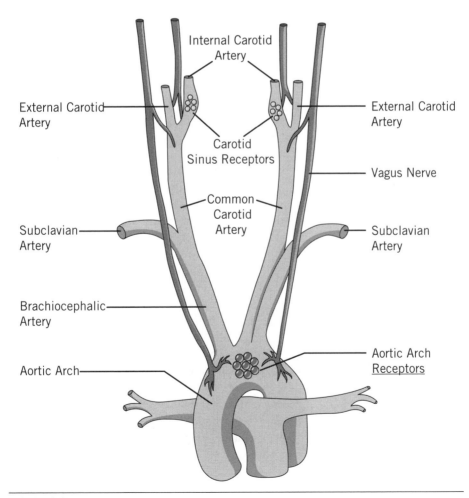

FIGURE 9.3
The Aortic Arch and Carotid Baroreceptors

sympathetic stimulation to peripheral vessels and decreasing parasympathetic stimulation of the heart. Peripheral vessels vasoconstrict, and the heart rate increases. An increased heart rate increases cardiac output while vasoconstriction increases venous return, which adds to the cardiac output. As the blood pressure rises, baroreceptor firing increases providing negative feedback to the medulla.

Preload. The loss of vascular compliance with age reduces the ability of older adults to accommodate an increase or decrease in blood volume. A stiff ventricle requires more time to relax after contraction. The additional time required for relaxation takes time away from filling. As the heart stiffens, the time required for the left

Each time the ventricle contracts, an average of 58% of the blood is ejected.

ventricle to fill also increases, and by age 80 the filling rate is half that of a younger adult. With less filling time early in diastole, the contribution of atrial kick to fill the ventricle in late diastole takes on added importance. In a young heart, 80% of filling of the ventricle is complete during the passive phase of diastole. In an older adult, atrial contraction is more important to ventricular volume. The loss of atrial kick due to atrial fibrillation can be tolerated in younger individuals, but is devastating for elders. Unable to fill the ventricle enough to eject a sufficient cardiac output, the older adult experiences chest pain, fatigue, and light-headedness.

An acute change in blood volume will have a more dramatic effect in older adults. As the venous vessels stiffen with age, their ability to maintain a constant preload is diminished. The loss is most noticeable when blood loss or peripheral pooling immediately follows spinal or epidural anesthesia and results in exaggerated hypotension.

Afterload. Age-related changes in the medial layer of the aorta create a stiff, noncompliant large vessel. The result is an elevation of systolic arterial pressure as the once elastic aorta is no longer able to absorb the energy created by the ejection of blood from the left ventricle. Isolated systolic hypertension is the most common form of hypertension in adults over 50 years. Diastolic blood pressure shows little change with healthy aging. The aim of afterload reduction to treat hypertension is to decrease vascular resistance. The use of angiotensin-converting enzyme (ACE) inhibitors is effective in decreasing large blood vessel inelasticity with aging. In addition to ACE inhibitors, diuretics also act to lower systolic blood pressure and pulse pressure. Nitrates also selectively lower systolic blood pressure.

Contractility. The ejection fraction of elders, a measure of contractility, is unchanged with age. However, elders have a reduced ability to increase the EF during exercise. With stroke volume fixed and the ability to generate an increased heart rate declining with age, elders lose cardiac reserve, or the ability to augment cardiac output. Adults over 85 years have lost nearly one-third of their cardiac reserve. While the lack of cardiac reserve does not affect the daily function of healthy elders, the diminished reserve becomes problematic when there is an increased need for cardiac output during physiological stress.

Nervous system influences. Aging is characterized by an increase in plasma levels of catecholamines (see Chapter 18). However, the beta-adrenergic receptor sites on the heart responsible for responding to catecholamines decline with age. The deficiency represents a beta blockade that limits the older adult's ability to respond during exercise or stress. When the demand for additional cardiac output occurs, the heart rate response is blunted and there is little increase in contractility. The maximal achievable heart rate declines with age. Under optimum conditions, older adult's ability to "fight or flight" is limited. However, the catecholamines remain available to trigger peripheral vasoconstriction in older adults as in younger adults.

The beta-adrenergic dysfunction limits the effectiveness of administered catecholamines. When isoproterenol is given, heart rate and cardiac output of elders is only half of that of younger adults.

The parasympathetic influence on the heart is reduced with age as a result of decreased vagal tone. Loss of parasympathetic response contributes to the decrease in heart rate variability of older adults compared to younger counterparts. Loss of vagal tone blunts the effectiveness of vagal agonist drugs such as atropine to speed up the heart.

Systolic blood pressure along with aging decreases baroreceptor responsiveness and the ability of stiff arteries and veins to constrict. Blunted baroreceptors fail to produce the change in heart rate response found in younger adults. Baroreceptors are less quick to respond to a fall in blood pressure when standing contributing to postural hypotension. Baroreceptors are also less responsive to the decrease in venous return and blood pressure caused by the Valsalva maneuver. Older adults who strain during defecation or coughing may experience a sudden drop in blood pressure. The decreased sensitivity of the baroreceptors results in labile blood pressure.

Postural hypotension. Older adults are at considerable risk for postural, or orthostatic, hypotension as a result of age-related changes in the cardiovascular system. Over one-third of adults over 75 years demonstrate postural hypotension, a greater than 20 mm Hg fall in systolic or 10 mm Hg fall in diastolic blood pressure when rising to an upright position. These changes are strongly associated with syncope and falls. Postural hypotension can be aggravated by diuretics, antihypertensive drugs, and hypovolemia.

> *Postural hypotension is found in over one-third of elders over 75 years.*

HEART FAILURE

Heart failure (HF), formerly called congestive heart failure, represents a problem with contractility. HF is progressive beginning in the middle ages, becomes more prevalent with age, and is the most frequent cause of hospitalization in adults over 65 years. The incidence of HF increases fivefold from the age of 40 to 70. Over 80% of all HF patients are over 65 years old. Morbidity from HF is high in the elderly. Between 30% and 50% of older patients hospitalized for HF will be rehospitalized within 3 to 6 months. HF is described as systolic or diastolic.

Systolic HF. Systolic HF occurs when the left ventricle is not strong enough to overcome afterload. Causes include weakened or damaged heart muscle, mitral valve incompetence, or aortic valve stenosis. When the left ventricle is inefficient, pressure builds up in the ventricle and ultimately prevents blood from emptying out of the atria and the pulmonary vessels. The EF in systolic HF is less than 50%. Over time, the increase in preload as a result of poor emptying will cause the ventricle myocytes to enlarge or hypertrophy and stretch or dilate.

Diastolic HF. In diastolic dysfunction, the heart is stiff and does not relax normally after contraction during diastole. The ventricle's inability to fully relax decreases chamber capacity and reduces the EDV. Unlike systolic HF, ventricular function is preserved with the heart able to contract normally. EF is normal. The heart fails in the ability to supply the body's oxygen needs due to reduced cardiac output. Stiff myocytes are unable to stretch but compensate by increasing in size, or hypertrophy. As the left atria tries to force blood into the stiff ventricle, the left atria also hypertrophies and enlarges. Left atrial enlargement can lead to pulmonary congestion and shortness of breath. Shortness of breath is often the first symptom of diastolic HF.

> *EF can discriminate systolic from diastolic HF.*

An important risk factor for HF is diabetes. For women with diabetes aged between 45 and 75, the likelihood of HF increases fivefold. For men with diabetes, the frequency of HF is 2.5 times that of healthy individuals.

The treatment for HF depends on the etiology. Diastolic HF requires careful fluid management. There is a narrow range between a stiff ventricle that is too full and one that is too empty. Treatment for systolic dysfunction involves the use of inotropic drugs, afterload reducing drugs, venous dilators, and diuretics.

CORONARY ARTERY DISEASE

Nearly 85% of the deaths from an MI occur in patients over 65 years old.

Eighty-five percent of individuals who die from CAD are over age 65. CAD is the leading cause of death in older adults. It is estimated that half of all adults over 70 years suffer from CAD, though less than one-third have been diagnosed. After age 75, women have a higher prevalence of CAD than men. Age is also a risk factor for hospital death due to CAD. Like the aorta and carotid arteries, the medial layer in coronary arteries thickens with age. The hyperplasia, or thickening, and the loss of NO increases the risk of atherosclerotic plaque development. Insufficient myocardial oxygen supply results in poor contractility of the ventricle.

Atherosclerosis usually causes no symptoms until middle age. However, age-related changes in the arterial endothelial wall promote further injury by substances such as nicotine, lipids, and sugar, which are elevated by comorbid diseases. Thus, diabetes, smoking, and high-serum low-density lipids (HDL) are identified as risk factors for CAD. Diastolic hypertension can further accelerate the intimal damage.

Angina. When the coronary arteries lose 50% to 70% of their inner circumference, they are unable to meet the need for increased blood supply during activity or stress. When sufficient oxygenated blood is not available to meet the myocardial muscle demand, anaerobic energy is produced with the byproduct of lactic acid. As lactic acid builds up, chest pain, or angina, occurs. Lack of sensory nerve endings on the heart means the brain has difficulty interpreting incoming stimuli. Descriptions of angina differs between patients but usually includes discomfort, heaviness, pressure, aching, burning, or fullness. It can be felt in the chest, shoulders, back, arms, neck, throat, jaw, or teeth. Angina represents a warning that coronary blood supply is unable to meet the demand. If the supply is not increased or demand does not decrease, the mismatch will result in cell death or myocardial infarction.

MI. The symptoms of angina can signal a MI. However, elders, especially women and older adults with diabetes, can experience unusual symptoms of a MI, which is a "silent MI," such as shortness of breath, fatigue, and weakness. Nearly 85% of the deaths from a MI occur in patients over age 65.

VALVULAR HEART DISEASE

Calcification of the annulus of the mitral valve is a chronic, degenerative process that is common among elderly patients; its occurrence increases with age, occurring more frequently in women than men. The formation of a ridge or ring of calcium is a long, slow process that eventually leads to a "lifting" of the leaflets of the mitral valve into the left atrium and/or a stretching of the leaflets. The changes result in mitral regurgitation. The accumulation of calcium in the mitral annulus extends into the surrounding ventricular septum, which affects the conduction system, blocking impulse spread down the bundle branches.

Mitral valve problems can also be caused by lack of blood flow to the myocardium in CAD. Hypoxia of the heart muscle impairs the mitral papillary apparatus. When the papillary muscles are unable to function, regurgitation of blood back into the left ventricle occurs.

With aging, the aortic valve becomes sclerotic as the aortic leaflets become fibrotic and calcium is deposited. Aortic sclerosis has been found in nearly 30% of elders over age 65 and nearly 40% in those over 75 years. As the sclerosis progresses, the valve narrows and becomes stenotic. Up to 10% of older adults develop aortic stenosis as a result of age-related stiffening, scarring, and calcification of the valve leaflets. The stenosis progresses slowly with patients often diagnosed with aortic stenosis between 70 and 90 years old. Syncope and chest pain are presenting symptoms.

CEREBRAL VASCULAR ACCIDENT (STROKE)

The medial layer of the carotid arteries nearly triples in thickness by age 90. When the stenosis of the carotid artery is 70% or greater, surgical intervention can decrease the risk of stroke compared to medical therapy. Most strokes occur postoperatively, a mean of 2 days following surgery. The risk of stroke increases with age with a 3% incidence over age 80. Risk also increases up to four times for patients with diabetes. There has been no link between anesthesia, intraoperative hypotension, and stroke. It is likely that hypercoagulability after surgery contributes to stroke risk (see Chapter 16). Perioperative stroke has been associated with atrial fibrillation in 33% of patients. However, the risk factors for perioperative stroke have not been identified.

> *Most strokes occur during the immediate postoperative period.*

Gerioperative Care

PREOPERATIVE CONSIDERATIONS

History

A comprehensive history includes identifying previous cardiac events and potential cardiac complications. Specific questions about hypertension, HF, heart attack, chest pain, syncope, and claudication provide a baseline for a more focused query. The elder or companion-coach should be asked about the duration of the hypertension, and if they have a record of their recent values or know the usual "numbers." Elders may be taking antihypertensive drugs without knowing the reason.

> *A pacemaker implant card should be reviewed during the preoperative visit.*

Older adults may not be told they have HF but a "weak heart." Questions related to their activity limitations can provide a baseline for postoperative activity. How many flights of stairs can an older adult climb before resting or becoming short of breath? How long have they been taking a diuretic?

Older adults can provide information about a heart attack though they frequently mislabel angina as a "heart attack." Identify the last admission for chest pain and the frequency of needing nitroglycerin tablets or spray in the past 6 months. Ask the patient if the nitroglycerin is effective or if redosing is required to reduce discomfort. A thorough history can provide information on the type of angina. Stable angina occurs during exertion and is predictable during periods of stress. Unstable angina occurs at rest or with minimal activity and is not well controlled. Unstable angina can occur frequently, feel more severe, and signals a critical imbalance between myocardial supply and demand. Less common is Printzmetal's angina caused by spasm of the coronary arteries. Spasm occurs at rest or when exposed to cold temperatures, but rarely during activity. Spasms can occur close to partial atherosclerotic blockages and lead to complete occlusion.

Patients with pacemakers should present their "Implant Card" during the preoperative visit. The card lists the device, implant date, and parameters including minimum heart rate. Document the last time the device was checked, or interrogated, to determine proper functioning. Inform the anesthesia provider of the presence of a pacemaker.

A history of vascular disease can include peripheral artery bypasses, transient ischemia attacks, or even stroke. The assessment of vessel integrity including pulses, skin color, temperature, and any ulcers should be documented preoperatively. Peripheral vascular disease includes any history of deep vein thrombosis.

Review the list of current medications and allergies. Ask the patient to identify the medications and their purpose. Medications for comorbid conditions can impact cardiac function.

Assessment

Blood pressure and apical heart rate are key parameters of a cardiovascular assessment. Blood pressure must be measured correctly, with the patient sitting, legs uncrossed, and arms supported. A correctly sized cuff must be available, especially for obese elders. Auscultation may be difficult if the environment is noisy; however, it is more accurate than noninvasive blood pressure devices. Listen carefully for the diastolic pressure, which helps determine pulse pressure. A diastolic blood pressure of 110 or higher requires control before surgery.

A diastolic blood pressure over 110 requires control prior to surgery and anesthesia.

Auscultation of the apical heart rate is directed at appreciating regularity. After auscultating the rate, listen for murmurs and identify their timing in the cardiac cycle by palpating the radial pulse. If the murmur occurs after feeling a pulse, it is a systolic murmur; before the pulse, it is a diastolic murmur. Aortic stenosis and mitral regurgitation murmurs are systolic, while mitral stenosis and aortic regurgitation murmurs are diastolic. If the older adult has a permanent pacemaker, assess the site over the pacemaker battery for any skin breakdown.

Peripheral pulses are assessed bilaterally. The carotid arteries are checked by auscultating for bruits. Radial, brachial, and pedal pulses are evaluated for strength and symmetry. If vascular surgery is planned, pulses are assessed and then their location marked with a permanent marker. Marking facilitates intraoperative and postoperative assessments.

Preoperative Testing

A 12-lead EKG is commonly requested for elders prior to surgery, particularly for those with a previous cardiovascular event or comorbid disease such as diabetes. An EKG provides information about rhythm, rate, conduction delays, the presence and functioning of a pacemaker, previous MIs, and signs of hypertrophy.

An EKG is useful to determine the degree of stenosis or regurgitation for elders with valvular disease. Hypertrophy in patients with a history of HF can also be evaluated with an EKG. An EKG provides a noninvasive measurement of EF and cardiac output, which can indicate the availability of cardiac reserve. A normal EF does not mean there is no HF. Diastolic HF will be reported in the findings but does not show up as a change in EF. Perioperative and particularly intraoperative interventions differ for systolic versus diastolic HF. For elders in chronic atrial fibrillation, an EKG may be ordered to identify the presence of blood clots in the atria. Clots

TABLE 9.1

Clinical Predictors of Cardiac Complications During the Perioperative Period

Major predictors
  Unstable coronary syndrome
  Decompensated heart failure
  Significant arrhythmias
  Severe valvular disease

Intermediate predictors
  Mild angina
  Prior myocardial infarction
  Compensated heart failure
  Diabetes

Minor predictors
  Abnormal electrocardiogram
  Non sinus rhythm
  Low functional capacity
  History of stroke
  Uncontrolled hypertension

can travel to the pulmonary artery or into the systemic circulation as emboli. Additional tests depend on the findings obtained during the preoperative history.

The American College of Cardiology recommends a stepwise approach to preoperative evaluation based on clinical predictors, surgical risk, and functional capacity. Clinical predictors are divided into three categories: major, intermediate, and minor (see Table 9.1). Functional capacity is based on energy expenditure and ranked on two levels. Poor functional capacity describes activities requiring 1 to 4 metabolic equivalents (METs), including eating, dressing, walking one or two blocks on level ground, and light housework. Moderate or excellent functional capacity, at 4 to 10 METs, includes climbing stairs, running a short distance, and participating in recreational activities. Surgical procedures are classified as high, intermediate, and low risk (Table 9.2).

TABLE 9.2

Surgical Procedures Ranked by Risk of Cardiac Complication

High risk
  Major emergency procedures
  Major vascular procedures
  Peripheral vascular procedures
  Prolong procedures with fluid shift or blood loss

Intermediate risk
  Carotid endarterectomy
  Head and neck procedures
  Intraperitoneal/intrathoracic procedures
  Orthopedic surgery
  Prostate surgery

Low risk
  Endoscopic procedures
  Skin and breast procedures
  Cataract

Preoperative coronary angiography is recommended for patients with major predictors. Revascularization may be needed prior to noncardiac surgery. For patients with intermediate predictors and poor functional capacity or minor predictors undergoing high-risk procedures, additional noninvasive testing is indicated. A stress test determines the ability of the elder to tolerate changes in heart rate and blood pressure with exercise. A treadmill, dobutamine stress test, stress EKG, or nuclear stress test will identify the areas of the heart that becomes hypoxic with activity, providing additional information about EF and cardiac reserve. Depending on the findings, further testing can include a cardiac angiography. The goal of preoperative testing is to identify unknown cardiac pathology that will impact the elder's response to perioperative stress.

Preoperative Interventions

Older adults with heart valve dysfunction are at risk of endocarditis due to bacterial infections. American Heart Association guidelines recommend antibiotic prophylaxis before any invasive procedure. Antihypertensive medications should be continued during the perioperative period as well as beta blockers.

INTRAOPERATIVE CONSIDERATIONS

Cardiac monitoring during anesthesia includes continuous blood pressure, heart rate, and pulse oximetry monitoring. Hemodynamic monitoring with a central venous or pulmonary artery catheter can be helpful for elders who are hemodynamically fragile and if the surgery is expected to interfere with vascular volume. In surgeries where blood pressure requires precise control, such as carotid endarterectomy or abdominal aortic aneurysm repair, an invasive arterial line is required. Prior to placement of an arterial line, complete an assessment of the arteries in the forearm and hand to assess collateral blood flow via the ulnar artery. Doppler ultrasound assessment is preferred as the traditional Allen's test is not a reliable assessment tool. Frequent assessment of the hand during surgery can avoid complications related to the arterial catheter. The pulse oximeter waveform can act to continuously assess the peripheral pulse.

The traditional Allen's test for ulnar blood flow is not reliable.

Fluid management. Age-related changes coupled with preoperative dehydration and anesthetics can result in significant blood pressure swings. Added events such as fluid shifts during abdominal surgery or blood loss during vascular surgery can potentiate an already labile blood pressure. Excessive amounts of inhaled anesthetics can cause cardiac depression and peripheral vasodilation. Narcotic administration during total intravenous anesthesia can also result in hypotension from peripheral vasodilation. Regional anesthetics interrupt sympathetic discharge resulting in vasodilation.

Fluid management in the older adult is critical to minimizing cardiac complications. If the blood pressure response to fluids is inadequate, alpha agonist vasoconstrictor agents such as phenlynephrine or norepinephrine will constrict arterial vessels, causing a temporary increase in blood pressure. Vasoconstricting agents may need to be continued intravenously for the duration of the anesthetic. Due to age-related changes causing premature ventricular and atrial beats and increased sensitivity to vasoconstrictors, phenylephrine, rather than ephedrine, is the vasoconstrictor of choice in elders with hypotension in the operating room. Ephedrine can result in additional cardiac irritability, resulting in more ectopic beats and tachycardia.

Hypotension induced by blood loss must be corrected with fluid administration. Blood loss is usually replaced with 3 mL of crystalloid for every 1 mL of blood loss. When the hemoglobin declines significantly, blood products may be indicated (see Chapter 16).

Fluid management is critical when caring for patients with a history of mitral or aortic stenosis. Patients with these valvular disorders may be normally asymptomatic. However, when faced with preoperative dehydration, the heart chambers have insufficient filling volume or pressure to open the tight valves. Attention to adequate hydration and slow heart rate allows for complete filling of the chambers and avoids hemodynamic instability.

Under- or overhydration can precipitate atrial fibrillation in older adults who have dilated atria- or age-related sinus node changes. A rapid ventricular response in the face of atrial fibrillation can reduce cardiac output by over one-third. Quick recognition and treatment can prevent cardiovascular collapse.

Ventricular arrhythmias are common in older adults but can also signal myocardial irritability due to acid-base imbalance, hypoxemia, or electrolyte disturbance. Treatment is dependent on the severity of the effect. Intravenous amiodarone 150 mg over 10 minutes followed by an infusion can convert ventricular tachycardia.

Patients with pacemakers or implantable cardioverter defibrillators are at risk for device damage or reprogramming when exposed to electrocautery. A magnet can be placed over the device to protect the programming and set the pacemaker rate to fixed. When removed, the pacemaker assumes the preoperative parameters.

Hypertension during the intraoperative period can be an indication that the patient is sedated but experiencing pain. Additional narcotics may be needed.

POSTOPERATIVE CONSIDERATIONS

Postoperative monitoring in the postanesthesia care unit (PACU) includes continuous cardiac rhythm monitoring with capability to evaluate the ST segment of the EKG. ST segment elevations reflect myocardial damage. Elevations in heart rate or pain can cause ST segment changes. Treatment with pain medication may resolve the ST segment changes. Blood pressure should be monitored at least every 15 minutes or more frequently as needed. However, frequent blood pressure monitoring can result in petechia on elders' fragile skin. Pulse oximetry will evaluate the peripheral pulse though waveform analysis. Elders should always be placed on supplemental oxygen in the PACU. Oxygen saturations in the low 90s can result in ST segment changes. Oxygen administration can return the ST segment to baseline. Any change in ST segment configuration requires notification of the anesthesia provider as further evaluation and testing may be required.

The incidence of an MI after surgery is increased among patients who have had a previous coronary event within the past 3 years. The incidence of an MI is nearly 50% in a patient who has reported a history of MI within the previous 6 months. The development of arrhythmias, pain unrelated to the surgical procedure, diaphoresis, anxiety, or an unexplained change in vital signs should alert the nurse to suspect a coronary event. Interventions include morphine, oxygen, and a nitrate (three parts of the mnemonic "MONA"). Aspirin, the fourth component of the "MONA" mnemonic, should not be administered unless approved by the surgeon. A postoperative 12-lead EKG should be compared to the preoperative EKG to detect ischemic or patterns of injury.

> *Over one-third of postoperative hypertensive episodes are idiopathic and will resolve in 3 hours.*

Careful fluid management during the intraoperative period is continued postoperatively. The PACU nurse should calculate the fluid balance considering all the perioperative fluids administered and fluids put out by the patient.

Postoperative hypertension is common during the immediate postoperative recovery. Etiology includes uncontrolled pain, ischemia, fluid overload, anxiety, or a distended bladder. Thirty percent of PACU hypertension is idiopathic and resolves within 3 hours. If treatment is required, calcium channel blockers or beta blockers can be administered, considering the appropriate dosage for older adults.

Postoperative assessment of the older adult with a pacemaker includes examining the site for skin integrity. The EKG rhythm strip is examined for pacing activity. If a magnet has been used during surgery, the pacemaker should be checked within the next 24 hours. Many manufacturers use remote telephonic systems that makes pacemaker checks easy and convenient.

The risk of stroke increases after orthopedic, carotid revascularization, and cardiovascular procedures. Neurological assessments, including cranial nerve checks, extremity movement, and strength, are conducted at least every 30 minutes. The six Ps of neurovascular assessment are documented after extremity surgery: pain, pallor, paresthesia, pulses, paralysis, and poikilothermia.

Older adults are at higher risk for postural hypotension. Blood pressure must be monitored as they are repositioned in the PACU. When assisted off the stretcher and into a recliner in phase II prior to discharge, the nurse should allow the elder to take extra time when sitting up.

Age-related changes increase the risk of decreased cardiac output for gerioperative patients. The decreased output occurs as the result of myocardial ischemia, hypertension, valvular dysfunction, arrhythmias, tachycardia, decreased fluid volume, or electrolyte imbalance. While signs of decreased cardiac output vary depending on etiology, the development of angina, new arrhythmias, EKG changes including ST segment depression or elevation, hypotension, or diminished pulses are findings of concern. Pulmonary symptoms of decreased cardiac output manifest as auscultated crackles, dyspnea, orthopnea, and cough. Neurological changes of dizziness, confusion, anxiety, or restlessness occur when cerebral perfusion is compromised by the decreased cardiac output.

Interventions for decreased cardiac output depend on the etiology. Laboratory analysis of electrolytes, renal function, and arterial blood gases assist in determining the etiology along with a 12-lead EKG. Intravenous inotropes may be required to provide a temporary increase in cardiac output.

PATIENT REPORT: Mr. Brookshire

Mr. Brookshire returns to the preoperative clinic 2 weeks before his planned surgery. The NP reviews his blood work, EKG, and results of his stress test. An old lateral wall MI was noted on the EKG with similar finding on the stress test. The remaining findings were negative, and Mr. Brookshire is cleared for surgery. The intraoperative period and general anesthesia was uneventful, and Mr. Brookshire is admitted to the PACU. His blood pressure is 94/50, heart rate 87, temperature of 36.0° C, respirations of 16, and oxygenation saturation of 90%. The ST segment showed no change from preoperative status. His fluid status indicates he received an adequate intravenous replacement for his 350 mL blood loss during surgery. The PACU nurse places a nasal cannula on Mr. Brookshire at 4 L; his oxygen saturation increases within a few minutes to his preoperative baseline of 96%, and his blood pressure increases to 104/55.

SUMMARY

While cardiovascular disease is not age-dependent, age-related changes limit cardiac reserve and the ability to respond to challenges requiring additional cardiac output. Attention to optimum fluid balance throughout the perioperative process is key to positive outcomes. Interventions to maximize oxygenation improve cardiac function. Careful attention to blood pressure changes will reduce safety risks during recovery.

KEY POINTS

- The maximal heart rate response to exercise is reduced by one-quarter in older adults.
- As arteries stiffen, the systolic pressure increases and diastolic pressure decreases, resulting in a wider pulse pressure. Pulse pressure is a useful indicator of arterial elasticity.
- Isolated systolic hypertension is the most common form of hypertension in adults over age 50. Diastolic blood pressure shows little change with healthy aging.
- Catecholamine response declines with age, limiting the older adult's ability to respond by increasing heart rate during exercise or stress.
- Loss of vagal tone blunts the effectiveness of vagal agonist drugs such as atropine to speed up the heart.
- The decreased sensitivity of the baroreceptors results in labile blood pressure and orthostatic hypotension.
- The treatment for HF depends on the etiology. Diastolic HF requires careful fluid management while systolic dysfunction involves the use of inotropic drugs, afterload reducing drugs, venous dilators, and diuretics.

TEN

Renal

Susan J. Fetzer, Jennifer V. Long, and Raelene V. Shippee-Rice

PATIENT REPORT: Mrs. Coburn

Mrs. Coburn, a 70-year-old obese woman (100 kg) with hypertension, coronary artery disease, diabetes, and a history of heart failure, arrives in the surgical holding area awaiting a diagnostic laproscopy to evaluate a bowel obstruction. Her medications include metformin, furosemide, and metoprolol. She has a nasogastric tube and has had nothing by mouth for 2 days. Her oral medications were changed to intravenous medications, and metformin was discontinued. She has been started on a sliding scale with insulin coverage. Her blood sugar is 120 mg/dL. Her vital signs are as follows: blood pressure 120/65, heart rate 60/minute, respirations 20/minute, temperature 98.0° F, and oxygen saturation 98%. Her mucous membranes are dry. The peripherally inserted central catheter has 5% dextrose in normal saline (D5NS) infusing at 125 mL/hr.

Fluid and electrolyte balance is vital to life. Too little or too much fluid in a patient can lead to serious complications made worse by the diminished reserves seen in elderly surgical patients. Normal age-related and pathophysiologic changes predispose the elderly to dehydration and can compromise fluid and electrolyte replacement. Complications of dehydration are serious. Dehydration in older adults is associated with cognitive changes, bowel obstruction, urinary tract infections (UTIs), orthostatic hypotension, and early death.

Likewise, fluid overload can destabilize a patient. Elders are predisposed to fluid volume overload secondary to cardiac impairment, chronic renal insufficiency, and medications.

In this chapter, the role of the aging kidney in maintaining fluid balance during the perioperative period is presented. The involvement of hormones, the influence of medications, and the considerations in fluid replenishment and maintenance are explored. Understanding normal function of the renal system and age-related changes allows the health care provider to better anticipate potential problems, take preventive action, and implement early and appropriate interventions to minimize the impact of problems on the immediate and long-term health outcomes in the gerioperative patient.

Renal Considerations

The genitourinary system is defined as the kidney, ureters, bladder, and urethra. At birth, the kidneys are formed with the number of nephrons already established. Growth involves enlargement of the functional areas of each nephron. The kidney reaches the maximal size early in adulthood, and then progressively decreases.

Age-Related Changes

Changes in the aging renal system begin long before an adult reaches geriatric status. Kidney growth may be measured by weight, with maximal weight being reached around age 30; by the age of 80, a kidney will have lost 20% to 40% of its maximum weight. The ability of the kidneys to meet body requirements, however, is not age- or weight-dependent but rather depends on blood flow and filtration ability of each functional unit of the kidney.

RENAL BLOOD FLOW

By early adolescence, nearly 25% of the cardiac output, 1.2 L/min, is destined for the kidneys. Each kidney normally receives 600 mL/min of blood by way of the aorta to the renal arteries. Kidney blood flow increases or decreases depending on physical demands or the condition of the vessels leading to the kidney.

The ability of the kidneys to meet body requirements depends on blood flow and filtration ability of each functional unit of the kidney.

The basic functional unit of the kidney is the nephron (Figure 10.1). A nephron eliminates wastes from the body, regulates blood volume and blood pressure, controls serum electrolyte and metabolite concentrations, and regulates blood pH. As blood enters the kidney, it is shunted into smaller arteries and finally passes through over 1 million arterioles. Each incoming (afferent) arteriole ends in a ball called a glomerulus and is encapsulated by tissue called Bowman's capsule (Figure 10.2). The glomerulus and Bowman's capsule together form the filtering structure of the kidney. The pressure inside the glomerulus is regulated by outgoing (efferent) arterioles, which are narrower than the afferent arterioles. The pressure differential between afferent and efferent arterioles forces plasma to be squeezed through the glomerular walls into the space made by Bowman's capsule. The filtrate passes into Bowman's capsule and then into the nephron tubules, a process known as ultrafiltration. Only one-fifth of the blood entering the glomerulus leaves via the efferent arteriole.

Age-Related Changes

Blood flow decreases consistently with age to the point that at 90 years old, renal blood flow is approximately 300 mL/min, half the volume of blood perfusing the kidneys of a 30-year-old. As with other blood vessels, the walls of the blood vessels leading to the kidney change with aging. These changes include atherosclerosis of the vasculature, a loss of muscle tissue in the middle layer of the arteries, and a thickening of the arterial walls. Aging changes compound and result in decreased blood flow to the functional units of the kidney.

Aging changes compound and result in a decreased blood flow to the functional units of the kidney.

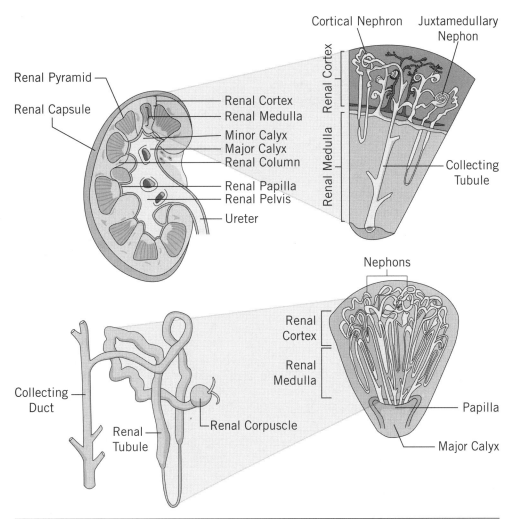

FIGURE 10.1
Internal Structure of a Kidney

Reduced blood flow from the renal arteries results in reduced blood flow through the glomerulus. In addition, sclerotic changes of the small arterioles of the glomerulus can lead to anastamoses (connections) being formed between the afferent and efferent arterioles. The anastamoses of the arterioles creates a shunting of blood from the afferent to the efferent arterioles. When the arteriole blood is shunted, the filtering surface of the kidney is reduced. Such arteriole sclerosis effectively decreases the number of functional glomeruli and the overall function of the kidney.

GLOMERULAR FILTRATION

The glomerular filtrate produced by ultrafiltration of the blood at the glomerulus enters the Bowman's capsule and then passes through to the proximal convoluted tubule. The amount of fluid passing from the glomerulus to the collecting tubule is referred to as the glomeru-

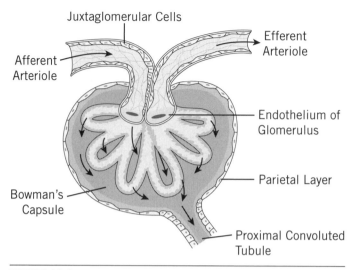

FIGURE 10.2
Bowman's Capsule

lar filtration rate (GFR), measured in volume per unit time per body surface area (mL/min/m²). Normal GFR is accepted as being greater than 90 mL/min/1.73 m². A GFR of greater than 60 mL/min/1.73 m², however, is considered adequate and is used as one of the breakpoints for estimating kidney function in many facilities.

Glomerular filtrate is similar to blood plasma but lacks the large blood proteins, blood cells, and platelets. The outgoing (efferent) arteriole contains concentrated blood plasma. Conversely, the filtrate in the proximal tubule is dilute and contains a large volume of water. The efferent arteriole and the proximal tubule pass down into the medulla of the kidney side by side. As a result of the concentration difference between the arteriole and the tubule, osmotic forces result in nearly 60% of the water in the tubule moving back into the arteriole (Figure 10.3). The tubule wall is not permeable to the urea that was initially filtered out of the blood while passing through the glomerulus. This urea, therefore, does not pass back into the arteriole, but remains in the tubule. The tubule walls are permeable to glucose, amino acids, and electrolytes. Active transport processes that require energy act to move these important substances back into the blood from the proximal convoluted tubule.

The filtrate moves through the proximal tubule into the descending and ascending convoluted tubules which, together, form a U-shape. The U-shaped tubule is described as the loop of Henle (see Figure 10.3). The descending tubules of the loop of Henle are permeable to water. Water that was not reabsorbed into the arteriole when the filtrate was passing down the proximal convoluted tubule will be reabsorbed into the arterioles from the descending tubule in the loop of Henle. Ascending tubules are permeable to electrolytes, which allows the regulation of sodium, chloride, and potassium ions. The electrolytes that still remain in the filtrate have the opportunity to be reabsorbed by the ascending tubules where they will move back into the interstitium of the kidney medulla. Permeability and reabsorption becomes an important aspect of fluid-electrolyte balance in the body. The filtrate that moves from the loop of Henle into the distal convoluted tubule is hypotonic, having lost most, but not all, of the original electrolytes.

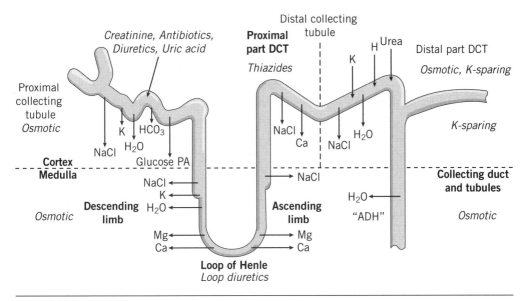

FIGURE 10.3
Renal Osmotic Forces With Site of Medication Actions

Cells in the distal convoluted tubule engage in active transport to reabsorb calcium into the blood and excrete phosphate into the tubule. The distal tubule is under the influence of endocrine control, particularly parathyroid hormone (PTH) and aldosterone from the adrenal gland. An increase in PTH causes the tubule to reabsorb calcium and excrete phosphate. Aldosterone and atrial naturietic peptide control sodium reabsorption in the distal tubule. As sodium is reabsorbed into the blood stream, the sodium ions are exchanged for potassium and hydrogen ions, which move into the tubule. The addition of the hydrogen ions increases the acidity of the filtrate. Thus, the distal tubule plays an important role in acid-base balance and serum calcium concentrations. After passing through the distal tubule, the filtrate is delivered to the collecting ducts.

The collecting ducts, with normally impermeable membranes, pass through the ion-rich interstitium of the medulla. Under the influence of antidiuretic hormone (ADH) in the medulla, the walls of the collecting ducts become permeable to water. The medulla has a high osmotic concentration, and in an effort to dilute the ion-rich interstitial medulla, water leaves the collecting tubule through passive osmosis. The loss of water in the collecting duct due to osmosis further concentrates the filtrate. The interstitial water from this osmotic process in the medulla is reabsorbed by the capillaries and re-enters the blood stream. Collecting ducts account for approximately 39% of water reabsorption, adding to the 60% of water reabsorbed earlier in the proximal tubule. In all, 99% of the water that was removed from the blood by Bowman's capsule is returned to the vascular system.

Age-Related Changes

The decrease in blood flow and the sclerotic changes to the afferent arteriole result in a loss of glomerular function with age. This results in a significant decline in GFR (approximately 8 mL/min/1.73 m^2) for each decade over 40 years old. The decline in glomerular function with age is also associated with changes in membrane permeability to protein. Normally, protein is not squeezed out of the plasma during filtration. Both the glomerular membrane and the membranes of Bowman's capsule thicken and become sclerotic with age, rendering them more permeable barriers. Proteins pass with the filtrate into the proximal convoluted tubule. From this point forward, any filtered proteins remain in the filtrate because they are too large to pass back through the tubule walls where the electrolytes are reabsorbed. As these proteins are unable to be reabsorbed, they pass completely through the nephron and are excreted.

The functional decline of the glomeruli with age parallels a decline in tubular function of the nephron. Over time, tubule walls become thicker, fat deposits accumulate, and the tubules shorten. All of these changes result in a decrease of the tubules' ability to reabsorb water and balance electrolyte concentrations. With age, the ability of the kidney to produce a concentrated filtrate as well as the ability to dilute the filtrate declines. In an attempt to compensate for these functional changes in the nephron, hormonal influences on the distal tubules also change with age.

KIDNEY FUNCTION AND HORMONAL INFLUENCE

The kidneys are the source of and the site of action of many hormones that affect the control of body fluids, serum electrolyte concentrations, drug and drug-metabolite elimination, and erythropoietin production.

The kidney produces hormones as well as being regulated by hormones to maintain homeostasis of fluid and electrolytes, serum calcium, and red blood cell production. Once produced by the skin's exposure to ultraviolet light, vitamin D is converted into calcitriol by the liver. In turn, the kidney produces the active form of vitamin D as a hormone. Decreased levels of vitamin D can occur due to low light exposure or liver or kidney disease. Table 10.1 summarizes the hormones involved in kidney function: their stimulus, source, site of action, function, effect, and changes that occur with aging.

RENIN

In the kidney cortex, located near Bowman's capsule and the distal convoluted tubule is a group of cells responsible for regulating filtration called the juxtaglomerular apparatus (JGA) (see Figure 10.2). The JGA is composed of cells located in the incoming and outgoing arterioles of the glomerulus and cells located in the walls of the distal tubule. This group of cells is responsive to several stimuli. A decrease in blood pressure, inadequate filtration rates, or ionic (charged) filtrate in the distal tubule results in the release of renin from the juxtaglomerular cells. The renin circulates in the blood and converts angiotensin I to angiotensin II. Angiotensin II causes arterial constriction, which increases blood pressure. The increased blood pressure caused by renin release ultimately increases glomerular pressure and glomerular filtration. Angiotensin II also acts to stimulate the adrenal cortex to release aldosterone.

Age-Related Changes

The response of the juxtaglomerular cells to stimulation declines with age. The decline is due to a reduced synthesis and impaired release of the renin peptide. Thus, the basal renin level declines with age. When less renin is present, there is a potential loss of angiotensin I and angiotensin II. However, to compensate, angiotensin II receptors located in the arterioles appear to increase

TABLE 10.1
Hormones Regulating Kidney Function

Hormone	Stimulus	Source	Action Site	Function	Effect	Change with Aging
Renin	↓ BP ↓ filtration ↑ Na$^+$ concentration	JGA	Blood stream	Convert angiotensin I to angiotensin II	↑ BP secondary to arterial vasoconstriction	↓ response of JGA to release of renin ↑angiotensin receptors
Aldosterone	↑ K$^+$ concentration	Adrenal cortex	Ascending and descending tubules	↑ reabsorption of Na$^+$ ↑ excretion of K$^+$	↑ serum Na$^+$ ↓ serum K$^+$	↓ amount of aldosterone ↑serum K$^+$ In the elderly, there is a longer response time to changes in K$^+$
ANH	Stretching of cardiac muscle cells	Atria of the heart	Adrenal cortex and distal tubules	↓ aldosterone ↑ Na$^+$ reabsorption	↑ Na$^+$ and H$_2$O excretion ↓BP	↑ ANH levels results in ↓ Na levels and ↑ response to Δ in fluid levels
PTH	↓ Blood Ca^{++} levels	Posterior pituitary	Distal convoluted tubules	Reabsorption of Ca^{++} Excretion of phosphorous	↑ serum Ca^{++} ↓ serum phosphorous	↓ tubular response to PTH leads to ↑ serum PTH levels; ↑ Ca^{++} loss leading to ↑ bone resorption
ADH	Δ Na$^+$ Δ BP Δ Blood volume Pain Nausea Stress	Posterior pituitary	Distal convoluted tubules	↑ permeability of distal tubules to H$_2$O	Concentration of urine	↓ ability to concentrate urine ↓ sensitivity to ADH resulting in more urine that is more dilute
Erythropoietin	Hypoxia	Tubular endothelial cells in the kidney	Bone marrow stem cells	↑ erythropoietin secretion	↑ RBC production	↑ resistance to EPO resulting in anemia

Δ, change; ↑, increase; ↓, decrease; ADH, antidiuretic hormone; ANH, atrial natriutic hormone; BP, blood pressure; Ca, calcium; EPO, erythropoietin; H$_2$O, water; JGA, juxtaglomerular apparatus; K, potassium; Na, sodium; PTH, parathyroid hormone; RBC, red blood cell.

with age. If renin can be synthesized and can be released, the ability of renin to raise blood pressure is improved as additional angiotensin receptors are available to be stimulated by the renin.

ALDOSTERONE

The adrenal cortex produces the steroid hormone aldosterone. Aldosterone release is triggered by elevated serum potassium concentrations. When serum potassium levels are high, aldosterone acts on the ascending and distal tubules to increase the active transport of sodium and potassium across the tubule membrane. High serum levels of potassium result in the reabsorption of sodium into the blood and potassium passes out into the tubule. For aldosterone to be effective in reducing serum potassium, functional ascending and distal tubules are required.

Age-Related Changes

The plasma concentration of aldosterone declines with age. The decline is not due to adrenal gland changes but is a result of the decrease in renin activity. Lower renin production results in lower serum aldosterone concentrations, which in turn result in a reduction of the distal tubule response to potassium. As a consequence of this lowered aldosterone level, the elderly are at risk for higher serum potassium concentrations and more time is required before such hyperkalemia can be resolved.

ATRIAL NATURIETIC HORMONE

Atrial naturietic hormone (ANH) is secreted by muscle cells in the heart's atria. When the cardiac muscle cells are stretched, ANH secretion is increased. The stretch of atrial cells occurs when blood volume in the atria increases. The release of ANH affects the adrenal cortex and the distal tubules of the kidneys. The release of ANH by the atrial cells inhibits aldosterone and promotes sodium reabsorption into the distal tubule. With aldosterone inhibited, potassium is saved and sodium remains in the filtrate. By increasing sodium excretion, water follows the sodium. As sodium and water are excreted, the circulating blood volume decreases. In turn, when blood volume decreases, the atrial stretch is reduced, and less ANH is secreted.

Age-Related Changes

Serum ANH levels increase with age. The ANH increase is independent of cardiac disease and is almost twice the levels seen in young adults. In addition to increased baseline levels of ANH, older adults are more responsive to physiologic and pharmacologic stimulation of ANH. Elevated ANH may contribute to the sodium loss seen among elders.

ANTIDIURETIC HORMONE

ADH or vasopressin is produced by the posterior pituitary. ADH is released in response to serum sodium levels, blood volume, and blood pressure. ADH release can also be triggered by nausea, pain, and stress.

The serum sodium level is monitored by the posterior pituitary. When the sodium level increases, ADH is released and acts on the distal convoluted tubules. ADH increases the permeability of the distal convoluted tubules to water. Increased tubule permeability results in more water being absorbed into the blood. The increase in water dilutes serum sodium levels, while the filtrate in the distal tubule becomes concentrated.

Under normal conditions, ADH secretion is diurnal, with more of the hormone present at night. Additional nighttime ADH results in water being reabsorbed into the blood and a higher filtrate concentration. Nighttime ADH secretion results in less urine production while sleeping. Under normal conditions, urine volume during the day is approximately twice what is produced by the kidneys at night.

Age-Related Changes

Age-related changes in the production and secretion of ADH are controversial, showing either no change or an increase in basal ADH levels. Age-related changes appear to cause a hypersensitivity of posterior pituitary receptors to ADH stimulants. Serum sodium levels in older adults trigger twice the response by ADH than do the same serum sodium levels in young adults. However, age appears to decrease the kidney's sensitivity to ADH. The decrease in sensitivity may be responsible for the decreased concentrating capacity of the aging kidney.

The diurnal rhythm of ADH secretion is absent or even reversed in some elders. Nighttime urine production can exceed the daytime rate. Coupled with sleep-wake changes and lack of ADH secretion to concentrate the urine, nocturia is a common problem among elders. It is estimated that up to 70% of elders experience regular nocturia.

PARATHYROID HORMONE

As bone is broken down, calcium and phosphate are released into the blood. Calcium and phosphate are filtered out of the blood at Bowman's capsule. A low level of blood calcium results in PTH stimulation. PTH acts at the distal convoluting tubule to actively reabsorb calcium from the filtrate into the blood and at the same time allows the excretion of phosphate into the filtrate.

Age-Related Changes

Aging decreases the sensitivity and responsiveness of the tubule to PTH. The decrease in PTH responsiveness results in a decrease in calcium reabsorption and an increase in calcium excretion. Aging is associated with increases in PTH, possibly in response to chronic low serum calcium. A sedentary lifestyle stimulates an increase in calcium breakdown. When coupled with decrease calcium reabsorption and increased renal loss, the result is a chronically low level of calcium among elders and further bone deterioration.

ERYTHROPOIETIN

While not involved in filtration, erythropoietin (EPO) is an important hormone secreted by the tubular endothelial cells in the kidney's cortex. The cells near the proximal tubules are sensitive to oxygen. The cells respond to cellular hypoxia by secreting EPO. The function of EPO is to increase red blood cell survival and stimulate the development of blood cell precursors by the stem cells.

Age-Related Changes

Among healthy elders, EPO levels increase. The increase is believed to be related to a resistance to EPO. Chronically ill elders, including individuals with controlled diabetes and hypertension, demonstrate a decreased response to EPO and can develop anemia quickly.

Fluid and Electrolyte Balance

Body fluid homeostasis influences every body system. Adjusting body water requires the ability to concentrate and dilute urine. While healthy elders are able to satisfactorily maintain fluid, electrolyte, and acid-base balance, the regulation of these parameters takes longer for the aging nephron.

SODIUM

Sodium is squeezed into the filtrate in Bowman's capsule and must pass through the tubule membrane to be reabsorbed into the vascular system. Sodium is an important ion for the regulation of water balance and in the propagation of nerve impulses.

Age-Related Changes

The aging kidney is slow at conserving sodium. A decrease in renal blood flow and the decline in filtration rate encourage sodium to remain in the vascular space. At the same time, when sodium is filtered out of the vascular space, the transfer of sodium from the distal tubule back into the vascular system is slower. Overall, serum sodium levels decline approximately 1 mEq/L for each decade of life. When placed on a low-sodium diet, elders' kidneys are slow to respond by decreasing sodium excretion. There is a longer period between reduced sodium intake and change in serum sodium. Older adults take more than twice the time to achieve the same degree of sodium retention as younger adults. The increase in aldosterone and ANH, which influences sodium excretion, may also play a role in delayed sodium conservation. It has been estimated that up to 11% of hospitalized elders and twice as many institutionalized elders experience hyponatremia, a serum sodium less than 136 mEq/L. Over half of long-term care residents over 60 years old experienced hyponatremia at least once a year. The low sodium content of tube feedings required by many elders contributes to the risk of hyponatremia. In addition, many of the drugs routinely administered to elders result in hyponatremia and associated electrolyte shifts. Sodium wasting is a recurrent problem in the elderly.

Hypernatremia can also occur in the elderly. Hypernatremia can develop with either normal or low total body sodium, but it is rarely the result of increased total body sodium. The usual cause of a high blood sodium levels is a loss of sodium-poor fluids or inadequate fluid intake. With a loss of body water, elders are unable to dilute a normal level of sodium. Body water can be lost through febrile illness, tachypnea with increased water loss from the lungs, and diabetes under poor control. Elders with impaired thirst mechanisms are at particularly high risk for hypernatremia. Poor water intake results in lower blood volume and lower blood pressure. Lower blood pressure reduces kidney filtration and sodium is not excreted. The amount of vascular water continues to drop, with sodium remaining stable. An aggressive use of diuretics, among other drugs noted in Table 10.2, also increases elders' risk of hypernatremia.

POTASSIUM

Despite 98% of the body potassium existing within the cells, the kidney is responsible for potassium balance. Potassium is filtered into the tubule by the glomeruli and is reabsorbed into the vascular system with active and passive transport through the tubule membrane. Secretion of aldosterone also affects potassium excretion.

TABLE 10.2

Medications Associated With Sodium Imbalance and Electrolyte Shifts in the Elderly

Medication	Effect on Renal Function and Electrolyte Balance
Thiazide	Decrease in serum potassium Increase or decrease in serum sodium
Loop diuretics	Decrease in serum potassium Increase or decrease in serum sodium
SSRI/SNRI	Increase in serum potassium Decrease in serum sodium
Tricyclic antidepressants	Anticholinergic properties
Anticonvulsants	Decrease in serum sodium
Lithium	Competes with sodium reuptake in the kidney tubules, which may lead to hyponatremia Alternatively, a low sodium status can lead to lithium toxicity
ACE inhibitors	Increase in serum potassium Decrease in serum sodium
Oral hypoglycemics NSAIDs	Electrolyte imbalance Affect kidney function, resulting in nephrotoxicity and an increase in BUN and serum creatinine

ACE, angiotensin-converting enzyme; BUN, blood urea nitrogen; NSAIDs, nonsteroidal anti-inflammatory drugs; SNRI, serotonin and norepinephrine reuptake inhibitors; SSRI, selective serotonin reuptake inhibitors.

Age-Related Changes

With age, body potassium declines. Age-related changes decrease muscle mass, which causes a decrease in the overall potassium content in the body. Potassium is lower in the elderly by approximately 20%.

With less potassium available, there is a tendency to retain more and excrete less potassium. Reduced excretion results in a risk of hyperkalemia. A decrease in aldosterone secretion with age means less potassium remains in the distal tubules. Elders tend to take more drugs that aggravate hyperkalemia. Angiotensin-converting enzyme (ACE) inhibitors, angiotension II receptor blockers, nonsteroidal anti-inflammatory drugs, and potassium-sparing diuretics can contribute to hyperkalemia. The risk of hyperkalemia among older adults is significant.

Similar to the response to hypernatremia, when the aging kidney is faced with hyperkalemia, it is slow to respond. The slow response is apparent when assessing the effect of diuretics on electrolyte levels. When elders are medicated with potassium-losing diuretics, the decrease in serum potassium and hypokalemia usually takes 1 to 2 weeks to appear.

Hypokalemia among elders is usually drug-induced and rarely the result of aging. Loop and thiazide diuretics, insulin, and beta-agonists are the frequent culprits. Any condition that results in diarrhea such as enteritis or excessive laxative use can quickly result in hypokalemia in the elderly.

ACID-BASE BALANCE

The distal tubule plays an important role in acid-base balance. Sodium is allowed to pass through the tubule membrane to the medullary interstitium in exchange for hydrogen ions. The hydrogen ions are excreted in the urine, making the normal pH of urine slightly acidic.

Age-Related Changes

With the ability of sodium reabsorption compromised in the aging distal tubule, hydrogen ions remain in the blood stream. Metabolic acidosis is common among the elderly. The time required by elders to excrete the acid load from metabolism is up to three times longer than a younger adult. When faced with a high acid load, such as lactic acidosis during shock states, an elder can remain in an uncompensated metabolic acidosis for a longer time than a younger individual.

BODY WATER

The amount of water in the vascular system, the cells, and the interstitium accounts for 60% to 75% of body weight in an adult. Gender differences in body weight are significant. Males have a greater percent of body water (63%) than females (52%). Two-thirds of the water is located in the cells. At any time, only a small percentage exists in the vascular system. Two mechanisms are primarily responsible for water balance: thirst and ADH.

The conscious perception of thirst, the need to ingest fluids, is believed to be the result of receptors in the thirst center located in the hypothalamus. As blood becomes more concentrated with particles, water is shifted out of the cells through osmosis. Hypothalmic osmoreceptors detect cellular dehydration and stimulate perception of thirst. When the plasma osmolality or the concentration of ions, sugar, and proteins in the blood is greater than 298.5 mmol/kg, a behavior response to drink is activated by the cerebral cortex.

A decrease in blood volume can also create thirst. When blood volume drops, pressure receptors in the carotid artery and aortic arch activate the thirst center in the brain. However, the pressure or osmotic thirst mechanism to restore fluid balance is far from perfect. There is poor response when the loss of fluid occurs rapidly.

Termination of the thirst stimuli occurs when plasma osmolality returns to normal. However, the desire to drink will diminish when the stomach becomes distended and sends feedback messages to the hypothalamus. Ingesting fluids as a result of thirst will gradually restore fluid balance. Some fluids and foods have been shown to influence thirst. Carbonated drinks dull the thirst response. Sweet fruity drinks and caffeinated liquids have mild diuretic effects, which can increase thirst. Despite popular opinion, water temperature does not appear to affect thirst perception. Meals high in protein require more water to filter byproducts than meals with fat or carbohydrates. The administration of high-protein tube feedings in patients with a compromised thirst response increases the risk of dehydration.

The second major regulator of water balance is ADH. One stimulus responsible for the release of ADH by the posterior pituitary is blood volume. When blood volume drops along with blood pressure, ADH release causes the distal tubules to increase the permeability of the distal tubules to water. The release of water by the tubules sends water back into the serum to increase blood volume and restore water balance.

Age-Related Changes

With aging, lean body mass decreases and body fat increases in both men and women. The change in body composition alters body water percentage. The percentage of body water in men drops from 63% to 60% and in women from 52% to 45%. The primary source of body water loss with aging occurs in the intracellular compartment. Plasma water, red blood cell mass, and interstitial fluid volumes are relatively unchanged in healthy elders. However, these fluid spaces are called on when electrolyte or water imbalances occur. While normal aging does not result in water imbalance, the lower percentage of body water places elders at higher risk for disturbances. When the total body water is depleted, dehydration occurs. Water losses (dehydration) and water gains (overload) have a more dramatic effect in elders.

Dehydration causes extracellular sodium to rise. The increase in sodium outside the cells pulls water from inside of the cells. The cells shrink and have difficulty maintaining their functional ability. Because elders' ability to respond to fluid and electrolyte changes is slower, mortality due to water imbalance is as much as 70% in the elderly.

When elders are exposed to conditions that waste salt and water, such as vomiting or diarrhea, the loss of water can be considerable. Volume depletion occurs when both water and salts are lost. Elders' intrinsic defect in thirst is a risk factor for dehydration. When exposed to 24 hours of water deprivation, younger adults experience less dehydration, lose less body weight, and perceive a higher level of thirst than older adults. Older adults reports of thirst are

> *Older adults have an intrinsic decrease in their thirst sensation, resulting in a greater tendency to dehydration.*

absent or diminished. After the period of deprivation, older adults take more than twice as long to correct their water imbalance when given free access to fluids.

The assessment of dehydration in the elderly is difficult. An evaluation of elders' risk factors for dehydration is essential. Patient age over 85, history of prior dehydration episodes, and infection are three major risk factors for dehydration. Other significant risk factors are living in an institution, a diagnosis of dementia, and dependency on others for feeding and eating.

The usual signs of dehydration seen in younger adults are often not present due to aging changes. Table 10.3 lists common signs of dehydration in older adults when compared to younger adults. The best indicators of dehydration are hemoconcentration, serum sodium, and serum osmolality values. Orthostatic hypotension caused by decreased circulating volume is a common indicator. Mucous membranes may be the best indication of hydration, with dry mucous membranes indicating dehydration.

Overhydration, on the other hand can lead to interstitial edema, poor wound healing, decreased pulmonary compliance, heart failure, and delayed return of bowel function. As noted previously, caring for the elderly surgical patient is a balance between too much

TABLE 10.3
Signs of Dehydration in Younger and Older Adults

Sign or Symptom	Younger Adult	Older Adult
Dry mouth, tongue	*	**
		Longitudinal furrows or folds in the tongue
Thirst	**	*
Sunken eyes	*	**
Poor skin turgor	*	Normal sign of aging
Muscle weakness	–	*
Decreased urine output	*	*
Postural hypotension	*	**
Compensatory tachycardia	**	–
Changes in mental status	–	*

Key:
–absent sign in most patients
*mild to moderate sign in most patients
**moderate to strongly notable sign in most patients

versus too little fluid. The fine line of fluid dehydration and overhydration is blurred by changes that take place in the aging urine system.

Urine Excretion

The collecting ducts of the nephron complete the formation of urine. From the collecting ducts, the filtrate from all of the nephrons is collected as urine in the renal pelvis. Urine passes from the renal pelvis and exits the kidneys through the ureters. The flow of urine from the renal pelvis to the ureters and ending at the bladder is continuous. The bladder is a muscular organ that can normally stretch to accommodate 400 to 700 mL of urine. When 100 to 200 mL has entered the bladder, a cognitive sensation of filling is experienced. The desire to void occurs when 200 to 300 mL or urine is in the bladder. Normally, approximately 50 mL remains in the bladder after voiding.

Bladder size is controlled by the detrusor muscle. The detrusor comprises of three layers of involuntary muscle fibers. During relaxation, when the bladder is being filled with urine passing down the ureters, the detrusor is under sympathetic nervous system control. The the internal sphincter, an involuntary band of muscle, is at the base of the bladder. The internal sphincter is a continuation of the detrusor muscle and is located at the top of the urethra. The internal sphincter prohibits urine flow from the bladder. Similar to the bladder itself, sympathetic stimulation results in contraction of the internal urinary sphincter. The bladder also has a secondary sphincter, the external sphincter. Also located at the base of the bladder at the top of the urethra, the external sphincter is composed of skeletal muscle. The skeletal muscle is under voluntary control by the pudendal nerve of the somatic nervous system.

When stimulated by the volume of urine in the muscular bladder, the number of nervous system impulses sent to the sacral spinal cord increases. The increase in impulses triggers the micturation reflex (urge to void). The micturation reflex allows parasympathetic activity to override sympathetic control. The loss of sympathetic control causes the detrusor muscle of the bladder to contract and the internal sphincter to relax. Once the external sphincter is consciously relaxed, urine passes from the bladder to the urethra and micturation occurs. Control over the voluntary micturation reflex is a learned response as a result of impulses to the hypothalamus and cerebral cortex of the brain.

Pelvic floor muscles are important in controlling the urethra. The urethra is composed of smooth muscle lined with epithelium. In women, it is shorter and averages 4 cm. In men, the urethra extends down the penis, 20 cm in length, also acting as a conduit for seminal fluid. Cessation of urine flow involves the voluntary contraction of the pubococcygeus muscle. The pubococcygeus muscle supports the pelvic organs. When the pubococcygeus muscle is contracted, the bladder neck is elevated and the urethra is compressed. In men, the pubococcygeus lies below the prostate to compress the urethra.

Age-Related Changes

Bladder capacity decreases with age, and the detrusor muscle becomes fibrous. As collagen deposits in the bladder wall accumulate, bladder compliance declines. As compliance declines, bladder capacity decreases and emptying can be impaired. The bladder capacity of an elder is approximately 250 mL, or half the volume of a younger adult. The result of these changes is a decrease in the amount of urine per void and an increase in the amount of urine remaining in the bladder. After voiding, residual urine, the amount remaining in the bladder, can be up to 100 mL in an elder. In addition to a decrease in the amount of urine per void and an increase in residual urine, the frequency of voiding increases. Decreased bladder compliance weakens the bladder contraction, and the rate of urine flow during the void also declines with age. The result in elders means frequent, small voids that require more time.

Neuromuscular changes with age result in the development of involuntary bladder contractions. While the prevalence of bladder spasms has been debated, up to 10% of women and 33% of men experience involuntary bladder contractions with no symptoms. However, for women, a combination of the loss of pelvic floor muscle strength with age and pregnancy, age-related involuntary spasms, and reduced bladder capacity can result in problems of urge incontinence.

GENDER DIFFERENCES IN VOIDING

Reproductive organs and function have a considerable influence on lower urinary function. In women, estrogen serves to maintain tissue tone in the pelvis and bladder neck. In addition, estrogen maintains the muscle tone of the female urethra.

Age-Related Changes

In postmenopausal women, the lack of estrogen weakens the pelvic floor tissues. The mucosa and muscle tone of the urethra decrease. A thinner urinary sphincter is less able to resist an increase in bladder pressure. Vaginal atrophy can affect urinary function. These changes contribute to a decline in urethral contractility. The drop in estrogen after menopause alters vaginal pH, placing women at higher risk for UTIs.

In men, the prostate gland surrounds the bladder neck and the top of the urethra. The bladder neck experiences an increase in collagen deposits with age. The deposits can thicken the bladder tissue and cause obstruction. Aging changes also occur in the prostate tissue as early as 40 years old. The outer prostatic tissue begins to proliferate, and by age 60 the entire gland undergoes hypertrophy. One-third of men over 30 years, half of men between 51 and 60 years, and 90% over age 80 have benign prostatic hypertrophy.

Hypertrophy of the prostate at any age constricts the urethra. The ability of the urine to flow through a constricted urethra causes urinary retention and bladder distension. Chronic distention weakens the detrusor muscle while thickening the bladder wall. When the bladder can no longer compensate by hypertrophy, it also loses the ability to contract. The result can be a backflow of urine into the ureters and renal pelvis, backing into the kidney leading to hydronephrosis and eventual kidney failure. Prostatic growth also displaces the bladder neck and lengthens the urethra. A common occurrence in older men is that they have incomplete bladder emptying and retained urine, which leads to an increased risk of UTIs.

CONTINENCE

Continence, the ability to control the storage and micturation of urine, is dependent on normal urinary function, intact nervous system function, and intact cognitive function. Urinary incontinence (UI), defined as an involuntary loss of urine, can affect quality of life in younger or older adults. While incontinence is not a normal part of aging, the normal changes in physical function as a result of aging can affect one or any of the many factors needed to remain continent.

Age-Related Changes

UI occurs in approximately one-third of noninstitutionalized elderly women and 20% of elderly men. Among institutionalized elders, the prevalence of UI increases to 60% to 80%, with women being affected twice as often as men. Yet, only one in every four women will seek treatment, relying instead on incontinence pads and undergarments. Over one-third of elders admitted to the hospital will develop UI. UI is categorized into four types depending on etiology. Each type of UI can occur in the elderly and displays characteristic signs and symptoms, as noted in Table 10.4.

Stress incontinence is the result of an increase in intra-abdominal pressure. An increase in pressure overcomes bladder neck sphincter tone, resulting in loss of urine. The weakened sphincter tone can be due to muscle stretching during pregnancy, hormonal deficits, or neuromuscular factors. Coughing, sneezing, or standing may increase the intra-abdominal pressure enough to overcome a weak sphincter and cause urine loss.

> *Among institutionalized elders, the prevalence of urinary incontinence is upward of 80%, with women being affected twice as often as men.*

Urge incontinence is the inability to delay voiding when the bladder is perceived as full. Urge incontinence is also referred to as unstable or hyperactive bladder. Urge incontinence has been associated with bladder spasms. When the bladder involuntarily contracts, the sphincters are unable to withstand the pressure and urine is lost.

Overflow incontinence is the result of an overdistended bladder. The overdistention can be caused by a failure to contract, a failure to empty, or both. More common in elderly men, the culprit is usually prostate enlargement causing obstruction to urine outflow. The bladder becomes distended and small amounts of urine pass the obstruction spontaneously, resulting in incontinence. The bladder may also fail to adequately contract when nerves have been damaged or are diseased, such as in diabetic neuropathy. In multiparous elderly women or those with estrogen deficits, a prolapse of the urethra into the bladder can be the cause of overflow incontinence.

Functional incontinence occurs when there is an inability to access toilet facilities. In the elderly, functional incontinence can be due to cognitive deficits or mobility problems. Apathy, anxiety, and dementia are associated with functional incontinence due to cognitive defects. Mobility problems such as weakness, lack of mobility aids, or a dark or unfamiliar environment can also contribute to functional incontinence.

TABLE 10.4

Type of Incontinence by Symptoms, Gender Differences, and Contributory Medications

	Urge Incontinence	Stress Incontinence	Overflow Incontinence	Functional Incontinence
Symptoms	Urgency Frequency Large volume of urine loss	Precipitated by laughing, coughing, sneezing Small volume of urine loss	Poor urine stream Continual urine dribbling Increased frequency Nocturia Postmicturation dribble	Desire to void without ability to access toilet Dementia Immobility
Gender differences	Men > Women	Women < 60 years Men after prostate surgery	Men > Women	No difference
Medications	Diuretics (furosemide, butmetanide)	Sympatholytics, alpha blockers	Anticholinergics, sympathomimetics, calcium channel blocker	

Mixed incontinence refers to the occurrence of two or more types of incontinence. Up to 55% of elderly women with complaints of incontinence will have a combination of stress and urge incontinence.

URINARY TRACT INFECTION

While age alone is not a causative factor for UTIs, changes in the urogenital system increase older adults' risk and vulnerability to UTIs. The prevalence of UTI among adults aged 65 to 96 is nearly 20% compared to an 8% incidence in persons 25 to 44 years old. It is estimated that over 10% of younger women experience an UTI annually, while older women have twice the prevalence. Elder men have one-third the incidence of UTI compared to elder women. To compound the risk, UTIs in older adults are more difficult to detect and treat. The classic symptoms of UTI found in young adults (fever, flank, or suprapubic pain, and hematuria) can be absent in elders. Instead, symptoms may be more generalized such as anorexia, nocturia, enuresis, or confusion.

> *The classic symptoms of UTI found in young adults (fever, flank, or suprapubic pain, and hematuria) can be absent in elders.*

Despite the normal physiological changes experienced by the kidney with aging, the decline in function is usually not evident until the body becomes stressed. Under periods of stress, the aging kidney is simply not as effective or efficient in filtering wastes, maintaining water balance, or regulating electrolytes. The kidney's response to demands posed by low blood volume or excessive blood volume is slow. The need to improve water balance is hampered by neurological and cognitive deficits. The impact of low blood pressure on the kidney's ability to filter is more significant. The challenge to remove excess concentrations of electrolytes is more complicated. When urine is produced by the stressed kidney, aging changes in the lower urinary tract can cause functional difficulty. Urine retention, incontinence, and UTIs in elders can mask renal problems while precipitating additional stressors.

Gerioperative Care

PREOPERATIVE CONSIDERATIONS

Assessment of renal and lower urinary function during the preoperative phase is essential to minimize kidney damage and promote the restoration of fluid and electrolyte balance disrupted by surgery and anesthesia. Preoperative renal status is the most accurate predictor of postoperative renal failure.

As previously described, elders can suffer from dehydration due to normal age-related changes such as decreased thirst mechanism, changes in renin and aldosterone secretion, along with reduced activity and fluid intake. Pathophysiologic mechanisms of diabetes, hypertension, and underlying renal disease along with medications such as hypoglycemics, antihypertensives, and diuretics can contribute to dehydration.

Attempts should be made to minimize the stress placed on the kidney. When possible, surgery for elders should be scheduled early in the morning to reduce fasting times that contribute to fluid imbalance and dehydration. Guidelines advocate that clear liquids can be consumed up to 2 hours prior to anesthesia. Limiting the duration of fasting will reduce the risk of fluid imbalance.

HISTORY

The preoperative medical and surgical history should include information pertaining to preexisting renal and urinary tract diseases. There are no age-specific renal or urinary tract diseases specific to elders. Information should be obtained on factors that would increase the risk of developing renal insufficiency and altered postoperative elimination. An assessment of risks includes ability to maintain renal blood flow during the stress of surgery and anesthesia, and the impact of stressors on the hormonal changes that effect filtration.

Obtaining information related to the patient's current fluid volume status is essential. A minimum of 1,500 to 2,500 mL from fluids and foods for adults who weigh between 50 and 80 kg adults is necessary to prevent dehydration. Dehydration prior to surgery can result in poor renal perfusion during and after surgery. Each 8-hour period a patient is not allowed to eat or drink increases the fluid volume deficit by approximately 1 L. Elders may eat their last meal and drink their last liquid hours prior to the required nothing-by-mouth deadline. When the patient has not had anything to drink after 6 p.m. the previous evening, and surgery does not commence until 10 a.m., the patient will begin surgery with a 2-L fluid volume deficit. If the patient completed a bowel preparation regimen, the history should include an assessment of the amount of preparation ingested and approximate amount expelled. Bowel cleansing regimens place elders at high risk for hypernatremia, hypokalemia, and dehydration.

Obtain a history of their normal fluid intake and voiding patterns. Assess for UI and obstruction. If an elder voids frequently preoperatively, urge incontinence may occur immediately on recovering from anesthesia. Chronic obstruction due to prostatic enlargement can be particularly troublesome if the patient is required to void before going home after ambulatory surgery.

The usual signs and symptoms of lower UTI are unlikely in an elder. Changes in voiding frequency, amount, and timing may be the only clues to an urinary infection.

A comprehensive drug history targets medications known to alter renal blood flow, blood volume, blood pressure, tubule permeability to electrolytes, and hormones influencing reabsorption such as those indicated in Table 10.2. The anesthesia provider makes the determination regarding which essential medications should be continued throughout the perioperative period. Ambulatory surgical patients are usually allowed to continue with antihypertensive and cardiac medications. Diuretics may be stopped for the day of surgery depending on the anticipated nothing-by-mouth duration, surgical time, and anesthesia recovery time. The timing and amount of the most recent dose of any medication is critical.

A comprehensive drug history targets medications known to alter renal blood flow, blood volume, blood pressure, tubule permeability to electrolytes, and hormones influencing reabsorption.

PHYSICAL ASSESSMENT

There are few outward signs of renal insufficiency or urinary tract dysfunction among elders. When conducting a preoperative assessment, attention should focus on lower urinary tract symptoms that will impact postoperative care and outcomes. Note the use of diapers or incontinence pads reflecting self-care of incontinence not mentioned in the patient history. Elderly patients are at risk for dehydration secondary to medications, disease processes, and age-related changes. A prominent sign of dehydration is dry mucous membranes.

PREOPERATIVE TESTING

Glomerular Filtration Rate

The GFR is one of the best estimates of renal function. While GFR can be directly measured, such measurements are time-consuming and invasive. Direct measurement of the GFR requires injection of a substance that is freely filtered by the glomeruli (not absorbed and not excreted). As a result, formulas have been developed to estimate GFR. A calculated GFR's ability to predict renal insufficiency is strongly debated. GFR calculations must account for serum creatinine, age, gender, and ethnicity.

Creatinine

Creatinine is a breakdown product of creatinine phosphate. Creatinine phosphate assists in producing adenosine triphosphate energy in skeletal muscle and the brain. The breakdown of creatinine phosphate is relatively constant, producing a stable level of creatinine in the healthy adult. Creatinine is filtered out by the glomeruli into Bowman's capsule. Once creatinine enters the tubules, it is not reabsorbed back into the interstitium or vascular system. The nephron's inability to resorb creatinine allows kidney function to be measured by monitoring serum creatinine concentrations, referred to as creatinine clearance (CrCl). Creatinine clearance measurement is a laborious although less invasive substitute for direct GFR measurement as a basis for kidney function.

CrCl is the amount of creatinine removed from the blood over a given time interval, usually measured over 24 hours. Three measurements are required for the determination of CrCl: the amount of urine produced in 24 hours, the amount of creatinine in the 24-hour urine volume, and the plasma creatinine. The factors influencing CrCl include nutritional status, protein intake, and muscle mass; each of these factors change as adults age. Thus, it is not surprising that fewer than two-thirds of elders will show a decline in CrCl. While CrCl is noninvasive, it is a difficult test for elders to complete at home. The variability of CrCl and difficulty of testing does not lend itself to a preoperative measure of assessing renal function in the elderly.

Serum creatinine is a fast, easy, and relatively noninvasive assessment of kidney function. Normal serum creatinine values are typically between 0.5 and 1.0 mg/dL. Because the serum creatinine values can be easily altered with muscle use or muscle damage, the creatinine value only offers an imperfect substitute for GFR measurements. Nearly 10% of patients over 40 years have elevated creatinine levels. Interpretation of the serum creatinine values should be undertaken with caution. The serum creatinine of a male body builder may be normal at 2.0 mg/dL, while the same value in a 60-year-old woman may indicate 50% loss of renal function. A decline in GFR with age parallels a decline in muscle mass. Decline in elders' muscle mass decreases the serum creatinine. Thus, despite renal function decline, in the elderly, serum creatinine may be within the normal range. The finding of a normal creatinine value during the preoperative assessment in an older patient can be misleading.

Serum creatinine will also be affected by drug therapy. Two common drugs prescribed for elders are ACE inhibitors and angiotensin II receptor blockers. Both increase serum creatinine. Therefore, evaluating the trend of serum creatinine level over time is a better indicator of renal status than a single value. Having access to past creatinine levels can provide a better preoperative assessment than obtaining a single creatinine the day of surgery.

Preoperative patients of any age who have a cardiac history, hypertension, diabetes, or renal insufficiency are all candidates for preoperative assessment of creatinine. Patients likely to have intraoperative hypotension, reduced blood flow, or those who take potentially nephrotoxic or renal-affecting medications should also have preoperative creatinine values evaluated. Some clinicians order creatinine testing for all patients over 40 or 50 years, though there is no evidence that these values change intra- or postoperative management.

Blood Urea Nitrogen

Serum creatinine values are often ordered along with an assessment of the blood urea nitrogen (BUN). The serum BUN is a measure of the amount of nitrogen in the blood in the form of urea. The typical normal value for BUN is between 7 and 21 mg/dL. Urea is filtered by the glomeruli. The tubule is not permeable to urea, and the amount filtered is the amount excreted in the urine. While it seems that BUN would be a good indicator of glomeruli function, the amount of urea in the blood is dependent on factors outside the control of the glomeruli. Any time an excessive amount of blood byproducts is processed by the liver, the amount of urea increases. Any time there is an increased metabolism of proteins, such as with steroid use, high protein diets, or burn injuries, the serum BUN will increase. Decreased renal blood flow will also result in a higher serum BUN. As a single value, the BUN, unless it is considerably elevated (> 60 mg/dL), offers little value is assessing renal function.

The ratio of BUN to serum creatinine is used as an indicator of renal function. The normal range of BUN:creatinine is between 10:1 and 20:1. Values greater than 20 may indicate reduced blood flow to the kidney. Values less than 10 may indicate damage to the nephron. However, because aging decreases muscle mass which results in a lower creatinine, the BUN:creatinine value may be elevated in the absence of renal dysfunction.

Cystatin C

Cystatin C is a small protein produced by the nucleus in all cells. As a protein, it is freely filtered through the glomeruli. Levels of cystatin C can be detected in the blood as an indicator of renal function. The typical normal value for cystatin C is between 0.57 and 1.12 mg/L. The advantage of cystatin C is a greater sensitivity of renal function. In addition, cystatin C does not appear to be strongly influenced by age. A major disadvantage is cost and availability of this relatively new test.

Urinalysis

Preoperative testing of urine is still required in facilities despite reports that abnormal preoperative findings can only be detected in up to one-third of all surgical patients. Studies indicate that asymptomatic UTIs do not require treatment, so despite these abnormal findings from routine preoperative urinalyses, less than 3% of all patients will be treated. Nearly 100% of elders with indwelling catheters will have bacteriuria without symptoms.

In general, preoperative urinalysis across the lifespan has not been found cost-effective and, therefore, is not routinely recommended. The evidence is less clear for the older surgical patient. The typical symptoms of dysuria, urgency, and frequency associated with UTIs are often absent in the older adult. Up to 36% of elderly patients who present for orthopedic surgery have previously unknown UTIs. It is known that patients with either a UTI or urinary tract colonization have higher rates of superficial wound infection than controls. In joint replacement surgeries, UTIs can lead to infections at the site of the prosthesis.

These findings bring into question whether all older adults should, indeed, be routinely screened for UTIs preoperatively. Urine cultures are indicated if the elder has symptoms of new onset urgency, burning, frequency, or confusion. All older adults having joint replacement must be screened preoperatively for UTI. Urine dipsticks to detect the presence of nitrites and leukocytosis may prove to be a cost-effective screening tool for UTIs in the gerioperative patient.

Electrolytes

Assessing serum electrolytes in elderly patients requires a consideration of the preoperative state and the surgical procedure. The incidence of preoperative electrolyte imbalance is nearly one in eight patients. A key concern during the intraoperative and postoperative periods is the development of arrhythmias secondary to hypokalemia or hyperkalemia. Serum potassium evaluation is appropriate for any patients with preexisting cardiac disease or renal insufficiency. Serum potassium values in elders taking hypertensive medications, diuretics, and antiarrhythmic medications may indicate the need for perioperative intervention. Because hyponatremia is a common finding among long-term care residents, preoperative assessment of electrolytes in this population may be warranted.

Unexpected postoperative electrolyte disturbances occur in up to 8% of surgical patients. Certain surgeries that are more common in the elderly population, however, increase the risk of electrolyte imbalances. Neurosurgical procedures on or near the pituitary, hypothalamus, thyroid, or parathyroid can disrupt hormonal function that regulates electrolyte reabsorption by the renal tubules. Transurethral prostate resections require high volumes of surgical irrigation, which can translate to the inappropriate secretion of aldosterone. Surgeries requiring the administration of intraoperative steroids or diuretics can result in altered fluid and electrolyte balance in the postoperative period. Baseline preoperative data is helpful in determining the effect of these drug therapies on kidney function.

Routine laboratory testing for renal or urinary tract problems in healthy elders does not add significant information to the data collected in the history. Routine laboratory testing is not recommended. Laboratory testing is indicated when the preoperative history and physical indicate preexisting renal disease, urinary tract problems, or use of nephrotoxic medications. Preoperative testing is also warranted when surgical procedures are likely to create hypotension, hypovolemia, or excessive bleeding. Vascular procedures of the heart or large vessels (e.g., abdominal aortic aneurysm) can significantly reduce renal artery blood flow for prolonged periods of time. Time-consuming orthopedic procedures conducted under intentional hypotension such as back procedures and joint replacements can reduce blood volume to the kidney. Surgery involving highly vascular organs such as the spleen or liver can result in unexpected hypotension, hypovolemia, and excessive blood loss. Plastic surgery procedures can require extensive intraoperative fluid replacements. Serum creatinine and BUN:creatinine ratio, though crude indicators of GFR, can provide baseline data to assess the intraoperative and postoperative recovery of the aging kidney.

INTRAVENOUS FLUID ADMINISTRATION

The goal of fluid administration is to promote hemodynamic stability during the perioperative period by maintaining or restoring blood volume. Dehydration can result in hypotension leading to decreased oxygen delivery and perfusion to the kidneys. Maintaining renal blood flow is essential for renal protection during surgery.

The goal of fluid administration is to promote hemodynamic stability during the perioperative period.

Preoperatively, the goal of normovolemia is maintained by hydration. Oral fluid hydration is preferred, though administration of intravenous fluids may be needed to supplement or replace oral intake. The risk of intraoperative hypotension may be reduced with preoperative clinical pathways for fluid management. It has been shown that 3 L of normal saline administered preoperatively over a 24-hour period to elders with femur neck fractures significantly reduces the risk of intraoperative hypotension. However, further research in preemptive fluid management in the preoperative period is needed.

Historically, fluid management of elderly patients has often been neglected. Perioperative fluids should be ordered with the same priority as perioperative prescriptions. It is the nurse's responsibility to ensure adequate hydration preoperatively by informing the health care provider of possible risks as well as any signs and symptoms of dehydration.

Intravenous Fluid Choices

Type of intravenous fluid is a function of the patient condition, circumstances, and the desired goal.

Intravenous fluids administered during the perioperative period may be colloids, crystalloids, or a combination of both. Colloids are large molecular weight solutions containing particles that do not easily cross the semipermeable cell membranes. The large particles create an oncotic pressure, drawing water into the vascular space. Colloids are plasma volume expanders and include albumin, hetastarch, and dextran. Colloids are replaced on a 1 mL:1 mL ratio of blood loss to replacement. The risks of colloids include a small but significant incidence of adverse reactions, and the ability to cause dramatic fluid shifts that can be dangerous if not monitored. The benefit of using colloids over crystalloids in acute fluid replacement has not been supported.

Crystalloids are clear solutions composed of water and electrolytes. Crystalloid solutions readily cross the semipermeable cell membrane, leaving the vascular space within 60 to 90 minutes. Common crystalloids include 0.9% normal saline (NS) and its variant 0.45% NS, lactated Ringer's solution (LR), and dextrose-containing solutions such as 5% dextrose solution in water (D5W), D5NS, and 5% dextrose in 0.45% NS. Many more specific variations of these crystalloid solutions exist and may be used, depending on the patient and the patient's electrolyte status and the goal of use. As a general rule, 3 mL of crystalloid is required to replace each milliliter of blood loss. The higher replacement ratio of crystalloids increases the risk of heart failure and pulmonary edema when they are administered to replace blood loss. Crystalloids have the advantage, however, of being easily available, less costly, and have a longer shelf life.

Crystalloids are selected for fluid replacement based on their osmolarity. Generally in practice settings, fluids are referred to in terms of their tonicity. Osmolarity and tonicity are closely related but different concepts, thus, the terms ending in -osmotic (isosmotic, hyperosmotic, hyposmotic) are not synonymous with the terms ending in -tonic (isotonic, hypertonic, hypotonic). The terms are different because osmolarity takes into account the total concentration of penetrating solutes and nonpenetrating solutes, whereas tonicity takes into account the total concentration of only nonpenetrating solutes. Penetrating solutes can diffuse through the cell membrane, causing momentary changes in cell volume as the solutes "pull" water molecules with them. Nonpenetrating solutes cannot cross the cell membrane, and therefore osmosis of water must occur for the solutions to reach equilibrium. Simply stated, osmolarity refers to the amount of solute in a solution, whereas tonicity refers to osmotic effect of the solution in relation to another solution across a semipermeable membrane. Tonicity, therefore, is dependent on the ability of the solute to pass through the cell membrane. The concept of tonicity in the body is complex as cell permeability varies with cell type and circumstances.

In this discussion, fluids will be described as hypertonic, hypotonic, and isotonic in relation to blood. Understanding fluid tonicity and composition is important for the perioperative nurse. Vascular volume is not only a function of quantity of fluid administered, but also dependent on the type of fluid a patient receives. Each intravenous fluid choice has a specific formulation that confers certain advantages based on its composition, and therefore, choice of fluid type is a function of the patient, the circumstances, and the desired goal. Tables 10.5 and 10.6 outline the composition of commonly used fluids in the management of surgical patients and their most common uses, respectively. Intra- and extravascular volumes vary considerably depending on the solute concentration of the administered fluid, as noted in Table 10.7.

TABLE 10.5

Composition of Common Crystalloid Fluids Compared to Blood Plasma

Solution	Na$^+$	K$^+$	Ca^{++}	Mg$^+$	Cl$^-$	Buffers$^-$	Glucose	Osmolality	pH
Plasma	142	4	5	3	103	27	0	290	7.4
NS (0.9%)	154	0	0	0	154	0	0	308	5.6
0.45% NS	73	0	0	0	77	0	0	154	5.6
D51/2NS	77	0	0	0	77	0	50 g	431	4.4
D5W	0	0	0	0	0	0	50 g	273	4.0
LR	130	4	3	0	109	28 (lactate)	0	274	6.5

Ion values expressed as mEq/L.
Ca, calcium; Cl, chloride; D51/2NS, 5% dextrose in half NS; D5W, 5% dextrose solution in water; K, potassium; LR, lactated Ringer's solution; Mg, magnesium; Na, sodium; NS, normal saline.

TABLE 10.6

Common Intravenous Fluids and Perioperative Use

Intravenous Fluid	Purpose
D5LR	Fluid maintenance
LR	Fluid replacement
D51/2NS	Fluid maintenance
D5NS	Fluid replacement

D5LR, 5% dextrose in lactated Ringer's solution; D51/2NS, 5% dextrose in 1/2 normal saline; LR, lactated Ringer's solution; D5NS, 5% dextrose in normal saline.

TABLE 10.7

The Effect of Administering 1 L of Fluid on Intra- and Extravasculature Fluid Volumes

Fluid Type (1 L)	Approximate Intravasculature Fluid Volume Increase in Milliliters (approximate fraction of the 1 L)	Approximate Extravascular Fluid Volume Increase in Milliliters (approximate fraction of the 1 L)
NS	1000 mL	0 mL
LR	900 mL	100 mL
D5NS	500 mL	400 mL
0.45% NS	700 mL	300 mL
D5W	300 mL	700 mL

NS, normal saline; LR, lactated Ringer's solution; D5NS, 5% dextrose in normal saline; 0.45% NS, 1/2 normal saline; D5W, 5% dextrose solution in water.

Hypertonic solutions (e.g., 3.0% NS) have a higher osmolarity than serum. When administered, the osmotic pressure difference across the vasculature cell membranes causes fluid to move from the cells and extracellular spaces into the blood stream. The movement of fluid stabilizes blood pressure and increases urine output by increasing intravascular volume. Three percent NS also effects hypotonic hyponatremia and decreases interstitial edema. When cells are already dehydrated, however, the administration of hypertonic crystalloids can cause cell shrinkage and death. Hypertonic solutions must be used with extreme caution.

Hypotonic solutions (e.g., 0.45% NS) have lower osmolarity than the serum. The reduced number of particles in the solution creates a lower osmotic pressure with water in the solution moving quickly from the vasculature into the cells and surrounding extracellular spaces. These solutions are helpful when cells are dehydrated such as in diabetic ketoacidosis. However, when the blood volume is already low, the risks of using hypotonic solutions include cardiovascular collapse and the creation of hyponatremia. Administration of hypotonic solutions can also increase intracranial pressure by a shift of water from the cerebral vessels to brain cells.

Isotonic solutions (e.g., 0.9% NS or LR) have an osmolarity similar to serum. Isotonic solutions remain in the vasculature for a few hours and can be administered for short-term volume expansion or maintenance hydration as required.

Dextrose-containing fluids are considered hypertonic on administration. However, the dextrose is quickly metabolized leaving the remaining solution. When D5W solution is administered, the remaining solution is hypotonic (water). When D5NS is administered, the fluid remaining after dextrose metabolism is isotonic NS. Dextrose solutions are used preoperatively to maintain water balance and provide an energy source for patients that cannot have anything by mouth. Care must be taken in patients with history of heart failure or increased intracranial pressure to avoid overhydration.

AGE-RELATED CHANGES

Compared with younger adults, elderly patients have a lower overall body fluid level. Preoperative dehydration is a common occurrence. Elders who are mildly dehydrated have lost fluid equivalent to more than 5% of body weight; those moderately dehydrated have lost about 10%; and those severely dehydrated have lost upwards of 15%. The type of fluid administered depends on the cause of the dehydration.

VASOPRESSORS

Renal blood flow can be increased with the administration of vasopressors. Dopamine is a naturally occurring catecholamine that causes sympathetic vasoconstriction and redistributes blood flow to the kidneys. However, tachycardia, dysrhythmias, and myocardial ischemia are problematic side effects. Ephedrine sulfate is a potent vasoconstrictor and often used when rapid effects are needed to increase blood pressure and maintain renal blood flow. Ephedrine, eliminated by the kidneys, also causes tachycardia and dysrhythmias. However, because of its short half-life, it can be repeated two or three times before a receptor resistance (tachyphylaxis) builds up. Phenylephrine is neither inotropic nor chronotropic and will increase blood pressure.

Age-Related Changes

Elderly patients often exhibit hypotension due to loss of fluid volume and blood. In the event the patient is severely dehydrated, overhydrated, or hydration is contraindicated, the administration of vasopressors can maintain renal blood flow during the pre-, intra-, or postoperative period. However, the tachycardia and dysrhythmias of dopamine and ephedrine sulfate can result in additional cardiac compromise for elders. Ephedrine should be used with caution as it can react with many medications taken by elders and result in severe hypertension. Phenylephrine is an excellent drug choice for short-term treatment of hypotension in the elderly. It causes a consistent increase in blood pressure, can be administered as an intravenous drip, and causes a reflex bradycardia that can be cardioprotective.

INTRAOPERATIVE CONSIDERATIONS

Care of the aging kidney during the intraoperative period focuses on maintaining water and electrolyte balance, ensuring renal blood flow, and avoiding nephron damage.

Fluid Balance

Most elective surgical patients begin surgery and anesthesia in negative fluid balance, their input has been less than their output. Status of having nothing by mouth creates a fluid deficit that is compounded by bowel cleansing preparations, diuretics, or medications that regulate blood sugar. Intraoperative intravenous fluid administration includes maintenance fluids and fluids to compensate for preoperative and intraoperative losses. Fluids must be meticulously managed in elderly patients. Hypotonic fluid administration (0.45% NS, D5W) can contribute to or worsen elders' risk for hyponatremia. LR can contribute to hyperkalemia, which can further acidosis. NS or packed red cells are preferred to manage volume replacement.

Renal Blood Flow

Anesthesia agents have little direct effect on renal function. However, anesthetic agents' impact on cardiac output, peripheral vascular resistance, and heart rate can impact mean arterial pressure (MAP), which affects glomerular filtration. After the induction of general anesthesia, peripheral vascular resistance decreases. In elders on cardiorhythmic medications, the ability to alter heart rate to compensate for a decrease in peripheral vascular resistance is limited. Elders are also unable to compensate if they are volume depleted. It is important to maintain MAP sufficient for renal perfusion throughout the perioperative period.

Renal blood flow and the filtration ability of the glomerulus can be compromised by the occurrence and duration of intraoperative hypotension. The likelihood of renal compromise is greater in intra-abdominal surgery and procedures involving the aorta. During surgery to repair abdominal aortic aneurysms, the renal arteries may be clamped for a short period of time. In elders, the lack of blood flow, even for short durations, may overwhelm the kidney's reserve. Vascular procedures also increase the risk of excessive bleeding, hypovolemia, and further risk of renal compromise. Monitoring of urine output is critical during procedures that can compromise MAP or carry a high risk of bleeding. A urinary catheter is necessary during the intraoperative period to insure that a urine output of at least 0.5 mL/kg per hour is maintained.

Nephrotoxicity

Reduced blood flow and the decline in glomerular filtration due to age alter the pharmacokinetics of anesthetic drugs. When a preoperative evaluation of CrCl is not available, calculation of medication doses for elders assumes renal impairment. An isolated serum creatinine level cannot be relied on to assess anesthetic drug metabolism.

Anesthetic agents bound to proteins are lipid-soluble. The agents are filtered by the glomeruli and are completely reabsorbed by the tubules back into the blood. The exception is muscle relaxants that are partially eliminated by the kidneys. Anesthetic drug toxicity is seen at lower doses in elderly patients. When renal filtration is impaired by aging or diseases, the metabolism of anesthetic agents is delayed.

Opioids are metabolized by the liver but require renal filtration for elimination. While most of the opioid metabolites are inactive, the commonly used morphine sulfate is an exception. Morphine sulfate, while not directly eliminated by renal filtration, requires glomerular function for the elimination of two active metabolites. Thus, morphine sulfate requires careful dosing in the elderly to minimize the risk of side effects produced by the poorly filtrated metabolites.

POSTOPERATIVE CONSIDERATIONS

Care of the elderly during the postoperative period is a continuation of the intraoperative period and is focused on maintaining water and electrolyte balance, ensuring renal blood flow, and avoiding nephron damage. Additionally, postoperative care requires ensuring that the lower urinary tract has returned to preoperative baseline and the patient is prepared to maintain adequate hydration.

Water and Electrolyte Balance

The stress of surgery, anesthesia, and pain causes the release of ADH from the adrenal glands in both younger and older adults. The "flight or fight" response is designed to conserve fluids in order to augment cardiac output. It is not uncommon for postoperative patients to experience weight gain from water retention. Within 3 days after surgery, when the stress response has abated, a postsurgical diuresis occurs. Elders may have a blunted stress response and/or a reduced postsurgical diuresis. Reestablishing fluid balance takes longer for elders.

Immediately postoperatively, perioperative fluid balance should be calculated. Output determinations, including preoperative deficits, blood loss, and estimates of third spacing of fluids, are combined with urine output. Intake considers all fluids and blood products. Once fluid balance is determined, a vital activity in the care of the postoperative patient is achieving and maintaining a balance between fluid overload and fluid deprivation. Monitoring of urine output in the presence of a urinary catheter includes assessment of urine volume and color, remembering that the aging kidney may be unable to dilute urine.

The intraoperative pharmacologic regimen is important during the immediate postoperative recovery as the infusion of large amounts of blood products can lead to electrolyte imbalance, particularly hyperkalemia. The intraoperative administration of diuretics can lead to hypokalemia. Fluid lost through excessive intraoperative irrigation, such as during large abdominal surgeries or transurethral resections of the prostate, can contribute to hyponatremia. Postoperative care requires knowledge of the perioperative events that have increased the risk of electrolyte imbalance. Elders' kidneys can be slow to respond to electrolyte shifts and slow to adjust to imbalance.

When the patient is able to take fluids by mouth, appropriate fluids should be offered. Fruit juices and caffeinated drinks should be avoided in the immediate postoperative period. Water or (diet) ginger ale is suggested. Patient and caregiver education regarding the need to resume adequate hydration will improve postoperative outcomes.

Renal Blood Flow

Maintaining an adequate MAP is as important postoperatively as intraoperatively. Vasoconstrictors may be required while the elder's intravascular volume is replaced. Postoperative blood pressure should remain within 15% to 30% of the patient's normal preoperative blood pressure.

Nephrotoxicity

Careful considerations are given to drugs administered postoperatively that may be potentially nephrotoxic. Morphine sulfate and muscle relaxants must be carefully titrated in the presence of renal insufficiency.

Diuretics

Diuretics such as furosemide and mannitol are often used during the perioperative period to stimulate urine output and prevent renal failure. Furosemide is a loop diuretic that stimulates the cells in the loop of Henle to reabsorb sodium and chloride and secrete potassium. Used to treat acute pulmonary edema, increased intracranial pressure, oliguria, and excessive fluid overload, furosemide side effects include hypokalemia and dehydration. Diuresis occurs within 2 to 10 minutes after intravenous administration.

Mannitol is a sugar that produces diuresis because it is filtered by the glomeruli and not reabsorbed in the renal tubules. The increased osmolarity of fluid in the renal tubule increases excretion of water. Mannitol also increases plasma osmolarity, which draws fluid from the intracellular spaces. Mannitol is used primarily in craniotomies to decrease intracranial pressure by redistributing fluid from intracellular to extracellular spaces, reducing brain size. A side effect of mannitol can be exacerbation of heart failure from an increase in intravascular fluid volume.

The postoperative nurse must be aware of the diuretics given intraoperatively in order to assess urine output. Electrolytes must be monitored closely when the urine output is greater than 500 mL after arrival to postanesthesia care unit (PACU).

Excretion

After a spinal anesthetic, the bladder muscles of the elderly patient can be the last to regain function. Once the bladder volume can be sensed, the urge for a bedpan may be immediate. Frequent small amounts of voided urine may be of concern in a younger adult but are a normal behavior in an elder. Knowledge of preoperative voiding habits is essential for postoperative evaluation. Bladder scanning is a noninvasive technique to detect residual volume. Residual volumes up to 100 mL are tolerable in the stretched older bladder. If needed, straight catheterization is preferred. Older men may need the abdominal pressure obtained by standing to urinate. A distended bladder in an older adult may manifest as acute delirium, which resolves when the bladder is emptied.

PATIENT REPORT: Mrs. Coburn

Mrs. Coburn arrives in the PACU following a 2-hour surgery for removal of a small section of her transverse colon in response to the laparoscopic findings. The intraoperative report indicates that vasopressors were necessary during surgery to maintain blood pressure. Her blood pressure in the PACU is 100/50 with a MAP of 65 mm Hg and a heart rate of 60 beats/minute. The blood sugar is 100 mg/dL. Other vital signs are stable. A Foley catheter is in place with yellow urine. Her fluid balance for the 2-hour surgery is calculated as −325 mL, as indicated in Table 10.8. During the first postoperative hour, her urine output is 30 mL of concentrated yellow urine, and her BP is 90/60 (MAP 60). What is Mrs. Coburn's fluid status, and what circumstances surround her fluid status? What should be the nurse's course of action?

Mrs. Coburn's history of hypertension, diabetes, and heart failure predispose her to dehydration from the chronic disease processes and use of diuretics. During

TABLE 10.8

Mrs. Coburn's Postsurgical Fluid Status

Input	0.9% normal saline	1,500 mL	
	Hetastarch	500 mL	
Output	Urine	50 mL	2,000 mL
	Blood loss (estimated)	50 mL	
	Nasogastric tube drainage	50 mL	
	Other fluid losses (bowel)	2,175 mL	
			−2,375 mL
Net fluid balance			**−325 mL**

surgery, the anesthesia team may have been hesitant to give excess intravenous fluids secondary to the history of heart failure. The low blood pressure and concentrated urine indicate dehydration, as does the report that vasopressors were necessary to maintain blood pressure in surgery. Why is it that her heart rate has remained 60? She is on metoprolol, which controls her heart rate. Should she be given a diuretic to increase her urine output? Her dry mucous membranes indicate that the problem is lack of fluid, not the need to hydrate her kidneys. Mrs. Coburn is dehydrated and needs intravenous fluids in order to prevent renal failure. The priority nursing action is to contact anesthesia or the surgeon and negotiate an order for a fluid bolus and to increase her intravenous fluids.

Nurses have a responsibility to review and analyze data from preoperative, intraoperative, and postoperative reports when formulating a plan of care for the gerioperative patient. Consideration of data from every level of care is important in planning current care needs and anticipating future needs. Knowing Mrs. Coburn's preoperative health history and intraoperative events are critical to preventing renal damage after her surgery.

SUMMARY

The kidney is a complex and highly vascular organ that is controlled by and controls many hormone systems. The basic functional unit of the kidney is the nephron. A nephron eliminates wastes from the body, regulates blood volume and blood pressure, controls serum electrolyte and metabolite concentrations, and regulates blood pH. Fluid and electrolyte balance is vital to life. Too little or too much fluid can lead to serious complications, complications that are increased by the diminished reserves of gerioperative patients. Normal age-related and pathophysiologic changes predispose the elderly to dehydration and can compromise fluid and electrolyte replacement. Complications of dehydration are serious and may be life-threatening. Likewise, fluid overload can destabilize a patient. Elders are predisposed to fluid volume overload secondary to cardiac impairment, chronic renal insufficiency, and medication side effects.

In this chapter, the role of the aging kidney in maintaining fluid balance during the perioperative period has been discussed. The involvement of hormones, the influence of medications, and the considerations for fluid replenishment and maintenance in the perioperative older surgical patient were explored, and the nursing implications and care management was discussed.

KEY POINTS

- Age-related changes in the renal system increase potential for impaired drug excretion, serum electrolyte imbalance, and altered fluid balance.
- Diuretic medications can cause either hyponatremia or hypernatremia in older adults.
- Older adults can have a urine output at night as much as three times higher than daytime output.
- Preoperative dehydration is a common occurrence. Up to 50% of older adults have chronic dehydration.
- Maintaining optimal fluid balance is critical throughout the perioperative continuum.
- Preoperative fluid balance influences intraoperative and postoperative risk for renal-related complications.
- Delirium is a common symptom of postoperative fluid and electrolyte imbalance requiring immediate intervention.

ELEVEN

Pulmonary

Jennifer V. Long, Raelene V. Shippee-Rice, and Susan J. Fetzer

PATIENT REPORT: Mr. Dawson

Mr. Dawson is a 73-year-old retired automobile mechanic who is scheduled to have a right total hip replacement. He has a history of chronic bronchitis secondary to a past and current smoking history equal to a pack of cigarettes a day for 50 years. He has kyphosis causing him to stand with his shoulders hunched forward. His medications include fluticasone/salmeterol, albuterol metered dose inhaler (MDI), and ipratroprium bromide MDI.

The pulmonary system develops throughout life, but maximal lung function is achieved by the age of 30. After age 35, pulmonary function deteriorates secondary to the changes in lung structure, function, and reserve, even in those who get regular aerobic activity. Although there is no evidence that age-related changes in the respiratory system disrupts day-to-day function, changes become evident when physiologic demands reach the limits of the supply and there is little or no reserve. When elders are physiologically stressed during the perioperative period, the risk of pulmonary complications is increased due to progressive loss of homeostatic reserves. Respiratory complications account for nearly 40% of the perioperative deaths in patients over the age of 65.

Years of smoking and exposure to pollutants or environmental toxins, together with changes in lung structure, contribute to postoperative respiratory complications. Pulmonary complications cause higher surgical morbidity and mortality in the elderly. Surgical procedures further diminish the respiratory system reserve secondary to positioning, anesthetic medications, pain, and changes in fluid balance. Understanding normal respiratory anatomy and function along with the changes that occur with aging allows health care providers to anticipate potential problems and implement appropriate interventions to minimize the impact of these problems on older adults.

This chapter reviews changes in the aging respiratory system. A review and discussion of respiratory compromise, early detection of complications, and immediate intervention is presented. The term *respiratory* refers to respiratory structure. Pulmonary refers to the overall function of the respiratory system and when discussing perioperative pulmonary care of the older adult.

Pulmonary Considerations

The respiratory system provides oxygen to tissues for metabolism and removes carbon dioxide (CO_2). It also serves several secondary functions including speech production, a site for the sensory organ of smell, warming and filtering of inhaled air to protect the alveoli, and facilitating acid-base and fluid balance.

Ventilation, diffusion, and perfusion all contribute to respiration, the cellular utilization of oxygen. Although often used interchangeably, these concepts are critically different. Understanding these differences is key to understanding pulmonary function. Ventilation is the mechanical act of moving air in and out of the lungs. Ventilation is affected by changes in both the lung structure and the musculoskeletal system. Diffusion is the exchange of oxygen and CO_2 across the alveoli capillary membrane. Perfusion refers to the delivery of blood to the alveoli allowing for gas exchange.

The respiratory mucous membranes begin in the nose and end in the smallest tubules of the lungs. Mucous membranes moisten the inhaled air to protect the airway. The mucous membrane of the respiratory tract is ciliated (covered with tiny hairs that move back and forth simultaneously, rhythmically, and continuously like a brush) to move foreign particles into the oropharynx, where they can be expectorated or swallowed. The mucous membrane goblet cells produce phlegm, a sticky substance that helps to trap foreign particles. The goblet cells produce up to 500 mL of mucous each day. The phlegm, cilia, and mucous membrane create a mucociliary blanket to protect the system from bacteria, allergens, dust, and pollutants.

The effects of the mucociliary blanket can be enhanced by coughing or inhibited by smoking, dry air, or decreased oxygen levels. Smoking slows or impairs ciliary motion and may permanently destroy cilia. Once cilia become damaged by cigarette smoke, allergens and dust accumulate in the airways decreasing the effectiveness of diffusion. Cigarette smoke also decreases diffusion by causing an overgrowth or hyperplasia of mucous membrane goblet cells. An increase in goblet cells increases mucous production resulting in thick secretions that are difficult to expectorate. The risk of respiratory infections increases as pathogens are trapped in the lungs and not removed. Immunoglobulin A (IgA) antibodies are present in the mucosal membrane. The immediate presence of antibodies in the respiratory tree increases the defense against inhaled viruses.

Submucosal cells secrete a thin watery substance that moistens the air taken into the respiratory tract. More moisture is added from the watery layer as air passes deeper into the respiratory tree. The capacity for the air to retain water vapor without condensation increases as the temperature increases from air to alveoli. The difference between the water content of the inspired air and the water content of air at the alveoli is contributed by the mucous membrane. The loss of moisture from the mucous membrane is known as insensible water loss and can be up to 500 mL per day.

Fever increases the amount of insensible water loss. The increased respiratory rate necessary to compensate for the increased metabolic demands of a fever causes additional water to be lost from the respiratory mucosa. As more water is lost, secretions thicken and cilia movement slows. Fever impairs the defenses provided by the mucociliary blanket.

Age-Related Changes

The mucociliary blanket changes with age. A loss of elastin fibers and an increase in collagen causes the mucous membrane to thin. Mucous cells atrophy leading to nasal dryness and epistaxis, dry mouth, and the potential for mucosal injury. With age, the number of submucosal cells decreases, resulting in a thicker mucous. Older adults often report a persistent "tickle" sensation and chronic cough as a result of the thick mucous that lodges in the nasopharynx.

Cilia decrease in number and are less functional with age, making them unable to move foreign particles up and out of the airway. The concentration of IgA antibodies found on the mucous membrane decreases with age, creating a decrease in the body's ability to defend against viruses. The combination of thicker mucous, fewer cilia, and immune system changes makes the elderly more susceptible to respiratory infections.

UPPER RESPIRATORY TRACT

The upper respiratory tract includes the nose and sinuses, mouth, pharynx, and larynx. The main function of the upper airway is to cleanse, moisturize, and warm the air entering the lungs.

The nose is a rigid, partly bony (upper third) and partly cartilaginous (lower two-thirds) structure. It is the first port of entry into the respiratory system. The nose, divided by the septum, is lined with thick hairs called vibrissae. Vibrissae act as the first line of defense by trapping large particles to prevent them from entering the lungs.

From the nose, air enters the turbinates or conchae. Three turbinates (superior, middle, and inferior) lie on each side of the internal portion of the nose. The nasolacrimal duct drains into the inferior turbinate, explaining why people develop nasal congestion when they cry. Turbinates increase the surface area of the mucous membrane so that air is heated, humidified, and filtered as it enters the nasopharynx. The heat provided by the extensive vascular network of the nasal septum and turbinates, as well as the vasculature, prevents damage to the sensitive tissues of the lungs. Olfactory receptors in the turbinates detect odor and communicate a sense of smell through the olfactory nerves.

The four sinuses (frontal, ethmoid, sphenoid, and maxillary) are air-filled structures surrounding the hollow bones of the nasal passages. The sinuses produce resonance during speech. A lining in the sinuses produces mucous that keeps the nose and sinuses moist. Sinuses decrease the weight of the skull and act as shock absorbers to reduce damage to the skull in the event of trauma.

The mouth is an alternative airway in the event that nasal passages are clogged or when exchange of a large volume of air is needed. However, important benefits of nasal breathing, moisturizing, heating, and filtering air to protect lung tissues are lost with mouth breathing.

Age-Related Changes

The least appreciated age-related changes in the upper airway are those to the nose. The nose becomes longer, the supporting structures become weaker, and the tip begins to droop. These changes increase resistance to nasal airflow. Minor septal deviations that did not cause obstructive symptoms earlier in life become problematic with age. Changes to the upper airway can lead to changes in quality of life. A diminished sense of smell contributes to loss of taste and can decrease appetite. Decreased appetite can lead to malnutrition, a significant risk factor for perioperative complications.

Older adults often increase their use of salt or sugar to compensate for the loss of the smell followed by loss of taste. The increase in salt and sugar can exacerbate high blood pressure, heart failure, and diabetes.

A diminished sense of smell can impact safety as fires and chemicals may not be noticed. Sensory deprivation resulting from loss of smell and taste is associated with depression possibly due to loss of familiar memory such as roses, coffee brewing, or a particular perfume.

Age-related changes cause thickened nasal secretions, atrophy of the nasal mucosa, and an increase in vascular rhinitis. The most common complaints of the elderly related to these changes include nasal drainage, postnasal drip, sneezing, coughing, and rhinitis. These may be a result of changes to autonomic control of the submucosal glands and goblet cells. Humidification of the air and prevention of dehydration can help alleviate these symptoms. Air humidification also helps prevent epistaxis secondary to dry mucous membranes. Changes in the nasal and sinus mucosa result in increased susceptibility to upper respiratory infections.

PHARYNX

The pharynx is a passageway for both the larynx in the respiratory system and the esophagus in the digestive system. The epiglottis is a flap of tissue that covers the entrance to the larynx to prevent food from entering the trachea and airway. The Eustachian tube extends from the nasopharynx to the ear canal and helps with sound conduction by equalizing pressure between the middle ear and the atmosphere. The adenoids are important lymphatic tissues located in the nasopharynx. They act as important defense mechanism, trapping organisms entering the nose and mouth. When a person opens the mouth, the oropharynx or back of the throat is visible. The tonsils reside on either side of the oropharynx and are part of the body's immune system, guarding against organisms entering through the mouth.

Age-Related Changes

With age, cartilage in the upper airway changes leading to loss of pharyngeal support. Loss of pharyngeal support can lead to upper airway obstruction and sleep apnea. Older adults with diabetes, obesity, a history of smoking, or a family history of sleep apnea are at a greater risk of developing sleep apnea. Repetitive episodes of upper airway occlusion occur in up to 75% of elderly individuals. Elderly patients with upper airway occlusion have a decreased respiratory response to hypoxemia and hypercapnia. Chronic hypoxemia can lead to cognitive impairment. Sleep apnea can further impair elders' oxygenation and ventilation. Altered sleep patterns lead to depression, memory problems, and heart failure.

Neurological age-related changes and diminished reflexes result in decreased sensation in the pharynx. Decreased sensation leads to a diminished gag reflex. Swallowing patterns of elders are slow. The combination of decreased sensation, changes in swallowing, along with the diminished cough force in the larynx increases the risk of aspiration in the older adult.

LARYNX

The larynx, or voice box, located above the trachea and below the pharynx at the base of the tongue, serves as an air passage to the lungs and controls phonation (voice production) and deglutition (swallowing). Several different types of cartilage in the larynx protect the air passages.

The epiglottis is a fold of cartilage that keeps food from entering the trachea during swallowing. The thyroid cartilage or Adam's apple is the largest laryngeal ring and protects the larynx from outside pressures. The cricoid cartilage lies below the thyroid cartilage and is the only cartilage that makes a complete ring in the air passage. The major purpose of the cricoid is to prevent the larynx from collapsing. The false and true vocal cords lie in the cricoid cartilage. The primary function of the false vocal cords (vestibular folds) is to prevent aspiration by forming a valve during swallowing. The true vocal cords are necessary for making vocal sounds. The larynx is innervated by the laryngeal nerves, which can be damaged during intubation, leading to changes in phonation as well as difficulty breathing, swallowing, and coughing.

Coughing protects the airway by forcibly expelling air from the lungs or upper airway to remove foreign objects. The cough begins with a short inspiration of air followed by closure of the glottis, the opening between the true vocal cords. A forcible exhalation of air opens the glottis and air rushes out of the lungs at approximately 600 miles per hour. The forceful cough explains the need to cover the nose and mouth when coughing or sneezing as a large number of bacteria can be spread quickly over a wide area. The cough reflex is impaired by chest muscle weakness, tracheostomy, or vocal cord pathology. Prolonged inactivity, surgery, bed rest, and damage to the nerves of the larynx can affect the cough reflex resulting in a weak cough that is ineffective in clearing the lungs of mucous or protecting the airways. Muscle weakness also can decrease oxygenation by limiting lung expansion.

Closure of the glottis can result in temporary breath holding as the intra-abdominal muscles contract causing an increase in intrathoracic and intra-abdominal pressures. This increase in pressures applies more pressure to the large veins in the abdomen, decreasing venous return to the heart, which results in a decrease in blood pressure with a rebound tachycardia. When the intrathoracic and intra-abdominal pressure is released, blood flow returns to the heart with a rebound bradycardia. Patients may feel faint or lose consciousness during these episodes, which can occur during Valsalva maneuvers. Causes of the Valsalva maneuver include coughing, heavy lifting, or strained defecation and urination.

The cricothyroid membrane in the larynx is the site for emergency airway access and is located below the vocal cords. A cricothyrotomy is an emergency airway created between the thyroid and cricoid cartilage that allows air to flow directly into the trachea if there is an obstruction above the thyroid cartilage. The need for an emergency airway often results in a tracheostomy.

Age-Related Changes

With age, loss of elastin and increased collagen cause changes in the larynx, altering the quality and pitch of the voice. The pitch of a woman's voice lowers while a man's voice becomes higher. The voice may become softer, breathier, and hoarser, making phonation more difficult and creating communication difficulties especially in noisy environments.

The cough reflex diminishes in the elderly secondary to a decrease in nerve receptor sensitivity. Weaker respiratory muscles make coughing less forceful. A poor cough combined with dry mucous membranes and diminished ciliary function promotes retention of secretions and foreign particles in the respiratory tree. These factors also increase the risk of aspiration and contribute to the likelihood of postoperative pneumonia in the elderly. It is important for health care providers to assess for changes in the older adult's upper airway and implement strategies to prevent poor outcomes. Upper airway changes can lead to perioperative complications and contribute to postoperative pneumonia.

LOWER RESPIRATORY TRACT

The lower respiratory tract includes the trachea and the lungs. Bronchia and bronchioles are a series of branching tubes extending from the trachea to the alveoli in the lungs.

Trachea

The trachea, anterior to the esophagus, is a continuous tube of 6 to 10 C-shaped cartilaginous rings that extend from the larynx to the sternal carina. The C-shaped rings open posteriorly toward the esophagus, preventing the trachea from collapsing when negative pressure builds in the thorax. The smooth muscle in the open portion of the C abuts the esophagus. Care must be taken to maintain low pressure in an endotracheal or tracheostomy cuff so as not to erode the smooth muscle and create a tracheoesophageal fistula.

At the sternal carina, the trachea divides into the left and right mainstem bronchus. Located at the level of the superior portion of the 5th vertebrae posteriorly and the angle of Louis anteriorly, the carina is heavily innervated with sensory neurons. Coughing and bronchospasm result when the neurons are stimulated with a foreign body such as dust, endotracheal tube, or suction catheter. The right mainstem bronchus is shorter, wider, and descends at a steeper slope than the left mainstem bronchus. Aspiration of foreign objects is more likely to enter the right mainstem than the left because of these differences.

Lungs

The lungs are the functional structures of the respiratory system. The primary function of the lungs is to bring air in and out of the alveoli for gas exchange. The lungs are cone-shaped, spongy, elastic organs made up of collagen and elastin that support lung expansion and contraction.

The larger right lung has three lobes while the left lung has two. The upper portion of the lung, behind the clavicle, is the apex, and the lower portion, against the diaphragm, is the base. The diaphragm is the major muscle of inspiration. The hilum, a slitlike opening in each lung, serves as the entry of the primary bronchus, pulmonary blood vessels, lymphatics, and nerves. The primary nerves of the respiratory system include the phrenic nerve that controls the diaphragm, the vagus nerve which innervates the thorax, and the thoracic nerves which serve the intercostals muscles.

A continuous smooth membrane, the pleura, completely encloses the lungs. The pleura is a large serous membrane that folds back on itself to form a two-layered structure. The pleural cavity is the space between the two layers. The pleural membranes continually secrete and reabsorb a serous fluid called the pleural fluid that acts as a lubricant to allow the two membranes to glide easily over one another during the act of breathing. The pleural fluid also creates surface tension, adhering lung surfaces to the chest wall to allow for optimal inflation of alveoli during inhalation.

The lining of the mediastinum, thoracic cavity, and superior surface of the diaphragm is the parietal pleura. The visceral pleura covers the lungs and surrounding structures such as blood vessels, bronchi, and nerves. Due to sensory innervations, the parietal pleura is sensitive to pain, while the visceral pleura is not.

Elasticity, Lung Compliance, and Surface Tension

Lungs distend with inspiration and recoil with expiration. Collagen and elastin fibers in the lungs have opposing roles in the lung tissue. Elastin fibers are like rubber bands that stretch easily to a certain point but then recoil to cause the lung to deflate. The property that allows the lungs to expand and then retract is called elasticity. Collagen tissue in the lungs makes the lungs stiffer, preventing overexpansion.

Lung compliance is the ease with which the lungs expand. Compliance is the difference between intra-alveolar and intrapleural pressures, which are the pressures necessary to inflate the lungs. A small change in pressure is required to inflate normal lungs, so normal lungs are said to be compliant. In certain disease states such as pulmonary fibrosis and pulmonary edema, more pressure is needed to inflate the lung. Lungs that require a larger pressure to expand are called noncompliant.

Overcompliance refers to lungs that are difficult to deflate because they have lost the elastic recoil. In emphysema, for example, overcompliance of the lungs means very little change in pressure is needed to inflate the lungs. At the same time, overcompliance makes it difficult for the lungs to deflate. Alveoli in overcompliant lungs can easily be overinflated and rupture during mechanical ventilation or when patients have a severe cough.

Surface tension in the alveoli is an important factor in lung compliance. The alveoli are lined with a thin layer of fluid. The interface between the fluid and the air in the alveoli is where surface tension develops. Forces that hold the fluid molecules together are stronger than the forces that hold the air molecules together. As an example, the force that holds the water molecules together in a raindrop is surface tension. An increase in surface tension in the alveoli causes the fluid molecules to contract, making lungs more difficult to inflate. In the alveoli, surface tension is decreased by surfactant, a substance that makes the lungs easier to inflate.

Age-Related Changes

The diameter of the trachea increases approximately 10% with aging. However, the round tube is distorted with cartilage calcification. The increase in size and shape creates a functionally insignificant increase in anatomic dead space. Of greater clinical significance is the decrease in tracheal cilia and sensitivity of the cough reflex. Loss of these protective functions creates the potential for pathogens and irritants to reach deeper lung tissues.

In the lungs, the total amount of collagen and elastin in the lungs does not change and there is little or no lung destruction. The greatest age-related change is a significant decrease in lung elasticity. Elastic recoil relies on the contraction of elastin fibers. With aging, the lung tissue loses an ability to return to its original position after expansion. The elastin fibers lose function, and the lungs become more compliant. The inability of the lungs to recoil and empty the air results in air trapping and hyperinflation. This trapping and hyperinflation syndrome, known as senile emphysema, reduces gas exchange.

BRONCHIAL TREE AND ALVEOLI

The function of the bronchial tree is to provide for air passage to and from the alveoli. An inverted treelike structure, the bronchial tree is a series of tubes composed of muscular, cartilaginous, and elastic tissue. Dichotomous branching, each branch giving rise to two smaller branches, begins with the trachea and ends in the alveolar sacs (Figure 11.1). The terminal bronchioles are located at the end of an air conduction pathway and give rise to respiratory bronchioles that then divide into alveolar ducts. Each alveolar duct contains five to six alveolar sacs with each alveolar sac containing approximately 17 alveoli.

As the bronchioles become smaller in diameter, the structure of the airway changes. The cartilage decreases as smooth muscle increases. The mucociliary blanket changes gradually until it becomes simple squamous epithelium in the alveolar ducts and alveolar sacs. Alveoli are cup-shaped structures that have a thin side and a thick side. The thin side, composed of flat squamous epithelial cells (Type I alveolar cells), allows for rapid transport of oxygen and CO_2 across the alveolar membrane to the capillary. The capillary wall–alveolar membrane, approximately 0.4 μm, is only as thick as the linings of the alveoli and capillary combined. The thick side of the alveoli abuts other alveoli. The thicker membrane includes a pulmonary interstitial space between the capillary and endothelial membranes. The interstitial space is made up of alveoli, the walls of alveoli, and the spaces around blood vessels and small airways. These spaces contain connective tissue made up primarily of collagen, elastic fibers, and macrophages.

The lungs have as many as 300 million alveoli surrounded by pulmonary capillaries. The surface area for gas exchange between alveoli and capillaries is extensive secondary to the sheer number of alveoli as well as the fact that many alveoli share common capillary walls.

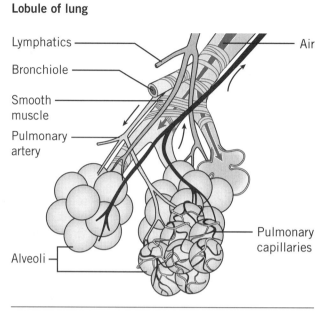

Lobule of lung

Lymphatics

Bronchiole

Smooth muscle

Pulmonary artery

Alveoli

Air

Pulmonary capillaries

FIGURE 11.1
Lung Lobule With Bronchioles and Alveoli

Alveoli are composed of two different types of cells. Type I alveolar cells provide for gas exchange, and Type II alveolar cells produce surfactant. Surfactant is a complex phospholipid protein that reduces surface tension in the walls of alveoli. This allows the alveoli to remain open and prevents the collapse of smaller airways. Surfactant decreases resistance to lung inflation, increases compliance, and prevents the collapse of alveoli or atelectasis. Atelectasis reduces gas exchange secondary to the decreased surface area of collapsed alveoli. Without adequate surfactant, the increase in surface tension would allow the alveoli to contract and water to be pulled out of the pulmonary capillaries into the alveoli. Surfactant helps to prevent pulmonary edema by keeping the surface tension low and the alveoli dry.

Age-Related Changes

The diameter of the conducting airways increases with age, causing a slight increase in the anatomic dead space of the respiratory tract. Compliance of the large and small airways decreases with age, resulting in compression of the airways during maximal exhalation (increased closing volume [CV]). Airway compression can lead to atelectasis due to reduced alveolar ventilation.

Weakened supporting structures that occur with age decrease the diameter of the small airways. The decrease in small airway diameter decreases the maximal expiratory flow as the narrower airways close sooner with aging. These changes lead to obstructive airflow patterns similar to those seen in lifetime nonsmokers, implying that these changes are characteristic of aging.

Elastin fibers anchor alveoli to the respiratory and terminal bronchioles to keep the alveoli open. Changes to elastin properties disrupt the anchoring fibers, allowing the airways to close before the CO_2 is removed from the alveoli. The air trapping in the alveoli results in poor gas diffusion. Elastin fiber changes also cause the alveolar lobules to enlarge and individual alveoli to flatten. Air remains in the larger alveolar also duct inhibiting gas exchange. Changes can be seen in Figure 11.2.

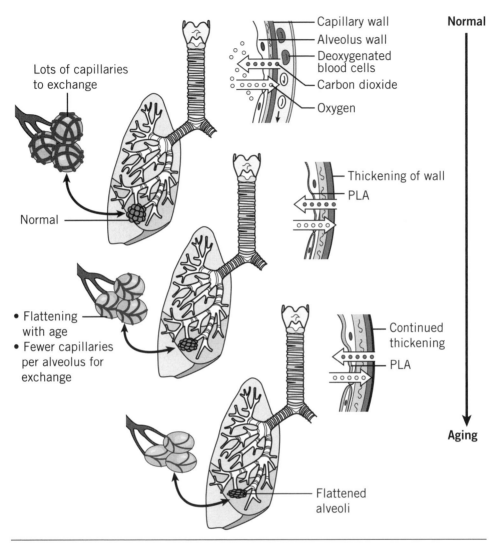

FIGURE 11.2
Comparison Young and Old Alveoli With Loss of Lung Tissue Due to Shrinking and
Flattening of Alveoli

Beginning around age 20, lung mass decreases as much as 50% with aging due to changes
in the alveoli. With aging, the number of alveoli diminishes and old structures become
dysfunctional. Chemical changes to the elastin fibers in alveolar walls causes the alveolar
diameter to widen. As the alveolar surface widens, the surface area per unit of lung volume
decreases. The decrease is at a rate of approximately 1 mm² every 4 years. The change in
alveolar shape and surface area results in capillary loss. The number of functioning capillaries
decreases, further compromising gas exchange and oxygenation.

The result of age-related changes in the pulmonary tree is a decrease in ventilation, diffusion, and perfusion, all potentiallycompromising tissue oxygenation. Yet, changes in the
alveoli have minimal clinical significance in healthy older adults. The remaining functioning
lung tissue provides adequate respiratory reserve. However, the physiological stress of surgery and anesthesia can overwhelm respiratory reserve, placing the older adult at risk for
pulmonary complications.

Surfactant dysfunction usually occurs in response to severe infection or injury and is not necessarily related to the aging process. Although research shows age-related changes in surfactant in animal studies, similar changes have not been identified in older adults. Research continues to investigate the effects of age-related changes in surfactant.

Mechanics of Ventilation

The act of ventilation requires inspiration, expiration, and a closed compartment. The thoraxis a closed compartment with only a single opening to the atmosphere: the trachea. The thorax consists of the chest wall sealed by neck muscles superiorly and the diaphragm inferiorly. The outer walls of the thorax consist of 12 pairs of ribs, the sternum anteriorly, vertebrae posteriorly, and intercostal muscles between the ribs.

The principal muscle of inspiration is the diaphragm, innervated by the phrenic nerve arising from the cervical spinal cord, usually at C4. The diaphragm accounts for approximately 75% of the change in chest volume. Contraction of the diaphragm (flattening) causes the lungs to expand by pulling the base of the thoracic cavity down, creating an increased negative pressure within the lungs from -5 cm H_2O to -9 cm H_2O. At the same time, the external intercostal muscles contract, lifting the rib cage upward and outward, causing air to flow into the lungs. In a normal inhalation, the diaphragm moves 1 to 2 cm but can increase to 10 cm with forced inspiration like that caused by mechanical ventilation. Expiration occurs when the diaphragm and external intercostal muscles relax, and the elastic recoil of the lungs and chest wall causes these structures to fall back into place. The return to the original position increases pressure in the lungs greater than atmospheric pressure and airflows out.

Accessory muscles of inspiration include the sternocloidomastoid that elevates the sternum, the scalene muscles, which elevate the first two ribs, and the trapezius and pectoralis muscles that fix the shoulders. Back and abdominal muscles as well as internal intercostal muscles all come into play in labored breathing to help with inspiratory and expiratory effort.

AGE-RELATED CHANGES

Musculoskeletal changes contribute more to age-related respiratory function than lung changes. Calcification of the ribs and vertebral joints decreases compliance of the chest wall. Kyphosis, flexion of the upper torso, and osteopenic loss in the height of the vertebral column further compress the thorax, decreasing chest compliance. The anteroposterior diameter of the chest increases slightly, causing a change in the shape and effective functioning of the chest wall.

By age 55, the major respiratory muscles such as the diaphragm and intercostal muscles begin to weaken. Respiratory muscle contraction can decrease as much as 35% primarily due to muscle atrophy and age-related decreases in nerve conduction. Poor nutritional status and lack of general conditioning further decrease respiratory muscle mass and strength.

The diaphragm flattens and becomes less efficient with age. Diaphragmatic strength can be reduced as much as 25%. Obesity and loss of abdominal muscle tone can compress the diaphragm limiting its movement.

Age-related changes in the musculoskeletal structure lead to an increase in resistance to lung expansion that increases the overall work of breathing and alters respiratory patterns. The work of breathing causes older adults to take more frequent and less effective breaths. Each breath results in a smaller tidal volume (TV). The overall effect is a decrease in respiratory reserve and function.

Changes in the respiratory system are not often considered when elders have decreased appetites and poor nutrition. Due to changes in the shape of the chest and diaphragm, many elderly experience early fullness as there is not enough room in the abdominal and chest cavities for food and air. Elderly often report being short of breath after eating. The act of breathing can fill the stomach with air, creating the sensation of bloating. Taking more time when eating improves nutritional intake by reducing feelings of breathlessness and decreasing energy expenditure. This is highly relevant after surgery in older adults. Providers need to ensure the gerioperative patient is encouraged to take time to eat and not feel rushed.

Dyspnea occurs with eating due to the stomach pushing up on the flatter, weaker diaphragm, affecting diaphragmatic excursion. Elderly individuals should be encouraged to eat five small meals a day rather than three larger meals. Gas-forming foods that apply pressure to the diaphragm should be limited. Elevating the head and thorax on pillows or use of a wedge to sleep at night also helps reduce gastric reflux and promotes diaphragmatic excursion, improving breathing and sleeping patterns.

Elders may eat more carbohydrates and less protein, as carbohydrates require less energy to chew and digest. Many older adults resort to canned soup as it easy to prepare and does not cause feelings of overfullness. Explaining to older adults how age-related changes in the pulmonary and gastrointestinal systems affects their comfort preparing and eating meals helps in understanding how changing to smaller, more nutritious meals can decrease oxygen and energy demands, increase their comfort at meal times, and improve their nutrition.

CONTROL OF VENTILATION

Ventilation is primarily an involuntary process controlled by the respiratory center in the brain medulla and pons. Central nervous system (CNS) stimulation causes contraction of the diaphragm and intercostal muscles. Afferent impulses from peripheral chemoreceptors, lung receptors, and central chemoreceptors trigger changes in ventilation rhythm, rate, and volume via the autonomic nervous system and respiratory center. Central chemoreceptors monitor levels of oxygen and CO_2 in the blood through changes in central spinal fluid pH. Peripheral chemoreceptors respond primarily to arterial blood oxygen levels. Lung receptors affect ventilatory rate and lung volume. Mechanical receptors in the upper airway control reflex responses that protect the airway through sneezing and coughing.

The limbic system, when triggered by emotions, is able to override the normal breathing pattern governed by the respiratory center. Voluntary control can be exercised for short periods of time via the cerebral cortex and control of intercostal muscles and diaphragm. Voluntary control of volume, respiratory rate, and rhythm is needed to support talking, singing, and other vocal activities or holding one's breath as in swimming underwater. Voluntary control is not absolute. When chemoreceptor input is of sufficient intensity, involuntary control takes over and controls ventilation. This can most readily be seen during voluntary breath holding that cannot exceed chemoreceptor sensitivity.

Age-Related Changes

Aging leads to attenuated response to mechanical and chemoreceptors. Diminished neural stimulation to respiratory muscles interferes with impaired ventilation. A loss of peripheral chemoreceptors leads to decreased sensitivity of respiratory centers to hypoxia and hypercapnia. The respiratory center loses the ability to monitor and integrate information from mechanical and chemical receptors contributing to the attenuated response. As a result, respiratory patterns do not adapt as quickly or efficiently during increased respiratory demand. The ventilatory response to hypoxia is reduced as much as 51% in aging men. The response to hypercapnia is reduced as much as 41%.

Surgical stress increases respiratory demands requiring rapid and effective responses to changes in oxygen, CO_2, emotional reactions such as fear and anxiety, and lung volume. When the respiratory system is incapable of quick or early detection of changes in oxygen and CO_2, older adults are more vulnerable to postoperative pulmonary complications. The loss of ventilation sensitivity and response creates an even greater impact during sleep. Sleep apnea resulting from the aging system's ability to detect and respond to changes in gases or in airway size occurs in up to 45% of older adults. Monitoring of respiratory function and respiratory response to increased temperature, diminished blood gases, infection, or to airway obstruction is needed for early detection of impending physiologic changes.

RESPIRATORY PRESSURES

Ventilation, the act of moving air in and out of the lungs, relies on changes in respiratory pressure, assisted by muscles of the respiratory system. The degree to which the lungs inflate and deflate depends on lung pressures, compliance, elastic recoil, and airway resistance. Air moves from areas of greater pressure to areas of lower pressure.

The pressure inside the airways and alveoli is known as intra-alveolar pressure. When the glottis is open creating an open system, the intra-alveolar pressure inside the alveoli is equal to the pressure in the atmosphere, which is 760 mm Hg. At end inspiration and end expiration, the intra-alveolar pressure is zero. On inspiration, the lungs are pulled down and out by respiratory muscles, creating a negative pressure in the lungs allowing air to flow in. With expiration, the release of respiratory muscles causes a passive increase in pressure in the lungs and forces the air out.

Intrapleural pressure, the pressure inside the pleural cavity, is always negative in relation to alveolar pressure, except when coughing or during forced expiration. The negative pressure is secondary to the elastic recoil properties of the lungs and chest wall. If the closed environment of the chest cavity was removed, the elastic recoil properties of the lungs would allow the lungs to shrink and the chest wall would expand to a larger size. However, in the closed chest cavity, the opposing forces of the constant tension between the chest wall to expand and the lungs to shrink creates a pull on the pleural cavity, creating negative pressure. Without the negative intrapleural pressure holding the lungs and chest wall together, the lungs would fall away from the chest wall during inspiration and collapse. Inspiration increases the elastic recoil property of the lungs and creates an increased negative intrapleural pressure.

Intrathoracic pressure is the pressure in the thoracic cavity and is similar to the intrapleural pressure. The intrathoracic pressure is the pressure to which the heart, lungs, and great vessels are exposed. Forced expiration against a closed glottis greatly increases the intrathoracic pressure and intrapleural pressure.

LUNG VOLUMES AND LUNG CAPACITIES

Lung volumes reflect the amount of air exchanged during ventilation and are measured with a spirometer. The TV is the amount of air exchanged during normal inspiration and expiration, which is approximately 500 mL. Inspiratory reserve volume (IRV) is the amount of air forcibly inhaled over and above the normal inspiration phase of TV, which is about 3000 mL.

The expiratory reserve volume (ERV) is the amount of air that can be forcibly exhaled after a normal TV exhale, which is about 1100 mL. The residual volume (RV) is the amount of air always in the lungs, even after forced expiration, about 1200 ml. The RV provides oxygen availability between inspirations. The sum of all the lung volumes (IRV + TV + ERV + RV) equals the maximum to which the lungs can be inflated or total lung capacity (TLC). Table 11.1 lists the lung volumes and capacities along with abbreviations, descriptions, and age-related changes.

CV is the volume of gas in the lungs when small airways begin to close during controlled maximal exhalation. Because the small airways lack cartilaginous support, they easily collapse with exhalation. CV is usually less than the RV, meaning that in normal situations there is enough air for the alveoli to remain open during inhalation and exhalation. CV increases with age, obstructive lung disease, and pulmonary edema. With higher CVs, air can get trapped in the alveoli causing atelectasis. Total lung volume is the amount of air the lungs and air passages can hold. Lung volumes are influenced by age, gender, race, lifestyle habits, and disease.

TABLE 11.1
Lung Volumes and Capacities*

Volume	Amount	Abbreviation	Description	Changes With Age
Tidal volume	500 mL	TV	Amount of air exchanged during normal inspiration and expiration	↓
Inspiratory reserve volume	3300 mL	IRV	Amount of air inhaled with maximal inspiration	↓
Expiratory reserve volume	1100 mL	ERV	Amount of air inhaled with maximal expiration	↓
Residual volume	1200 mL	RV	Amount of air left in the lungs after maximal expiration	↑
Closing volume	150 mL	CV		↑
Capacity				
Total lung capacity	6000 (IRV + TV + ERV + RV)	TLC	The volume of air contained in the lungs at the end of a maximal inspiration	↓
Vital capacity	4800 (IRV + TV + ERV)	VC	Greatest amount of air expired after a maximal inspiration; often used as an index of pulmonary function	↓
Inspiratory capacity	3800 (IRV + TV)		Amount of air maximally inhaled	↓
Functional reserve capacity	2300 (ERV + RV)	FRC	Volume of air in the lung at the end of a normal exhalation	↑
Closing capacity	1350 (CV + RV)	CC	The volume of air at which the alveoli collapse	↑

*As measured in men.

Lung capacities are clinically useful measurements based on the combination or equivalent of the sums of two or more lung volumes. The vital capacity (VC) represents the amount of air that can be exhaled after maximal inhalation, which is about 4800 mL. VC equals IRV + TV + ERV. Asthma can decrease VC when air cannot be forced out of the lungs easily. Inspiratory capacity is the TV + IRV and equals the amount of air that can be maximally inhaled after a normal exhalation, approximately 3500 mL. Functional residual capacity (FRC) equals the lung volume at the end of a normal exhalation, about 2200 mL (ERV + RV). Several factors decrease FRC: obesity, supine or prone positioning, and restrictive lung disease.

Closing capacity (CC) is the point at which the alveoli collapse. It is equivalent to the CV plus the RV. CC is important because any process that increases CC and lowers FRC can lead to hypoxemia secondary to air trapping and atelectasis.

AGE-RELATED CHANGES

Increased chest wall stiffness, decreased lung elasticity, and muscle weakness combine to decrease ERV and increase reserve volume. The ability to "squeeze" air out of the lungs is diminished. VC is also decreased in the elderly as the reserve volume increases. TLC does not change. FRC is increased due to the increase in reserve volume.

CV increases due to changes in alveoli and small airways structures, causing them to close earlier in exhalation. Clinically, the change in CV is the most important lung volume change. The increase in RV and increase in CV (CC) often surpasses the FRC in a sitting healthy 65-year-old or a supine 44-year-old. In individuals whose CC exceeds FRC, small airway closure can occur during normal tidal breathing, leading to faster onset of atelectasis and hypoxia. Understanding age-related changes in RV and their effect on air exchange and oxygenation is critical to understanding the older person's susceptibility to postoperative pulmonary complications.

Pulmonary Circulation

Two separate circulatory systems, the pulmonary and the bronchial, provide blood flow to the lungs. The bronchial arteries divide and subdivide alongside the respiratory tree and provide blood, oxygen, and nutrients to the conducting airways and supporting parenchyma of the lung. The bronchial circulation system does not participate in gas exchange. In addition to meeting the lungs' metabolic demands, the bronchial circulation warms and humidifies air in the conducting airways.

The pulmonary circulation provides the blood necessary for gas exchange and is composed of a highly vascular capillary network. The pulmonary blood vessels are thinner, more compliant, and offer less resistance than blood vessels in the systemic circulation. Pressures in the pulmonary circulation are much lower than in the systemic circulation (22/8 mm Hg pulmonary versus 110/70 mm Hg systemic). The pulmonary circulation can accommodate a large flow of blood without signs of congestion because of low resistance and low pressure in the pulmonary system. The flow of blood through the pulmonary capillary bed requires that the mean pulmonary arterial pressure exceeds the mean pulmonary venous pressure. This pressure difference keeps blood flowing forward through the capillaries.

The pulmonary circulation also acts as a reservoir for blood for the systemic circulation. Capillary volume remains relatively constant. However, total pulmonary blood volume can range between 500 and 1000 mL. Passive dilation of pulmonary blood vessels and recruitment of collapsed pulmonary vessels accommodates large increases in cardiac output or blood volume. Systemic venoconstriction shifts blood into pulmonary circulation, and systemic vasodilation shifts blood from the pulmonary circulation to the systemic circulation.

AGE-RELATED CHANGES

The intima and medial layers of the pulmonary artery thicken with advancing age. There is an increase in pulmonary vascular stiffness and pressures, which increases vascular resistance. The effect is a decrease in pulmonary capillary blood volume. Pulmonary vasculature changes in the absence of disease do not seem to have a significant negative impact at rest. However, as the vasculature becomes less distensible under conditions of physiological stress, there is a rise in pulmonary vascular resistance followed by impaired circulation and potential hypoxemia.

Pulmonary Processes

VENTILATION

Ventilation, the movement of gases, has a usual TV of 500 mL per breath. In an individual breathing 15 times per minute, the total amount of air entering and leaving the lungs is 7500 mL/minute, known as minute volume or total ventilation per minute. Not all of this inspired air reaches the alveoli for gas exchange. The air left in the conducting airways and exhaled without participating in gas exchange is the dead space. Anatomical dead space is air in the conducting airways. There is no oxygen–CO_2 exchange of air in the anatomical dead space. Alveolar dead space occurs when alveoli are well ventilated but not perfused, that is, there is no capillary circulation and no oxygen–CO_2 exchange. The sum of anatomical dead space and alveolar dead space is the physiologic dead space and is the total amount of air inspired that does not participate in gas exchange. Physiologic dead space increases with age, upright position, neck extension, emphysema, and mechanical ventilation. Physiologic dead space decreases in the supine position, with neck flexion, and after a tracheostomy.

For each 500 mL of inhaled air, 150 mL remains in the conducting airways as anatomic dead space and never reaches the alveoli. The amount of air reaching the alveoli for diffusion is called alveolar ventilation. Alveolar ventilation is the actual amount of air available for the exchange of gases across the alveolar capillary membrane.

DIFFUSION

The movement of gases across the alveolar-capillary membrane is known as diffusion. The alveolar-capillary membrane includes the epithelial lining of the alveolus, a potential interstitial space (formed in pulmonary edema and pneumonia), basement membrane, and endothelial lining of the arterial capillary. From the alveoli, oxygen diffuses into the capillary lumen, then into the red blood cell across the red blood cell membrane. Finally, the oxygen binds to hemoglobin for transport to the rest of the body. Diffusion of CO_2 is reversed. CO_2 is released from hemoglobin, diffuses across the red cell membrane and out of the venous capillary into the alveoli, where the CO_2 is exhaled. CO_2 has a higher solubility than oxygen and is 20 times more soluble in blood. This means that CO_2 diffuses across the alveolar capillary membrane much faster than oxygen.

> **BOX 11.1** Fick's Law:
>
> $V = D(A/T) \times (P1 - P2)$
>
> The formula reflects that V is equal to the volume of the gas, D is the permeability coefficient of the membrane, A is the area, and T equals the thickness of the membrane. $P1$ and $P2$ are the partial pressure of the gas on either side of the membrane.

Fick's law is the physiologic principle relating to diffusion (see Box 11.1). This formula represents the ability of oxygen and CO_2 to exchange across the alveolar membrane. The volume of exchange is directly related to the partial pressure of the gases in the space, the surface area for gas exchange, and the diffusion coefficient.

As the partial pressure of oxygen or CO_2 increases, such as an increased fraction of inspired oxygen, the ability of the gas to diffuse across the alveolar capillary membrane increases. Oxygen supplementation with nasal cannula or face mask increases the oxygen available for diffusion across the membrane in the alveoli. Increased CO_2 in the blood secondary to exercise, lactic acidosis, or sepsis increases the partial pressure of CO_2 in the blood, driving the ability to get rid of the excess CO_2 via diffusion across the alveolar capillary membrane into the alveoli and elimination with increased respiratory rate.

As the surface area available for diffusion increases, the ability to diffuse across the membrane increases to a certain point. Like everything else in the human body, too much of a good thing can be bad. If you increase the surface area of the alveoli or blood vessel too much, the diffusion capability actually decreases.

The thickness of the alveolar capillary membrane is inversely related to the rate of diffusion. If the thickness of the membrane increases as it does in pneumonia and pulmonary edema, there is more tissue or fluid to diffuse across. Hence, the diffusion capability decreases, leading to hypoxia and possible acidosis.

Age-Related Changes

Diffusion capacity and the ability of oxygen and CO_2 to cross the alveolar capillary membrane decreases with increasing age. Diffusion capacity begins to decreases at a rate of 17% (2.03 mL/min/mm Hg) per decade after age 50. This age-related decline diffusion results from a loss of alveolar capillary membrane surface area described previously. Thickening of pulmonary vasculature increases the distance required for diffusion, further contributing to diminished diffusion capacity.

PERFUSION

The primary purpose of the pulmonary circulation is to perfuse the lungs for oxygen–CO_2 exchange. Blood flows through the lungs at a rate of approximately 5 L per minute. Alveolar ventilation occurs at the alveolar-capillary membrane. At any given moment, there may be only 70 to 100 mL of blood in the pulmonary capillaries undergoing gas exchange. At the alveolar-capillary membrane, this small volume is only one red blood cell thick. To ensure optimal gas exchange, each capillary perfuses more than one alveolus.

Exchange of gases between the air in the alveoli and blood in pulmonary capillaries depends on matching ventilation and perfusion, measured as the V/Q ratio. A V/Q ratio of 1 occurs when ventilation and perfusion are perfectly matched. However, in healthy adults usual ventilation approximates 4 L/min and normal perfusion equals approximately 5 L/minute. This results in a

V/Q ratio of 0.8 (4 L/5 L), a normal physiologic mismatch. When the V/Q is higher than 0.8, ventilation exceeds perfusion. A V/Q lower than 0.8 occurs when there is a decrease in ventilation.

A pulmonary shunt refers to blood in pulmonary capillaries that does not participate in gas exchange. During a pulmonary shunt, the alveoli are perfused but there is a decrease in alveolar ventilation. Blood flows through the pulmonary capillary bed without gas exchange across the alveoli allowing unoxygenated blood to enter systemic circulation, as seen in Figure 11.3. The V/Q ratio is zero. Physiologic shunting is the most common cause of hypoxemia. As a result of no ventilation, the blood blow diverts from the unventilated alveoli.

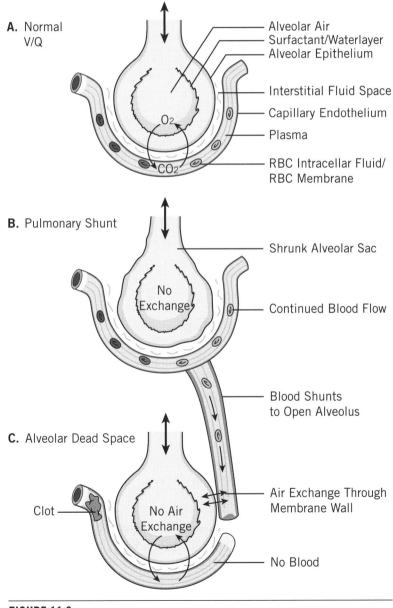

FIGURE 11.3
A. Ventilation/Perfusion Mismatch; B. Pulmonary Shunt; and
C. Alveolar Dead Space

In alveolar dead space, the alveoli are ventilated but not perfused such as occurs in pulmonary embolus. Gas enters and leaves the alveoli having no contact with capillary blood flow, therefore gas exchange does not occur.

Pulmonary blood flow is not uniform and is subject to change as a result of gravity and body position. Gravity exerts a force that allows the lower (dependent) regions of the lung to receive greater blood flow than the upper (nondependent) region of the lung. Pulmonary vasoconstriction allows shunting of blood away from regions of the lung that are not being ventilated.

Body position changes the V/Q ratio to influence mismatch and gas exchange. When the body is upright, the apex of the lung has optimal alveolar ventilation but poor perfusion. In the lung base, there is good perfusion but poor ventilation. In the supine position, there is optimal perfusion to the dependent area (posterior) and good ventilation to the anterior lung segment. Therefore, the upright position is the best position for optimal ventilation and perfusion. During surgery, older adults in prone, supine, lateral, or lithotomy positions for extended periods can develop more severe V/Q mismatch than younger adults.

Age-Related Changes

Age-related changes in V/Q mismatch occur primarily in response to increased physiologic dead space and collapse of peripheral airways. In healthy older adults at rest, a V/Q imbalance is not clinically significant. However, reserve capacity diminishes with age. Ventilation and perfusion changes that pose no problem during everyday activities become risk factors for decreased alveolar ventilation and shunting during physiologic stress.

Disease and lifestyle factors have a greater impact on V/Q mismatch than changes related to aging. Factors decreasing ventilation include smoking, chronic obstructive pulmonary disease (COPD), or pulmonary edema. Factors decreasing perfusion include heart failure, pulmonary hypertension, and atherosclerosis. In caring for the gerioperative patient, the combined effects of age-related changes, disease factors, and body position during and after surgery challenge optimal gas exchange.

Gerioperative Care

Patient- and procedure-related factors influence risk for postsurgical pulmonary complications, as shown in Table 11-2. Higher odds ratios indicate a stronger relationship between the risk factor and postoperative pulmonary complications.

Table 11.2 provides a list of risk factors and the associated odds ratios. Increasing age, beginning around age 60 and escalating at age 70, increases risk for postoperative pulmonary complications, remaining true even for healthy older adults. COPD and heart failure are also significant patient-related risk factors. Functional limitation as reflected in the American Society of Anesthesiologists (ASA) composite scores constitutes a patient-related risk factor. A composite score of greater than 2 on the American Anesthesia Association preoperative scale indicates a high risk for postoperative pulmonary complications. An important point to consider with the gerioperative patient is that some anesthesiologists use advanced age of 75 or 80 as a criterion for listing an older adult as a grade 2, by definition a risk factor for pulmonary complications. The ASA classification scale is described in greater detail in Chapter 8.

Advanced age is an independent predictor of postoperative pulmonary complications even in healthy older adults.

While patient-related risk factors are contributory, procedure-related factors are more significant in predicting postoperative pulmonary complications. Procedure-related factors

TABLE 11.2

Risk Factors for Postoperative Pulmonary Complications

Risk Factor	Odds Ratio
Age	
60–69	2.09
70–79	3.04
Currently smoking	1.26
Chronic obstructive pulmonary disease	1.79
Heart failure	2.93
Serum albumin (< 3.5 g/dL)	2.53
American Society of Anesthesiologists classification ≥ 2	4.87
General anesthesia	1.83
Type of surgery	
Thoracic	4.24
Any abdominal	3.01
Upper abdominal	2.91
Neurosurgery	2.53
Prolonged (2.5–4 hrs)	2.26
Emergency surgery	2.52

Adapted from: Smetana, Lawrence, and Cornell, 2005.

include length of surgery, type of surgery, site of incision, and anesthesia type. Patients having surgery near the diaphragm have a higher risk of postoperative complications due to incision site. Chest and upper abdominal incisions cause painful respirations. Patients are more likely to "splint" respirations, that is, take shallow breaths with small tidal volumes. This is a special concern in the gerioperative patient. Older adults are likely to have more rapid, shallow respirations as a typical breathing pattern resulting from age-related musculoskeletal changes. Adding the insult of an upper abdominal surgical incision results in even less exchange of air in the gerioperative patient.

Identifying modifiable risk factors and maximizing respiratory function before surgery along with systematically monitoring the gerioperative patient throughout the perioperative period is critical to preventing morbidity and mortality caused by postoperative pulmonary complications. Prevention, early detection, and rapid intervention are key to maintaining optimal respiratory function across all phases of the perioperative continuum. Table 11.3 lists preoperative, intraoperative, and postoperative assessment, prevention, and intervention strategies shown to decrease pulmonary complications in older adults.

PREOPERATIVE CONSIDERATIONS

The most fundamental and important step in evaluating pulmonary risk is a thorough history and physical examination. A plan of care with preventive strategies and interventions can be developed and implemented for use across the perioperative continuum based on preoperative assessment findings. Key areas for assessment include current

TABLE 11.3

Perioperative Assessment, Risk Identification, and Prevention Strategies for Decreasing Pulmonary Complications in Older Adults

Perioperative Phase	Assessment	Preventative Interventions
Preoperative	Assessment Lung sounds Presence of COPD, cardiovascular, lung cancer, neurological disease Sputum production Nutritional status Albumin levels Exercise Capacity Obstructive sleep apnea Smoking history Fluid status	Pulmonary prehabilitation: Health coaching • Type of surgery and incision site • Postoperative pulmonary toilet • Use incentive spirometry • Pain relief • Hydration and nutrition Physical exercise plan Breathing exercises schedule Incentive Spirometry schedule Stabilize comorbid disease Optimize medication regimen Smoking cessation Fluid intake
Intraoperative	Review history and physical Assess lung sounds Assess oxygenation and end title carbon dioxide Ease of ventilation	Bronchodilators Hydration Careful positioning Short acting muscle relaxants Reverse muscle relaxants Prevent aspiration Analgesia management
Postoperative	Airway Lung sounds Hydration Oxygen saturation Pain severity Ventilation effectiveness Respiratory rate and depth Nutritional status Frailty, respiratory fatigue Cognition	Health coaching Prevent hypoventilation Maintain airway patency Oxygenation Encourage deep breathing, coughing Incentive spirometry Oral care at least twice daily Elevate head of bed Pain relief Optimum Hydration Optimum Nutrition Systematic monitoring: lung sounds, cognition In bed exercises Early ambulation

level of respiratory comfort, functional status, past and present pulmonary and comorbid disease history, lifestyle habits such as smoking and alcohol use, hydration, and nutritional status.

The preoperative assessment begins when first meeting the older adult. The initial observation of the patient's respiratory patterns and the effect on speech or movement provides clues to guide the history and physical assessment. Posture can indicate potential problems with pulmonary effectiveness and serve as clues to disease states.

RESPIRATORY COMFORT AND FUNCTIONAL STATUS

Asking the older adult about respiratory comfort and effects of respiratory changes on every-day activities are key indicators of respiratory function. Exhibit 11.1 presents a set of questions used to assess respiratory discomfort. Questions about the older person's ability and respiratory comfort in carrying on everyday activities such as dressing, toileting, eating, walking, shopping, or visiting with friends provides information on how well the older adult will be able to manage postoperative recovery activities.

HEALTH HISTORY

Past and current health and surgical history can identify risk factors associated with postoperative pulmonary complications. History of occupational exposures can identify lung problems not yet evident. For elders over age 70, questions about occupational exposures can uncover to be significant predictors of perioperative pulmonary complications.

Chronic Disease
Past and current health history is highly relevant in identifying comorbid and lifestyle factors that contribute to changes in the older person's pulmonary function. Table 11.4 lists health history and associated postoperative pulmonary complications. Assessment should address duration of disease, and number and severity of exacerbation episodes of chronic pulmonary diseases such as emphysema, bronchitis, asthma, and mycobacterial and respiratory infections. The presence of chronic diseases including heart failure, obstructive sleep apnea (OSA), gastroesophogeal reflux, and neurologic changes should also be evaluated. Questions about current vascular disease or previous thromboembolic events are important in establishing risk for pulmonary emboli.

Cough and Sputum Production
Cough and sputum production are important indicators of changes in pulmonary function. Questions related to cough focus on frequency, duration of coughing, triggers associated

EXHIBIT 11.1 Assessing Respiratory Discomfort

- Does the patient have any problems or difficulty with breathing at rest (e.g., sitting in a chair)? At night? During activity? If so, what kind of activity?
- What words does the patient use to describe breathing difficulty or problems?
- Do the problems with breathing make it interfere with or make it difficult to carry out any other physical activities? Hobbies or leisure activities? Social activities?
- How does the person feel or react when difficult breathing episodes occur?
- What makes the problems with breathing more difficult? What does the person do to make breathing easier?
- How long do difficult breathing episodes last?
- How long has the patient had problems with difficult breathing?
- Have the episodes of difficult breathing always been caused by the same problem?
- What has the patient been told by a health care provider about possible causes or diagnoses for the difficult breathing?

TABLE 11.4

Postoperative Pulmonary Complications Associated With Chronic Diseases

Health History	Postoperative Pulmonary Complications
Chronic obstructive pulmonary disease	Respiratory failure Atelectasis Pneumonia V/Q mismatch
Respiratory infection	Pneumonia
Obstructive sleep apnea	Upper airway obstruction
Gastroesophogeal reflux	Aspiration
Neurologic disease	Atelectasis Pneumonia Aspiration
Heart failure	V/Q mismatch
Vascular disease	Pulmonary emboli V/Q mismatch

with a specific type or duration of activity, and cough relief. An important consideration is the effect of coughing on the older adult, specifically level of fatigue generated by the cough, shortness of breath, headache, or rib fracture.

Assessment of cough characteristics includes productive or nonproductive, hacking, tickling, congested, or harsh. A cough test provides additional information for follow-up questioning. The cough test is an efficient way to screen for pulmonary secretions and complication risk. The patient should be asked to cough. The test is positive if the patient continues to cough repeatedly after the first cough. A positive cough test is an independent predictor of postsurgical pulmonary complications. If the cough is productive, sputum color and quantity should be assessed. Observation of the patient is not considered a part of the cough test. However, observation provides important information for teaching related to effective postoperative deep breathing and coughing.

Sputum production is a more significant risk factor for pulmonary complications than history of smoking without productive cough. Older adults with chronic respiratory disease, history of smoking, or exposure to occupational hazards often have increased sputum. Current infection can also trigger increased sputum production. All gerioperative patients should be asked about current status of pneumonia and influenza vaccination.

Comorbid Diseases

Unstable heart failure is associated with postoperative pulmonary complications. Asking about weight gain, orthopnea, dyspnea at rest or on exertion, fatigability, cough, and wheezing allows for an evaluation of the severity and level of disease control. Presence of symptoms calls for a consideration of further evaluation and intervention prior to surgery.

Gastroesophageal reflux is a gastrointestinal condition that can predispose to respiratory problems intraoperatively and postoperatively due to danger of aspiration. Gastroesophageal problems often go undiagnosed in older adults. Asking the patient about heartburn or indigestion, symptom frequency, and duration can provide indications of a problem that needs further evaluation. Older patients who smoke have a greater risk for gastroesophageal reflux due to weakening of the lower esophageal sphincter. Antidepressant, anticholinergic, beta-adrenergic agonist, and bronchodilator medications can increase gastroesophogeal reflux. Obesity increases intra-abdominal pressure and forces stomach contents into the esophagus in the supine position. Obese patients may benefit from receiving prokinetic or proton pump inhibitors preoperatively to reduce risk of vomiting and aspiration.

OSA secondary to upper airway obstruction occurs in 45 to 75% of older adults with higher rates at older ages. Older patients often are not aware they have OSA. Asking patients about snoring, waking abruptly in the night, not feeling rested, and somnolence can identify possible problems. Older adults who demonstrate sleep apnea may need additional testing prior to surgery as OSA poses a significant risk in the perioperative period.

Two neurologic risk factors predispose patients to pulmonary complications: history of cerebrovascular accident and impaired cognition. A history of stroke or neurologic disease such as Parkinson disease can impair swallowing with an associated risk for aspiration. Changes in cognition predispose an elder to respiratory complications in the perioperative period secondary to inability to follow directions about respiratory recovery activities. Aspiration risk is increased due to changes in swallowing effectiveness.

Lifestyle Habits

Questions about smoking are directed to the frequency and duration of cigarette smoking and the use of inhaled street drugs. Information about previous smoking cessation efforts is important as it can guide decisions about programs to consider for more effective smoking cessation.

Preventing alcohol withdrawal should be planned before surgery for implementation during and after surgery.

Extensive alcohol use predisposes the older adult to pulmonary complications due to its effect in reducing lower esophageal sphincter tone (see Chapter 15) and impairment of the immune system. Alcohol cessation prior to surgery improves outcomes. A major concern postoperatively is alcohol withdrawal. To prevent postoperative problems, alcohol use should be discussed preoperatively to plan for appropriate intervention during and after surgery.

Medications

A thorough review of current medications assists in determining patients' respiratory status and overall health. Important areas to consider are frequency of rescue inhaler use and if and when steroids have been required. It is important to identify prescription medications used by the patient, as distinct from medications prescribed, as well as eliciting information on over-the-counter and herbal remedies.

Older adults taking steroids for exacerbations of asthma or COPD will need to be considered for an additional dose of steroids. Asking a detailed medication history about the use of CNS depressant medications, narcotics, and sedatives provides important information for prevention of intraoperative complications as these medications can alter the normal ventilation response to hypoxemia and hypercapnia. In addition, CNS depressant medications increase the tendency for upper airway collapse. Both CNS depressant and narcotic effects can be more severe in persons with OSA as decreased arousal can lead to prolonged apnea and cardiovascular or respiratory arrest.

Nutritional Status and Hydration

Poor nutrition increases postoperative complications secondary to effects on respiratory muscles and overall patient deconditioning. Nutrition history and albumin levels are important indicators for identifying malnutrition in older adults. A more detailed discussion of nutrition assessment is included in Chapter 15.

Improving nutritional status can be difficult in the elderly especially if the reason for the surgery is related to the cause of malnutrition, such as colon cancer. Options for preoperative intervention include parenteral nutrition, enteral nutrition, or anabolic agents. However, there is little agreement on the effectiveness of the available options.

Questions about fluid intake and assessment of mucous membranes can help identify dehydration and its effects on upper and lower airway mucosa. Dry oral mucous membranes, caked secretions, and open mouth lesions can be sites for bacterial invasion and increase infection risk. Dry mucous membranes can make swallowing difficult. Pills or food can get stuck in dry, caked areas, increasing potential for aspiration. Dehydration thickens lung secretions, making it more difficult to expectorate, especially in the presence of an ineffective cough. Ineffective coughing results in retained lung secretions, creating a risk for intraoperative and postoperative atelectasis. Dry mucous membranes contribute to difficulty during intubation. Placement of the intubation blade and endotracheal tube is more likely to cause trauma if membranes are dry.

PLANNING FOR DISCHARGE

Planning for the older patient's discharge to home or alternative agency after surgery begins during the preoperative assessment. Asking the older adult who will be assisting with preoperative care and postoperative support identifies what person(s) should be included in the postdischarge teaching plan. Asking family caregivers about their knowledge and comfort in encouraging older adults to carry out recommended therapies such as deep breathing, coughing, adhering to medication regimen, and exercise is important. An important area for assessment is family beliefs and attitudes about administering pain medications. This can be especially important in decreasing pulmonary complications after surgery.

PHYSICAL ASSESSMENT

Breath Sounds

Auscultation of breath sounds is the most reliable method for assessment of the respiratory system. Auscultation provides information about ventilation and the presence of mucous, fluid, or obstruction in the tracheobronchial tree and lung fields. When evaluating breath sounds in older adults, it is important to remember that age-related decreases in tidal volume results in diminished breath sounds throughout all lung fields.

Neurological and Neuromuscular Changes

Neurologic and neuromuscular changes such as mouth drooping, hemiparesis, slurred speech, and confusion suggest swallowing difficulties. Voice sounds provide information about changes in the larynx and pharynx. Hoarseness may be a sign of gastric reflux, smoking, or normal voice changes of aging. Assessment of muscle strength, cough, and swallowing reflexes, along with gastroesophageal reflux is necessary when assessing aspiration risk.

An efficient determination of activity tolerance is to ask how many flights of steps the patient can climb before having to stop. In a study of 63 patients aged 39 to 84, patients who were able to climb four flights of steps (18 steps per flight) had half the rate of complications as patients able to climb two flights or less (Girish, Trayner, Damman, Pinto-Plata, & Bartolome, 2001). Study participants unable to climb any steps due to physical limitations had an 89% postoperative complication rate. The authors concluded that the ability to climb two or fewer flights could identify patients who have an increased risk for developing postoperative complications after chest or upper abdominal surgery.

PREOPERATIVE TESTING

Albumin and Prealbumin

Testing preoperative albumin levels is a national guideline for all older adults who show evidence of malnutrition or who have one or more risk factors for perioperative pulmonary complications. Preoperative protein depletion is a clinical indicator for postoperative pneumonia.

> *Albumin and prealbumin levels should be available on all gerioperative patients with evidence of malnutrition or identified risk factors for perioperative pulmonary complications.*

Pulse Oximetry

A pulse oximetry check should be conducted on room air as tolerated. Pulse oximetry establishes a preoperative baseline of oxygen diffusion and carrying capacity. Chest radiograph is necessary only when signs and symptoms of pulmonary compromise have been identified. A nonsmoking healthy older patient with no change in health status does not require a preoperative chest radiograph. Preoperative arterial blood gasses are needed only if acute respiratory problems are evident.

Pulmonary Function Testing

Conducting pulmonary function testing as a standard procedure to assess perioperative pulmonary risk is controversial. There are no standards for lower levels of forced expiratory volume in 1 second, which is the maximal amount of air the patient can forcefully exhale in 1 second, at which pulmonary complications will occur in older adults. Older adults, by virtue of age, have an increased risk of pulmonary complications even with minimal to no changes in pulmonary function.

Pulmonary testing is recommended for advanced age adults, who are usually defined as those over 75 years of age. Testing is also recommended for older adults who smoke more than one pack per day, who have any pulmonary disease, chronic productive cough, obesity, or kyphoscoliosis. Older adults who are having thoracic or abdominal surgery, pulmonary surgery, or expected to have prolonged anesthesia are also recommended for pulmonary testing. The type and extent of testing depends on the patient's demonstrated respiratory function and the degree of airway obstruction.

Spirometry measures lung function. The test requires patients to exhale into an instrument to calculate airflow. The accuracy of the test is highly dependent on the patient's ability to cooperate and participate. Test results can be inaccurate if the patient is unable to do the test as instructed.

Bronchial Challenge Testing

Bronchial challenge tests and postbronchodilator tests are useful in identifying stimuli that lead to bronchospasm and determining potential benefits of nebulizer treatments in the preoperative or postoperative period in improving outcomes.

PREOPERATIVE INTERVENTIONS

Prehabilitation

The outcome for preoperative pulmonary interventions is to ensure maximum respiratory function and decrease intraoperative and postoperative pulmonary complications. Preoperative pulmonary prehabilitation utilizes an interdisciplinary team approach. A prehabilitation program can emphasize one or more of the following: physical exercise, smoking cessation, respiratory exercises, disease and medication management, nutrition, hydration, and vaccination.

Physical Exercise

Physical exercise such as walking, swimming, and water aerobics is one of the most effective ways to increase pulmonary function. Yoga and tai chi are low-impact ways to maximize breathing capacity and assist in relaxation, further contributing to respiratory function. Frail, bed-bound, or wheelchair-bound patients can perform deep breathing exercises and upper and lower mobility exercises. The exercise must be consistent with the older persons' physical ability, health status, available resources, and heath care provider recommendations.

Smoking Cessation

Smoking cessation is critical in preventing perioperative complications. Patients who smoke should be counseled on the risks of smoking in relation to surgery and the benefits obtained by not smoking during the preoperative period. Surgery can be a trigger for helping older adults consider smoking cessation. The preoperative assessment offers a teachable moment when the risks of smoking before surgery are more relevant. Lauerman (2008) conducted a literature review on patient education about smoking cessation and found that although surgical patients are asked about their smoking behaviors, few patients receive follow-up information on what to do about their smoking behaviors or how to access assistance with smoking cessation.

Asking the older adult about experiences with previous smoking cessation can help develop a more effective preoperative smoking intervention strategy. Smoking cessation pre-operatively decreases the risk of pulmonary complications in the postoperative period. At least 4 to 8 weeks is needed for smoking cessation to decrease postoperative pulmonary complications. While 4 to 8 weeks has been suggested, the minimum period of cessation prior to surgery has not been established. Smoking cessation less than 4 weeks prior to surgery can stimulate the mucociliary blanket, resulting in increased sputum production. Increased sputum increases the risk for ventilation and diffusion complications intraoperatively and postoperatively. Practice guidelines for patients undergoing lung surgery or anesthesia advocate for preoperative smoking cessation regardless of timeline to surgery. Short-term smoking cessation, less than 4 weeks, has shown an increased risk of complications from increased sputum production.

There is a lack of consensus on the length of time most beneficial for smoking cessation. There is consensus that older adults should be encouraged to stop smoking at the earliest possible time prior to surgery. Smoking cessation programs should be initiated as early as possible as longer periods of cessation have greater benefit and result in lower risk of complications.

Documenting the length of preoperative smoking cessation is important for managing intraoperative and postoperative care. Older adults who stop smoking a short time before surgery may require additional monitoring to assess for increased sputum production and adverse effects on pulmonary function.

Smoking cessation programs use different methods with varying degrees of effectiveness. Two programs used for preoperative smoking cessation are the 5As program and the Ask, Advise, Refer (AAR) model. The 5As program was initially developed for community-based smoking cessation programs (Fiore, Bailey, & Cohen, 2000; Exhibit 11.2). The As stand for *a*sk, *a*dvise, *a*ssess, *a*ssist, and *a*rrange. The model is designed for use with patients who are willing to stop smoking.

The AAR model is an abbreviated version of the 5As. The ASA Smoking Cessation Initiative Task Force (Warner, 2009) initiated AAR as a model to facilitate preoperative smoking cessation counseling. Although anesthesiologists who tested the model found it useful for talking preoperatively with patients about smoking cessation, more research is needed to evaluate the effectiveness of the model in getting patients to stop smoking.

EXHIBIT 11.2 **5As Smoking Cessation Guidelines**

Ask	• Ask every gerioperative patient about tobacco use • Identify current smoking behaviors • Assess readiness to stop smoking
Advise	• Strongly urge all gerioperative patients who smoke to stop prior to surgery • Identify strategies the patient will consider ways to change specific behaviors • Set a date for smoking cessation
Assess	• Assess patient's willingness to stop smoking • Assess type of program patient will accept
Assist	• Support patient's commitment • I dentify barriers and facilitators to patient's progress • Help patient find informal and formal resources
Arrange	• Establish short-term follow-up dates • Support successes • Conduct discharge follow-up to reinforce smoking cessation benefits after surgery

Adapted from Fiore, Bailey, and Cohen, 2000.

Managing Sputum Production

Older adults with chronic pulmonary diseases often produce excess sputum secondary to underlying pulmonary infection. When excess sputum is identified preoperatively, a sputum culture should be obtained to determine effective antibiotic treatment. Steroids to decrease the inflammatory response may be prescribed to decrease sputum production. Bronchodilators are helpful in clearing respiratory secretions as well as decreasing hyperreactivity of the airway and alleviating bronchospasm. Ipratropium bromide is a perioperative bronchodilator of choice and should be started several days prior to surgery. If the older person has wheezing on lung auscultation, a combination of albuterol and ipratropium or similar treatment preoperatively may prevent intraoperative bronchospasm. Fever associated with an upper or lower respiratory infection is an indicator to reschedule surgery until the infection is cleared and respiratory function optimized.

Patient Coaching

Preoperative education improves understanding, feelings of competence and comfort, and improves adherence for prehabilitation and postsurgical rehabilitation. The gerioperative patient should identify a family member or friend who can be a coach and support person to serve as another "ear" when listening to information and instructions and to help in carrying out preoperative activities. The family member or friend should be included when the gerioperative patient is receiving preoperative education or instructions.

Both the patient and companion-coach should receive information, experience demonstration, and practice on use of incentive spirometry (IS) and deep breathing. Patients should receive a prescription for exercise based on ability and function. If the patient is chair- or bed-bound, the patient should be shown chair or in-bed exercises.

Preoperative teaching should include information on how increasing fluid intake improves secretion mobilization, prevents oral dehydration and formation of dried membranes, and contributes to a faster recovery. Fluid intake recommendations should remain within limitations set by cardiac or kidney disease.

Older adults with sleep apnea should be instructed to have their continuous positive airway pressure (CPAP) or bilevel positive airway pressure (BiPAP) machines available for use on the day of surgery. These machines assist airway management during sedation, anesthesia, and immediately postoperatively. A drop in oxygen saturation can be detrimental to the older adult. CPAP/BiPAP devices maintain airway patency and ventilation, preventing airway compromise. Depending on agency policy, the biomedical department or respiratory therapy must conduct a safety check on a patient-owned CPAP/BiPAP machine prior to use in a health care facility.

Epidural Analgesia

Surgical procedures on older adults lasting more than 2.5 hours and surgeries involving upper abdominal or thoracic incisions have a significantly greater risk of pulmonary complications after surgery. Epidural analgesia provides the patient with wound and incision pain control, allowing for greater diaphragmatic excursion and improved participation in deep breathing. Epidural pain control offers the patient the ability to provide a more forceful cough while minimizing the need for systemic narcotics and the associated side effects. Thoracic epidurals for pain control should be offered to older adults having long surgeries or upper abdominal incision sites. A clear explanation of the benefits of epidurals in preventing postoperative pulmonary complications as well as potential risks of the procedure assists the older person in making an informed decision.

INTRAOPERATIVE CONSIDERATIONS

Nursing interventions are needed to prevent pulmonary complications during intubation or extubation.

Anesthesia is a major pulmonary stressor for the older adult. The gerioperative patient is highly vulnerable to pulmonary complications during anesthesia induction, intubation, anesthesia emergence, and extubation. A quiet, therapeutic environment is needed during these periods to allow the nurse and anesthesia provider to monitor for airway compromise. The nurse needs to remain with the older patient throughout the induction and emergence of anesthesia to prevent, detect, or intervene in the event of a pulmonary complication. Hypoxia, hypoxemia, aspiration, and medication effects are major areas of respiratory concern.

Intraoperative management of the older adult's respiratory status requires continuous monitoring and attention to the older adult's respiratory status. Pulse oximetry is monitored continuously to detect threat of hypoxemia. Hypoxemia can lead to serious intra- and postoperative complications. For example, an older patient with cardiovascular disease who experiences a single event of severe hypoxemia ($< 85\%$ oxygen saturation) of 5 minutes or more of mild hypoxemia is more likely to suffer a silent ischemic event. Blood pressure, end-tidal CO_2, and cardiac electrocardiogram monitoring are additional measures used to continually evaluate the older person's respiratory stability and maintain patient safety. Interventions to decrease risk of hypoxemia during surgery include 3 minutes of preoxygenation prior to induction of anesthesia and adequate fluid administration to loosen and mobilize secretions.

Intubation using rapid sequence induction is used to prevent aspiration in patients who have a history of gastroesophogeal reflux or who are having emergency surgery when the contents of the stomach are unknown. In this procedure, cricoid pressure or the Sellick maneuver is applied to prevent gastric contents from entering the trachea in the event the patient regurgitates. Cricoid pressure requires the circulating nurse to exert 4 kg of pressure (approximately 8.5 lbs) on the cricoid cartilage of the anterior larynx. The pressure is applied with the thumb and forefinger on the front of the neck toward the sixth cervical vertebrae posteriorly as the patient is induced for anesthesia and paralyzed. The pressure begins at the beginning of induction and continues until the patient is anesthetized and paralyzed, the endotracheal tube is placed, the cuff is inflated, and endotracheal tube placement is verified with bilateral breath sounds and monitored positive end-tidal CO_2. Only upon ETT verification is the pressure released. This procedure can easily be performed incorrectly by applying the pressure laterally rather than posteriorly. The effectiveness of cricoid pressure, once a mainstay of trauma anesthesia, has recently come into question. However, many anesthesia providers still request nurses to assist with this technique during intubation.

In older adults with gastroesophogeal reflux, a Salem sump gastric tube is inserted after intubation to empty stomach contents and prevents aspiration on extubation. Salem sump tubes are contraindicated in any patient who has a history of alcohol abuse or with increased risk of esophageal varices.

Older adults are highly sensitive to narcotics. CNS depressant medications such as narcotics and sedatives are used with caution as they can alter the ventilatory response to hypoxemia and hypercapnia in older adults. In addition, CNS depressant medications increase the tendency for upper airway collapse. The effects of CNS medications on altered ventilatory response and upper airway collapse are even more significant in the older adult with OSA as the arousal response to breathing is diminished resulting in prolonged apnea.

Positioning can change ventilatory effectiveness and pulmonary blood flow. Attention to positioning of the older adult during surgery is critical in maintaining optimum respiratory function. Older patients who have kyphosis have restricted lung expansion. Additional head support with pillows is needed to minimize neck and back strain and improve ventilatory function in the supine position. The bed or table can be placed in a reverse Trendelenburg position to help the patient feel more upright and relieve abdominal pressure that prevents diaphragmatic excursion. If the head is supported on pillows or blankets, the arms must also be supported to prevent stretching of the brachial plexus.

Older adults who are obese or have a history of chronic respiratory disease are often short of breath, uncomfortable, or anxious when in a supine position and report feeling they cannot "get enough air." Placing these patients in a reverse Trendelenberg position will take pressure off the diaphragm to helpoptimize ventilation and comfort.

POSTOPERATIVE CONSIDERATIONS

Pulmonary Compromise

Pulmonary compromise can present as a single entity or in combination with other systemic alterations. Hypoventilation is a consistent concern across the perioperative continuum as a result of age-related changes that compound disease and trauma. Common pulmonary complications that occur early in the postsurgical period are upper airway obstruction, bronchospasm, laryngospasm, and aspiration. Atelectasis is an intraoperative or early postoperative complication. Pneumonia, the most common postoperative pulmonary complication, occurs several days after surgery. Pulmonary edema, pulmonary embolism, and pneumothorax are less common potentially life-threatening pulmonary complications.

Respiratory considerations for the postoperative management of older adults are similar to preoperative and intraoperative considerations. Priorities include adequate oxygenation, ventilation, and protection of the airway. Postoperative monitoring includes pulse oximetry, auscultation of lung sounds, monitoring of respiratory rate and depth, electrocardiogram, and blood pressure monitoring. Monitoring cognition is critical when assessing for potential pulmonary complications in the gerioperative patient. A change in cognition is a frequent yet atypical symptom that may be the first sign of hypoxia in older adults.

After surgery, patients are often drowsy, and supplemental oxygen is necessary to maintain an oxygen saturation above 95%. Older adults have as much as a 50% decrease in their response to hypoxia and hypercapnia over younger patients. As a result, the oxygen saturation may dip below 70% before the CNS stimulates the older patient to waken and breathe spontaneously. Close monitoring with pulse oximetry is mandatory to detect a drop in oxygen saturation.

Pulse oximetry must be monitored continuously in the operating room and during transport to the postanesthesia care unit. Pulse oximeter wave forms should be tall and wavy. The wave form can be affected by a number of factors. If the wave form for the pulse oximeter is not adequate, the pulse oximeter may not be reading accurately. If the oxygen saturation is low, it is critical to assess the patient by examining skin color, respiratory rate and depth, breath sounds, pulse, and blood pressure. Only if the patient appears to have no symptoms of distress should pulse oximeter dysfunction be considered. Figure 11.4 shows three common types of pulse oximetry wave forms.

Three common factors contribute to pulse oximetry inaccuracy: patient movement, peripheral vasoconstriction, and low blood pressure. If the patient is restless, placing the pulse oximeter on the toe can sometimes provide an adequate wave form. In the older adult, peripheral circulation can be poor in response to surgical hypothermia. Vasoconstriction with poor blood flow to the fingers will decrease oximeter accuracy. Placing warm blankets on the patient and wrapping the oximeter can promote circulation to the extremities. Low blood pressure affects perfusion and accuracy of oximetry readings.

Auscultation of breath sounds is critical to the identification and treatment of pulmonary concerns. If the lungs are clear, the patient may be overnarcotized or may be weak from the muscle relaxant and not ventilating well. Supporting findings include not being able to

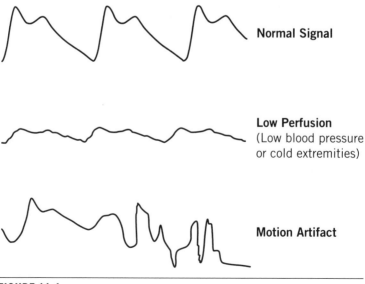

FIGURE 11.4
Pulse Oximetry Waveforms

hold arms up, not able to respond to voice commands, or not able to speak above a whisper. If wheezing is heard, bronchoconstriction is suspected. If no breath sounds are heard and the patient's chest and stomach are moving asynchronously, the airway may be obstructed. The presence of rales can be indicative of pulmonary edema. Each of these changes can result in hypoxemia and hypoventilation. The anesthesia or health care provider must be notified whenever there are changes in the older adult's pulmonary status.

Hypoxemia and Hypoventilation

Hypoxemia and hypoventilation are common in the perioperative period secondary to age-related pulmonary changes and the effect of anesthetic and narcotic medications. Hypoxemia is defined as a pulse oximeter reading of less than 90%. Hypoventilation is defined as decreased gas exchange in the alveoli that results in hypoxemia and/or hypercapnia. Risk factors include anesthesia, abdominal incisions, narcotics, or airway obstruction. Use of oral and nasal airways to maintain airway patency, adequate reversal of muscle relaxants to allow restoration of muscle tone, and good narcotic balance that prevents splinting and allows for adequate respiratory rate can avert hypoxemia and hypoventilation.

Treatment begins with assessment to determine the cause. If the patient's oxygen saturation is less than 90% and the patient is not responding to commands, it may be necessary to use a bag mask system to ventilate the patient, even if the patient is breathing spontaneously. The most common device is the bag valve mask. When using an bag valve mask, long, infrequent sustained inflations should be used. Rapid "bagging" with large tidal volumes is ineffective. Rapid inflations also can lead to hyperventilation, respiratory alkalosis, and gastric distention.

If the patient is alert, supplemental oxygen may be all that is necessary to keep the oxygen saturation over 95%. Frequent reminders asking the patient to cough and deep breathe may also be necessary. Table 11.5 shows methods of oxygen administration with associated oxygen liter flow and suggests oxygen flow for different types of oxygen support.

Older patients can be sensitive to anxiolytics. If hypoxia or hypoventilation is related to sedation, naloxone can be used to reverse narcotic influences; flumazenil is used to reverse midazolam effects. If the patient had midazolam prior to surgery, the midazolam should be reversed prior to narcotic reversal to ensure pain relief.

Gerioperative patients require postoperative pain relief; however, this can be a balancing act between achieving pain relief and maintaining adequate ventilation. Achieving a balance is a particular problem when older adults are receiving opioids, especially if they have sleep apnea. Opioids can further depress ventilation in patients with sleep apnea. Inadequate ventilation also can occur as a result of inadequate pain relief and respiratory splinting. Administering oxygen at 2 L to all older adults receiving opioids can help decrease medication-related hypoxemia. Careful monitoring of both pain and ventilation is critical to the safety of the older adult.

Postoperative patients with a history of OSA require close monitoring with a pulse oximeter, blood pressure monitoring, and electrocardiogram to prevent hypoventilation. Sedating medications are given sparingly. CPAP/BiPAP are utilized to optimize respiration.

Lying in bed for long periods in poor posture can cause postoperative hypoventilation. Movement and getting the older person out of bed to a chair or ambulating will improve ventilation. The older person should be monitored closely to maintain movement and activity within the tolerance of respiratory function and conditioning. Moving the patient to a more upright position in bed and raising the head of the bed can improve ventilation for older adults on bed rest.

TABLE 11.5
Oxygen Support and Liter Flow

Flow Rate	Percent Oxygen Delivery	Clinical Use	Advantage	Disadvantage
Nasal cannula				
1–6 L a minute Each 1 L ↑ in flow rate = 4% ↑ in oxygen concentration		Supplemental, not for patients in distress	Well tolerated	Drying to nares/ not humidified
0 L/min	21% = Room air			
1 L/min	25%			
2 L/min	29%			
3 L/min	33%			
4 L/min	37%			
5 L/min	41%			
6 L/min	44%			
Face mask				
6–10 L/min	35–60%	Supplemental, better for mouth breathers	Mixes with room air Moderate to high concentration of oxygen	Poorly tolerated by children
Partial rebreather				
6–10 L/min	35–60%	Moderate hypoxia	High percentages available	Must have reservoir bag inflated
Venturi mask				
4–8 L/min	25–60%	Controlled delivery: Each colored piece provides specific air flow and oxygen delivery	Variable setting available	Drying to nares if not humidified
Non-rebreather				
10–15 L/min	90–95%	Most oxygen delivery without positive pressure ventilation	Close to 100% oxygen	Must have bag reservoir inflated

Severe cases of hypoventilation that do not respond to interventions may require reintubation. An anesthesia provider should be notified, and equipment must be readily available. Equipment required includes mask, ventilation equipment, oxygen, reintubation supplies (blade, handle, endotracheal tube with stylet), and suction. Nurses are called upon to assist with reintubation, administer necessary medications, and manually ventilate the patient.

Bronchospasm and Laryngospasm

Bronchospasm is an involuntary contraction of smooth muscle that precipitates airway closure. A medical emergency, bronchospasm is caused by stimulation of reflexes or airway irritation to aspiration, laryngoscopy, intubation, or extubation. Airway edema, inflammation, and increased bronchial secretions occur in response to bronchospasm. The closure of the airways increases airway resistance to the point where ventilation may not be possible. Bronchospasm can also be secondary to a latex or medication anaphylactic reaction. In a patient who is intubated, bronchospasm is evidenced by increased airway resistance and ventilation difficulty. Airway pressures increase in response to airway resistance.

Signs of bronchospasm include expiratory wheezing or absent breath sounds, prolonged expiration, and an increase in airway resistance. Patients who are awake and not intubated may exhibit use of accessory muscles, dyspnea, and tachypnea. Smoking, COPD, asthma, tracheal or oropharyngeal suctioning, and aspiration are risk factors that can trigger bronchospasm. Interventions designed to minimize airway stimulation, prevent aspiration, or increase bronchodilation can prevent bronchospasm.

Treatment of bronchospasm involves identification of the cause and removal of the offending stimuli. In the case of airway stimulation, beta-adrenergic agonists are the first-line treatment to open alveoli. If bronchospasm is secondary to anaphylaxis, all medications are stopped temporarily. Epinephrine and antihistamines are administered along with intravenous fluids. Glycopyrrolate may be added to dry secretions. Steroids are used to decrease inflammation.

Laryngospasm, also known as laryngeal obstruction, is a medical emergency. This type of obstruction is more often seen in children and young athletic adults but can occur in the elderly. Laryngospasm occurs when stimulation of the glottis by secretions causes the extrinsic muscles of the larynx to contract closing the vocal cords. Prior to laryngospasm, there is often a high-pitched crowing sound or stridor. Laryngospasm makes ventilation impossible but often lasts less than 60 seconds. Treatment is high-pressure ventilation to relax the vocal cords. If this is ineffective, a small dose of succinylcholine may be required. While laryngospasm is unsettling, it is rarely fatal in the geriatric patient. However, prevention and vigilance are key to quickly resolving the spasm. The need for the perioperative nurse to remain quietly at the bedside during intubation and extubation cannot be overemphasized.

Aspiration

Aspiration is inhalation of foreign matter into the lungs such as gastric juices, blood, or oropharyngeal secretions. Aspiration occurs most often in intraoperative and immediate postsurgical phases of the perioperative continuum. Aspiration pneumonitis, the inhalation of gastric contents, changes the pH of the parenchyma of the lungs, causing inflammation and edema to the lung tissue. The lungs become "burned" by the gastric juices. Aspiration pneumonitis usually occurs during the intraoperative period, and the extent of the insult is directly related to the volume and acidity of the aspirated fluid. Causes are related to increased abdominal pressure while lying supine under intraoperative sedation, vomiting during intubation or extubation, or reflux in the presence of a laryngeal mask airway. Aspiration can also occur at any time in the postoperative period. The risk is generally lower in the geriatric population, as this age group experiences less nausea and vomiting after surgery. However, after bowel surgery, gastric aspiration can cause serious respiratory complications

The primary treatment for gastric aspiration is prevention by restricting oral intake (NPO) and providing antinausea medications as needed. Ranitidine may be useful in patients with history of reflux. Medical bromide is recommended for use prior to some surgical procedures. However, it should be used with extreme caution in older adults. A risk–benefit ratio should be conducted prior to administrating the medication.

If aspiration is suspected, immediate suctioning of the airway and oxygen supplementation is necessary. Symptoms of aspiration, including bronchospasm, hypoxemia, and atelectasis are treated on the basis of severity. Reintubation may be considered to suction the lungs. Monitoring the patient for 24 to 48 hours after surgery may be necessary. Antibiotics are not indicated unless the patient is taking antacids that have changed the gastric pH, the patient has a small bowel obstruction with increased stomach bacteria, or the pneumonitis does not resolve within 48 hours. Mortality for uncomplicated pneumonitis approaches 5%. When pneumonitis is accompanied by empyema, mortality is increased to 20%. Mortality from massive pneumonitis is 70%.

Aspiration pneumonia occurs secondary to inhalation of blood after upper airway surgery or trauma. The lack of anesthesia reversal leads to an inability to swallow adequately. Age-related changes resulting in a decrease in gag and cough reflexes, diminished swallowing mechanism, or changes in the mucociliary blanket increase the risk of aspiration pneumonia.

Prevention of aspiration includes reversal of muscle relaxants and assessment of swallowing function after anesthesia recovery. Proper positioning in an upright position in a bed or a chair prior to eating or drinking facilitates swallowing. It is important to monitor cognitive assessment throughout the postoperative period as changes in cognition can increase aspiration risk.

ATELECTASIS

Atelectasis is defined as a lack of gas exchange due to collapsed alveoli. Older adults are vulnerable to atelectasis due to age-related changes in the respiratory system. Up to 90% of anesthetized patients develop atelectasis even if they are spontaneously breathing. Atelectasis typically begins during anesthesia and continues into the postoperative period. Preoperatively bed-bound gerioperative patients are at risk for developing atelectasis prior to surgery as a result of poor positioning in bed causing decreased ventilation. Patients with preoperative abdominal pain are at risk for developing atelectasis before surgery secondary to "splinting" of respirations to minimize abdominal discomfort. Diminished or absent lung sounds and hypoxemia are the most common signs of atelectasis. Fever that develops within 24 hours after surgery is often due to atelectasis. A change in cognition or delirium resulting from hypoxia can be one of the first signs of atelectasis in older adults.

Few strategies are available to prevent atelectasis intraoperatively. Adding positive end-expiratory pressure may be helpful. Using some air rather than 100% oxygen intraoperatively and during extubation appears to decrease the amount of atelectasis that occurs.

Prevention of preoperative and prevention of postoperative atelectasis is similar: humidified oxygen, encouraging coughing, deep breathing exercises, IS, hydration, turning and moving in bed, and ambulation. Intermittent positive pressure ventilation (with CPAP/BiPAP) may be necessary to re-expand collapsed alveoli. Prevention of perioperative atelectasis decreases the risk of postoperative pneumonia.

PNEUMONIA

Postoperative pneumonia is the most common postoperative pulmonary complication. It is also the third most common surgical complication after urinary tract and wound infections. A single case of postoperative pneumonia can cost up to $40,000 in additional health care costs and increase mortality rate up to 50%. Risk factors for acquiring postoperative pneumonia include age greater than seventy, malnutrition, surgery lasting over 2.5 hours, surgery requiring upper abdominal or thoracic incisions, altered mental status, positive cough test, and preexisting lung disease.

Postoperative pneumonia usually develops 48 to 72 hours after surgery secondary to hypoventilation, decreased lung expansion from splinting due to pain, poor posture in bed, decreased ambulation, and poor mouth care. The lungs develop postoperative atelectasis and fluid enters the alveoli, forming consolidations.

In older adults, the signs and symptoms of pneumonia can be subtle. Rather than cough, sputum production, and fever seen in younger patients, older adults often exhibit normal to low body temperature, change in mental status, and falls. Complaints of general malaise and fatigue with increased respiratory rate should prompt suspicion of pneumonia. Onset of delirium is a major presenting symptom of postoperative pneumonia in older adults that requires immediate intervention (see Chapter 21).

The most effective intervention for pneumonia is preventing hypoventilation. Hypoventilation is prevented by regular and systematic cough and deep breathing exercises, and correct use of incentive spirometry (IS). Although IS has a demonstrated effectiveness in pneumonia treatment, the evidence supporting the ability of IS to prevent pneumonia is less compelling. However, postoperative guidelines recommend IS as part of a pneumonia prevention program (Qaseem et al., 2006). Correct use of IS is critical to its effectiveness. Exhibit 11.3 provides directions on the correct use of IS.

Diligent nursing and interdisciplinary team care prevents postoperative pneumonia.

Interventions to prevent pneumonia also include mouth care at least two times a day with chlorhexidine swabs, ambulation with optimal pain relief, elevation of the head of

---

EXHIBIT 11.3 **Correct Use of Incentive Spirometer**

- Assist older adult to upright position unless contraindicated.
- Hold the incentive spirometer in an upright position.
- Place the mouthpiece in the patient's mouth and make sure his or her lips are sealed tightly around it.
- Ask the patient to breathe in slowly and as deeply as possible, raising the piston toward the top of the column. The coach indicator should be in the blue outlined area.
- Ask the patient to hold his or her breath as long as possible (or at least 5 seconds). Allow the piston to fall to the bottom of the column.
- Allow the patient to rest for a few seconds.
- Repeat steps one to five at least 10 times every hour when the patient is awake.
- Position the indicator tab on the left side of the spirometer to show the patient's best effort.
- Use the indicator as a goal to work toward during each repetition.

EXHIBIT 11.4   Checklist for Prevention of Postoperative Pneumonia

Patient-centered care interventions
- Cough and deep breathing exercises
- Incentive spirometry
- At least twice daily mouth care with chlorhexidine swabs
- Optimal pain relief that allows patient movement and ambulation
- Elevating head of bed 30 degrees
- Sitting up for meals with head of bed elevated or in chair
- Bed-bound patients: Reposition every 1–2 hours
- Maintain hydration
- Optimal nutrition
- Handwashing protection

Interdisciplinary team interventions
- Staff education
- Documentation of completed interventions
- Handoff communication: Risk factors
- Computerized pneumonia prevention orders
- Quarterly staff update and review
- Monitor pneumonia data to assess prevention effectiveness

Adapted from Wren, Martin, Yoon, & Bech, 2010.

---

bed greater than 30 degrees, and getting the patient out of bed or sitting upright in bed for meals. Patients unable to be out of bed must be encouraged to change positions or assisted with repositioning on a regular schedule every 1 to 2 hours. Hydration helps keep airways moist to facilitate sputum production and decrease airway irritation. Nutrition helps meet the increased metabolic demands posed by surgical stress and promotes increased resistance to infection.

Prevention depends on nursing and interdisciplinary team education with regularly scheduled discussions of prevention effectiveness, documentation of pneumonia bundle care, and computerized pneumonia prevention order sets. Establishing a pneumonia alert checklist and early implementation of prevention protocols must be a routine part of postoperative care (Exhibit 11.4). Effective nursing care after surgery is one of the most significant factors in preventing postoperative pneumonia in older adults.

Antibiotics and expectorants are used to treat pneumonia unresponsive to nursing and interdisciplinary team nonpharmacologic interventions. Antitussives must be used cautiously as they suppress the cough reflex. However, for elders with a severe cough, it is important to consider the need for rest and energy conservation. Administering antitussives at bedtime can prevent sleep interruption and conserve energy. Close monitoring of the older adult is needed as suppressing the cough reflex can further impede responses to decreased oxygenation levels already compromised by age-related changes and sleep-related loss of receptor sensitivity.

Pulmonary Edema, Pulmonary Embolus, And Pneumothorax

Pulmonary edema is the accumulation of fluid in the alveoli. Causes of pulmonary edema are decreased interstitial pressure, increased hydrostatic pressure, or an increase in capillary permeability. Decreased interstitial pressure may be a result of prolonged airway obstruction. Fluid overload, left ventricular failure, and cardiac ischemia can cause an increase in hydrostatic pressure. Increased capillary permeability can occur in response to aspiration, anaphylaxis, shock, or disseminated intravascular coagulation.

The risk of developing pulmonary edema is higher in patients with a history of heart failure or myocardial infarction. The elderly are particularly at risk. Older adults with a cardiac history may not tolerate the required amount of surgical fluid replacement. Feeling short of breath, anxious, or not feeling well are early indicators of pulmonary edema. The older person may appear "puffy." Auscultation reveals rales or crackles. The older adult can rapidly become hypoxic and exhibit respiratory distress. Because pulmonary edemain the elderly is notable, a high index of suspicion can identify early signs and symptoms. The handoff from the perioperative nurse to the postanesthesia care unit nurse must include information on the older patient's fluid balance during surgery with data that provides a baseline assessment of respiratory function. Monitoring fluid balance, anticipating potential problems, and remaining alert to early onset of signs and symptoms contributes to early intervention of pulmonary edema and prevention of adverse events.

Pulmonary embolism is a relatively rare but serious complication of surgery. More likely to occur after orthopedic surgery, a low oxygen saturation accompanied by tachycardia and hypotension is an ominous sign that must be responded to immediately. Rales may be heard on auscultation, or the lungs may be clear or diminished. Pulmonary embolism can be deadly, but the signs and symptoms are nonspecific and require a high index of suspicion for a diagnosis. The patient may complain of shortness of breath or chest pain, but typically may have no symptoms. Pulmonary embolus is one of the most life-threatening of all respiratory complications and must always be considered when patients complain of dyspnea.

A pneumothorax is a collection of air or gas in the pleural cavity between the lung and the chest wall. It may be a secondary complication of central line insertion, positive pressure ventilation, or a nerve block (i.e., interscalene block, brachial plexus block, and supraclavicular block). Signs and symptoms of pneumothorax vary according to the extent and location but can include patient statements of chest pain and dyspnea. Symptoms are vague and range from none to hypoxemia, restlessness, and respiratory distress. Auscultation may reveal decreased breath sound on the affected side or there may be no change in breath sounds. Patient history and risk factors can assist in identifying this complication. Older adults with a history of COPD have a high risk for pneumothorax. An upright chest radiograph can confirm the diagnosis as well as the extent and location of the pneumothorax. Treatment depends on the size of the pneumothorax and symptoms. A small pneumothorax, less than 20%, can resolve with little to no intervention beyond supplemental oxygen and monitoring. A larger pneumothorax with persistent and severe hypoxemia requires a chest tube to reinflate the lung. The presence of a pneumothorax without a chest tube is a contraindication to general anesthesia with positive pressure ventilation. Positive pressure ventilation will increase the size of the pneumothorax. Communicating information about preoperative chest trauma, central line insertion, or intraoperative block is essential during all perioperative handoffs.

Discharge Considerations

Transition from ambulatory or hospital surgery requires knowledge of the patient history, living situation, support systems, and surgically related postdischarge care. Reviewing the preoperative assessment and the proposed discharge plan developed preoperatively is important in developing the postoperative discharge plan. Of special significance to prevention of pulmonary complications is the availability of a caregiver. Caregivers can be a significant support in helping the patient carry out postdischarge activities targeted at preventing pulmonary complications. Among these is adequate pain relief, getting out of bed, ambulation, hydration, coughing, and deep breathing. These postoperative activities have a more critical and immediate need for attention in older adults discharged from ambulatory or day surgery.

Older adults who have had inpatient surgery usually have a postoperative stay that allows for detection of pneumonia prior to discharge. Pneumonia, one of the most common and most serious postoperative pulmonary complications, has a usual onset of 48 to 72 hours, and occurs after the older person has been discharged home. Surgery is a stressor that affects immunity and overall health condition, making the older person at risk for community-acquired pneumonia as well as hospital-acquired pneumonia.

Interventions used to prevent postoperative pneumonia in the hospital should be taught to the gerioperative patient and all caregivers for use at home. Strategies include pain relief, coughing, deep breathing, sitting up, ambulating, hydration, nutrition, and depending on timeframe and pulmonary status, IS. Teaching older adults and caregivers about the correct use of medications is important in preventing pulmonary complications. Medications important to preventing pulmonary complications include bronchodilators, analgesia, and antibiotics. Pain medication is a major issue for older adults at home. Studies consistently indicate that older adults are hesitant to take "pain pills" at home. Reinforcing the importance of pain relief to prevent splinting, prevent barriers to ambulation and movement, and eating is critical in supporting the need for patients to attend to this critical area of pulmonary complication prevention. Smoking cessation continues to be a priority in discharge teaching. Reinforcing strategies for older adults who ceased smoking preoperatively is important in continuing cessation after discharge. Older adults who did not cease smoking prior to surgery should receive the 5As or AAR program. A critical point is to provide advice and counsel on smoking cessation resources.

Handwashing is as important in the home as in the hospital. Older adults have an increased risk of changes in immunity after hospital discharge due to the stress of surgery and hospitalization. Family members out in the community can transfer pathogens from the community to the older adult in the home. Reviewing and reinforcing the discharge information and teaching that was included during the preoperative assessment helps gerioperative patients and their families remember the information and feel more comfortable instituting recommended treatment plans. Providing new information on treatment or findings from hospital or ambulatory surgical events should build on the preoperative information and not be seen as a different or contradicting discharge plan. Helping the older person and family integrate care needs contributes to the understanding and adherence needed to maintain the safety and well-being of the gerioperative patient.

Having the older adult demonstrate interventions such as IS and use of an inhaler prior to discharge assists in a smooth transition from hospital or ambulatory surgery to home. Older adults are able to carry out treatments such as IS, hydration, regular ambulation, and nutrition in the hospital with nursing and other staff assistance. Carrying out the same interventions at home or other new environment can be difficult and create barriers to adherence. Providing written instructions and reviewing the instructions with the older adult and caregivers and companion-coach several days prior to discharge allows time for questions and follow-up teaching as needed. Giving written instructions at the time of discharge can result in misunderstandings and lack of adherence due to misunderstanding.

PATIENT REPORT: Mr. Dawson

For Mr. Dawson, the first step is to conduct a health history. Important questions for Mr. Dawson are about his exercise tolerance, smoking cessation, and past medical history. Mr. Dawson reports he continues to smoke close to a pack of cigarettes a day, although he has tried to "cut down." He wheezes on exertion and uses his albuterol inhaler several times a week with relief. He reports no recent upper respiratory infections. His pneumonia and influenza vaccines are current. He coughs up clear sputum in the morning. He has not needed any steroids in the past year. On auscultation, his lung sounds are diminished with wheezes in all lung fields. Mr. Dawson has a positive cough test and says he gets short of breath walking up two flights of stairs. He drinks coffee several times a day, uses alcohol one or two times a day always with meals, and reports a good appetite.

Based on the preoperative assessment data, Mr. Dawson has an elevated risk for postoperative pulmonary complications. Risk factors include age, smoking, body habitus, chronic bronchitis, positive cough test, low exercise tolerance, and poor hydration. Modifiable risk factors include smoking, exercise, hydration, and nutrition. His bronchi are restricted secondary to age-related changes (Figure 11.5); chronic bronchitis decreases them even further by inflammation and sputum production. Although his chronic pulmonary disease is moderately severe, maximizing his respiratory function and preventing pulmonary complications across the perioperative continuum become major goals.

An interdisciplinary health team develops a plan with Mr. Dawson for pulmonary prehabilitation. When asked, Mr. Dawson states he would like his wife to participate in learning the prehabilitation program with him. A review of his medications and inhaler shows correct use of both. He receives verbal instruction, written directions, and demonstration on correct use of the incentive spirometer and deep breathing exercises. He is given a written scheduled regimen for using them.

Improving Mr. Dawson's exercise tolerance begins with walking as far as he can within his comfort level and increasing gradually to tolerance. He is having hip repair because he has pain on ambulation. He is instructed that when walking is too difficult,

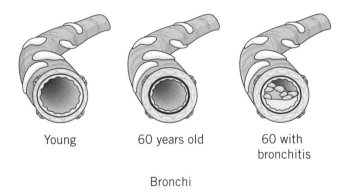

Young   60 years old   60 with
                                     bronchitis

Bronchi

FIGURE 11.5

Comparison of Young, Aged, and Diseased Bronchus
Mr. Dawson's bronchus is narrowed by age when compared with bronchus in a healthy, young adult. Air exchange is further restricted due to inflammation and sputum production caused by chronic bronchitis. The combination of age and disease significantly increase his risk of postoperative pulmonary infection.

he is to do upper and lower extremity chair exercises to improve respiratory volume and function. The exercise program is to begin immediately.

Mr. Dawson is given information on maintaining fluid intake and improving nutrition. Mr. Dawson is offered a smoking cessation program and encouraged to start the program immediately. Smoking cessation efforts continue until just before surgery.

Although chest radiographs are not a routine preoperative screening test, Mr. Dawson is a good candidate for a preoperative chest radiograph. He is given a combination albuterol and ipratropium treatment prior to surgery.

After surgery, Mr. Dawson is placed on a pulmonary complication alert checklist. He receives systematic pulmonary monitoring and regularly scheduled preventative pulmonary care. He and his wife receive a review on the correct use of the incentive spirometer and deep breathing exercises with written directions, demonstration, and written schedule.

A pain relief plan is established incorporating his ice packs and heating pad used preoperatively. A pain assessment with follow-up pain relief intervention as needed is scheduled before ambulation and pulmonary toilet. He is given a schedule for ambulation combined with bed exercises and positioning. He is assisted out of bed or assisted to an upright sitting position in bed as allowed within postoperative guidelines for hip surgery. He is placed on a warfarin regimen per standard guidelines. Mr. Dawson is on a hydration schedule and regular diet. He is given respiratory therapy as ordered.

Ongoing, systematic monitoring for early detection of symptoms includes lung auscultation, pulse oximetry, and observation for changes in cognition. Medication reconciliation reveals his preoperative medications should begin as soon as possible after surgery to prevent onset of acute bronchitis.

Mr. Dawson remains free of pulmonary complications and is discharged on schedule. The discharge team develops a postdischarge care plan in collaboration with Mr. Dawson and his wife. The plan emphasizes pain relief as needed, deep breathing exercises, exercise schedule, smoking cessation, correct use of his medications, hydration, nutrition, and follow-up care appointments. Mr. Dawson is provided information on whom to call if he or his wife has questions after discharge.

SUMMARY

Pulmonary complications remain one of the most serious causes of surgical morbidity and mortality in older adults. While the majority of age-related changes in respiratory anatomy, physiology, and function are not clinically significant in everyday activities, they become highly significant when the older adult is placed under the stress of anesthesia and surgery. A major outcome is the prevention of perioperative pulmonary complications.

A systematic, patient-centered preoperative assessment identifies patient-related risk factors for intraoperative and postoperative complications. Developing a preoperative plan of care focusing on prehabilitation and patient education can maximize pulmonary function prior to surgery. Postoperative pulmonary alerts and implementation of prevention guidelines can prevent many complications. The majority of prevention strategies require nursing intervention. Continuous, systematic monitoring and prompt intervention minimizes morbidity and mortality in the event a complication occurs. Nurses are critical players in protecting older adults from postoperative pulmonary-related adverse events. Gerioperative care is critical in maintaining optimal pulmonary function and preventing complications in the older adult before, during, and after surgery.

KEY POINTS

- Age-related changes in respiratory anatomy, physiology, and function are not clinically significant for everyday activities; the changes are highly significant in the gerioperative patient.
- Increasing age is an independent predictor for postoperative pulmonary complications, even for healthy older adults.
- Pulmonary prehabilitation decreases postoperative pulmonary complications and improves gerioperative outcomes.
- Preoperative smoking cessation improves pulmonary function regardless of time to surgery.
- Delirium is a red flag, atypical, but frequent symptom of hypoventilation, atelectasis, and pneumonia in the gerioperative patient and requires a rapid response.
- An interdisciplinary treatment bundle based on aggressive prevention, systematic monitoring, early detection, and rapid intervention improves pulmonary outcomes in gerioperative patients.
- Diligent nursing and interdisciplinary team education and collaboration prevent postoperative pneumonia in older adults.

TWELVE

Neurological

Raelene V. Shippee-Rice, Jennifer V. Long, and Susan J. Fetzer

PATIENT REPORT: Ms. Summitt

Ms. Summitt attends the preoperative clinic prior to her scheduled mastectomy. While reviewing the medical record prior to the appointment, the nurse practitioner notes that Ms. Summitt is 81 years old and lives in an assisted living facility. Her niece and family live nearby. Her primary care physician diagnosed breast cancer during Ms. Summitt's visit for incontinence complaints and getting up at night to use the bathroom.

The nervous system is the central control system for everything the older person does, thinks, and feels, as well as for regulating the functioning of all body systems. Every anesthetic drug and medication exerts a direct or indirect effect on central and peripheral neurologic function. The neurologic system in older adults is highly sensitive to the effects of anesthesia and surgical stress in ways that are not well understood. Anesthesia and surgical stress trigger inflammatory processes that precipitate short- and long-term cognitive changes in the aging brain.

This chapter provides an overview of age-related changes in the neurological system and the effect of these changes on functional status. An important consideration is the effect of aging and disease on the perioperative care of the older adult. Understanding age-related changes in the neurological system allows health care providers to remain "ahead of the curve" in anticipating potential gerioperative problems, to take preventive action, and to implement early, targeted interventions to optimize gerioperative patient outcomes.

Neurological Considerations

The human nervous system is composed of the central nervous system (CNS) and the peripheral nervous system (PNS). The CNS, composed of the brain and spinal cord, is connected to body systems by the PNS that extends from the spinal cord to end neurons in all tissues. The PNS relays information to the CNS (afferent information) and from the CNS (efferent information) to end organs throughout the body via somatic and auto-nomic pathways. The somatic system controls sensory and voluntary motor innervations, whereas the autonomic nervous system manages control of involuntary systems such as the visera, smooth muscle, and glands. Parasympathetic and sympathetic pathways in the autonomic nervous system maintain homeostasis. Figure 12.1 presents a schematic of the CNS and PNS.

The somatosensory system connects the outside world with the CNS and protects the body from harm through sensation and interpretation of touch, vibration, temperature, pro-prioception, and pain. The autonomic nervous system maintains homeostasis by regulating functions of visceral organs, heart, lung, and glands through parasympathetic and sympa-thetic pathways. The parasympathetic system conserves energy and maintains continuing function of organ systems, while the sympathetic system protects the organism through an arousal of the "fight or flight" response when there is an internal or external threat to the integrity of the system.

Transmission of information throughout the nervous system to all end organs is through a neural network composed of cell bodies, dendrites, and axons. Neurons connect through electrical- or chemical-mediated synapses. The majority of synapses are chemical in nature controlled by neurotransmitters.

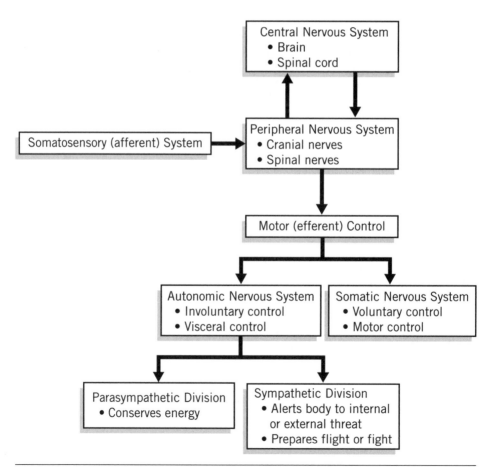

FIGURE 12.1

Schematic of the Central and Peripheral Nervous System

Central Nervous System

AGE-RELATED CHANGES

The brain grows quickly from birth achieving its maximum size and weight by the early 20s. Loss in brain weight and size occurs slowly, beginning around age 40, at a rate of approximately 2% per decade with significant variability across individuals. By age 90, the aging brain has lost between 5 and 10% of its weight primarily in the frontal, parietal, and temporal lobes. Initially, the loss in size and weight was thought to result from the decreased number of neurons. More recent evidence suggests the loss is due to changes in the size of neurons, primarily in the dendrites.

By the sixth decade, anatomical changes in the brain have started, and they progress slowly with time. The cortical sulci, or valleys in the brain, widen. The gyri, or ridges and bumps surrounding the sulci, narrow. The ventricles of the brain dilate. Senile plaques composed of hard clusters of damaged neurons and neurofibrillary tangles, twisted masses of degraded proteins within the neuron, begin to form in the aging brain in late middle age.

Brain size begins to decrease around age 40.

As people age, nerve cells decrease in number and size, with regions of the brain differentially affected. The rate and degree of change within and across individuals varies considerably. Due to the brain's ability to adapt and to create new neural networks, the functional effect of age-related changes is minimal in healthy, older adults until very late ages. Age-related changes in brain anatomy and physiology become markedly increased causing severe damage in dementia. Figure 12.2 illustrates a young adult brain compared with an aged brain.

NEUROTRANSMITTERS

Neurotransmitters, chemicals synthesized by neurons, transfer impulses across a synaptic gap from one neuron to another neuron or to a muscle or organ (see Figure 12.3). Neurotransmitters produce an excitatory or inhibitory response to promote or inhibit nerve transmission.

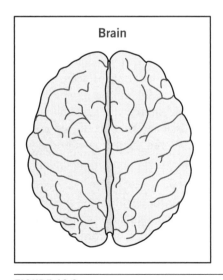
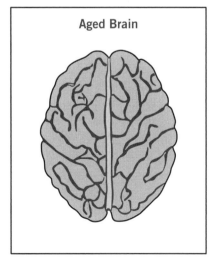

FIGURE 12.2
The Adult and Aged Brain

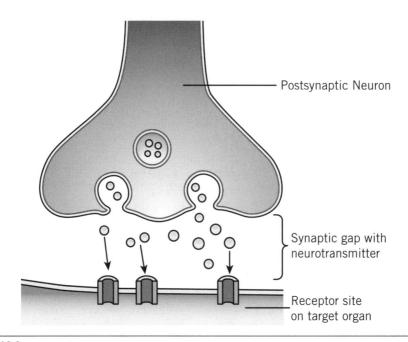

FIGURE 12.3

Synapse With Neurotransmitter

Neurotransmitter synthesis occurs in the presynaptic neuron. The neuron releases the neurotransmitter into the synaptic gap. Receptors on the postsynaptic or target organ bind the neurotransmitter to continue signaling process. Neurotransmitter action is terminated by removal from the synapse via reuptake into the transmitting neuron, breakdown by enzymes, or diffusion from the synapse. Acetylcholine is destroyed by the enzyme acetylcholinesterase while norepinephrine, serotonin, and dopamine are removed through reuptake.

CNS neurotransmitters have excitatory and inhibitory functions.

There are over 100 human neurotransmitters, with the possibility of more to be discovered. The functions and age-related changes in serotonin, acetylcholine, norepinephrine, and dopamine, four of the major CNS neurotransmitters, are outlined in Table 12.1. The ability of neurotransmission to manage neural messaging systems is dictated by the amount of neurotransmitter available, the number of available neurotransmitter receptor sites, and the ability of receptors to take up the neurotransmitter. Disruption in any of the neurotransmitter mechanisms reduces neural function and signal transfer. Loss of neural transmission results in slowed cognition and motor function, changes in memory and mood, and altered regulation of body systems.

Age-Related Changes

Aging is associated with reduced numbers of neurotransmitter receptor sites, reduced neurotransmitter production, and impaired neurotransmitter reuptake. Age-related changes in neurotransmitter function occur over time, affecting different neurotransmitters and neurotransmitter availability at different rates. The variability creates an imbalance between neurotransmitters as well as changes in the quantity of individual neurotransmitters. The imbalance between excitatory and inhibitory neurotransmitters contributes to a variety of health conditions such as depression, anxiety, and insomnia. For example, with age, the number of

TABLE 12.1

Central Nervous System Neurotransmitter Action and Age-Related Changes

Neurotransmitter	Action	Age-Related Changes
Acetylcholine	Mediates consciousness Attention processes Cognition especially memory Rapid eye movement sleep	Decrease in synthesis Loss of receptor sites in cerebral cortex
Norepinephrine	Fatigue Depression Reactions to stress Sleep patterns	Fewer receptors Decreased reuptake
Dopamine	Depression Anxiety states Influences acetylcholine	Reduced levels Reduced receptors Increase in dopamine breakdown
Serotonin	Thermoregulation Sleep Mood states including depression and anxiety states	Decreased number of serotonin receptors in the cortex, up to 30% loss

dopamine receptors is decreased, causing alterations in body positioning. Arms become flexed with decreased arm movements. Similarly, in Parkinson's disease, a greater dopamine deficiency produces marked change in body positioning and motor function. Age-related changes in acetylcholine availability result in minor changes in cognitive function and speed of information processing. A severe loss of acetylcholine availability is associated with Alzheimer's disease. Changes in CNS neurotransmitters alter sleep patterns, impair cognition, and contribute to geriatric depression. Postoperative delirium is most likely caused by an imbalance in dopamine and cholinergic neurotransmitters (see Chapter 21).

> *Alzheimer's disease is associated with a loss of acetylcholine which is responsible for changes in cognition.*

Effect on Function

The link between changes in neurotransmitter and functional loss is indirect. The brain is able to adapt to significant alteration in neuronal loss and neurotransmitter availability before a change is seen clinically apparent. The brain has more cells than are needed for day-to-day function. The "reserve" of brain cells compensates for age-related changes, so there is minimal initial effect on function. Chapter 19 discusses cognitive reserve and resilience, the ability of the brain to adapt under conditions of stress and changes in biochemistry. Cognitive reserve allows the brain to adapt for a prolonged period of time before showing signs and symptoms of alterations in function.

CEREBRAL BLOOD FLOW AND METABOLISM

The brain receives 750 mL of blood per minute or 15% of the resting cardiac output. Yet the brain makes up only 2% of body weight and accounts for up to one-quarter of the body's oxygen consumption. In addition to a constant rate of blood flow to the brain, local blood flow to specific areas

> *The brain at 2% of body weight requires up to 25% of available oxygen.*

of the brain varies in response to the level of neuronal activity. Increased neuronal activity increases metabolic demand for oxygen and glucose, requiring an increase in blood flow. Brain function is highly dependent on a consistent and considerable supply of oxygen and glucose. Decreased blood flow from any cause that disrupts oxygen or glucose availability quickly leads to brain dysfunction.

The brain's capacity to autoregulate its blood supply in response to metabolic needs is a complex process mediated by intrinsic nerve innervations, neurotransmitter function, and intracerebral and vasculature conditions. Cerebral blood flow is also influenced by blood pressure, cardiac output, pulmonary function, acid-base balance and extracerebral vasculature. Nutrition is critical in maintaining adequate glucose availability.

Age-Related Changes

Older adults are vulnerable to changes in cerebral oxygen, glucose, and blood flow. Any loss in blood flow decreases neuronal function up to 20%. Cerebral blood flow is diminished due to age-related changes, which are not fully understood. The change in flow affects the ability to meet metabolic demands.

BLOOD-BRAIN BARRIER

The blood-brain barrier (BBB) maintains the brain's chemical environment by preventing fluctuations in essential nutrients and protecting neurons from unwanted or toxic substances. The BBB separates the interstitial fluid surrounding neurons from systemic circulation. The barrier is created by a specialized system of capillary endothelial cells that create physical and enzymatic barriers at the interface of blood and brain cells. The interface allows essential nutrients to permeate the BBB. Harmful or toxic substances and large molecules such as proteins and peptides are blocked. Lipid soluble compounds permeate the BBB at varying rates with high lipid compounds transported more quickly. Water-soluble compounds have difficulty crossing the BBB. As a result, the BBB deters the therapeutic effects of many water-soluble drugs. At the same time, the BBB protects the brain from harmful effects of substances. Alcohol, heroin, and some narcotics are fat-soluble and easily cross the BBB.

A second barrier, the blood-cerebrospinal fluid (CSF) barrier, separates the systemic circulation from the CSF. The choroid plexus of the cerebral ventricles secretes CSF and serves as the site of the barrier. Although permeable to more substances than the BBB, the choroid plexus blood-CSF barrier provides a critical role in monitoring CNS homeostasis, neuroendocrine regulation, and preventing CNS infections (Zheng & Choodobski, 2005). Age-related changes in the blood-CSF barrier function may contribute to the development of CNS disorders such as Alzheimer's and Parkinson's disease.

Age-Related Changes

With aging, the increased permeability of both the BBB and the blood-CSF barrier make the aging brain more vulnerable to toxic substances. Age-related changes in blood-brain permeability contribute to the increased sensitivity of older adults to the adverse effects of drugs.

SPINAL CORD

The spinal cord is composed of millions of nerve fibers that transfer data to and from the brain and all body systems. Through 12 cranial and 31 spinal nerves, the spinal cord links the CNS with the PNS. Afferent fibers of the PNS send signals to the spinal cord and brain to direct systems to maintain homeostasis in response to internal and external environmental demands. Efferent fibers transmit messages from the CNS to the PNS, activating organ response.

The spinal column and the vertebral bodies protect the spinal cord. Spinal nerves, or nerve roots, branch from the spinal cord, exit the spinal column through the foramen in the vertebral body, and travel to the rest of the body sending signals to and from the brain. Spinal nerve roots are protected and held secure by the spinal vertebrae.

The reflex arc is a stimulus-response mechanism within the spinal cord that occurs without direct input from the brain. Peripheral sensory stimulation triggers an immediate message to the spinal cord with an immediate response back to the motor neurons eliciting a protective motor response. From the spinal cord, the stimulus is transmitted to the brain and interpreted. By the time the brain registers a cognitive response of "ouch," the motor response has already occurred. The stimulus-response can be understood most readily through the "hot stove" response. A finger touching a hot stove is jerked back before the brain recognizes that "it is hot, it hurts, act now." The action is already completed; the finger is removed from the stove. The cognitive sensation of pain is understood after the finger is removed.

Age-Related Changes

Age-related changes influence the protective function of the spinal column. The bony spinal canal becomes narrow with age, increasing the risk of spinal cord compression. Vertebrae become harder and brittle with increasing age. There is a loss of vertebral cushioning and increasing risk of vertebral collapse with the breaking off of bony fragments. Injured vertebrae compress the spinal cord and spinal nerve roots. Spinal cord or nerve root compression causes decreased sensation, loss in muscle strength, impaired balance, tingling, numbness, and pain. Vertebral degeneration is a major cause of neuropathic pain in older adults.

Transmission speed from periphery to the spinal cord and back is slowed with age.

Age-related changes slow transmission speed from the periphery to the spinal cord and back to the periphery. The reflex arc is slowed by changes in neurotransmitters, myelin sheath changes in the PNS and in the CNS. As a result of age-related neurological changes, older adults are at risk for a greater degree of injury than a younger adult for the same amount of trauma.

Peripheral Nervous System

The autonomic and somatic networks are major divisions of the PNS. The somatosensory system controls motor and sensory pathways, providing information to the brain from the external environment and protecting the brain from sensory overload.

The autonomic nervous system is a self-regulating system composed of the sympathetic and parasympathetic neural networks. Although many functions can be controlled consciously, the autonomic nervous system operates outside of conscious control but is highly responsive to emotional and environmental influences. The parasympathetic system maintains body function during periods of rest and inactivity. The sympathetic system regulates body systems to prepare and respond to perceived potential or actual threat in the classic "fight or flight" response. While the parasympathetic system "slows down" and conserves body functions, the sympathetic system stimulates functions. The parasympathetic and sympathetic nervous systems balance each other in response to internal and external demands, thus promoting homeostasis.

The somatic nervous system controls skeletal muscles, skin, and sensory organs. The system is composed of long neural networks covered with myelin sheaths. Myelin, a lipid-protein substance, covers the nerve cell axon. A white substance responsible for the brain's "white matter," myelin increases electrical resistance to promote conduction speed along the axon. The size of the neural fibers and the amount of myelin sheathing around the fibers determine the speed at which nerve impulses are conducted. Motor, touch, and proprioceptive networks contain large heavily myelinated fibers that rapidly conduct impulses. Pain, temperature, and autonomic fibers are smaller fibers with little or no myelin, resulting in slower conduction. Myelin degenerates with age, causing slowed transmission of nerve impulses.

Age-Related Changes

The parasympathetic nervous system is the predominant regulator of body systems. The sympathetic nervous system responds when internal or external demands increase. With increasing age, parasympathetic stimulation decreases with a subsequent increase in the influence of the sympathetic nervous system. Despite the increase in sympathetic stimulation, the beta receptors for sympathetic neurotransmitters are less responsive. Referred to as age-related autonomic dysfunction or autonomic neuropathy, changes in the autonomic nervous system have major effects on cardiovascular control (see Chapter 9).

With increasing age, parasympathetic control decreases and sympathetic control increases.

SENSORIPERCEPTUAL

Sensory processing involves reception, perception, and response to a stimulus. Reception depends on an intact sensory organ and neural transmission system. Perception is the conscious mental acknowledgment that a sensory stimulus has been received. Response is the cognitive interpretation and motor reaction to the stimulus. Sensory function includes vision, hearing, smell, taste, and touch. Tactile sensation includes vibration, thermal, pain, proprioception, and kinesthesia. Although related to sensory stimuli, proprioception and kinesthesia are distinct. Proprioception is the coordination of sensory data within the CNS in relation to movement and where body parts are in relation to each other. Kinesthesia integrates data to locate where the body is in relation to the external environment. Proprioception and kinesthesia integrate and coordinate signals from the sensory organs such as vision, hearing, stretch receptors, and tactile sensation.

Intact sensory structures and neural mechanisms are needed for sensory processing. For example, hearing involves ear structure as well as the auditory nervous system that transmits signals from the inner ear to the cerebral cortex. The auditory nervous systems discriminates location, strength, type of sound, and, eventually, definition of the sound.

Age-Related Changes

Age-related sensoriperceptual changes are the result of changes in the physical structure of the sensory organ as well as nervous system changes. Structural age-related changes interfere with stimulation of sensory receptors. For example, yellowing and thickening of the lens in the eye prevents light waves from reaching the retina. Damage to hair cells in the inner ear interferes with the ability to detect sound waves. Slowed neural transmission interferes with sensory integration and inaccurate interpretation of information received through nerve stimulation. For example, older adults with delirium have difficulty interpreting sensory input. Sensory misinterpretation causes panic, discomfort, and inaccurate response to the environment.

Disease further impairs sensory function. Diabetes mellitus damages peripheral nerves in the lower extremities and eyes. Cardiovascular disease interrupts blood supply to nerves interfering with neural transmission. Parkinson's disease and Alzheimer's disease impair sensory integration and the ability to screen out or interpret incoming sensory stimuli. Medications can cause ototoxicity while others interfere with sensory integration and interpretation.

Attention to sensoriperceptual age-related changes is critical to maintaining patient safety. Sensorineural changes in vision and hearing interfere with a patient's understanding or interpretation of provider information or with the patient providing misinformation due to misunderstanding questions asked. Changes in proprioception and kinesthesia create a fall safety risk caused by impaired balance and slowed reaction time.

> *Proprioception and kinetic age-related changes increase fall risks.*

Age- and disease-related changes occur slowly in older adults, allowing the older adult to adapt to diminished acuity. Older adults who have assistive devices such as glasses or hearing aids often are unaware that sensory loss has increased and that the devices have not kept pace with functional losses.

PSYCHOMOTOR SPEED

Psychomotor speed is the time necessary for a stimulus to reach the brain and a response to a stimulus. In the elderly, psychomotor speed slows a result of slower axonal conduction by myelinated fibers and loss of excitatory neurons. Aging increases processing time, including the time it takes to receive, interpret, and respond to stimuli. Older adults require more time to process and respond to questions. A decreased ability to screen out unwanted stimuli further increases processing time.

Slowed psychomotor response increases the risk of injury due to slower reaction times. It takes longer for the afferent signal to reach the CNS and for a response to be transmitted to the end organ. For example, incontinence can be the result of slowed signals regarding bladder fullness and the ability to get to the bathroom in time. Decreased receptors causing ineffective signal transmission slow gastric emptying, reduce peristalsis, and slow colonic transit.

SLEEP

Sleep is a required biologic activity. With age, quality and quantity of sleep changes. The normal sleep cycle has four stages divided into two components. The first component is non-rapid eye movement sleep, divided into Stages 1 through 3. The second component is rapid eye movement (REM) sleep. A sleep cycle begins when a person enters Stage 1 sleep and progresses through Stages 2 and 3. At Stage 3, the cycle reverses and sleep progresses back to Stage 2. Upon re-entering Stage 2, the person transitions to REM sleep and completes a sleep cycle. The cycle begins again with completion of REM sleep. Table 12.2 shows progression of the sleep cycle. A complete sleep cycle requires 90 to 110 minutes.

Stage 1 sleep or drowsiness, lasting 5 to 10 minutes, is the onset of sleep. Light sleep is transient and people are easily awakened. The eyes begin to move slowly and muscles begin to relax. Breathing is slow and regular. People awakened during this stage may say they have not slept. Stage 2, true sleep, lasts about 20 minutes. The brain demonstrates rapid, rhythmic brain waves, body temperature drops, and breathing and heart rate slow. There is little eye, muscle, or body movement. Fleeting thoughts and images may occur. Stage 2 sleep is known

TABLE 12.2

Sleep Cycle

Sleep Cycle	Description
Non-rapid eye movement sleep	
• Stage 1	Enters sleep cycle Transition from wakefulness to sleep Light sleep Drifting in and out of sleep Awakens easily
• Stage 2	Slow brain waves Slow muscle activity Body temperature begins to decrease Heart rate slows
• Stage 3	Slow brain waves (delta waves) extending to extremely slow delta waves No muscle activity No eye movement Restorative sleep
• Return to Stage 2	Transition to rapid eye movement sleep
Rapid eye movement (REM)	Breaths increase and become more shallow, irregular Heart rate increases Blood pressure increases Body temperature cools
• Return to Stage 2	New sleep cycle begins

as the transition stage; the transitions to REM sleep occur from Stage 2. Stage 3 is a transition from light to deep sleep. Brain waves slow with bursts of rapid activity in early Stage 3. Stage 3 sleep is known as deep sleep or restorative sleep. Deep slow brain waves, called delta waves, are the hallmark of this sleep stage. There is no eye movement or muscle activity. It is difficult to awaken someone from Stage 3 sleep.

The sleep cycle transitions back through Stage 2 to REM sleep and paradoxical sleep begins. The brain is active but the muscles are inactive. During REM sleep, breathing becomes rapid, shallow, and irregular. Eyes jerk faster and muscles are temporarily paralyzed. Brain waves are similar to those in awake individuals. Heart rate and blood pressure increase. Dreams occur during REM sleep.

A typical sleep period consists of three to five sleep cycles. REM sleep increases in duration as sleep periods lengthen, while sleep in Stage 3 shortens.

Age-Related Changes

With age, sleep patterns change. Shorter, interrupted, unsatisfactory sleep is a problem common in the elderly. Most changes in elder sleep patterns occur because of changes in sleep stages. However, despite age-related changes in sleep patterns, elders require as much sleep, 6 to 8 hours per night, as younger individuals. Insomnia is defined as difficulty falling asleep or maintaining sleep and is not a considered a normal age-related change. Other definitions of insomnia include nonrestorative sleep or a feeling of having not slept. In the general population, up to

Half of older adults suffer from insomnia.

30% of individuals suffer from insomnia. The rate of insomnia increases with age and affects more women than men. Insomnia occurs in over 50% of elders aged 65 and above and in over two-thirds of institutionalized elders.

Disruption in sleep patterns and insomnia are underrecognized and undertreated in the elderly. Lack of sleep and poor sleep quality is particularly problematic in the gerioperative patient. Sleep efficiency diminishes in older adults. Older adults spend less time sleeping when in bed. Inadequate sleep quantity and quality are positively correlated with alterations in immune function, musculoskeletal safety, coping capacity, mood, and cognition.

Circadian rhythm is a cycle of biological, chemical, physiological, and behavioral activity based on a 24-hour period. Circadian rhythms are endogenous to the organism but are governed by environmental cues called zeitgebers. Light is a primary zeitgeber. The regular variations in the environment, such as the alteration of night and day, or light and dark, influence the circadian rhythm and the sleep-wake cycle.

Melatonin is a molecule synthesized and secreted by the pineal gland in response to environmental light. Changes in melatonin secretion signal information to the brain regarding light/dark and day length. Melatonin is virtually nonexistent in the blood during daylight. As the day wanes and there is less light, melatonin is secreted. As days get shorter, darkness signals melatonin release earlier in the day. Melatonin secretion signals nighttime sleepiness and participates in the sleep-wake cycle.

Melatonin synthesis and secretion decreases with age. In addition, optical changes to the lens of the eye such as senile meiosis and increase in lens thickness and opacity decrease the amount of light to the retina. The elderly often leave lights on all night to improve visibility when going to the bathroom at night. In the hospital, assisted living facilities, and long-term care facilities, lights remain on 24 hours a day. Vision changes combined with changes in lighting alter the normal dark-light, day-night cycle as the environment becomes varying shades of gray, alters the circadian rhythm, melatonin secretion, and the sleep cycle.

With increasing age, sleep becomes irregular with early evening sleepiness leading to earlier bedtimes. Elders wake earlier in the morning, between 2 and 4 a.m.

Sleep patterns become irregular, reducing sleep quality and quantity. Changes in sleep patterns include increased time in Stage 1 or light sleep with less time in Stage 3 and REM sleep. Overall, the time spent in restorative sleep is reduced and is responsible for feelings of not having slept or increased fatigue upon awakening. Poor sleep at night increases time spent in unintended daytime napping and loss of energy. Unintended napping is linked with increased cardiovascular events.

Comorbid diseases and medications exacerbate sleep changes in the elderly as well as disease processes that affect patient comfort. The severity of the discomfort affects the degree of sleep pattern change. Similarly, poor quality of sleep can exacerbate chronic health problems.

Causes of insomnia and disrupted sleep patterns are varied and include environmental, physical, medical, pharmacological, emotional, psychosocial, psychological, and functional factors. A positive correlation exists among hours of sleep, quality of sleep, and subsequent health. Inadequate sleep causes fatigue, short tempers, inattention, change in cognitive function, poor physical performance, and reduced sense of well-being and quality of life. Elders often suffer from the effects of the insomnia as well as from side effects of medications prescribed to treat the condition. Psychosocial despair, chronic obstructive pulmonary disease, obstructive sleep apnea, diabetes, dementia, delirium, depression, pain, Parkinson's disease, urinary problems associated with benign prostatic hypertrophy, and incontinence influence the amount and quality of sleep in older adults (see Table 12.3).

TABLE 12.3

Impact of Comorbidity on Sleep

Cormorbid Conditions	Impact on Sleep
Obstructive sleep apnea	
Hypopnea—shallow, slow respiration	Decreased oxygenation
Apnea—complete cessation of respiration	Decreased sleep time
Dementia	Delay in sleep onset Increase in daytime sleepiness Prolonged wake time after arousal from sleep Increase in activity during periods of wakefulness
Chronic pain	Decrease in sleep time Increase in nighttime awakenings Delay in sleep onset
Chronic kidney disease and incontinence	Restless leg syndrome Sleep apnea
Diabetes	Increase in incidence of obstructive sleep apnea Autonomic neuropathy during sleep leading to ventilatory disorders Increase in incidence of sleep-disordered breathing
Chronic obstructive pulmonary disease	Exaggeration of respiratory frequency Reduction in oxygenation Decline in baseline oxygen saturation, more pronounced in rapid eye movement sleep
Parkinson's disease	Decrease in sleep efficiency Decrease in total sleep time Increase in nighttime wakening
Benign prostatic hyperplasia	Increase in frequency of urination leading to increased awakenings
Depression	Insomnia Increase in number of awakenings

INTERVENTIONS

Nonpharmacologic interventions for improved sleep include avoidance of stimulants such as nicotine and caffeine. Alcohol use before bedtime causes changes in sleep patterns. Increasing exposure to natural light and bright light during the day can make the day-night difference more profound improving the sleep cycle. Some medications cause insomnia. A change in dose or administration times may decrease insomnia affects.

Over-the-counter self-medication is common among elders. Antihistamines may be used for sedation but are associated with changes in cognitive function, daytime drowsiness, and anticholinergic effects. Motor impairment and driving skill changes have been noted with diphenhydramine 75 mg available over the counter. Antihistamines should be discouraged in the elderly due to hangover and other side effects.

Melatonin has been shown to have moderate success in treatment of insomnia in the elderly. Taken 2 hours before desired bedtime, melatonin causes drowsiness, quicker onset of sleep, and longer sleep times. Melatonin 1 mg extended release is generally well tolerated by elders. As in many over-the-counter products, there is variability in quality control, and care must be taken in selection of these agents. Doses vary between 0.5 mg to 10 mg depending on the product. Larger doses have not been found to be more effective. The lowest effective dose may be sufficient to induce sleep benefits in elders. Herbal preparations such as valerian, chamomile, and kava-kava are touted as sleep aids in the herbal medicine arena. The side effects of these products in the elderly are not well documented. However, herbal products are known to interact with anesthetic agents. If it is learned that these products are being used, the anesthesia provider must be notified.

There are four basic principles of medication prescription for insomnia: lowest effective dose is all that is necessary, intermittent dosing (every other day), short-term prescribing (not longer than 4 weeks), and gradual medication discontinuation to prevent rebound insomnia. Prescription medications include benzodiazepines (BZDs), BZD receptor agonists, antidepressants, and mood stabilizers. Many of these medications have side effects that are compounded in the elderly.

BZDs are discouraged in the elderly (see Chapter 5, Table 5.2). However, many elderly patients have been on diazepam or other BZDs for many years. Sudden discontinuation of BZDs after long-term administration can result in withdrawal symptoms and seizures. It is important to avoid prescribing BZDs, but it is more important to not discontinue them suddenly when patients have a history of taking them preoperatively. BZDs are well known causes of postoperative delirium, falls, dizziness, and oversedation (see Chapter 5).

BZD receptor agonists known as the "Z" drugs include zolpidem, zaleplon, and eszopiclone. These pharmacologic agents are effective in the elderly in reduced doses and have few side effects. However, recent studies have indicated that changes in cognition and increased fall risk may be side effects.

Antidepressants have been utilized to assist with sleep in the elderly with varying degrees of success. In general, side effects of antidepressants in the elderly have not been well studied. Nontricyclic antidepressants such as trazodone are relatively effective, but produce side effects of daytime sleepiness and dizziness. Paroxetine has been shown to improve sleep in the elderly. Antidepressants can react with agents used during anesthesia, and the anesthesia provider must be made aware of any antidepressant medications.

Mood stabilizers are increasingly being used as sleep promoting agents in older adults. Gabapentin is used in treatment of restless legs and helps sleep by decreasing leg movements and sensations. Topiramate and carbamazepine help with pain control and thus assist with sleep. Side effects are a major concern and need to be carefully monitored.

Clinician recognition of sleep disturbances as a common health problem in the elderly, and the benefits of nonpharmacologic treatment contribute to improving sleep patterns with minimal side effects. Nonpharmacologic interventions can be initiated without a provider order.

COGNITION

Cognitive impairment is among the most devastating diagnoses encountered by the older adult and their significant others. The mind, as the repository of the self, is highly vulnerable to the effects of surgery and anesthesia. Mild cognitive impairment, Alzheimer's disease and vascular dementia, stroke, and Parkinson's disease are the most common preexisting cognitive impairment in the gerioperative patient. Delirium and postoperative cognitive dysfunction are the most common postoperative neurocognitive disruptions (see Chapter 21). Depression is a major preoperative and postoperative event affecting cognitive function.

In consideration of the significant interactive effects of age, disease, surgery, and anesthesia on cognition and personhood of the older adult and the care challenges presented by threats to cognitive function in perioperative care, cognitive changes are discussed in detail in separate chapters. The effect of a stroke on perioperative care of the older adult is discussed in Chapter 9. Depression, mild cognitive impairment, and Alzheimer's and vascular dementia are described as preexisting conditions in Chapter 20. Prevention, early detection, and rapid intervention in care of older adults at risk for delirium and postoperative cognitive dysfunction is discussed in Chapter 21. Care of the older adult with Parkinson's disease is presented in this chapter under gerioperative care.

NEUROPATHIC PAIN

Preexisting neuropathic pain is caused by damage to the CNS, PNS, or injury to nerve fibers themselves. Spinal stenosis and vertebral disc collapse are common sources of preexisting central neuropathic pain in older adults. Preexisting peripheral neuropathic pain can be caused by age-related changes, diabetes, vascular disease, or chemotherapy. Medications used to treat neuropathic pain can interact with preoperative medications and anesthetic agents. Postoperative neuropathic pain is common in patients with limb amputation, breast, thoracic, or abdominal surgery. Direct pressure on nerves caused by poor positioning or inadequate protection of superficial nerves during surgery also results in neuropathic pain.

Gerioperative Care

PREOPERATIVE CONSIDERATIONS

Preoperative assessment requires more time and energy in older adults due to psychomotor and sensoriperceptual age-related neurological changes.

Assessment of neurological changes in the older adult is important in considering preoperative medication management, choice of anesthesia, surgical positioning, and perioperative care. During the preoperative assessment, elders must rely on information processing that involves information registration (input), storage (retention), and retrieval (process input for response) to answer questions and provide data to health care providers. Information registration requires attention to focus on stimuli and process input. Sensoriperceptual changes affect the older patient's ability to pay attention and to register and retrieve information during the preoperative assessment process. Ensuring that information materials are available in large, dark, and easy-to-read fonts improves the review of information and the eliciting of information from the patient. Excessive noise interferes with the ability of older adults to attend, process, and respond. Distracting noise makes it difficult for older adults to retain and retrieve information that requires thought and recall.

Due to the slowed psychomotor response time, the interviewer must allow time for the patient to respond before the next question is considered. More time is needed to conduct a preoperative evaluation with an older adult than with a younger adult. Additional time for the preoperative interview is needed as older adults tend to have longer and more complex histories that must be validated with the medical record review.

HISTORY

A neurological health history begins with a review of current signs and symptoms associated with changes in function. Ask the older adult about current problems with memory;

problem solving, changes in hearing, vision, or touch, or musculoskeletal problems. Ask about specific diagnoses related to neurological dysfunction such as dementia, depression, stroke, seizure disorders, or Parkinson's disease. Neurological changes occur with nonneurologic disease conditions such as diabetes, vascular disease, hypothyroidism, renal disease, spinal stenosis, osteoporosis, or osteoarthritis, especially of the spinal column or vertebral discs. The presence of persistent or neuropathic pain is important when evaluating postoperative pain severity and the need for pain relief intervention. Ask about location, intensity, duration, and characteristics of any persistent pain.

Review recent changes in vision, hearing, taste, smell, or touch. Ask when the most recent vision and hearing evaluations were completed, who conducted the evaluation, and the results. Many older adults with hearing impairment have never had a hearing evaluation. Changes in vision due to cataracts, glaucoma, and macular degeneration occur slowly without the patient recognizing changes in vision. Sensory changes in smell and taste are often ignored as "old age."

Conduct a sleep assessment asking about hours of sleep, number of times that sleep is interrupted at night, sleep routine, daytime napping, and levels of fatigue. Asking about meal times and about type and amount of food and fluid during the evening and immediately before bedtime provides cues to sleep interruptions. Assess medication and herbal remedies used by the patient to help promote sleep and their effectiveness. Inquire as to elder's preference for sleep aid or sleep routine while in the hospital.

MEDICATIONS

Medications used to treat persistent neuropathic pain interact with anesthetic agents, increase bleeding times, and influence blood pressure control. Medication for pain relief must remain constant to keep pain controlled throughout the perioperative continuum. Decisions to terminate or continue pain medications preoperatively should be based on pain severity, effect of drugs on bleeding times, and interacting medications such as prednisone. Information on duration of medication use is needed as well as the name, dose, and scheduling of the medication. Medications such as chemotherapeutic agents, amitriptyline, and cimetidine increase distal sensorimotor peripheral neuropathy. Nonsteroidal anti-inflammatory drugs increase bleeding times.

PHYSICAL EXAMINATION

Physical examination centers on sensoriperceptual integrity, cognitive status, musculoskeletal function, and peripheral neuropathy. Sensoriperceptual integrity evaluates vision and hearing with assistive devices. Glasses and hearing aids will be required during the perioperative period. Attention to spinal vertebral integrity is important in older adults to evaluate spinal disease and identify special attention to intraoperative positioning and protection.

Evaluating spinal integrity is accomplished by asking the patient to bend backward, forward, and to each side. Standing next to the older adult or having a support available is essential to maintain patient safety while carrying out bending procedures. Palpation and tapping of vertebra helps determine spinal integrity. Areas of tenderness require further evaluation including radiographs to assess presence of vertebral fracture, which is common in older adults with osteoporosis. Osteoarthritis causes erosion and breaking off of vertebral cartilage, a common cause of neuropathic pain.

Examine the lower legs for evidence of hair loss, pallor, decreased temperature, and capillary refill. Inspect the feet for evidence of sores and nail changes. Test lower extremities for sensitivity to light touch, pinprick, position sense, and vibration. Ask the patient to stand with the eyes closed to determine stability and balance. Stand next to the patient during the maneuver to ensure patient safety.

INTERVENTION

Maintaining safety is a major issue in patients with neurological changes. Document safety issues related to sensoriperceptual function, sleep (particularly nighttime wakening), orthostatic hypotension, gait, ambulation, and changes in cognition.

Older adults learn more efficiently when they are able to learn and respond at their own pace. Environmental influences, age-related sensoriperceptual changes, and pacing of instruction affect the processing of information. Environmental influences produce negative responses from the elderly because older adults are less comfortable in unfamiliar settings with unfamiliar people. The ability to block out extraneous information and to focus on multiple instructions decreases with age.

Sleep interferes with patient safety by slowing cognitive function and physical reaction time. Loss of sleep impairs immune function. Resolving sleep problems before surgery is important in helping older adults obtain physical and psychological well-being. Bedtime routines, consistent bed and rising times, adequate physical and cognitive exercise during the day, and decreasing psychosocial stress are important elements to improving sleep patterns. Anticipating surgery can be a major source of stress in the gerioperative patient. Providing information, responding to questions, listening actively, and focusing on the patient contribute to allaying perioperative concerns.

PARKINSON'S DISEASE

Older adults with diagnosed Parkinson's disease require additional preoperative evaluation. Parkinson's disease is a degenerative neurological disease characterized by decreased levels of dopamine. Impaired swallowing and difficulty managing saliva predispose the patient with Parkinson's disease to aspiration. Kyphosis, increased rigidity of thoracic muscles, bradykinesia, and uncoordinated movement of chest muscles increase risk of postoperative atelectasis and pneumonia. Evaluating severity of dysphagia and level of difficulty with salivation management provides a risk estimate for postoperative complications. Assessing pulmonary function preoperatively provides a baseline for postoperative comparison. Physical examination focuses on breath sounds, lung excursion, and kyphotic chest changes. Autonomic dysfunction results in orthostatic hypotension. Orthostatic hypotension is also a side effect of the key medication used for Parkinson's disease, levodopa. Gastrointestinal changes associated with Parkinson's disease include constipation and weight loss. Weight loss results from dysphagia, saliva management and loss of appetite from disease, depression, medications, and inactivity. Older adults with Parkinson's disease are frail and at risk for deconditioning.

Urinary tract infections (UTIs) are common in patients with Parkinson's disease. Risk for UTI is due to difficulty initiating urination, resulting in urine stasis. Symptoms are atypical and often not recognized by patients or providers. A urinalysis will rule out UTI with follow-up treatment as needed (see Chapter 10).

Patient safety is a major concern in older adults with Parkinson's disease. Minimizing preoperative and postoperative infections, avoiding drug-drug interactions, preventing falls, and preventing aspiration are among the most serious concerns. Aspiration pneumonia is a major cause of death in older adults with Parkinson's disease.

Pulmonary prehabilitation helps to prevent pneumonia. A swallow evaluation is needed in patients who have not previously had one or if the evaluation is over a year old. Training in swallowing techniques and strategies to manage saliva contribute to safety and nutrition. Encouragement in nutrition using small frequent meals with foods

Pulmonary prehabilitation reduces the increased risk of pneumonia for patients with Parkinson's disease.

that do not increase salivation helps to minimize weight loss. Encouraging activity alternating with rest periods and social interaction in a safe environment with family and friends helps to decrease stress, increase cognition, and improve mood. Exercise is important in maintaining neuromuscular function and conditioning in patients with Parkinson's disease. Preoperative prehabilitation requires collaboration, attentive planning, and ongoing evaluation by the interdisciplinary care team and gerioperative care facilitator.

Medication management is critical in preventing excessive muscle rigidity and autonomic instability. The established medication regimen should be reviewed to determine if any drugs should be discontinued before surgery and to ensure there is a mechanism for restarting drugs after surgery. Levodopa is continued until the morning of surgery and restarted immediately after surgery. Delayed administration of levodopa results in autonomic instability and severe muscle rigidity, increasing the risk of hypoxia due to poor respiratory effort. Tremors increase, resulting in higher levels of postoperative pain. Management of levodopa is carefully evaluated if surgery is expected to extend beyond 6 or 8 hours.

INTRAOPERATIVE CONSIDERATIONS

Neurological monitoring is a major intervention in patients with neurological dysfunction. Depth of anesthesia is important in minimizing risk of postoperative cognitive impairment and in preventing increasing dementia severity in patients with preexisting disease.

Older adults are unable to regulate body temperature due to age-related changes in the autonomic nervous system, skin, and blood vessels. Intraoperative hypothermia predisposes older adults to wound infections and delirium. Antihypertensive, antidepressant, and analgesia medications interfere with thermoregulation. As a result, older adults have inadequate heat production and conservation, with increased heat loss. In general, geriatric patients neither vasoconstrict nor shiver in response to cold until their temperature has fallen to levels below 35.2°C.

Injury to superficial nerves during surgery is a major patient safety issue. Older adults are often placed in awkward positions, depending on type of surgery. Chapter 8 provides an extensive description of surgical positions and patient safety concerns. Postoperative pain increases in severity, depending on surgical position and length of surgery. Older adults with preexisting neuropathic pain, peripheral neuropathy, or preexisting neurological disease are more vulnerable to pain and discomfort from surgical positioning and inadequate or incorrect padding.

Parkinson's Disease

Anesthesia management in older adults with Parkinson's disease centers on avoiding interactions with levodopa. Anesthetic agents have the potential to increase muscle rigidity, produce dysrhythmias, increase hyperkalemia, and cause dystonic reactions depending on the type, amount, and duration of the anesthetic and underlying

Anesthesia management of elders with Parkinson's disease focuses on avoiding levodopa interactions.

physiology of the patient. The ability to respond physiologically to hypovolemia and vasodilation are reduced for patients with Parkinson's disease.

POSTOPERATIVE CONSIDERATIONS

Postoperative care of patients with neurological impairment depends on the type of surgery, preexisting disease, and the level of preoperative function. The most common concerns in the postoperative period are prevention of delirium and postoperative cognitive dysfunction, maintaining hemodynamic stability and homeostasis, maximizing patient function, and paying attention to patient safety.

Patients requiring assistive devices for vision and hearing must have them in place immediately after surgery. Patients' ability to follow instructions depends on being able to hear the instructions, retain the information, and respond as needed. Poor vision can be distracting, interfering with attention and ability to integrate instructions. Impaired proprioception and loss of muscle strength increase the risk of postoperative falls. Loss of smell or taste interferes with nutritional intake.

Sleep is a major issue after surgery. Disrupted sleep is a risk factor for delirium, impairs wound healing, interferes with mobility, and heightens pain severity.

REM sleep is decreased immediately after surgery for the first 24 hours. When combined with poor preoperative sleep patterns, older adults have a high risk for sleep deprivation. REM sleep increases or rebounds by the second to fourth postoperative night. The autonomic variability associated with REM sleep intensifies during rebound sleep, decreasing hypoxic drive, increasing irregular breathing, and exaggerating unstable hemodynamics. Rebound sleep can result in adverse cardiorespiratory events in vulnerable older adults. Opioid medications further disrupt REM sleep and depress respirations. Increased levels of opioids increase dysfunction in sleep pattern and increase hypoxia. Disrupted sleep patterns subsequently intensify pain, requiring use of additional opioids. Focusing on multimodal pain relief methods, sustaining sleep protocols, along with increased oxygen use, minimizes the negative outcomes of REM rebound–opioid interaction.

Environmental factors including noise, lights, care disruptions, stress, and pain interfere with the older person's sleep, both with getting to sleep and staying asleep. Modifying the environment and implementing sleep protocols contribute to helping the gerioperative patient get to sleep and remain asleep.

Pain is a major neurological complication that affects the older adult's ability to participate in postoperative exercises and activities. Providing adequate pain relief is a major responsibility of the interdisciplinary care team. Preexisting neuropathic and persistent pain increase severity of postoperative pain. Caring for older adults with complex pain patterns is challenging and often frustrating. Achieving effective pain relief, while preventing adverse events, depends on astute clinical judgment and a solid understanding of the complex nature of surgical pain in older adults. Chapter 22 offers an extensive overview of pain physiology, pain assessment, and pain relief methods in the gerioperative patient.

Implement a postoperative sleep protocol similar to the one described in Exhibit 12.1. Sleep protocols serve as a general guideline but must be adapted to the surgical care situation, patient's functional status, clinical condition, and perioperative care needs. The protocol in Exhibit 12.1 describes daytime activities, bedtime routine and preparation, and strategies for maintaining sleep while in the hospital. The patient and companion-coach should work with providers to adapt the protocol to the older adult. Sleep quality measured by patient feedback and sleep quantity determine protocol effectiveness. The sleep protocol is adapted after discharge to the patient's needs and care context.

EXHIBIT 12.1 Postoperative Sleep Protocol

Daytime activities
- Establish activity/rest/nap schedule during day.
- Activity to include range of motion, alternating chair-bed routine, walking, chair yoga depending on the older adult's functional status and clinical condition
- Balance rest and activity by alternating being out of bed with bed rest
- Uninterrupted quiet time morning and afternoon or per patient's clinical condition
- Pulmonary hygiene, deep breathing, spirometry

Thirty to sixty minutes before expected sleep time
- Organize nursing care, procedures, dressings, intravenous fluids, medications, urinary drainage, and other interventions to prevent sleep interruption during night.
- Warm drink
- Short slow walk or gentle range of motion
- Bathroom routine: toileting, evening hygiene
- Oral hygiene
- Acetaminophen 500 mg if discomfort or ordered analgesic as needed
- Back rub or nonpharmacologic pain relief method of patient's choice
- Few minutes gentle breathing with relaxation
- Provide soft music of patient's choice
- Integrate home routine or bedtime practices as applicable
- Turn down lights, close door, or make door ajar depending on patient preference and noise levels
- Redo patient preferred elements of sleep protocol if patient wakes during night

Nighttime monitoring
- Establish nighttime monitoring schedule and inform patient
- Maintain monitor alerts as low as possible, balancing safety and noise level
- Have same person familiar with patient conduct nighttime monitoring
- Ensure equipment, furniture, and items needed for patient care are organized and stored safely to prevent injury
- Limit monitoring to that required for patient safety and to meet patient needs

Patients With Parkinson's Disease

Levodopa increases the risk of postoperative orthostatic hypotension, exaggerated fluctuation in blood pressure, hallucinations, and delirium. Parkinson's disease increases the risk for aspiration pneumonia. Drugs to be avoided include phenothiazines (prochlorperazine, promethazine, droperidol) and haloperidol—due to antidopaminergic properties—and meperidine—due to accumulation of metabolites and potential delirium. Postoperative intermittent airway obstruction and laryngospasm increase the risk of respiratory dysfunction in older adults with Parkinson's disease. Fall risk is increased due to muscle weakness, rigidity, and motor fluctuations associated with levodopa. Postoperative ileus is common in patients with Parkinson's disease due to diminished gastrointestinal motility associated with disease processes combined with anesthesia-induced reduction in motility. Prevention of complications rests with vigilant monitoring, intense pulmonary rehabilitation, and early ambulation. Involvement of the interdisciplinary care team improves patient outcomes.

PATIENT REPORT: Ms. Summitt

Ms. Summitt undergoes general anesthesia and an uneventful surgery. She is placed on patient-controlled analgesia of morphine after surgery for pain control. On the second postoperative day, Ms. Summitt expresses her frustration at continuing discomfort and pain. Her morphine is increased and she is placed on acetaminophen, but her pain remains moderate to moderately severe. She states she is too tired to get out of bed and walk and is irritable when disturbed and angry at the nurses and anyone who bothers her to do anything. The nursing assistant says that when sitting in the chair, she sleeps most of the time with occasional jerking movements. When anyone enters the room, she startles and wakens with irritability. She needs strong encouragement to use the incentive spirometer, often refusing to do so, and is sometimes found asleep with the spirometry unit in her hand. One of the nurses suggests that she is overmedicated and the morphine should be reduced or even discontinued. Ms. Summitt becomes very upset and weepy when the nurse informs her about discontinuing her patient-controlled analgesia. The nurse explains that Ms. Summitt is not doing her recovery activities and spending much of her time sleeping. The staff thinks it is due to the morphine. By changing to another medication perhaps she will not be as tired, do more walking, and spend more time out of bed. Ms. Summitt explains she has been having a lot of trouble sleeping at night since surgery. She further explains that she has not been sleeping well for several weeks prior to her surgery due to worrying about her diagnosis. Her friends at the assisted living facility had started to call her "Sleeping Sal" because she fell asleep during the afternoon lectures and while waiting for dinner. Since surgery, she has not slept a wink and cannot understand why those nurses think she was sleeping all the time.

The nurse recognizes that Ms. Summitt has been sleep deprived for several weeks. On reflection and discussion with Ms. Summitt, the nurse further determines that surgery, the hospital environment, postoperative recovery demands, and treatment interruptions such as changing intravenous bags and monitoring checks have compounded the problem. While sharing the observations with Ms. Summitt, the nursing student caring for Ms. Summitt enters the room. Overhearing the discussion, the nursing student comments that anesthesia disrupts sleep and that morphine also interferes with sleep, increasing the problem even further. The nurse, Ms. Summitt, and nursing student review what they have learned. Ms. Summitt has been sleep deprived for several weeks before surgery. Surgery and anesthesia cause sleep disruption. The stress caused by pain, discomfort, being in the hospital, numerous postoperative recovery activities, frequent nighttime interruptions, and continued distress about her diagnosis adds to the sleep loss. Her weepiness, irritation, and lack of participation in postoperative recovery has resulted, to a large degree, from sleep loss. The nursing student states she just read a recent article on sleep interventions. The student asked Ms. Summitt if she was willing to try some of the suggested interventions. Interventions included decreasing the morphine, adding acetaminophen to the pain relief regimen, and using nonpharmacologic interventions. The student asked the nurse about introducing staff and environmental changes. The nursing student further suggested that Ms. Summitt and the nurse develop a schedule of recovery activities, uninterrupted rest periods in bed with the door closed, and soft music. When asked what she thought would help, Ms. Summitt stated in a somewhat embarrassed voice that if someone could bring her the pink elephant pillow from her apartment, she would be able to sleep much better. She added, "if I could just talk to someone about my cancer. No one at the assisted living wanted to hear about it." The nurse suggested a referral to the breast cancer center.

The sleep plan was put into effect, and although she continued to have problems with early morning awakening, Ms. Summitt reported she felt rested, her irritation disappeared, and she became an active participant in her postoperative recovery. Upon discharge, the nurse gave Ms. Summitt a copy of the sleep plan prepared by the nursing student.

SUMMARY

Age-related changes in neuron structure and neurotransmitters increase the older adult's response to anesthesia. Demyelization slows nerve transmission of sensory stimuli and motor responses. The impact on neurological function, especially in cognition, results in a continuum of change from mild to severe dysfunction. Autonomic dysfunction results in delayed responsiveness to stress. Sleep deprivation, underrecognized and undertreated, further impedes the older adult's ability to cope with the stress of surgery and postoperative recovery. Age-related changes in the neurological system slow response rates which, when added to anesthesia effects, increase safety risks. Slowed response rates require nurses to be patient with elders who need more time to process, communicate, and react to interventions designed to improve gerioperative outcomes.

KEY POINTS

- Cognitive reserve allows the brain to adapt for a prolonged period of time before showing signs and symptoms of alterations in function.
- Elders require as much sleep, 6 to 8 hours per night, as younger individuals.
- Sleep deprivation is a risk factor for postoperative complications.
- Sensoriperceptual changes increase safety risks.
- Levodopa is continued until the morning of surgery and restarted immediately after surgery.
- Patients requiring assistive devices for vision and hearing must have them in place immediately after surgery.

THIRTEEN

Musculoskeletal

Raelene V. Shippee-Rice, Jennifer V. Long, and Susan J. Fetzer

PATIENT REPORT: Ms. Augsten

Ms. Augsten is a 75-year-old retired waitress admitted for a laparoscopic cholecystectomy. Due to gallstones in the common bile duct found during the surgery, the laparoscopic surgery was converted to open cholecystectomy. The change in surgical approach will affect her postoperative course.

She lives alone in a second floor condominium. Her medical history includes well-controlled hypertension, gastrointestinal reflux, and moderate osteoarthritis in the right knee, which has increased in severity over the past few months. She is 5′5″ tall, weighs 176 pounds, and considers herself to be in "pretty good health," except for the last few months. Ms. Augsten says she did not want surgery, but her abdominal pain "kept getting worse until I couldn't stand it anymore."

Ms. Augsten describes her preoperative pain from her knee and the stomach pain as moderate when she is taking medication. She spends most of her time playing cards, visiting with friends, and taking her small dog for short walks twice a day. Before her osteoarthritis and stomach pain became so severe, she enjoyed grocery and incidental shopping with her neighbors. Over the past month, the neighbors have helped with grocery shopping and taking the dog for walks. She started using a cane just prior to admission. In addition to her regular medications, she admits to taking acetaminophen and oxycodone 5/325 mg two to three times a day for the past 2 months. The acetaminophen and oxycodone increased to three to four times a day when her stomach pain increased. Ms. Augsten further admits to increasing her alcohol use to one to two glasses of wine or beer a day with her friends in order to take her mind off her pain, "but I never drank with my pain pills." She has been "eating a lot of soups lately because they are easy to fix" and they do not upset her stomach. Her serum albumin at 3.5 g/dL; all other values are within normal limits.

Mobility, the ability to move from place to place or to have purposeful movement of any part of the body, is fundamental to maintaining daily activities and quality of life. Activity limitations increase with advancing age, from 36.8% in elders 65 to 69 years of age to 57% in those over age 85 (Kraus, Stoddard, & Gilmartin, 1996). In the acute care setting, impaired mobility of older adults ranges from 16 to 32% (Brown, Friedkin, & Inouye, 2004). Preserving mobility is critical in preventing the loss of the functional capacity to conduct basic activities of daily living and instrumental activities of daily living. However, impaired mobility remains one of the most misunderstood and least attended functional impairments among hospitalized older adults.

Although as much as one-third of overall strength and endurance can be lost as a result of age-related changes, most healthy older adults continue to climb stairs, rise from a squatting position, and perform the majority of their leisure activities and activities of daily living. Many older adults continue to ski, run, play tennis, and do moderately heavy yard work. Age-related changes in the musculoskeletal system slow the overall pace and level of activity. After surgery, the impact of disease, illness, environmental factors, and nutritional status can be more significant than biologic or chronologic age in influencing the older adult's ability to maintain mobility.

Activity and mobility are critical in the recovery from anesthesia and surgery. Mobility impairment and inactivity in the perioperative period delay recovery and interfere with rehabilitation. Even in healthy older adults, postsurgical immobility quickly progresses to deconditioning. Postoperative deconditioning is a functional decline resulting from inactivity and poor nutrition after surgery. Deconditioning creates a downward spiral as the initial loss of function limits mobility, resulting in further deconditioning. Up to 35 to 45% of older adults will experience a functional decline as a result of hospitalization (Inouye et al., 1993).

Deconditioning leads to anemia, depression, fatigue, poor sleep patterns, and increased pain. Skeletal muscle strength can decrease as much as 1.5 to 2% per day of bed rest (Gillis & McDonald, 2005; Vollmer, 2010). Baecker and colleagues (2003) studied bone resorption in healthy young adult males. Within 24 hours of bed rest, urinary calcium excretion increased; by the second 24 hours, bone resorption markers increased. Table 13.1 lists the effects of deconditioning.

Kortebein and colleagues (2008) studied the effects of bed rest on 11 healthy men and women ranging in age from 60 to 85 years. Results indicated that study participants had a significant loss of muscles strength equal to 10 years of aging after 10 days of bed rest. Lean tissue loss was greater in elders after 10 days than the loss experienced by young individuals after 28 days. In addition, older adults demonstrated a significant decline in protein synthesis despite meeting the recommended daily dietary allowance for protein. Aerobic capacity decreased by 12%. Interestingly, the deconditioning effects lasted beyond the study period with elder subjects, continuing to decrease their physical activity and increase inactivity time. These findings have important implications for teaching older adults and their caregivers about postdischarge physical activity.

Postoperative morbidity and mortality is higher in older adults with deconditioning. In addition to impeding mobility, deconditioning increases incontinence and falls, prolongs hospital stay, contributes to unnecessary discharge to long-term care, increases health care costs, reduces the ability to carry out leisure activities and activities of daily living, causes depression, and diminishes quality of life. Attention to age-related and disease-related changes in the musculoskeletal system can help improve physical conditioning prior to surgery, minimize postoperative deconditioning, maximize postoperative mobility, and decrease fall risk. The musculoskeletal system, composed of muscles, bones, joints, ligaments, and tendons, supports both mobility and activity.

Musculoskeletal Considerations

SKELETAL MUSCLE

The primary function of skeletal muscle, also known as striated muscle, is body movement and power generation. The human body has over 600 muscles that make up 40% of

TABLE 13.1

Acute Deconditioning Effects

System Tissue	Effect
Muscle	• Atrophy • Decreased strength and endurance • Decreased innervation • Decrease protein synthesis
Bone	• Increased rate of bone demineralization • Decreased synovial production • Loss of cartilage water • Cartilage friability • Increase in joint stiffness
Cardiovascular	• Increased heart rate • Decreased plasma volume • Reduced cardiac output • Postural hypotension • Decreased cardiac output • Increased risk venous thromboembolism
Respiratory	• Decrease in lung volume • Loss of respiratory muscle strength • Decreased maximal oxygen consumption
Gastrointestinal	• Decreased bowel function • Constipation • Loss of appetite • Decreased nutritional status
Kidneys	• Decreased fluid volume • Shift in fluid volume • Increase in urinary bladder retention

body mass. The muscles, attached to bones by tendons, help to maintain posture, balance, locomotion, voluntary movement, and activity. Skeletal muscle is made up of striated fibers that contract and relax in response to voluntary control via central and peripheral nervous system stimulation. The strength of skeletal muscle and the ability to power locomotion and movement depend on the size and density of muscle fibers. Skeletal muscles vary in size and number, ranging from extremely tiny, as in the muscle of the middle ear, to huge masses, as in the muscles of the thigh. Muscles contain thousands of muscle fibers wrapped in bundles covered by connective tissue. Muscle fibers increase and maintain their size and density in response to exercise, neurological stimulation, and hormonal influences.

Muscle contraction depends on an intact motor neuron unit composed of neuron, muscle fiber, and acetylcholine, a neurotransmitter released into the myoneural junction. The presence of calcium, sodium, potassium, and magnesium are required to activate a contraction. Contraction of muscle fibers begins with stimulation and transmission of nerve impulses from the central nervous system to the targeted myoneural junction. At the myoneural junction, acetylcholine transfers the nerve signal across the synaptic gap to muscle cells, as shown in Figure 13.1. When stimulated, calcium is released from the muscle cells, triggering a series of events that result in muscle contraction. Muscle contraction ceases when nerve stimulation ceases or when the muscle is too fatigued to respond to stimulation.

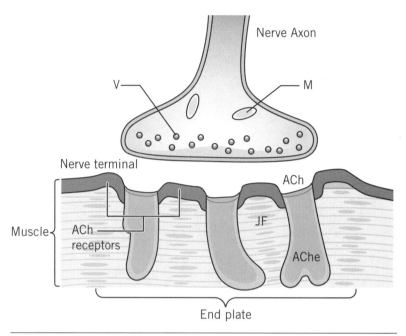

FIGURE 13.1

Myoneural Junction: ACh, acetylcholine; V, vesicle; M, mitochodria

Changes in electrolyte balance or neurotransmitter availability, or decreases in the number of motor neurons, lead to muscle dysfunction or weakness. Loss of motor neuron function results from fewer neurons or fewer muscle fibers per neuron. Electrolyte imbalance results from altered renal function, dehydration, disease, or metabolic disturbances. Increasing age and disease alter neurotransmitter availability. Loss of neurotransmitter such as acetylcholine impairs muscle function. Muscles adapt to meet the level of demand placed on them. Regular exercise increases muscle fiber size and strength, whereas disuse leads to muscle atrophy and weakness. In older adults, inactivity is a major cause of loss of muscle strength.

Age-Related Changes

Table 13.2 lists musculoskeletal age-related and associated functional changes. Aging is marked by senile sarcopenia, defined as a loss of muscle mass. Loss of muscle mass and strength begins slowly in early adulthood, between the ages of 25 and 30. Around 50 years of age, skeletal muscle is lost at a rate of 12 to 14% per decade. By 80 years of age, muscle mass is reduced 30 to 50%, due to loss in size and number of muscle fibers.

Lost muscle fibers are replaced with fibrous tissue and intramuscular fat storage, limiting the availability of functional muscle tissue. Altered hormone levels, particularly decreases in estrogen, testosterone, and growth hormone, further contribute to diminished muscle fiber density and muscle strength. Motor neuron depletion and altered blood circulation in muscles secondary to muscle fiber reduction add to the development of senile sarcopenia.

Although regular exercise and physical activity can maintain and even increase muscle fiber size and muscle mass, the density or number of muscle fibers cannot be regained. Strength performance declines with increasing age, despite maintenance of physical activity levels.

Diminished muscle strength leads to muscle shortening and postural changes. Common postural changes in elders include flexion of the elbow, knee, hip, and spine. Neck flexion,

TABLE 13.2

Age-Related Musculoskeletal and Neuromuscular Changes and Effects

Age-Related Changes in Musculoskeletal and Neuromuscular Function	Musculoskeletal and Neuromuscular Functional Effect
Decrease in number of muscle fibers and size of muscle fibers	• Diminished capacity to carry out activities of daily living and leisure activities • Sarcopenia • Loss of muscle strength and endurance • Women lose more muscle mass < 70 years • Men lose more muscle mass > 80 years
Decrease in bone density	• Increased risk of injury • Increased risk of falls • Increased risk of fall fracture
Increased fat, loss of fibrous tissue in muscles	• Increased risk of injury: fractures, sprains, strains, contractures
Loss of tendon flexibility	• Decreased restorative ability • Reduced flexibility and range of motion • Problems with balance
Decrease in ligament strength, stiffness	• Decrease in work/activity capacity • Increased joint instability • Increased recovery time
Water loss in articular cartilage	• Muscle, joint stiffness • Increase joint pain • Gait changes
Development of adhesions in articular collagen	• Increased pain
Loss of motor neurons	• Loss of muscle contractility
Decrease in neurotransmitter (acetylcholine) availability	• Slowed neurotransmission
Loss of neuronal innervations	• Decline in muscle innervations • Decreased muscle strength • Increased response time
Altered interaction of parathyroid hormone, calcium, vitamin D absorption, and renal function	• Loss of bone density
Changes in growth hormone, testosterone, estrogen levels	• Decreased muscle mass • Loss of bone density • Increased body fat • Skin atrophy
Neural and ligament changes in proprioception	• Alterations in balance and coordination • Increase risk of falls • Gait alterations

combined with an upper curvature of the spine, thrusts the head forward. Figure 13.2 shows the postural changes that commonly occur in older adults. The combined effect of reduced muscle strength, postural changes, and slowed reaction time makes it more difficult to maintain balance or regain balance once lost. Gait changes, including wider stance and shortened step length, are adaptations to retain balance.

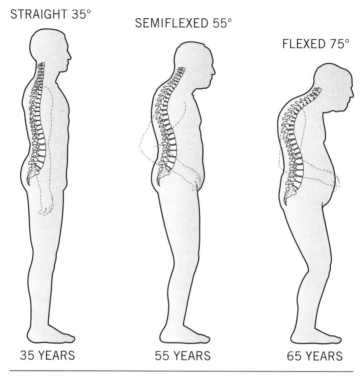

STRAIGHT 35°   SEMIFLEXED 55°   FLEXED 75°

35 YEARS   55 YEARS   65 YEARS

FIGURE 13.2
Postural Changes With Aging

Physical inactivity and poor nutrition exacerbate the rate and extent of muscle loss and strength. Muscle loss contributes to fatigue, weakness, and reduced activity tolerance. Muscle stiffness and contractures occur readily with inactivity. The adage "Use it or lose it" reflects the risk of inactivity in gerioperative patients. Inactivity rapidly escalates the loss of muscle tone and strength in older adults. After surgery, regaining muscle strength and function takes longer and requires significantly more energy for the gerioperative patient than younger surgical patients.

TENDONS, LIGAMENTS, AND ARTICULAR CARTILAGE

Tendons and ligaments are connective tissues that hold the musculoskeletal system together and support the movement of muscles and joints. Articular cartilage, found in joints, is a specialized and compressible connective tissue. Damage to any tendon, ligament, or cartilage can interfere with movement by limiting joint mobility.

Tendons, ligaments, and cartilage are composed of collagen, elastin, and water. Collagen and elastin are proteins that provide stability and flexibility in ligaments and tendons. Elastin assists ligaments and tendons to return to their original shape after stretching. Collagen provides strength and rigidity.

Tendons connect the end of a muscle to a bone. It is through the tendon that muscles exert force, allowing for movement and the ability to maintain posture. Tendons are composed mostly of collagen. The elastic property of tendons allows them to function as springs, providing and releasing tension during ambulation and movement, while collagen increases stiffness that prevents overstretching. Physical and mechanical loading (e.g., walking, running) stimulates the collagen synthesis that helps maintain elastin. Due to decreasing collagen turnover, inactivity markedly decreases the tendon's elastic properties.

Ligaments attach bone to bone and stabilize joints. Ligaments also serve a kinesthetic and proprioceptive sensory function. Monitoring sensory information is key when maintaining joint stability and motor control. Sprains and repeated microtrauma in the ligament can interfere with the sensory processing system, further increasing joint instability and movement. Ligament damage can cause a loss of proprioception and kinesthetic sense in the lower extremities, particularly the knee and foot. As a result, gait and balance are compromised, increasing risk of injury from falls. If an injury occurs, sensory processing may not be fully restored.

Although flexible and stretchable, ligaments are not highly elastic. Ligament elasticity enables a return to resting to its original length after movement or loading but does not allow for significant stretching. Overstretching leads to ligament tearing. Ligaments help hold bones together through stiffness, not through elasticity. Ligaments depend on repetitive loading and limited stretching to maintain tensile strength. Inactivity or immobilization can quickly cause a loss of ligament strength.

Articular cartilage is a specialized hyaline cartilage found between bony surfaces in long bones and between intervertebral discs. The extracellular matrix is composed of collagen, elastin, and proteoglycan gel. The stiff but flexible nature of cartilage allows it to act as the joint's weight-bearing cushion. Water is the major compressive component of cartilage. The proteogylcan gel, made up of carboyhyrate-protein molecules, holds and restores water in the cartilage, which is critical to its cushioning and shock-absorbing function. The proteoglycan gel also maintains nutrient exchange.

Cartilage is composed of water (70–80%), collagen (10–20%), and proteoglycan (5–10%). Cartilage has almost no blood vessels and little nutrient exchange, inhibiting the ability of the cartilage to self-repair. Synovial fluid is a slippery, thick substance with egg-white consistency that covers cartilage in synovial joints. Oxygen and other nutrients diffuse from the synovial fluid into the cartilage. Carbon dioxide and waste products are removed from the cartilage via the synovial fluid. In addition to serving as a transfer station for cartilage, synovial fluid provides the joint with additional lubrication and shock absorption.

Age-Related Changes

The effect of aging on tendons and ligaments in humans is not well documented. The few studies on tendons and ligaments in human aging indicate decreased water absorption in the collagen, causing tendons and ligaments to become rigid and lose elastic recoil. When the tendon loses elastic recoil, the ability to transmit forces from muscle contraction to the bone is impaired. The inability to move and recover quickly after tripping or losing balance increases the potential for falls.

Ligaments lose stiffness, strength, and elasticity with advancing age. As a result, the joint loses range of motion, increases laxity, and decreases stability. Laxity increases the risk of falling and injury from strains and sprains. Additionally, loose ligaments in the knee and ankle interfere with proprioception, further contributing to the potential for falling.

Articular cartilage loses cushioning and shock-absorbing capacity. Collagen makes up almost two-thirds of cartilage. With aging, the amount of collagen does not change, but the collagen and elastin in the cartilage become stiffer and less absorbent. The amount of water in the cartilage decreases, causing the collagen to become brittle. Microfractures roughen the cartilage surface. Production of synovial fluid decreases with age, interrupting oxygen and nutrient supplies to the cartilage and contributing further to deterioration.

As cartilage deteriorates, it loses the ability to cushion and absorb shock. Friction between the bones of the joint increases, and movement becomes increasingly painful. Decreased chest compliance caused by stiffening in costovertebral joints, changes in intercostal cartilage, and development of kyphoscoliosis impedes lung expansion and inspiratory volume.

DEGENERATIVE OSTEOARTHRITIS

Osteoarthritis is degeneration of synovial cartilage that results in pain and limited motion in the affected joint. Primary osteoarthritis is idiopathic in that there is no known cause of the tissue degeneration. Secondary arthritis results from trauma or disease to the joint tissues. The distinction between primary and secondary conditions is somewhat arbitrary, as weight bearing is a form of trauma that causes wear and tear on the joint. Degeneration in intervertebral cartilage can damage nerve roots and neuropathic pain due to collapse of vertebral discs.

In the gerioperative patient, osteoarthrisits is the most common cause of preexisting pain and can severely limit prehabilitation activities and mobility after surgery. While almost all older adults have evidence of cartilage degeneration on x-ray, not all older adults with degenerative disease have symptoms.

Osteoarthritis has long been considered a normal consequence of aging. Recent evidence suggests that inflammatory mechanisms trigger cartilage degeneration in addition to age-related changes. When osteoarthritis is considered "normal aging," patients and providers have diminished sensitivity to the seriousness of the condition on pain severity, functional ability, and quality of life. In older adults, osteoarthritis is a major cause of mobility impairment, functional loss, and deconditioning.

Hands, feet, spine, and large weight-bearing joints, such as the hips and knees, are the most common sites for osteoarthritic changes. Osteoarthritis of the knee is the most common symptom of osteoarthritis, occurring in approximately 34% of adults over age 65. The incidence of osteoarthritis increases with age.

Figure 13.3 shows osteoarthritic changes in the knee joint and cartilage. Osteophytes or bone spurs can develop within the joint and cause localized inflammation and pain. Pain severity and joint impairment caused by increased bone friction or joint inflammation can range from mild pain with minimal functional impairment to severe, incapacitating pain and immobility.

Pain and loss of cushioning by the cartilage alters gait patterns. Changes in gait alter joint alignment, which further contributes to cartilage erosion, exacerbating pain and limitations in joint movement. Ligaments and tendons lose elasticity and stiffness, causing the joint to become unstable. A downward spiral of cartilage deterioration, joint misalignment, and joint instability leads to increasing pain and disability, beginning a reconditioning cascade. Limited activity from pain and joint instability results in loss of muscle strength and restricted ligament and tendon function. The loss of ligament and tendon elasticity and stiffness leads to joint stiffening, further restricting movement. Interrupting the deconditioning cascade can preserve function and improve quality of life. Exercise, nutrition, and physical therapy can prevent reconditioning.

BONY SKELETON

The skeletal system serves as the structure for the body and provides protection for internal organs. Availability of calcium, phosphorous, and vitamin D, needed to maintain bone

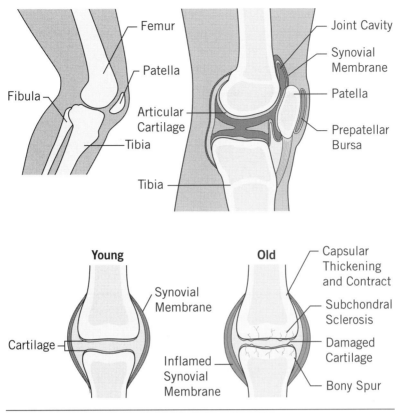

FIGURE 13.3
Osteoarthritic Changes in the Knee

density and strength, is controlled by parathyroid hormone (PTH), intestinal absorption, and renal function. Continuous bone remodeling prevents osteoporosis, a major factor contributing to postoperative patient falls.

Bone is composed of osteoclasts, osteoblasts, osteocytes, and an extracellular matrix made up of collagen. and makes up approximately 12 to 15% of body weight. The greatest increase in bone strength occurs during teenage years. Bone strength peaks around age 30, after which bones slowly start to lose density. Bone density is affected by numerous factors: age, sex, heredity, nutrition, level of physical activity, and medications.

Bone remodeling is a normal process that adds and removes bone throughout the life span. Remodeling removes old bone through a process of resorption by the osteoclasts, and new bone is created through an ossification process by osteoblasts. Bone resorption can be completed in 10 to 13 days. Bone formation takes much longer, up to 3 months.

Bone remodeling is necessary for ongoing and episodic bone repair. Bone homeostasis, the ratio of bone resorption to bone formation, helps maintain adequate levels of serum calcium. Calcium is essential to neurotransmission function, in addition to maintaining bone density and strength.

Calcium, PTH, and vitamin D interact to regulate the amount of calcium stored and released from bone to maintain serum calcium levels. Figure 13.4 shows the complex relationship that regulates bone remodeling. When serum calcium is low, PTH levels increase. The release of PTH stimulates bone calcium release, increases reabsorption of calcium by the kidney, and increases calcium absorption from the intestine. Vitamin D is needed for the

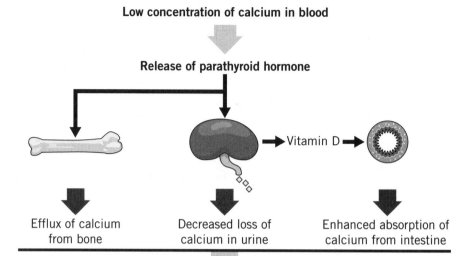

FIGURE 13.4

Low Calcium, Parathyroid Hormone, and Vitamin D

Used with permission of Richard Bowen. http://www.vivo.colostate.edu/hbooks/pathphys/endocrine/thyroid/pth.html. Downloaded March 21, 2011.

intestinal absorption of calcium and is converted to an active form by the kidney under PTH stimulation. Chapter 18 provides a more complete description of PTH.

Age-Related Changes

Bone remodeling slows with increasing age. In women, bone resorption with loss of calcium, phosphorous, and other minerals begins to outpace bone formation, leading to bone demineralization at around age 30. The resulting demineralization leads to diminished bone density and strength. During menopause, the ratio of bone resorption to bone formation increases at a rate between 3% and 7% per year, tapering to 1 to 2% per year after menopause. Men lose bone at a rate of 1 to 2% beginning around age 70.

PTH levels increase with advancing age, causing bone demineralization. Vitamin D is low in older adults due to inadequate intake and age-related changes in renal function lowering the rate of vitamin D conversion to an active form. Changes in any of three critical elements of bone mineralization PTH, calcium, or vitamin D can trigger a cascade of events. Table 13.3 presents an overview of age related changes in PTH, calcium, and vitamin D.

Estrogen

The presence of estrogen slows bone resorption to maintain bone strength. When estrogen production decreases with aging, bone resorption increases, causing bone demineralization and decreased bone density. Women experience the greatest bone loss in the first 10 years after menopause. Although the rate of loss slows in late menopause, bone demineralization continues. Men lose bone at a rate similar to that of late menopausal women, beginning around age 70. The early stage of bone demineralization is called osteopenia. More advanced bone demineralization results in osteoporosis.

TABLE 13.3

Age-Related Changes in Parathyroid Hormone, Calcium, and Vitamin D

- Increased parathyroid secretion
- Low serum calcium in response to:
  - Age-related renal changes decreasing calcium reabsorption and Vitamin D activation
  - Age-related gastrointestinal changes decreasing Vitamin D absorption
  - Decreased calcium intake
- Vitamin D availability secondary to
  - Low vitamin D dietary intake
  - Inability to absorb Vitamin D from intestine
  - Age-related changes in skin
  - Use of antacids interfering with Vitamin D absorption
  - Decreased sun exposure

Osteoporosis

Osteoporosis is a systemic, progressive skeletal disease characterized by severe loss of bone mass and deterioration of bone tissue. Osteoporosis can cause debilitating pain and immobility. Bone fragility from bone deterioration can be so severe in the gerioperative patient that changing positions or coughing causes spontaneous fractures.

Intrinsic causes of osteoporosis include estrogen depletion and age-related changes in the calcium absorption. Lifestyle habits, environmental influences, and medications are contributing extrinsic factors.

Disuse, or deconditioning osteoporosis, results from inadequate weight bearing resulting from inactivity or lack of exercise. Direct weight bearing (e.g., walking) stresses bone and creates muscle tension that pulls against bones, stimulating calcium retention and promoting bone formation. Bone demineralization results when inactivity and immobility decrease direct weight bearing and muscle force.

Gerioperative patients experience disuse osteoporosis due to low levels of preoperative activity and mobility. Postoperatively, pain and energy depletion make it difficult for older patients to do weight-bearing activities such as standing and walking.

Long-term use of glucocorticoids, proton pump inhibitors, and H_2 receptor antagonists can lead to induced osteoporosis or exacerbate bone demineralization in patients with preexisting osteoporosis. Glucocorticoid-induced osteoporosis is caused by an inhibition of calcium absorption and slowed estrogen production. The action of proton pump inhibitors and H_2 receptor antagonists decreases calcium absorption. Some chemotherapeutic agents and antiepileptic medications also interfere with calcium metabolism, causing osteoporosis.

Osteoporotic changes create a safety risk by impeding mobility and activity, increasing risk of falling, and increasing risk of spontaneous or traumatic fractures. Safety concerns in older adults are based on age-related changes in strength and endurance, flexibility, balance, and gait.

STRENGTH AND ENDURANCE

ss of muscle strength and disuse :reases risk of deconditioning.

Muscle fibers are classified as type I endurance (slow twitch fibers) or type II strength and speed (fast twitch fibers). With age, there is a greater loss of type II fibers, resulting in decreased muscle mass, while the number of type I fibers remain relatively stable.

Muscle changes affect strength and power more than endurance. Muscle strength and power decline as muscle mass declines. Muscle power also is reduced through loss of tendon function. With age, fat deposits and fibrous tissue begin to replace muscle fibers, decreasing muscle mass. Muscle fiber endurance, the ability to sustain action, is influenced more by impaired oxygenation due to alterations in cardiovascular and pulmonary function than by age-related changes in muscle.

Changes in thoracic muscles and skeletal structures contribute to pulmonary complications. Reduced muscle endurance causes a loss in pulmonary capacity. Coughing is impaired due to weakness of the intercostal muscles, making it difficult to clear airways.

FLEXIBILITY

Joint stiffness inhibits joint flexibility and decreases range of motion. The decrease in range of motion occurs so slowly that the older adult may not be aware of the loss. Joint stiffness in ankles, knees, neck, and spine causes changes in gait and balance, increasing the risk of falling. Joint stiffness also causes joint pain and discomfort. Physical inactivity and immobility further increase joint stiffness. Stretching, massage, range of motion, and postural awareness help maintain joint flexibility and gait stability. Attention to stretching exercises is essential for maintaining the flexibility needed for safety and balance.

BALANCE

Maintaining balance requires integrating visual, vestibular, and proprioceptive sensory processes with musculoskeletal flexibility. Without integration, balance is disrupted when changing position, turning, reaching, or going up and down stairs. Distractions in the external environment and inattention can cause imbalance by interrupting sensory input and processing. Atrophic changes in cartilage, muscle, ligaments, tendons, and neurotransmission slow reaction time, making it more difficult to recover once balance is lost.

GAIT

Walking integrates muscle and tendon action guided by sensoriperceptual coordination. In healthy older adults, walking is accomplished without conscious thought or awareness. As people age, walking becomes more difficult due to muscle weakness, stiffening of ligaments and tendons, loss of motor neurons, and decreased proprioception. To compensate for these physiological alterations, gait patterns change. Gaits in older adults rely on a wide base of support, small steps, short strides, slowed ambulation velocity, minimal ankle motion, and decreased arm swing. The altered gait pattern helps to prevent falling and minimize energy expenditure.

The rate of change in musculoskeletal structures and the effects on strength, balance, and flexibility are unpredictable. Many older adults retain high levels of musculoskeletal function and remain physically active. Others of the same age find it difficult to meet basic activities of daily living without assistance. Surgery can precipitate sudden changes in musculoskeletal function, creating challenges for postoperative recovery. Musculoskeletal changes and mobility impairment create risk factors contributing to decreased patient safety, deconditioning, and postoperative pulmonary and cardiovascular complications. Diligent nursing care, systematic monitoring, and early intervention must be consistently applied to maximize the patient's preoperative and postoperative function, as well as to ensure patient readiness for discharge.

Gerioperative Care

PREOPERATIVE CONSIDERATIONS

Evaluating the musculoskeletal system before surgery helps to develop a picture of the potential impact that activity and mobility strengths and limitations will have on the older adult's postoperative functional capacity. Musculoskeletal assessment involves compiling a history of musculoskeletal illness and injury, conducting a focused physical examination of mobility and activity levels, identifying patient safety and complication risk factors, and reviewing results of diagnostic testing.

HISTORY

The musculoskeletal history asks the patient to describe current and past musculoskeletal disease and disability. An important aspect of the history is the affect of any disease or disability on the patient's functional capacity and quality of life. The history focuses on the presence, site, severity of current joint and muscle pain and tenderness, muscle paralysis or paresis, muscle spasms or cramping, limitations in joint movement, and level of sensation in lower legs and feet. A detailed assessment of pain, tenderness, and muscle spasms will include location, cause, duration, length of time the patient has had symptoms, triggers, and alleviating or aggravating factors.

Identifying and documenting limitations in physical function provides a baseline for postoperative evaluation of the patient's physical function and ability to ambulate postoperatively. Knowing the source of musculoskeletal impairment, pain, or disability helps in identifying primary and secondary interventions. A musculoskeletal history includes the information needed for conducting a fall risk assessment.

MEDICATION HISTORY

Medications used to treat musculoskeletal discomfort can influence the type and amount of anesthesia and the analgesics for postoperative pain relief. It is not unusual for older adults to have multiple physicians or providers. Potentially inappropriate medications (PIMs) are medications that should be avoided in older patients, require dose modifications, or need a cautionary note (Fick, Cooper, Wade, Waller, Maclean, & Beers, 2003). Many muscle relaxants and analgesics are designated as PIMs due to their anticholinergic effects. Anticholinergics increase discomfort due to dry mouth, increase urinary retention, and increase risk of falls. Dry mouth after surgery is a major complaint, and it is most often caused by anticholinergic medications used during surgery to increase muscle relaxation. The medication history should be carefully evaluated for PIM use (see Chapter 5).

A sensitive issue for many patients is the use of prescribed and self-initiated medications. Medication information includes patient's knowledge of the name, dose, schedule, route of administration, and the purpose of the medication or the reason for taking it. Medication history includes prescribed and over-the-counter medications, as well as herbal or medicinal teas the patient drinks. Medicinal teas used in many cultures to treat musculoskeletal pain and discomfort often contain ingredients that negatively interact with anesthesia and allopathic medications. Patients also should be asked the names of any herbs, roots, leaves, or plants they use for self-treatment.

Patients with severe persistent pain often use illegal substances and alcohol to cope. Being aware of the amount, frequency, duration of use, and type of substances patients use is important for safe management of anesthesia and postoperative analgesia. Assessing the therapeutic/risk ratio of analgesics used to treat musculoskeletal pain is important for determining whether use should be continued before, during, and after the surgical procedure. Ask how long the older adult has been taking analgesics and if any analgesia was recently discontinued. Some analgesics used to treat musculoskeletal pain, such as nonsteroidal anti-inflammatory drugs (NSAIDs), can prolong bleeding and alter equianalgesic dosing for postoperative pain relief.

Older adults are often hesitant to share information about the use of opioids, illegal drugs, alcohol, or herbal remedies obtained from unlicensed or natural doctors. The person obtaining the patient's history must establish a trust and rapport that makes gerioperative patients comfortable in sharing this information. One approach is to reinforce that information about all medications and substances used to treat pain is important, but it is especially important to know about non-prescription drugs.

NSAIDs have been a mainstay for treating arthritis-related pain and inflammation. The American Geriatrics Society recommends that prescription opiates replace NSAIDs in order to avoid proton pump inhibitors and H_2 receptor antagonists used to minimize the risk of gastrointestinal bleeding. However, older adults who have taken NSAIDs and found them effective may prefer to remain on a familiar drug and continue to take medications to decrease gastrointestinal side effects. Ask the patient about the use of NSAIDs, proton pump inhibitors, and H_2 receptor antagonists. Long-term use of proton pump inhibitors can lead to osteoporosis and risk of fractures. Documenting the length of time the patient has been taking proton pump inhibitors or H_2 antagonists alerts providers to the potential for osteoporosis and fall safety risk.

Sedatives, hypnotics, antidepressants, and benzodiazepines, commonly prescribed for older adults, are associated with increase in fall rates. The use of any of these medications creates a patient safety alert due to the potential for increased fall risk.

SOCIAL SUPPORT

Older adults with musculoskeletal limitations often need adaptive equipment to manage home and community environmental barriers. Depending on the surgical procedure, patients may need to begin using adaptive equipment after surgery. Asking the patient to demonstrate the use of adaptive devices provides information about safety and fall risk.

Obtaining information about the level of social support and safety of the home environment helps to make advance plans for postdischarge care that will promote recovery and prevent hospital readmission. Patients and family members should receive written and verbal information and demonstrations on environmental and patient safety. Having this information helps the family to consider the need for modifications that help ensure home safety before the patient returns home.

PHYSICAL EXAMINATION

Assessing the musculoskeletal system begins as soon as the patient enters the room, through observation of the patient's posture, gait, balance, symmetry, and coordination. The screening musculoskeletal examination includes tests of muscle strength; palpation of joints, muscles, and bony areas; evaluating joint range of motion; and testing of proprioception, flexibility, balance, and gait. Exhibit 13.1 provides an outline for musculoskeletal assessment for the gerioperative patient.

EXHIBIT 13.1 **Preoperative Musculoskeletal Assessment**

- Mobility: gait, balance
- Pain level, joint palpation
- Range of motion: upper and lower extremities including wrist and ankle
- Range of motion: cervical and thoracic spine
- Muscle strength: hand grip, leg, arm
- Getting in and out of a chair
- Ability to carry out activities of daily living, areas of impairment
- Self-reported fatigue or decreased energy level

Severe joint pain or pain with movement, history of immobility and inactivity levels, and onset of new musculoskeletal pain or impairment unrelated to the surgery requires a focused evaluation. Older adults are apt to dismiss aching muscles, sore and inflamed joints, and restricted mobility as signs of "old age." A careful physical examination can identify new or emerging mobility problems or disease.

Range of Motion

Older adults demonstrate reduced flexibility and range of motion. These changes occur slowly over an extended period of time, allowing the older adult to adapt and continue with everyday activities. Older adults may be unaware of changes in their range of motion until attempts to complete an activity are unsuccessful. Assessment of range of motion asks the patient to bend, extend, and abduct and adduct their arms, legs, shoulders, hips, wrists, and ankles. Extending, flexing, and tilting the head evaluates neck flexibility, which is important for endotracheal intubation during anesthesia induction.

Proprioceptionn, Gait, and Balance

Balance is maintained through sensory organization of proprioception, vision, and vestibular function. Proprioception compensates when there is a loss of vision or vestibular function, allowing the older adult to maintain posture and remain standing. Ligaments in the hands, knees, and feet have been found to have sensory nerve endings that facilitate proprioception in response to ligament stretching and position. Age-related changes in knee ligaments interfere with upright proprioception.

Sensory receptors on the plantar surface of the foot and in the joints of the ankle help to maintain position awareness and perception. Peripheral neuropathy disrupts proprioception in the feet and ankle by altering sensorineural receptor function and neuroconduction. Cardiovascular disease, diabetic neuropathy, and age-related changes, often called idiopathic neuropathy, are the most common causes. Older adults with peripheral neuropathy who have not been diagnosed are often unaware they have lost sensation in the feet and ankles.

Among community dwelling elders, over one-quarter of 65- to 74-year-olds and over one-half of those over 85 years with diminished sensation will not have a diagnosis to explain the sensory loss. Peripheral neuropathy is a contributing factor in gait and balance disruption and should be assessed whenever a patient shows evidence of altered gait or balance.

Gait and balance can be reliably assessed with the "timed up and go" (TUG) tool (Podsiadso & Richardson, 1991). The TUG assesses overall gait and balance patterns.

Documenting TUG findings preoperatively provides a baseline for postoperative comparison and evaluation of changes in a patient's functional status. Assessing and documenting preoperative gait and balance is needed to develop a safe postoperative ambulation plan that optimizes patient mobility and function.

To conduct the TUG, the patient is asked to get up from a chair without using the armchair or other support, unless the need for assistive devices has been previously established. The patient walks 10 feet, turns around, walks back to the chair, and resumes a seated position. The examiner walks beside the older adult to ensure safety.

Observe the patient for ease with initiating movement, length of stride, width of stance, degree of arm swing, posture, and movement coordination. Alterations in gait are associated with an increased risk of falls. Older adults with no mobility impairment are able to complete the TUG in 19 seconds or less, with many completing the test in less than 10 seconds. Taking 13 seconds or longer is associated with increased fall risk, with a predictive ability of 90% in community dwelling older adults (Shumway-Cook, Baldwin, Polissar, & Gruber, 1997). General guidelines suggest that longer than 20 seconds indicates moderate mobility impairment, while more than 30 seconds indicates mobility dependency. Test results of more than 20 seconds should be flagged in the medical record as a safety alert. Older patients requiring more than 30 seconds should have an interdisciplinary musculoskeletal assessment. Standardized scores to determine fall risk using the TUG test on postoperative older adults have not been established.

Muscle Strength

Evaluate muscle strength using a scale of 0 to 5 with 0 unable to move and 5 indicating adequate strength. Documentation includes the level of bilateral symmetry in muscle strength. Lower extremity muscle strength is important when considering ambulation and mobility levels. Upper muscle strength is needed for using crutches, walkers, and getting out of bed.

ASSESSING FALL RISK

Instituting a fall risk assessment is important in evaluating patient safety. Gerioperative fall risk factors can be divided into three categories: patient, iatrogenic, and environmental concerns. Patient-related factors include advanced age, age-related physical and physiologic changes, use of assistive devices, toileting frequency, and comorbid illness. Iatrogenic factors include surgery, anesthesia, medication, and postoperative therapies, such as intravenous equipment, catheters, and drains. Sensory overload, unfamiliar environment, toileting facilities, and space layout constitute environmental factors. Staffing and availability of safety resources are additional system concerns. Exhibit 13.2 identifies common patient, iatrogenic, and environmental risk factors to assess prior to ambulation. The risk of a fall is in older adults living in the community who have no risk factor or a single risk factor is estimated at 27%. The risk increases to 78% when there are four or more risk factors identified (Tinetti, Doucette, & Claus, 1995).

Fall risk assessments should be completed routinely at strategic points throughout the perioperative continuum: preoperative assessment, admission to the surgical facility, postoperatively, predischarge, and postdischarge. Falls in the hospital have been linked with increased falls in older adults postdischarge. Fall risk should also be evaluated when there is a change in the patient's clinical condition that increases the number or severity in fall risk factors. Assessment tools used to evaluate fall risk should be targeted to the individual clinical situation. The Hendrich Fall Risk II scale (Hendrich, Bender, & Nyhuis, 2003) was designed specifically for use in the acute care setting. The scale has been labeled robust with

EXHIBIT 13.2 **Gerioperative Fall Risk Factors: Ambulation Considerations**

Intrinsic factors:
  Use of sensory assistive devices
  Cognitive function, alertness
  Attention span
  Comorbid illness (e.g., peripheral neuropathy, osteoarthritis)
  Standing balance, muscle strength
  Gait
  Need for mobility aids
  Safe foot wear
  Peripheral edema
Iatrogenic factors:
  Type of surgery
  Anesthesia effects
  Pain relief effectiveness
  Medication effects (e.g., time since diuretic, opioid analgesic administration)
  Dehydration, postural hypotension
  Toileting for incontinence or urgency
  Anabolism, catabolism
  Muscle strength
  Fatigue and energy level
Environmental factors:
  Medical tubes and tethers, equipment
  Equipment arrangement
  Furniture arrangement
  Noise and light levels
  Floor conditions
  Distractions
  Staffing Patterns
  Availability of safety resources

75% positive predictive value (Currie, 2008). A fall protocol that includes the Hendrich II Fall Risk is available in Appendix I.

PREOPERATIVE TESTING

Routine preoperative testing in older adults is based on disease history and clinical indicators, with additional tests recommended for specific surgeries or clinical conditions. Prothrombin time and activated partial thromboplastin time are required for patients with a history of liver disease, alcoholism, bleeding tendencies, or who are receiving medications that increase coagulation or bleeding time such as warfarin, aspirin, and NSAIDs. Patients having orthopedic surgery should have a preoperative sedimentation rate and C reactive protein. Sedimentation rate and C reactive protein determine active systemic inflammation that can cause prosthetic failure in total joint replacements.

Urine Culture

Monitoring urine culture results is critical in older adults having joint replacement surgery, as urinary infection can lead to prosthetic joint infection. Laboratory results must be reviewed before the surgical procedure. The presence of nitrates or leukocyte esterase is a positive indicator of a urinary tract infection. The surgeon should be notified immediately if nitrates or leukocyte esterase are found in the urine sample.

Imaging Studies

A bone mineral density scan is not routine for preoperative care. However, the patient should be asked when the last bone mineral density scan was done. The results should be reviewed to determine presence and level of osteoporosis and to evaluate fracture risk. In high-risk patients, bone fracture can occur spontaneously during movement or intraoperative positioning.

Radiology

Gerioperative patients with undetermined bone pain, previous osteoporotic fracture, or strong family history of osteoporotic fractures should be considered for x-rays. Osteoporotic bone changes can be detected when 25% of bone is lost, a level consistent with risk of bone fracture.

In a retrospective review of chest x-rays from 500 older adults who had a chest x-ray in an emergency department, results indicated that 16% had an osteoporotic vertebral fracture (Majumdar et al., 2005). Only 60% of the found fractures were reported. Of the patients with fractures, only 25% had received a diagnosis of osteoporosis. Evidence of current or past fracture is highly correlated with risk for future fracture. Gerioperative patients who have had a recent x-rays should be reviewed for evidence of vertebral fracture, especially if the patient complains of back pain or reduced flexibility.

DOCUMENTATION

Documenting findings related to patient safety, pain, and comfort enable the interdisciplinary care team to take precautions that will prevent injury, promote comfort, ensure safety, and improve care quality. Documentation is important for intraoperative care and patient safety. Documentation includes history of osteoarthritis, osteoporosis, and previous osteoporotic fracture; range-of-motion limitations; joint pain and discomfort; and muscle paresis or paralysis. Length of use and dose of opioids and adjuvant medications should be highlighted.

Postoperative alerts include mobility limitations, gait or balance impairment, use of assistive devices, and analgesic medications. Establishing an alert system that notifies providers in the next stage of the continuum about special needs or potential problems the gerioperative patient may encounter due to preexisting condition provides an immediate safety net. An alert system prompts prevention and focused monitoring when coached by the preoperative team through documentation and highlighted cues.

PREOPERATIVE INTERVENTION

Prehabilitation: A Primary Intervention

Physical prehabilitation is designed to improve functional capacity before surgery, prevent postoperative loss of functional ability, and increase the rate of postoperative recovery. Positive postoperative outcomes associated with physical prehabilitation include increased muscle strength, decreased complications, diminished pain, increased patient satisfaction, and reduced length of inpatient rehabilitation after perioperative discharge. Physical prehabilitation has been found effective with patients undergoing colon

Preoperative walking is a highly effective intervention for decreasing postoperative complications.

surgery, knee arthroplasty, orthopedic surgery, hip arthroplasty, and spinal surgery (Carli & Zavorsky, 2005; Carli, Charlebois, Stein, Feldman, Zavorsky, & Kim, 2010; Ditmyer, Topp, & Pfier, 2002; Nielsen, Jorgensen, Dahl, Pedersen, & Tonnesen, 2010; Rooks et al., 2006; Topp, Ditmyer, King, Doherty, & Hornyak, 2002).

Activities that can prevent unnecessary muscle atrophy are central to the coaching of older patients on how to prepare for postoperative recovery demands. Prehabilitation promotes maximum musculoskeletal function through conditioning exercises and diet. Prehabilitation programs incorporate strength training, flexibility training, and range of motion. However, it is important to keep the older person's needs and functional ability at the center of the prehabilitation program. Conducting a patient review with the interdisciplinary care team identifies specific therapeutic exercises and activities and prevents the development of a program that may be too taxing. Exercises should be designed at the level of the abilities and limits of the individual patient and directed to the type of surgery. Walking is one of the most effective muscle strengthening activities for older adults.

A prehabilitation protocol is based on individualized goals congruent with the older adult's clinical and physical condition and functional limitations. The individualized protocol uses a written exercise prescription with goals established in collaboration with the patient. Prior to initiating the prehabilitation program, all exercises and activities should be carefully reviewed and demonstrated to the older adult with a reverse demonstration or "repeat-back" by the patient and, if available, a companion-coach or family member. Encouraging the patient to keep a daily log of the prehabilitation activities and personal response to them is strongly recommended. The daily log helps to maintain motivation by showing evidence of the patient's progress.

Although prehabilitation programs can benefit any older adult preoperatively, not all older adults are candidates for extensive prehabilitation. The presence of risk factors and the possibility of adverse effects reinforce the need to stage the exercises and activities to the ability and clinical status of the individual. Frail older adults with severe limited mobility can benefit from passive range of motion with active range of motion and activities targeted to their level of function and ability.

INTRAOPERATIVE CONSIDERATIONS

Poor body alignment, poor joint positioning, and inattention to the patient's musculoskeletal status can lead to impaired mobility, alteration in neuromuscular function, overstretching of joints, fracture, unnecessary postoperative discomfort, and long-term disability. Avoiding intraoperative and postoperative discomfort and pain from surgical positioning of the geri-operative patient is a major musculoskeletal consideration. Reviewing preoperative alerts for intraoperative care can facilitate communication, promote comfort, and avoid injury.

Musculoskeletal changes of greatest concern when positioning older adults are kyphosis, lumbar/cervical disc disease, limited range of motion, brittle tendons and ligaments, osteoporosis, and arthritis. Joints and

Attention to positioning and correct padding decreases risk of nerve and joint damage.

extremities require protection and support during patient transfer to minimize risk of injury. Positioning for surgery requires keeping muscles and joints within the individual patient's range of motion when moved and maintaining optimal body alignment without excess flexion, extension, or rotation.

General anesthesia relaxes muscles, causing a loss in protective tone. The loss in tone makes it more difficult to determine when muscles and joints are overstretched. When muscles relax, additional strain is placed on tendons and ligaments if joints are not adequately supported. Older adults undergoing spinal or local anesthesia cannot report discomfort or pain from poor positioning or poor body alignment. Careful observation, both during and after positioning, can prevent injury.

Older patients with severe osteoporosis or vertebral disc disease are susceptible to lumbosacral strain and vertebral fracture. Severe neck strain can occur when a patient has kyphosis and the head is unsupported. Thoracic distortion increases the distance from the head to the table, requiring the use of higher pillows. When the head is elevated and an arm board is used, the shoulder joint should be checked for overstretching. Prolonged arm extension contributes to muscle and joint strain. Bending the elbows slightly and supporting the forearm on pillows can minimize strain.

Incorrect placement and inappropriate use of padding devices creates a potential for nerve injury. When padding is applied incorrectly, superficial nerves and blood vessels are compressed, causing numbness and paresthesia, muscle paralysis or paresis, limb deformity, and pain. The resulting loss in muscle function can be permanent. The risk of injury due to prolonged pressure increases with the length of surgery.

Proper positioning of the patient in the operating room, attending to optimal body alignment, avoiding joint overextension, having adequate number and type of padding devices and support, and correct usage of padding devices and support can all prevent musculoskeletal injury and ensure patient safety.

POSTOPERATIVE CONSIDERATIONS

Preoperative comorbidities and functional levels are stronger predictors of postoperative immobility and deconditioning than chronologic age. Acute loss of function is common after exposure to surgical trauma and stress. Browning, Denehy, and Scholes (2007) found that patients recovering from colorectal surgery spent an average of 3 minutes per day out of bed on postoperative day one, increasing to 34 minutes per day on postoperative day four. The variable "uptime" was operationally defined as the length of time the patient spent standing or walking as measured by a battery-powered activity logger. In a study on the effects of multimodal postoperative mobilization, Gatt et al. (2005) found that patients in the control group recieving standard care spent an average of 8 minutes out of bed on the first postoperative day.

Even healthy, older adults become easily deconditioned when under activity restrictions or bed rest. A study by Brown and colleagues (2009) indicated that ambulatory older adults spent 83% of hospital time in bed, 13% of their time sitting, and slightly less than 4% of hospital time standing or walking. The authors concluded that environmental factors contributed to the amount of time spent in bed and nonphysical activity. Environmental factors include design of patient rooms that encourages patients to lie in bed to view the television. Cluttered floor spaces in rooms and corridors make it difficult to safely and easily walk in the room or on the hospital unit.

"Get the patient moving" is a well-established "golden rule" of postsurgical care. Balancing the gold standard of mobility with the need to conserve patient energy and maintain homeostasis requires astute clinical judgment, a focus on patient-centered care, and integrated interdisciplinary care planning.

Immediate postoperative goals are the prevention of complications that limit mobility while preventing the complications that occur secondarily to immobility and inactivity. In addition, it is important to maintain mobility and activity within the limits of patient's condition and postoperative restrictions. The long-term goal is to return the patient as quickly as possible to preoperative levels of function or to optimal postoperative function. Knowing the older adult's preoperative ability, activity, goals, and treatment expectations serves as a guide for postoperative interventions.

PATIENT SAFETY

Attention to patient safety is paramount when assisting the gerioperative patient with positioning, transfers, and ambulation. Attention to joint support, body alignment, and positioning is as important after surgery as during surgery. Even though the older adult is capable of indicating when joints are overstretched or range of motion is exceeded, the potential for injury remains. Poor alignment and inadequate support can cause joint stiffening, contracture, and pressure on nerves and blood vessels. Using a team to help position or ambulate the older adult prevents unnecessary pressure on extremities and joints, promotes safety, and increases psychological and physical comfort.

PAIN

Pain is a major safety risk. Unrelieved surgical or musculoskeletal pain prevents the patient from moving, increasing postoperative risk for complications. Unrelieved pain also is distracting and slows response time, increasing fall risk. Medications used to relieve pain create a safety risk due to side effects of sedation and slowed response time. Patient safety depends on clinical judgment and best practice guidelines to achieve pain relief at a level consistent with the patient's comfort zone for activity and ambulation without causing safety risk secondary to sedation and slowed response time.

Hospital falls are most likely to occur when the patient is getting in or out of bed, transferring from chair to bed, or ambulating to the bathroom (Amador & Loera, 2007). Falls result when the patient hurries or is being hurried to move to a different location. A typical example is the need to get to the bathroom quickly especially when faced with poor mobility and a distant bathroom.

Older adults move at a slow pace after surgery, secondary to pain, fatigue, and stiffness. Providing the older adult sufficient time to "get situated" before moving allows for cognitive appraisal of the task to be performed and neurosensory mechanisms to prepare and adapt to position changes. Table 13.4 identifies assessment and intervention strategies to promote safe postoperative ambulation.

Coaching before the patient begins to move increases the patient's feelings of security and promotes safety. Explain the activity, such as transfer to a chair or walk to the bathroom, indicating the direction the patient is to go. Provide detail consistent with patient's level of comprehension, medication effects, discomfort, or anxiety.

Refer to or demonstrate any safety precautions that are needed and how the patient can move within the limitations of the surgical procedure and equipment to decrease discomfort and prevent injury. For example, taking time to clearly explain that the patient is to stand, walk to the door, turn around, and return to bed or stand, turn, and sit in the chair provides both direction and a goal that increases feelings of competence and confidence. Describing

TABLE 13.4

Assessment and Intervention for Safe Postoperative Ambulation

Activity	Assessment/Intervention
Assess clinical condition	
Cognition	Level of alertness Cognitive function
Comorbid factors	Hydration Musculoskeletal limitations Disease effects Clinical status
Medications	Diuretic Sedatives Hypnotics Benzodiazepines
Fall risk	Previous falls Postural hypotension
Patient concerns, fears	Fallophobia (fear of falling) Pain
Coach patient	
	Provide adequate time Avoid hurrying either by implicit or explicit nonverbal or verbal behavior Review activity goals Set expectations about activity to be completed, including activity duration or distance Provide clear directions Demonstrate ways patient can move to minimize discomfort, injury
Organize assistive devices	
Patient clothing	Safe footwear, clothes
Assistive devices	Cane, walker Glasses, hearing aid Orthotics
Lifting aids	Transfer belt Transfer lifts
Supportive devices	Chair available for bed to chair activity or if needed for support Provide foam cushions, support pillows
Organize environment	
	Arrange and organize patient treatment equipment (catheters, intravenous lines, drains, dressings, oxygen) Arrange or remove ancillary equipment Moderate noise, lighting Ensure safe floor condition: ensure nonslip, nonglare surface Arrange furniture to avoid tripping and to facilitate support Provide time for patient preparation and education

(continued)

TABLE 13.4
Assessment and Intervention for Safe Postoperative Ambulation *(continued)*

Activity	Assessment/Intervention
Enlist support as needed	
Interdisciplinary staff **Unit staff**	Physical therapy, physiatry, occupational therapy Support staff Providers Companion-coach, family
Evaluate patient comfort	
Monitor response	Monitor physiological, physical, and emotional response Negotiate next steps Assess level of pain and discomfort: Physical, emotional, fatigue Provide support and nursing action
Document preambulation activity	Assessment data Expected activity: time or distance Completed activity: time or distance Patient coaching, demonstration Patient's physiological, physical, and emotional response Level of fatigue, pain during and after activity Patient concerns Next steps

and demonstrating how to stand and get balanced, as well as indicating the correct use assistive devices, helps maintain balance when making positional changes.

Asking the patient to explain the activity and safety precautions helps the patient focus on the activity and provides opportunity for clarification if needed. Companion-coaches and family members can participate in helping the patient prepare for ambulation or transfer in anticipation of assisting the patient after discharge.

Catheters, drains, and intravenous equipment are known risk factors for limiting patients' activity and contributing to patient falls. Rearranging tubes and drains that limit movement before helping the patient move improves patient comfort, security, and safety.

Organizing the environment and removing environmental barriers limits fall risk and creates a visual path that decreases patient anxiety about tripping and falling. Noise, activity distractions, and inadequate lighting contribute to inattention and anxiety. Limiting noise and distractions by closing the door; turning off the television, radio, and unneeded equipment; and having adequate lighting creates a safer, user-friendly environment.

ASSISTIVE TECHNOLOGY

Canes, walkers, and wheelchairs are the most common assistive devices used by older adults with temporary or permanent mobility impairments. Other assistive devices include seat or chairlifts that work to help the person stand. Armchair bars help to push to a standing position and can be adjusted to a height that is easy for the older adult to access. Air or memory foam cushions decrease pressure on buttocks when sitting, and pillows alleviate arm and leg strain. Ensuring availability of appropriate assistive devices in the hospital and at home can increase the older adult's independence and mobility. Informal caregivers and patients should have training in correct use of assistive technology to prevent injury and ensure patient safety.

ASSESSING MOBILITY AND FUNCTION

The immediate postoperative assessment includes the evaluation of range of motion, muscle strength, and joint pain. Results should be compared with preoperative findings. Surgical positioning can result in musculoskeletal strain and discomfort. Compression and hypotension can result in injury to muscle and nerve cells. Longer surgeries in fixed positions on hard surfaces escalate the risk of musculoskeletal injury. Some positions, such as lithotomy, have higher rates of postpositioning adverse effects.

Reviewing the preoperative and intraoperative medical record provides needed information about the patient's preoperative level of function, positioning during surgery, and length of surgery. This information is needed to determine the level of risk and potential site location for postoperative discomfort and complications due to intraoperative positioning. Asking the patient about joint and muscle discomfort, assessing for changes in sensation, monitoring capillary refill, and evaluating presence of vascular impairment promote early detection and immediate intervention needed to improve patient outcomes.

A fall risk assessment is important after surgery to determine the effect of surgery on patient's mobility and function. The assessment should use the same tool as the one used during the preoperative fall assessment. Using the same tool supports a more reliable comparison between preoperative findings and postoperative results.

Balance and gait should be evaluated at the beginning of each transfer or walking activity to preserve safety. Physiological, mental, and physical changes, as well as reactions to new or routine medications affecting mobility safety, are common postoperative responses to heightened physiological and psychological stress.

INTERVENTION

Approximately 25 to 50% of hospitalized older adults lose some level of functional ability. A major focus of postoperative care is getting the older patient moving and ambulating as soon as possible, within the individual's musculoskeletal limitations and clinical condition. Early activity and ambulation contribute to optimal respiratory, bowel, cardiac, neurological, and renal function. Activity is critical in maintaining muscle strength, energy, and range of motion. Immobility promotes contracture development, deconditioning, and functional limitations.

When developing a plan of care to prevent deconditioning, the value of an interdisciplinary team that includes physiatry, physical therapy, occupational therapy, recreational therapy, and nutrition, in addition to nurses and physicians, cannot be overemphasized. The team approach with an emphasis on exercise and activity improves function and mood, reduces in-hospital length of stay, and increases the likelihood of direct discharge to home. Mobilizing includes repositioning when in bed, active and passive range of motion, getting into and out of bed, standing, and walking. Any level of movement or activity increases blood flow, stimulates muscle innervations and function, improves bone metabolism, and improves mood.

PREVENTING CONTRACTURES

Contractures are temporary or permanent stiffening of body joints that limits normal range of motion. Surgical trauma, poor positioning during and after surgery, impaired circulation, immobility, muscle weakness, poor nutrition, and edema contribute to postsurgical contracture development.

Contractures are a major concern because they limit the patient's functional ability and interfere with recovery activities and mobility. Contracture develops more quickly in older adults due to the altered structure of muscles, ligaments, and tendons. Extensive physical rehabilitation is needed to return joints with significant contracture to normal function. Immobilization causes initial changes in connective tissue around the joint that eventually results in changes within the joint muscles, tendons, and ligaments. Contractures result from lack of joint movement or from maintaining a joint in a fixed position. Contractures can begin to form after 8 hours of immobility. Early joint contractures can be relieved with stretching and range of motion. Significant joint contractures from bed rest or immobility can occur in as little as 2 weeks and require intense physical therapy to reverse.

Most contractures result in joint flexion with loss of extension ability. Severity of a contracture ranges from minor loss of movement in a single joint to severe loss of movement in multiple joints. The degree of motion a joint loses in response to a contracture depends upon the joint location, type, and function. Older adults often have some permanent loss of joint range of motion and some flexion contracture in upper and lower extremities due to the muscle shortening and tendon changes that occur with aging. These preexisting changes in joint position increase vulnerability to more severe contracture development after surgery unless the patient receives range-of-motion exercises.

RANGE OF MOTION

Active and passive range of motion helps to relieve muscle aches and joint stiffness and prevent contractures. Range of motion increases blood flow, improving oxygenation and removal of waste products in joint tissues. Physical and occupational therapy should conduct an initial evaluation before initiating range of motion in patients with severe osteoarthritis, osteoporosis, or age-related changes in joint function. The companion-coach and family can assist with active and passive range of motion after receiving coaching from a member of the interdisciplinary team or the gerioperative care facilitator.

PROMOTING ACTIVITY

A postoperative goal is to progress activity levels as quickly as possible within the limitations of the patient's physical and clinical condition. Recent studies on older adults undergoing colorectal surgery document the effectiveness of enhanced recovery programs in decreasing lengths of hospital stay and postoperative complications. Enhanced recovery programs recommend standardized daily goals.

Mobilizing requires more activity than sitting in a chair for an extended period.

Specialty surgeries such as orthopedic, neurologic, ocular, and cardiac surgery often have specific protocols dictating postsurgery activity levels and mobility. Standardized recovery programs and protocols help to ensure consistency and measure outcomes of care. However, they do not address the heterogeneity in older adults and the need for variability in care adjusted to the older adult's ability. The "one size fits all" model of mobility protocols must be adapted to the individual patient's clinical condition and unique needs. Clinical judgment and interdisciplinary collaboration are critical to achieving an effective, safe mobility, and activity treatment plan.

INCREASING ACTIVITY LEVELS

Transferring and sitting in a chair is often the initial activity level for older adults after surgery. However, sitting in a chair should be limited to short intervals. Older adults with limited

EXHIBIT 13.3 Hazards Associated With Prolonged Reclining

- Inhibits turning and repositioning
- Increased pressure on superficial nerves
- Decreased lung expansion
- Decreased cough effectiveness
- Decreased intestinal motility
- Exacerbated rate of bone demineralization
- Decreased in muscle strength
- Increased skin pressure on sacrum and shoulder pressure points
- Difficulty engaging in cognitive stimulating activities

strength or flexibility have difficulty shifting positions when sitting in a chair. The resulting fixed position increases the risk for pressure ulcers, joint stiffness, and impaired circulation in the extremities.

Sitting in reclined chairs decreases oxygen saturation and impairs cardiovascular function.

Sitting in a recumbent position in a reclined chair limits movement even further and interferes with cardiorespiratory function. Reclined positions decrease oxygen saturation, systolic and diastolic blood pressure, and heart rate (Nitz, Hourigan, & Steer, 2007). Exhibit 13.3 lists hazards associated with a prolonged recumbent position. The risk of postural hypotension is greater when rising from a prolonged reclined position. Lung expansion and coughing effectiveness are impaired in reclined sitting. Patients in a reclined chair have higher pressure on superficial nerves as well as on sacral and shoulder pressure points.

Progressing to ambulation is a primary intervention for preventing postoperative complications and promoting psychological and physical well-being. When gerioperative patients are unable to ambulate, encouraging multiple transfers between bed and chair increases activity and improves function more effectively than sitting in a chair for extended periods. Preventing falls becomes a major concern as patients become more active, transferring between bed and chair and progressing with ambulation.

FALL PREVENTION

Anesthesia and surgery add to the risk of falls in the gerioperative patient. Pain, fatigue, deconditioning, cognitive changes, and the presence of tubes, catheters, and drains contribute additional risk. Hospital environments are not mobility friendly. Rooms are filled with treatment equipment, over-the-bed tables, side tables, chairs, and other furniture that become potential barriers and hazards during ambulation. Cluttered spaces are difficult for older adults to navigate, especially if the patient has problems with balance, gait, or muscle strength or is using an assistive device. The unfamiliar environment can be distracting due to the presence of noise, lighting, and fast-paced hospital activity.

Dykes and colleagues (2010) documented a decrease in hospitalized patient falls after implementing a fall prevention program using bedside alerts, patient education, and a fall prevention plan tailored to the individual and the results of the patient's fall risk assessment. The authors noted that a key component of the program was ensuring that all fall prevention and intervention information was readily available to the patient, family, companion-coach, and providers. Information was made available through an alert poster, patient- and family-friendly education handouts, a provider care plan, and intervention materials. Study findings indicated that the adjusted fall rate for older adults in the intervention group was 2.08 per 1000 patient days compared with 4.18 in the older age control group.

Although studies have examined fall prevention and intervention strategies, few have specifically addressed falls in the gerioperative patient. Most of the studies on postoperative falls have investigated general fall risk factors.

Stenvall and colleagues (2007) tested the effectiveness of a geriatric interdisciplinary, multimodal intervention after femoral fracture repair. Interventions focused on individual care planning, prevention and treatment of postoperative complications, nutrition, and rehabilitation with early mobilization and functional retraining. Staff training on fall prevention and use of interdisciplinary team meetings were important system components of the intervention. Results showed a crude postoperative fall rate of 6.29 per 1000 days in the intervention group, compared with 16.28 per 1000 days in the control group.

Table 13.5 identifies fall risk factors, contributing factors, and suggested preventive interventions.

PROMOTING SELF-CARE

Allowing older adults to perform self-care is as important as providing support and encouragement for regaining or maintaining functional capacity. Given the time constraints in the hospital environment, it is often easier for care providers to "do for" the older person rather than support the patient's self-care activities. Self-care con-

Avoid "doing for." Allowing older adults time to do self-care contributes to recovery.

tributes to feelings of competence and confidence and demonstrates the patient's progress. Providers can enlist the assistance of the companion-coach or family members in helping the older adult engage in self-care activities. Occupational, recreational, and physical therapy can help the older adult manage self-care and improve functional status.

Providing the patient with a schedule of exercises, activities, and ambulation written as a prescription promotes self-care and management. An activity prescription with "dose" and "schedule" provides weight or value to an intervention, similar to that associated with a medication prescription. The patient can use a checklist to document the activity along with a checklist to indicate the response and a space to write notes.

Suggesting that patients document their activity progress levels promotes self-care and evidence of progress toward recovery. Using a white board in the room to document a patient's progress provides evidence of improvement, serves as a benchmark for measuring discharge readiness, and helps the patient and companion-coach or family members participate in planning postdischarge activity levels. Providers, companion-coach, and family members can reinforce the progress and encourage ongoing activity.

Documenting the patient and provider perspectives on activity, progress toward recovery, and emotional response in the medical record provides data to the interdisciplinary team regarding plans for postdischarge care.

DECISIONAL SUPPORT

Providers are often faced with competing principles in the postoperative care of older adults. On the one hand, postoperative recovery depends on gaining cooperation or participation to

TABLE 13.5

Fall Risk Factors With Interventions

Risk Factors	Contributing Factor	Preventative Interventions
Drug toxicity	Medication side effects Anticholinergic medication Benzodiazepines	Medication review Reconciliation Revise as needed
Postural hypotension	Dehydration Diuretic medication Antihypertensive medication	Monitor orthostatic blood pressure Avoid prolonged bed rest Avoid prolonged chair recumbent position Modify medication regimen
Delirium	Medication Surgery Sleep disturbance Dehydration or electrolyte imbalance Unrelieved pain	Modify drug regimen Monitor cognition and alertness Treat underlying cause Provide calm, reassuring environment
Balance or gait impairment	Age-related changes Medication side effects Unrelieved pain Osteoarthritis	Prehabilitation Correct use of assistive devices Physical and occupational therapy Modify drug regimen
Muscle weakness	Age-related changes Electrolyte imbalance Inadequate nutrition	Prehabilitation Physical therapy Dietary consult Range-of-motion exercises
Incontinence	Cognitive changes Fluid imbalance Medication side effects Gait changes Fatigue Delirium Unfamiliar environment Inadequate staffing	Regular voiding schedule Monitor fluid intake Increase fiber Assess toileting need regularly Review medications Post diuretic attention

Adapted from Amador & Loera, 2007.

prevent complications and promote recovery. Activities such as getting out of bed, range-of-motion exercises, or walking in the hallway can be uncomfortable, increase fatigue, and be unwanted by the patient.

The principle of autonomy argues that patients have a right to refuse treatment (intervention), and providers should honor that right even when the intervention promotes the person's best interest and stated goals. The provider who values best evidence regarding movement and mobility may experience a conflict when facing an older adult who resists mobilization intervention. While recovery and preventing complications depend on activity and moving, at the same time, patients can refuse. Providing accurate information and leaving the decision to the patient, even if the decision interferes with the patient's recovery, is a form of consumer advocacy.

Providers have a moral responsibility to go beyond providing information and then leaving it to the patient to decide. This assumes special importance when caring for older adults postoperatively. Pain, discomfort, fatigue, and medication effects can interfere with the older patient's ability to carefully consider the long-term outcomes of short-term decisions. In addition, older adults can experience undetected postoperative cognitive dysfunction or depression after surgery. The resulting alterations in cognitive function and mood, although not meeting the criterion for incapacity, can interfere with the patient's ability to attend to and interpret information. Such interference can cause the patient to make decisions that are inconsistent with the patient's usual decisions, values, and stated long-term goals. Ms. Ester provides an example of how iatrogenesis can result in poor decision-making.

Ms. Ester was comfortable taking medications and adhered to her prescriptions quite assiduously. She had rheumatoid arthritis that went undiagnosed for several months. She attributed her increasing pain severity to her longstanding osteoarthritis.

After being diagnosed and starting on medication, she had severe side effects. As a result, she refused to take any medication. Her condition deteriorated until she could not walk or stand without assistance. She spent all her time in a chair. Three months previously, she was hiking with her grandchildren, mowing the lawn, and traveling around the country.

In frustration, her family told her she was irrational and making "stupid" decisions. Surprised by their reaction, Ms. Ester agreed to medication. Once her pain was under control, she couldn't believe she refused medication. She said she had not understood that rheumatoid arthritis was different from osteoarthritis even though she could describe both conditions correctly and the treatment. She appeared cognitively intact and even passed her Mini-Mental Status Exam. However, her persistent severe pain interfered with her inability to "take in" information leading to decisions inconsistent with her intent.

Decisional support depends on patient-centered, relationship-centered care. Informed refusal is as important a concept as is informed consent. Both depend on the patient's ability to understand, interpret, and apply the information to his or her life and health situation. Disease, pain, and iatrogenesis can interfere.

Although providers must honor the patient's right to refuse treatment, they have a moral responsibility to evaluate if the decisions the patient is making are consistent with the patient's preferences, values, and future goals. Evaluation of a refusal to participate in postoperative recovery begins with exploring the patient's clinical situation and the context in which the decisions are being made. Providing decisional support can identify the older adult's desires and needs and identify inconsistencies. Decisional support is a critical element in best practice. Best practice means weighing the evidence (guidelines, literature, protocol) in the context of the individual situation. The goal is always the best interest of the older adult. When confronted with what appears to be competing principles, providers must rely on listening to the patient and engaging in patient-centered, relationship-oriented decisional support. Clinical judgment and ethical decision-making are equally important.

DISCHARGE CONSIDERATIONS

Continuing the recovery trajectory after discharge depends on the patient's understanding and ability to maintain optimal mobility. Share knowledge with the patient and family about patient safety, activity, and ambulation within the limits of the clinical condition, functional ability, and postsurgical restrictions. Discussing long-range functional and activity goals with the patient and family, as well as planning for short- and long-term interventions in order to meet those goals, decreases anxiety and contributes to the patient's security and well-being. The prescription model can motivate the patient to continue exercise, nutrition, and meaningful activity regimens.

EXHIBIT 13.4 **Discharge Coaching to Improve Musculoskeletal Function**

Maintaining daily routine
Increasing physical activity to tolerance within postoperative limitations
Balancing physical activity with rest and energy conservation
Potential outcomes of over- and underactivity
Facilitating ambulation and active or passive range of motion
Avoiding prolonged sitting, especially in reclining position
Promoting independence
Maintaining adequate nutritional status
Adequate vitamin D and calcium intake
Effects of medication on mobility and function
Maintaining hydration
Encouraging social interaction and engagement
Monitoring activity for safety and fall prevention
Conducting a self-home safety assessment
Completing follow-up visits with physician and surgeon
Attend physical, occupational, or recreational therapy as recommended

It is important to ask older patients about the home environment to identify factors that can facilitate recovery or identify safety hazards that can impede recovery. Once factors are identified, hazards can be removed, and safety measures and environmental supports are added.

Formal and informal community resources can be mobilized to help the older adult return to the home environment and recover. Formal resources that can be mobilized are interdisciplinary occupational, physical, or recreation therapy, and home health care. Informal supports are family, friends, and neighbors who supply instrumental and emotional support. Regardless of resource availability, coaching of the patient, as well as a significant support system, remains the mainstay of discharge planning. Exhibit 13.4 provides a checklist of items related to activity, mobility, and exercise to promote recovery and maintain physical capacity after discharge.

PATIENT REPORT: Ms. Augsten

On preoperative examination, Ms. Augsten shows decreased strength in both lower extremities and decreased range of motion in her right knee. Her gait is slow with halting steps and an uneven pace. She is unable to balance without the use of a cane. It takes her 26 seconds to complete the TUG test. Analysis of preoperative history and physical examination indicates Ms. Augsten has multiple factors that increase her risk for intraoperative and postoperative complications. Risk factors include being overweight, limited activity level, impaired gait and balance, decreased muscle strength in the lower extremities, preexisting persistent and acute pain, increasing alcohol use, inadequate nutrition, opioid use, and that the surgery involves the upper abdomen. The following discussion focuses only on those risk factors that pertain to her musculoskeletal status.

Ms. Augsten needs prehabilitation to improve her musculoskeletal function and nutritional status. Due to her emergent cholecystectomy, prehabilitation is not an option. The preoperative nurse discusses early postoperative ambulation with Ms. Augsten. On talkback, Ms. Augsten explains the importance of getting out of bed and walking around, followed by the comment, "but my knee hurts so much, I don't know if I will really be able to do much." The nurse restates how the interdisciplinary team will work with Ms. Augsten to see she has maximum pain relief and follows by coaching Ms. Augsten on how to talk to her care providers about her pain relief needs before getting out of bed and ambulating.

The preoperative alert checklist includes acetaminophen and oxycodone dose and duration of use, severity of right knee osteoarthritis, and impaired gait and balance, suggesting increased risk for a fall.

Her intraoperative care plan focuses on preventing injury to the right knee joint and minimizing pain from positioning during surgery. The care plan calls for supporting the right knee joint during each patient transfer, providing support for the right knee throughout the surgical procedure, and managing intraoperative pain medication in light of her history of increased alcohol, acetaminophen, and oxycodone use. Ms. Augsten's postoperative care demands attention to her activity level and mobility. Early ambulation is a major intervention for preventing general deconditioning, postoperative hospital-acquired pneumonia, deep vein thrombophlebitis, and pressure ulcers.

Ms. Augsten's mobility status is a challenge. Her gait and balance create a risk for falls. Her decreased muscle strength and severe joint pain limit movement in bed, mobility, and ambulation. Her poor nutritional status contributes to diminished energy levels that interfere with postoperative ambulation.

The interdisciplinary care team meets with Ms. Augsten and develops a plan for managing Ms. Augsten's mobility and early ambulation. The plan incorporates a high nutrition diet with multivitamin supplementation as soon as she can be started on oral fluids and food, physical therapy to conduct range-of-motion and physical exercise, occupational therapy for coping with the challenges of postoperative mobility, and initiation of nonpharamacologic and pharmacologic pain relief. The care plan protocol calls for Ms. Augsten to be out of bed in a chair the evening of surgery and to begin ambulating a short distance to tolerance. Ambulation increases each postoperative day by distance and number of times per day as tolerance increases. An important part of Ms. Augsten's plan of care is maintaining her safety during activity. Risk factors for her safety include orthostatic hypotension, balance changes, muscle weakness, pain, knee instability, weight support, and fear of pain. The patient safety plan of care includes increasing bed and chair range of motion and exercise, use of adaptive equipment, nursing assistance, and use of a transfer belt until she is stable when walking. A critical aspect of her safety program is to give her the time to ambulate without being hurried. Hurrying increases the risk of falls. Older adults are sensitive to how much time they take and attempt to get things done so they will not be a burden or take too long. Reassuring Ms. Augsten that as a safety issue she needs to take her time and not hurry can help relieve the feeling of having to rush. Clearing the area where she walks of clutter, equipment, furniture, and other impediments encourages ambulation and minimizes potential for tripping and falling. Ms. Augsten should be encouraged to keep a log of her activity level in a diary. Entries should include time of day, activity, length of activity, and reaction or response to the activity. Results of her diary should be posted on the white board in her room. Making the evidence of her progress visible encourages her to maintain her diary and serves as reinforcement for her continued progress.

Ms. Augsten regains mobility status and prepares for discharge. Ms. Augsten receives information about the correct use of her cane and walker. She is able to demonstrate the upper and lower extremity chair exercises, stating she will continue them and start taking short walks with her dog. Her pain relief plan is revised to incorporate acetaminophen and nonpharmacologic interventions. A consult is scheduled with the orthopedist to discuss a total knee replacement. A dietician meets with her to discuss postdischarge nutrition.

SUMMARY

Maintaining musculoskeletal function in the gerioperative patient promotes patient safety, prevents deconditioning, and enhances surgical recovery in the older adult. Deconditioning is a major risk factor for most postoperative surgical complications and can be avoided through diligent attention to activity, nutrition, hydration, and safety. Prehabilitation is a little used but highly effective intervention in preparing the gerioperative physically and psychologically to manage the stressors of surgery and in decreasing risk of postoperative deconditioning. Interdisciplinary team collaboration and coordination is key in maintaining patient safety and achieving progressive mobility and activity goals needed for rapid recovery. Elements of fast track surgery, when applied judiciously to musculoskeletal function and fitness, significantly enhance pre- and postsurgical physical health and functional capacity in the gerioperative patient.

KEY POINTS

- Exercise, gait, balance, and muscle training counteract the negative effect of age-related changes in muscle and bone strength, flexibility, gait, and balance.
- Providers underestimate the value and importance of adequate musculoskeletal function and the benefits of perioperative activity and mobility to the surgical recovery of the gerioperative patient.
- Interdisciplinary prehabilitation programs improve surgical outcomes.
- Diligent intraoperative interdisciplinary team care prevents positioning-related musculoskeletal and neurological injuries.
- Patient deconditioning diminishes functional capacity in all physiological and psychological systems resulting in poor patient outcomes, frailty, and dependency.
- Recumbent positions are detrimental to cardiorespiratory function and increase patient deconditioning.
- Balancing adequate postoperative pain relief, mobility progression, energy conservation, and patient safety depends on best practice, clinical judgment, and collaborative interdisciplinary planning and intervention.

FOURTEEN

Skin

Jennifer V. Long, Susan J. Fetzer, and Raelene V. Shippee-Rice

PATIENT REPORT: Mr. Kilty

Mr. Kilty, a 68-year-old retired police captain, has a 20-year history of osteoarthritis. He is admitted for a total right hip replacement under general anesthesia. He admits to drinking a six-pack of beer per day. He has a medical history of hypertension and has recently been told he has a "high sugar." He recently quit smoking but has a history of 50 pack-years. His body mass index is 22. He exercises daily by walking his dog.

The skin is the largest organ of the body, accounting for 16% of total body weight. Nerve endings and receptors on the skin respond to touch, pain, pressure, and changes in temperature. The skin forms a protective barrier as well as an interface between the internal organs and the environment. Because the skin is the first line of defense between the body and the environment, it demonstrates outwardly what is happening within the body. Skin eruptions may be a result of change in the dermal layer but may also be a sign of internal changes.

The skin is very important in the social aspects of human interaction, reflecting the emotional state of the individual. When people meet, first impressions are often based on appearance. The sense of touch and smell also convey strong emotional messages between people.

The skin is a window into the body and conveys messages of illness, well-being, health, beauty, integrity, and growing old. The most obvious manifestations of aging appear on the skin. Human beings emphasize the skin and the preservation of youthfulness as evidenced by the billions of dollars spent on creams, lotions, beauty aids, and retinol products. Plastic and cosmetic surgery is expanding. Americans spent 10 billion dollars on 13 million plastics and cosmetic procedures in 2010. Changes in the skin are important not only for obvious physiological reasons but also for the sense of body image that accompanies those changes. As such, the condition of an individual's skin can be the cause of emotional and psychological stress in the elderly.

Understanding the normal anatomy and physiology of the integumentary system, along with the changes that occur with aging, allows the health care provider to anticipate potential problems, as well as implement appropriate interventions to minimize the impact of these problems on the gerioperative patient. In this chapter, normal anatomy and physiology of the skin is presented with the normal physiologic changes associated with aging, and how these changes impact gerioperative care.

Skin Considerations

The integumentary system consists of the skin plus the accessory organs of hair, nails, and sweat glands. The skin is made up of three tissue layers: the epidermis, the dermis (or connective tissue), and the subcutaneous fat layer. As a protective barrier between the internal organs and the environment, the skin protects against ultraviolet light, toxins, injury, bacterial invasion, and dehydration. The hair and nails also serve as protection.

The integumentary system has several functions that maintain homeostasis: organ protection, thermoregulation, sensation, blood storage, metabolism of vitamin D, excretion of wastes and salts, and immunologic surveillance. Organ function is maintained by regulation of body temperature. Regulation of body temperature occurs by changes in the size of blood vessels in the skin. Blood vessels constrict to conserve heat when cold and expand to bring blood vessels closer to the surface, losing heat via radiation, when hot. The skin also perspires to cause the body to lose heat by convection as sweat is evaporated.

Sweat is composed of water, salts, and several organic compounds such as urea and ammonia. In addition to producing sweat for temperature regulation, sweat glands can excrete toxic waste products. When the body has an abundance of waste compounds, they are released by the sweat glands explaining the oily feeling on the skin of renal patients.

The dermis and epidermis have many nerve endings that sense heat, cold, pain, pressure, and touch. The sensors allow the skin to respond to stimuli that may be harmful to the body. It also allows humans to interact with one another by allowing us to feel the touch of another being.

The dermis of the skin acts as a blood reservoir by housing an extensive network of blood vessels that store 8 to 10% of the body's blood volume. During moderate exercise, blood vessels expand to help with heat loss, but during strenuous exercise or other stress, the blood vessels constrict to keep the blood central to muscles and vital organs.

Cells in the epidermis of the skin, Langerhan's cells, are active in the immunologic function of the skin. The lipid bilayer of the epidermis has antimicrobial characteristics. There are also macrophages and T-cells in the dermis that provide immunologic protection against bacterial invasion of the body.

Epidermis

The epidermis (shown in Figure 14.1) is the functional unit of the skin. Keratinocytes are specialized cells in the epidermis that produce keratin, a complex, protective, fibrous protein that forms the dead outer layer of the skin. Hair, nails, and glands are made of a keratin that is rich in cystine. Keratin waterproofs and protects the skin and underlying tissues of the body. The epidermis is avascular and consists of four to five cell layers depending on the body area. Epidermal nutrition is obtained by diffusion from blood vessels in the underlying dermis below.

Epidermal nutrition is obtained by diffusion from blood vessels in the underlying dermis below.

Keratinization is the transformation of live keratin cells (keratinocytes) into the dead cells (corneocytes) of the stratum corneum, a dynamic and ongoing process.

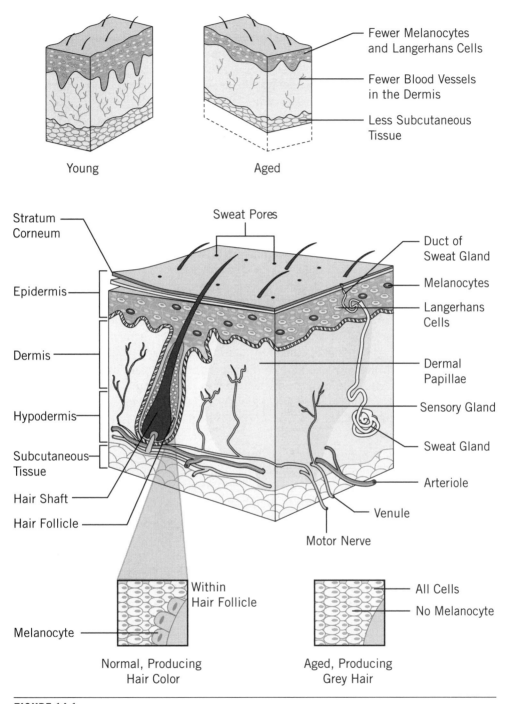

FIGURE 14.1

Skin Layers With Age-Related Changes

The skin is continually repairing and regenerating itself as dead cells are shed and replaced with new ones.

The *Stratum germinativatum (basale)* is the deepest level of the epidermis. It is made up of a single layer of basal cells that produce keratinocytes by mitosis. The migrating keratinocytes move up through the skin layers to replace cells lost by normal wear and tear of the skin.

The Stratum germinetivatum layer also contains Merkel cells and melanocytes. Merkel cells are mechanoreceptors associated with touch sensation. They are dense in the oral mucosa and on the bottom of hands and feet, lips, and outermost sheath of hair follicles. Melanocytes produce pigment granules called melanin. Melanin gives skin its color and protects the skin by absorbing and scattering ultraviolet rays of the sun. Darker skinned individuals differ from light skinned individuals in the size of the melanocytes.

Stratum spinosum is a thin layer of cells that is formed as the keratinocytes migrate toward the skin surface. The keratinocytes change from hexagonal to polygonal and are called prickle cells because of their spiny appearance. The appendages of these spiny cells, called desmosomes, act as anchors that hold the cells together, forming a mesh that retains water and prevents skin shearing. The prickle cells also begin to produce keratin, a fibrous protein filament that helps support and protect the skin.

The skin is an endocrine organ with vitamin D synthesized in the stratum spinosum and stratum germinivatum. When exposed to ultraviolet light, the skin releases a vitamin D precursor (7-dehydrocholesterol) that is transported to the liver where enzymes modify the molecule into vitamin D_3 (cholecalciferol). Vitamin D_3 then passes to the kidneys where it is converted into the most active form of vitamin D (calcitrol). Vitamin D is necessary to aid absorption of calcium in the small intestine. The main action of vitamin D, along with parathyroid hormone, is regulation of calcium and phosphorous homeostasis for bone formation and mineralization. If an individual is in the sun just until the skin turns pink, the body produces significant quantities of vitamin D necessary for calcium absorption. Melanin absorbs ultraviolet light; hence, dark-skinned individuals produce less Vitamin D in response to sun exposure than light-skinned individuals.

> *Melanin gives skin its color and protects the skin by absorbing and scattering ultraviolet rays of the sun.*

The *Stratum granulosum* contains the most differentiated cells of the human skin. In this layer, special keratinocytes, called lamellar bodies, produce a waxy substance made up of free fatty acids and ceramides (a type of binding protein). As the lamellar bodies move up toward the surface, the outer membranes of the cells disintegrate and release the waxy substance. The waxy substance acts as a mortar to bind the dying keratinocytes together and defends against moisture loss. Intercellular spaces through which keratinocytes receive nutrients become sealed off, causing cells to die. Other keratinocytes lose deoxyribonucleic acid structures and cytoplasm while producing keratin. The dying cells, filled with keratin (keratinizing), become anucleated and flat. The dead, keratinized cells, called corneocytes, rise to become part of the next level of epithelium, the stratum corneum.

Langerhan's cells comprise 3 to 5% of cells in the stratum corneum, compared to 95% of keratinocytes. Langerhan's cells are derived from precursor cells in the bone marrow and continuously repopulate the epidermis. The immunologic role of Langerhan's cells is to recognize foreign antigens and bind to the surface, migrating with the attached antigen from the epidermis to the lymph nodes where they present the antigen to the lymphatic system. Langerhan's cells are innervated by sympathetic nerve fibers, which may explain changes in skin secondary to stress as seen in psoriasis of elders. Keratinocytes play an important immunologic role by communicating and regulating the Langerhan's cells as well as secreting cytokines and inflammatory mediators.

The *Stratum lucidum* is a thin transparent layer found only in areas of thick skin such as the palms of hands, soles of feet, and over knees and elbows. The stratum lucidum is a transition zone composed of live and keratinized cells. The purpose of this layer is to protect the skin against friction and shear forces that occur between the stratum granulosum and stratum corneum.

Stratum corneum is the outer most layer of skin composed of dead keritinocytes and is 8 to 20 cells thick. Cells in levels 8 to 15 continually change from keritinocytes to corneocytes by filling with keratin and forming flattened anucleated cells. The cells of the uppermost layer of the stratum corneum, levels 1 to 8, are corneocytes. The structure of the stratum corneum is similar to a brick and mortar arrangement. The corneocytes are the bricks, made up of many tiny threads of keratin that are layered into an organized protein matrix that can hold large amounts of water between layers. The mortar is the waxy substance released from the lamellar bodies that forms a lipid bilayer essential to the barrier properties of the skin. The waxy substance also has antimicrobial properties that protect the skin from infection.

The cells in the strateum corneum layer are held together by desmosomes. The desmosomes begin to disintegrate as the cells move closer to the outer layer of the epidermis, a process called desquamization. As the cells move, the corneocytes with the protective lipid-rich cementing substance form the tough, protective, waterproof barrier. Cells are sloughed off and new ones are replaced from the bottom to the top. It takes 20 to 30 days for a keratinocyte to migrate from the stratum germinivatum to the stratum corneum, and each layer of the epidermis has a role in the progression of the keritinocyte to corneocyte.

A majority of changes to the epidermis are explained by pollutants, smoking, chemicals, and sun damage from ultraviolet light.

All keratinized cells migrate from the bottom to the top. Keratinocytes change shape and function as they migrate from the stratum germinavatum (basale) to the stratum corneum. The keratinocyte changes from a round cell to a prickle cell in the stratum spinosum, then to a flatter cell in the stratum granulosum. In the stratum corneum, it becomes a flattened elongated cell (corneocyte). The cell changes from a viable structure with cytoplasm and a nucleus to a nonliving structure filled with keratin and encompassed by the lipid bilayer, forming the protective, waterproof top layer of the skin.

Other keratinocytes, melanocytes, and Langerhan's cells do not migrate. In the lower levels of the epidermis, the desmosomes keep these cells from detaching during migration. These keratinocytes provide the skin with support.

AGE-RELATED CHANGES

Changes in elders' skin are caused by many factors. Among the elderly population, 70% have skin conditions. A majority of changes to the epidermis are explained by pollutants, smoking, chemicals, and sun damage from ultraviolet light. In non–sun-exposed areas, changes to the epidermis are less dramatic and are the result of normal age-related changes rather than external factors.

The loss of keratinocyte "mortar" compromises skin integrity as microscopic fissures are formed.

Age-related change to the epidermis is a complex phenomenon combining cumulative environmental insults with progressive internal changes resulting in structural and functional disturbances. Normal age-related changes alone do not account for the extent of changes seen in the integumentary system among elders. Skin changes vary based on skin care history, genetics, sun exposure, smoking, medications, and nutrition. Changes to the epidermis are much more dramatic in sun-exposed areas, indicating that sun damage is a prominent cause of cumulative age-related changes.

Increased dryness and roughness are two of the most notable age-related changes to the epidermis. Due to a decrease in corneocyte turnover, the rate of keratinocyte proliferation decreases, and the number of keratinized cells on the surface increases. These changes, combined with reduced production of stratum corneum lipids, contribute to increased skin dryness and flakiness. The loss of stratum corneum lubrication can result in decreased flexibility of this layer, causing an increase in fragility. The loss of keratinocyte "mortar" compromises skin integrity as microscopic fissures are formed. The compromised epidermal barrier increases susceptibility to irritant reactions from lotions, skin patches, and adhesives.

Over time, the overall thickness of the skin decreases, resulting in a transparent appearance. The reduction of fat that occurs all over the body also occurs in the subcutaneous layer of the skin, causing it to become thinner. The connective tissue of the dermis thins secondary to diminished amounts of testosterone and growth hormone. Although the number of cell layers remains the same, cells within the epidermis become smaller and thinner. Thinning of the epidermis leads to increased vulnerability to mechanical trauma, especially shearing and friction that causes skin tears. Thinning of the epidermis is exacerbated by sun exposure.

The risk of benign or cancerous skin lesions increases with age. The reduced epidermal proliferation rate and slower turnover also means that epidermal cells are exposed to potential carcinogens longer, increasing the risk of skin cancer. Continual basal cell mitosis over time increases the risk of malignant and benign lesions of the skin due to potential errors in division.

Another quality of aging skin is skin discoloration as the number of melanocytes decreases. After the age of 30, the number of melanocytes decreases up to 8 to 20% per decade in sun-exposed and non–sun-exposed areas. The functional melanocytes can be variable in shape and size. The uneven decrease and distribution of melanocytes results in the uneven pigmentation of the elderly known as "age spots." The decrease in the number of melanocytes results in the inability to tan as deeply as younger individuals. Medication reactions together with fewer melanocytes make elders more susceptible to sun exposure and sunburn, which increases the risk of skin cancer.

Vitamin D production decreases with age. The vitamin D precursors decrease by 75% with the aging process. Individuals over the age of 65 have a fourfold decrease in the ability to make vitamin D_3. With age, the gastrointestinal tract has a decreased ability to absorb vitamin D from foods and supplements. Lack of sun exposure and changes in diet add to elder's vitamin D depletion. The reduction in vitamin D production leads to bone loss and exacerbates osteoporosis, increasing the risk of fractures.

With aging, the number of Langerhan's cells and Merkel's cells decreases. The decline in Langerhan's cells leads to a decreased immune response. There is a greater reduction of Langerhan's cells in areas exposed to ultraviolet light, decreasing the cell-mediated immune response in the skin. The reduction of melanin combined with the decreased immunity and decreased inflammatory warning signs intensify the risk of developing skin cancers. The reduction of Langerhan's cells slows the body's inflammatory response to antigens and allergens, which may lead to delayed topical allergic reactions in the elderly. The decline in Merkel's cells explains why elders' have decreased tactile sensation.

The decline in Merkel's cells explains why elders' have decreased tactile sensation.

Dermal-Epidermal Junction

The dermal-epidermal junction is a transitional zone of attachment from the basal layer of the epidermis to the papillary dermis. Hemidesmosomes secure the epidermis to the dermis, providing adherence and support to the epidermis. The dermal-epidermal junction is a membrane that provides selective filtering of molecules between the two layers. This junction is the weakest part of the skin. Blistering of the skin, caused by shearing forces, heat, cold, and blistering disorders, occurs at the dermal-epidermal junction.

Dermis

The dermis, the connective tissue of the skin, is made up of collagen, the major stress-resistant protein of the body. The dermal layer contains the pilar (hair) and glandular structures. The dermis also supports and nourishes the epidermis. There are two dermal layers: the papillary dermis and the reticular dermis.

The papillary dermis consists of collagen and a gel-like matrix made up of proteins, enzymes, mucopolysaccharides, immune chemicals, metabolites, and other substances. Conical projections called dermal papillae extend from the papillary dermis into the epidermis (see Figure 14.1). The basal cells of the epidermis project down into the papillary dermis and form ridges. The basal layer ridges along with the dermal papillae valleys help to minimize separation of the dermis and epidermis. These ridges create the fingerprint. Dermal papillae contain capillaries, end arterioles, and venules that nourish the epidermal layers of the skin via diffusion. Lymph vessels and nerve tissue, nociceptors and thermoreceptors, are also found in the papillary dermis.

The reticular dermis contains blood vessels, immune cells, elastin and collagen fibers, nerves, hair follicles, and glands. There are two arterial blood supplies to the dermis, one between the dermis and the subcutaneous layer and one between the papillary and reticular layers. The pink color of light-colored skin comes from blood seen in this plexus. The capillary flow of blood extends up into the epidermis, supplying nourishment by diffusion.

Arteriovenous anastomoses in the skin allow for blood to flow directly between a vein and an artery, bypassing capillary circulation. These anastomoses are important for temperature regulation, opening when necessary to allow additional blood flow to dissipate heat or closing to conserve blood flow and body heat. The vascular network of the dermis is a storage area for blood that can be redirected to the vital organs in the event of blood loss. When blood is redirected from the dermis, the result is cool, pale skin, as seen in shock. The vascular network is assessed when measuring capillary refill time.

Fibroblasts in the dermis produce collagen and elastin fibers. Elastin is a stretchy fiber that allows the skin to stretch and then "bounce back" to its original state. Elastin accounts for the skin's strength, extensibility, and elasticity. Collagen is a fibrous protein that forms a support and strengthening component of the dermis. Darker-colored dermis contains more collagen and is more compact than lighter dermis. This accounts for less wrinkling in darker-skinned individuals.

Once believed to be primarily made up of fibroblasts, it is now known that dermal dendrocytes account for most of the dermal cells. Dermal dendrocytes possess both phagocytic and dendritic properties. These properties are thought to play a part in immune function, wound healing, blood clotting, and inflammation properties of the dermal layer.

Macrophages, T-cells, and mast cells are found in the dermis. The macrophages and epithelial cells provide antigens to the dermal T-cells. Most of the T-cells are memory cells that have been previously activated. The major type of immune response to an antigen in the skin is a delayed-hypersensitivity response. Mast cells located in the dermis respond to antigens with an immediate hypersensitivity response that is usually immunoglobulin E-mediated. These cells interact with antigens that come in contact with the skin and cause urticaria and the flushing seen in allergic reactions. The lymphatic system found in the dermis is responsible for combating skin infections.

The dermis is well supplied with afferent and efferent nerves to receive and respond to sensory information from the environment. Sensory receptors for pain, touch, heat, cold, and pressure are distributed throughout the dermis. Pacinian corpuscles are pressure-sensitive receptors that detect pressure and touch. Touch receptors known as Meissner's corpuscles are flat, encapsulated nerve endings found on the palmar surfaces of the fingers and hands and plantar surfaces of the feet. Ruffini's corpuscles are spindle-shaped mechanoreceptors that register tension in the supporting collagen fibers. The sympathetic nervous system provides control of blood vessels, sweat glands, along with cholinergic fibers, and arrector pili muscles that cause elevation of the hairs on the skin.

The lymphatic system found in the dermis is responsible for combating skin infections.

AGE-RELATED CHANGES

The epidermis, dermis, and dermal-epidermal junction thin with age. The dermal density decreases with fewer cells and blood vessels. The dermal-epidermal junction begins to flatten, weakening the adhesion of the dermis to the epidermis. The weakness of the dermal-epidermal junction allows for easy abrasions, shear-type injuries, and blister formation. Overall, elders' dermal layer is more friable.

Collagen production decreases 1% per year in adulthood, causing the thickness of the skin to decline each year after the age of 20. Thinner skin offers less cushioning and support. With age, collagen becomes thicker, less soluble, and more resistant to breakdown by collagen enzymes. These changes combined with changes in the number and type of cohesive bonds make collagen stronger and more stable. The increased collagen strength results in decreased elasticity and less give when stretched. These changes place elders' skin at higher risk for tear-type injuries.

The elastic fibers of the dermis change and become less elastic, causing loss of resilience and stretch. The loss of elasticity leads to sagging skin, wrinkles, and further predisposes the skin to injury. Solar elastosis is the leathery, weather beaten appearance of skin caused by years of sun exposure and damage to the elastin fibers.

Vascularity and supporting structures of the dermis decline resulting in fragile, easily broken blood vessels, decreased capillary growth in wounds, and decreased wound healing. Decreased dermal blood vessels create the pale skin of the elderly. With age, a benign proliferation of weak capillaries forms cherry angiomas, visible on the skin surface as tiny cherry red papules.

A decrease in dermal mucopolysaccharides along with decreased extracellular matrix allows for "breaks" in the skin and increased susceptibility to skin irritation from environmental factors. The viscosity of the dermal fluids is increased leading to a decreased rate of dermal clearance of substances. The slow clearance prolongs episodes of contact dermatitis. There is a reduced ability to move water from the dermis to the epidermis, causing epidermal dehydration seen in dry skin.

The immune response of the dermis is impaired in elders secondary to reduced production of cytokines, delayed hypersensitivity reaction, and decreased inflammatory response. These changes predispose the elderly to impaired wound healing, more intense reaction to skin irritants, and an increased risk of infection.

The number of Pacini's and Meissner's corpuscles, along with other nerve endings responsible for pain, heat, and cold sensations, decrease with age secondary to decreased blood flow and vitamin B_1 levels. Altered touch receptors make it more difficult to perform fine touch maneuvers with the hands. The decreased number of nerve endings responsible for hot, cold, and pain sensations predispose the elderly to thermal injury.

TOPICAL MEDICATION PATCHES

Percutaneous absorption refers to absorption of topical medications such as fentanyl patches, nitroglycerin paste, and clonidine patches through the epidermal layer to the dermis and into the bloodstream for systemic circulation. The advantage of this delivery system is a constant rate of absorption with prolonged action that avoids the need for gastrointestinal function and the first pass effect. Percutaneous medications have fewer side effects secondary to steady peak concentration levels and increased patient compliance.

The rate and amount of topical medication absorption is regulated by the stratum corneum. The pharmacokinetic characteristics for topical medications rely on the features of "normal" skin. Changes in the stratum corneum that lead to increased or decreased moisture content, changes in epidermal integrity, and environmental moisture alterations affect percutaneous drug absorption. When the moisture level or integrity of the stratum corneum is compromised, medication absorption can become erratic, compromising patient safety.

With aging, the lipid layer of the stratum corneum is diminished. Because many topical drugs are lipophilic, the reduction of lipids on the surface of the skin affects absorption. Flattening of the dermal-epidermal junction with aging, along with the reduction in capillaries, decreases transdermal absorption of drugs. However, there is limited research concerning the few transdermal medications available and absorption in the elderly. Kaestli et al. (2008) concluded that in practice, the age-related changes do not affect transdermal medication absorption. Yet, the study of fentanyl patch application, comparing young and older subjects, had a dropout rate of 100% of the elderly patients due to side effects. However, the younger subjects were successfully treated with very few side effects. It could not be determined if the higher serum drug concentration in the elderly was due to changes in topical absorption or drug clearance.

Many patients have discontinued the use of clonidine patches due to skin irritation. Alternating skin application sites can reduce the incidence of irritation. Transdermal medication systems may appear to have clear benefits to elderly patients with fewer first-pass effects, fewer drug interactions, and a more steady state. However, the fentanyl patch study raises many questions. Whether medication patches will prove to be safe and beneficial as more transdermal medications are formulated remains to be seen.

> *When the moisture level or integrity of the stratum corneum is compromised, medication absorption can become erratic, compromising patient safety.*

Subcutaneous Tissue

Describing the subcutaneous tissue as an actual layer of skin is controversial. However, because skin structures extend into the subcutaneous tissue, some pressure ulcers are classified by depth of wounds, and some skin diseases manifest in this tissue, it can be considered the third layer of skin. The subcutaneous layer consists of fat and connective tissue. These structures lend support to the nervous system and vascular components of the skin and anchor the skin to muscle and bone. Deep hair follicles, some bursae over joints, adipose cells, and macrophages are found in the subcutaneous tissue. The function of the subcutaneous layer includes fat storage, protection of internal organs, and thermoregulation.

AGE-RELATED CHANGES

The subcutaneous layer thins with age, and blood flow to the skin is decreased, making it more difficult for elders to stay warm. The loss of subcutaneous fat increases the risk of injury to the body, especially from pressure necrosis. There is a redistribution of fat that allows for the associated look of aging. Bags form under the eyes and chin (double chin); cellulite forms on thighs, stomach, and arms; and fat deposits in the abdomen. The thinner subcutaneous tissue provides less support to the other skin layers contributing to wrinkle formation.

Skin Appendages

SWEAT GLANDS

There are two types of sweat glands: eccrine and apocrine. Eccrine sweat glands, located throughout the body, are tubular structures originating in the dermis and opening on the skin surface. The sweat glands help control body temperature by sweating. The evaporation of sweat from the skin lowers body temperature. Apocrine glands are less numerous, larger, and located in the dermis. They open through hair follicles in the groin and axillary regions and secrete an oily substance that produces "body odor" when mixed with bacteria on the skin.

SEBACEOUS GLANDS

Sebaceous glands are located throughout the body except the palms of the hands and the soles and sides of the feet. The purpose of these glands is to secrete "sebum" to lubricate hair and skin with a mixture of lipids, cholesterol, wax, and triglycerides. The sebum prevents undue evaporation and heat loss in cold environments.

HAIR

Hair follicles originate in the dermis in the pilosebaceous unit. The pilosebaceous unit is made up of a hair follicle, sebaceous gland, arrector pili muscle, and an apocrine gland. Hair is keratinized and grows from the hair follicle similar to the way skin is pushed out of the epidermis (see Figure 14.1). The hair follicle bulb is nourished and maintained by a vascular network. The color of the hair is determined by melanocytes in the bulb. Located near the bulb, arrector pili muscles provide a thermoregulatory function by causing muscular contraction that wrinkles the skin, decreasing the surface area and the amount of exposed skin. These "goose bumps" reduce heat loss.

NAILS

The fingernails and toenails are hardened plates of keratinized cells made from cystine that protect the digits and facilitate dexterity. The nails grow from the floor of the nail groove or nail matrix. Like hair and skin, the nail is the end product of the dead keratinized cells pushed out from the nail matrix.

Age-Related Changes

Atrophy of sweat glands is a normal age-related change in the elderly. The loss of eccrine glands causes a decreased ability to sweat when overheated. The loss of apocrine glands contributes to decreased oil production. Though sebaceous glands increase in size, sebum and wax production is decreased causing reduced oil production; dry, scaly skin; and pruritis. Body odor decreases with age secondary to fewer apocrine glands and changes in sweat production.

With age, the number of body hair follicles declines, and there are fewer melanocytes, leading to loss and graying of body hair. In women, hair becomes coarse and more visible around the chin and upper lip. While in men, coarse hair grows from the ears, nose, and eyebrows.

With age, hair on the head becomes thinner, and hair growth slows. Atrophy of hair follicles result in baldness in men and women. Male pattern baldness around the temples and top of the head is the result of hereditary atrophy of hair follicles. Female pattern baldness occurs with a more general atrophy of follicles, resulting in thinning of hair and often making the scalp visible.

Age-related changes to the nails include decreased rate of growth. Alternating hyperplasia and hypoplasia of the nail matrix creates longitudinal ridges and thicker nail beds. The nails become thicker, more brittle, dull, opaque, and easily split, especially the toenails.

WOUND HEALING

A wound is a disruption in the continuity of cells. Wound healing begins with a trauma and ends with a scar, restoring the continuity of cells. There are two types of wounds: partial thickness and full thickness. Partial thickness wounds involve the epidermis and superficial dermis. Full thickness wounds involve the deep dermis, dermal blood vessels, and subcutaneous tissue.

Wound healing is accomplished by a complex series of overlapping events that begin with the injury and continue for days, months, or years depending on severity. The length of each phase is determined by the type of injury as well as the environment in which healing takes place. There are two types of wound healing: primary intention and secondary intention.

Primary intention occurs with partial thickness wounds. Surgical wound closure is an example of healing by primary intention. Primary intention replaces parenchymal tissue along with minimal connective scar tissue. Healing by primary intention is usually predictable.

Secondary intention wound healing is the result of a deep tissue wound that cannot be sutured. A primary wound that becomes infected may be reopened and allowed to heal by secondary intention. Secondary intention wounds heal from the inside out via granulation tissue. For surgical purposes, a health care provider may want a wound to heal by secondary intention due risk of infection or inability to close the wound. The surgeon may only close the fascia and leave the subcutaneous and other skin layers to heal by secondary intention. Secondary intention healing takes longer and requires larger amounts of connective tissue scar formation, which is not as strong or flexible as the surrounding normal skin tissue and is more susceptible to future injury. Regardless of wound type, there are four phases of wound healing: hemostasis, inflammatory, proliferative, and remodeling.

> *Wound healing is accomplished by a complex series of overlapping events that begin with the injury and continue for days, months, or years depending on severity.*

Hemostasis begins immediately with the injury and lasts until blood loss is controlled. Hemostasis consists of the vasoconstriction of blood vessels to decrease blood flow. Platelet activation and aggregation begin the clotting process. After approximately 10 minutes, the blood clot forms, and the body begins the inflammatory phase.

The inflammatory phase lasts 3 to 5 days and is critical to wound healing. This phase prepares the wound bed for healing. The inflammatory phase begins with vasodilation and increased capillary permeability. Plasma and plasma proteins leak into the surrounding area. White blood cells, neutrophils and macrophages, migrate into the wound. These white blood cells ingest bacteria and cellular debris. Macrophages release tissue growth factors that stimulate tissue regeneration, the formation of new capillaries, and attract fibroblasts.

The difference between normal wound healing and signs of infection is primarily determined by the exudates.

Clinically, the influx of plasma and white blood cells manifests as redness, warmth, and edema seen in the initial stages of wound healing. The difference between normal wound healing and signs of infection is primarily determined by the exudates. Serosanguinous drainage is normal, whereas purulent drainage represents infection.

The proliferative stage begins within 2 to 3 days of injury and lasts 2 to 4 weeks. The key cells in this phase are the fibroblasts, which produce new tissue to fill the gap left by the wound. Fibrin strands provide a framework to which the fibroblasts attach and begin to divide, stimulating the formation of collagen and glycoproteins. At the same time, capillaries surrounding the wound bed are stimulated by growth factors and begin to form new capillaries to serve the healing wound. The new capillaries and collagen fibrin network form the granulation tissue necessary for scar tissue formation.

Epithelialization occurs during the proliferative phase. Epithelialization is the migration, proliferation, and differentiation of epithelial cells from the edges of the wound into the wound bed. A new surface layer of cells, similar to those destroyed by the injury, is formed. By the end of the second week, white blood cells have migrated from the area, and edema has decreased.

The last phase, the remodeling phase, begins 3 weeks after the injury and continues until the wound is healed. During this phase, collagen is synthesized, reorganized, degraded, and stabilized, forming scar tissue. The newly differentiated epithelial cells continue to grow over the granulation tissue bed, while fibroblasts continue to produce collagen necessary for healing. Even after a year, the healed wound is not as strong as the original skin due to the decreased tensile strength of the scar tissue.

Abnormally dry skin, or xerosis, is the most common dermal problem in the elderly.

Surgical wounds are often stapled, sutured, or held together by surgical strips to approximate wound edges, allowing for healing to occur by primary intention. Carefully sutured skin has a tensile strength of 70%, which allows patients to move around without fear of wound dehiscence. Sutures or other means of wound approximation are usually discontinued within the first week to 10 days. The tensile strength of the wound is approximately 10% at the time of suture removal. The patient must be careful to avoid trauma or injury to the surgical site. Dehiscence (disruption of the wound scar) and evisceration (protrusion of wound contents) can occur if there is inadequate wound healing or injury to the wound. Wound edges may separate secondary to infection, coughing, sneezing, or edema. The risk of dehiscence or evisceration is increased in obese as well as elderly patients.

Age-Related Changes

The numerous changes in elders' skin affect wound healing: thinning and flattening of the epidermis, decreased epidermal proliferation, decreased vascularity of the dermis, loss of collagen, and compromised vascular responses. Age-related changes hinder the healing process by decreasing the influx of neutrophils and macrophages to the wound, slowing production of collagen and epithelial cells, and decreasing blood flow to new tissue being formed by the fibroblasts. Despite these changes, healthy elders often heal wounds without complications.

When age-related changes are combined with disease processes, healing can be compromised and slowed. Malnutrition and low albumin levels are a problem of the elderly, as they limit the amount of building blocks necessary for collagen synthesis. Cardiac and peripheral vascular disease decrease blood flow needed to transport white blood cells. Oxygenation, needed for cell growth, is affected by changes in circulation, pulmonary disease, and smoking.

The best opportunity for the promotion of healing in the gerioperative patient is to understand inherent risk factors. Complete assessment of the patient is essential for predicting and effectively managing barriers to wound healing. The patient should be assessed for impediments to wound healing such as poor nutrition, poor hydration, poor perfusion, poor glucose control, poor oxygenation, and risk for infection.

XEROSIS

Dry skin is a normal age-related change secondary to the decreased production of natural lipids and decreased water-binding capacity of the stratum corneum. Abnormally dry skin, or xerosis, is the most common dermal problem in the elderly. Prevalence can be as high as 85%, and by age 70, almost all individuals are affected.

Xerotic skin is dry, scaly, and can crack, forming fissures in the stratum corneum in a cracked porcelain pattern or "eczema craquele." Occurring mainly on the lower legs, the fissures can be deep enough to cause bleeding. Xerotic skin can cause intense itching, causing scratching that may lead to secondary skin lesions.

Often brought on by low humidity, xerosis is aggravated by home heating in the winter months, earning the term "winter itch." Hot showers as well as high alkaline soap and other cleansers, such as alcohol-based products, can aggravate the condition. Xerosis delays healing and increases the risk of postoperative wound infections.

Intervention

Treatment for xerosis centers on providing and maintaining hydration. A relative humidity of 60% is required to supplement hydration by the stratum corneum. Patients should be advised to use room humidifiers, especially during the winter months. Bathing in tepid water for 10 minutes allows the stratum corneum to absorb water. However, bathing or showering more than once a day can cause the skin to become drier. Soap use should be discouraged, and if soap must be used, mild cleansers are suggested. The skin must be liberally lubricated with moisturizers, which is most effective after bathing. The lipid barrier of the moisturizer seals the water against the skin allowing the keratinocytes to absorb the water. The application of petroleum jelly also helps seal moisture in the skin. Lotions containing ammonium lactate are effective, and treatment with steroid creams can be helpful in severe cases. Patients should be informed that ammonium lactate may cause mild burning with application and that sun exposure, real or artificial, should be avoided.

Chlorhexidine is a long-lasting antiseptic liquid used to disinfect patients' skin prior to surgery. Patients are often advised to take chlorhexidine showers or use chlorhexidine wipes prior to surgery. The literature is contradictory as to whether the chlorhexidine should be rinsed off, but most references advise against moisturizing skin after an application. Patients and health care workers should be aware that chlorhexidine can be very drying to the skin and aggravate xerosis. Unfortunately, there is little discussion about chlorhexidine for elderly skin in the literature. Clinical judgment would suggest that it would be reasonable to educate patients and nurses to rinse off chlorhexidine and moisturize skin after surgery. Health care workers bathing patients with chlorhexidine pre- or postoperatively should moisturize the patient's skin after the bath with a hospital-approved moisturizer that does not interfere with the action of the chlorhexidine.

PRURITIS

Pruritis, or itching, is an unpleasant sensation that creates the desire to scratch. In the elderly, pruritis can be a chronic problem with prevalence as high as 30%; it is more common in men than women. The itching can be intense and may be accompanied by pain, tingling, or burning. The itching often intensifies at night, a finding likely caused by a nocturnal rise in body temperature.

The etiology of pruritis is diverse and multifactorial. Pruritis can be the result of skin lesions or may occur without any visible signs of skin lesions. The itching can become all consuming to the point of suicidal ideations. Known causes include medication reactions, eczematous disorders, insect bites, skin infections, and neuropsychiatric disease. The most common cause of pruritis is xerosis. Other causes include underlying systemic diseases such as renal failure, diabetes, and edema of the extremities that stretches skin. Medications such as diuretics, calcium channel blockers, and nonsteroidal anti-inflammatory drugs can also cause pruritis. Many cases of pruritis are idiopathic, and the incidence with severity of idiopathic pruritis increases with age.

Interventions

Information about pruritis requires asking pertinent health history questions regarding onset, progression, provocation, precipitating event, palliation, quality, radiation, severity, timing, interventions, associated signs, and pertinent negatives. Pruritis is associated with histamine release that can exacerbate the cycle. Sudden onset of pruritis should be fully evaluated. Information related to the health history, family history, surgical and social history, medications, and review of systems is important. Physical inspection of the pruritic area may reveal chronically scratched skin that can become thickened and hyperpigmented.

The cause of pruritis may not be attainable, so treatment is provided to control symptoms. Treatment includes use of topical or oral steroids. Other treatments include antihistamines, cooling agents, lotions, and other palliative treatments.

SKIN LESIONS

The elderly develop skin lesions many of which are benign: moles, skin tags, keratoses, lentignes, and vascular lesions such as cherry angiomas, venous lakes, and telangiectasis. Lesions that are open, dry, scaly, red or dark pigmented, or uneven require closer attention. Open blistering lesions that track along a dermatome may indicate herpes zoster and should be reported to the care provider.

Gerioperative Care

PREOPERATIVE CONSIDERATIONS

During the preoperative interview, it is important to include questions about the skin. Pertinent questions of onset, progression, and timing are necessary to determine any pathologic processes that may be reflected by skin changes. The nurse should ask about any changes in the skin or chronic conditions such as pruritis, psoriasis, edema, or skin lesions. The nurse should also inquire about easy bruising or tearing of skin. During the interview process, inspection of the patient's skin color and general health can be observed. Patients that look pale may be anemic. Light-skinned, blue-eyed, or red- or blonde-haired individuals are at higher risk for cancerous lesions. While helping the patient to change into hospital garb, a quick physical inspection of exposed usually covered areas can prompt questions regarding any lesions or scars. Care must be taken regarding the patient's self-esteem, as many elderly are sensitive about skin changes and lesions.

> *Care must be taken regarding the patient's self-esteem, as many elderly are sensitive about skin changes and lesions.*

The health care provider should be informed of any new or suspicious lesions. The anesthesia team should be notified of topical or oral steroids and dose and frequency of use, as supplemental steroids may need to be administered to prevent an adrenal crisis during surgery. The anesthesia team should also be made aware of antihistamine use.

Moles, lesions, scars, or open areas should be documented preoperatively. To avoid a mole or skin lesion becoming inadvertently traumatized during surgery, the lesion should be covered with a transparent dressing. Fragile skin can be easily torn or abraded by tape used to secure dressings or intravenous lines. Minimal use of tape with skin-preserving securing devices and transparent dressing is preferred.

Record signs of edema as they may signal preexisting illness. Lower extremity edema can indicate cardiovascular or renal problems. Edema stretches the skin, increasing the risk of skin tears and abrasions.

Preoperatively, a multisystem approach enhances postoperative healing in the gerioperative patient. Providing proper nutrition is essential to wound healing. Vitamin supplements such as zinc and vitamin C have been shown to boost collagen formation, fibroblast function, and aid the immune system in resisting infection. Vitamin A is necessary to promote epithelialization and enhance macrophage function. Vitamin B is necessary for protein synthesis. Protein supplements can increase albumin levels and promote wound healing. Adequate fluid intake allows for hydration of tissues. A nutrition assessment questionnaire can assist in determining nutritional needs.

Preoperative instructions related to wound care and activity should be provided to the patient and any family members during the preoperative assessment and on the day of surgery. Instructions should be oral and written. In the event that the elder does not have anyone to assist with complex wound care, the surgeon should be notified that a home health referral may be necessary.

> *Providing proper nutrition is essential to wound healing.*

INTRAOPERATIVE CONSIDERATIONS

Elderly patients with fragile, dry, or edematous skin must be handled carefully during surgery. Moving patients from stretcher to the operating room (OR) table with a slide board can cause friction and shear injuries to the back, sacrum, and legs. Prior to moving, the lift sheet should be tight to prevent sudden pulling and shearing of skin against the sheet. Light elderly patients should be picked up with lift sheets and placed gently on the OR table.

Special care must be taken with positioning. Padding must be provided for all bony or pressure-exposed prominences to prevent pressure areas and nerve injuries. When securing the arms or legs and securing the patient to the OR table, padding must be provided under all belts and straps to prevent skin tears. Use of plastic tape to close the eyes and secure the endotracheal tube can result in skin tears, bruising, and other injury to fragile skin. The use of paper tape or securing devices is recommended. Tape or devices applied too tightly can cause edema to fragile skin, apparent only at the end of the procedure.

Elder's skin is dry and scaly. Electrocardiogram and cautery electrode pads may need to be taped in place to prevent dislodgement during the case. Thin skin and blood vessels provide little support, placing the intravenous line at higher risk of dislodging than in younger patients. The intravenous line should be secured and checked regularly as intravenous lines can infiltrate quickly and create severe damage to underlying aged tissue. The cautery electrode pad is strongly adhesive and applied to the fleshy part of the patient's body before surgery in order to decrease risk of fire or tissue damage when surgical electrocautery is needed. The pad must be carefully removed after surgery, with the area under the pad assessed and documented (i.e., no change in skin, red area noted under pad, small dime-sized area of skin removed with cautery pad, no bleeding noted, and clear dressing applied).

The loss of subcutaneous fat predisposes elders to intraoperative hypothermia (see Chapter 8). Prior to bringing elderly patients in to the OR, the room heat should be turned up to a bearable temperature. A warmed blanket or other warming device should be placed on the patient by the circulating nurse or anesthesia provider as soon as the patient is placed on the surgical table to prevent heat loss. However, due to sweat gland atrophy, overheating is a concern. Elders' skin and temperature should be checked frequently intraoperatively to maintain normothermia and assess for sweating, which creates a moist environment that predisposes elders to pressure ulcers.

The best dressing for elders to take care of is a simple dressing that requires little attention or instruction.

Special needs regarding wound care or dressing changes should be brought to the attention of the surgical team. If the patient lives alone, a longer-lasting dressing may be necessary so as not to require attention until the patient returns for the postoperative visit. The best dressing for elders to take care of is a simple dressing that requires little attention or instruction.

At the end of the procedure, care must be taken when removing any devices affixed to the patient as well as the surgical drapes. Elders' epidermis is fragile and can easily peel off or tear as a result of pulling or pushing on the skin. The patient's skin should be assessed after surgery to ensure that red areas, abrasions, or skin tears have not occurred. Bony prominences are extremely vulnerable, especially after a long procedure on the OR table, and should receive careful scrutiny. Any difference in skin condition from the preoperative assessment requires documentation. The patient should be moved gently to the hospital bed or stretcher, with care to avoid friction or shear injuries.

POSTOPERATIVE CONSIDERATIONS

Wound Care

Postoperatively, the wound and surrounding areas must be assessed on a regular basis. The choice of surgical dressing and wound care considers the type of surgical wound, type of healing (primary or secondary intention), and the ability of the patient to change the dressing. The size of the dressing should be kept to a minimum to prevent secondary harm to the wound from pressure. Tape should be kept to a minimum to prevent skin tears. There are many types of tape; one should be chosen that will cause the least trauma. The patient should be taught not to stretch the tape to secure it "better," as this can cause shearing injury to the skin. The patient should be educated about surgical strips and how to care for them. Clear dressings and surgical strips can be left on until they "fall off." However, due to dry, scaly skin, the patient should be coached that the dressing or surgical strips may fall off too soon. If this occurs and the incision appears open in areas, the patient should inform the surgeon.

The role of the gerioperative care nurse includes determining whether the patient or care provider has any questions regarding postoperative nutrition, wound, or skin care. The gerioperative care nurse should assess whether the patient or caregiver is able to provide dressing changes and adequate wound care, including wound inspection and cleaning. If it is determined that adequate wound care cannot be performed due to changes in eyesight, range of motion, or other factors, the nurse should inform the health care provider to ensure closer postoperative follow-up. A home health care referral for wound care may also be necessary.

Pressure Ulcers

Surgical pressure ulcers are created by trauma from mechanical forces exerted to or on the skin. The forces of pressure, friction, and shearing can lead to direct or ischemic tissue damage. Pressure ulcers that develop in surgical patients have a more complex etiology and may present differently than pressure ulcers occurring in medical patients. During surgery, circulatory and metabolic changes result in decreased oxygenation. Tissue nutrient delivery, as well as metabolic waste removal, is reduced. Combined with decreased blood pressure and unrelieved pressure due to surgical immobility, surgical pressure compresses superficial tissue between a hard surface and bony prominences. The pressure is exacerbated by muscle relaxants that remove the natural muscle tension that supports the bone.

Development of pressure ulcers during surgery is influenced by the patient's position, the duration of pressure, and the hardness of the surface. The OR table has a thin mattress and a hard surface. The body weight is distributed over a small surface area, resulting in a high interface pressure. Pressure ulcers may occur anywhere on the body. However, the heels, elbows, and sacrum are particularly vulnerable. Different body areas become more susceptible depending on surgical position (see Chapter 8). Equipment, such as Kraus arm rests and sand bags used to position patients, adds additional pressure points and must be thoroughly padded.

Intraoperative pressure ulcers usually develop deep in the muscle tissue layer and progress outward. The ulcer presents as a burn-like lesion or erythema that undergoes ecchymotic changes and may blister or become necrotic. Ulcers caused intraoperatively may not become apparent for 3 to 5 days after surgery, making the etiology of the lesion difficult to identify postoperatively.

The gerioperative population is particularly vulnerable to pressure ulcers secondary to normal age-related changes in the skin as well as comorbidities, medications, and nutritional changes.

Some ulcers may present as a stage 1 or 2 pressure ulcer and are noticed immediately after surgery. These ulcers may soon progress to stage 3 or 4 secondary to reperfusion damage. Reperfusion damage occurs when blood flow is returned to an area of ischemia and occurs in cells that are viable when reperfusion starts. Damage may be due to superoxide anions formed when oxygen is returned to muscle tissue deprived of oxygen for a period of time. The superoxide anion causes damage to capillaries and infiltration of neutrophils (Schouchoff, 2002).

The gerioperative population is particularly vulnerable to pressure ulcers secondary to normal age-related changes in the skin as well as comorbidities, medications, and nutritional changes. Diabetes and peripheral vascular disease cause blood vessel changes that decrease blood supply to tissues, increasing the risk of pressure ulcers. Medications such as corticosteroids cause thinning of the skin, which increases the risk of skin tears. The changes in elastin and collagen cause stiffening of tissue and decreased pressure resistance. Less sub-cutaneous fat combined with decreased muscle tone and slower regeneration of skin cells predispose elders to pressure. Body rinses such as chlorhexidine are drying and may exacer-bate skin problems.

In an elderly patient already compromised by risk factors, nutritional deficits can further predispose to pressure ulcers during the perioperative period. Several days prior to the pro-cedure, the patient's nutritional intake can be altered secondary to testing or blood work. After surgery, nutritional intake decreases secondary to anorexia and the stress of surgery.

In addition to age-related changes, risk factors for perioperative pressure ulcer forma-tion have been identified. Factors that increase risk include patient physical condition, length of surgery, intraoperative hypotension, American Society of Anesthesiologists classification of 3 or greater, and body habitus (see Exhibit 14.1). Research is needed to identify effective strategies to prevent perioperative pressure ulcers.

Prevention of pressure ulcer development during surgery is focused on risk assessment and pressure relief. Several tools are available to assess risk for potential development of pres-sure ulcers in medical patients such as the Norton scale and the Braden scale. However, these tools have not been validated for use in perioperative patients. A perioperative risk assess-ment for the gerioperative patient should include the variables identified in Exhibit 14.2 in addition to blood pressure, anticipated length of surgery, body positioning requirements, medications, and Ameri-can Society of Anesthesiologists classification.

Shearing forces and friction occur from improper handling of patients, poor positioning, poor lifting techniques, and moisture from perspiration, urine, or skin preparation solutions.

As part of a pressure ulcer risk assessment proto-col, every gerioperative patient should have a full body assessment prior to surgery. Many elders live alone or have mobility issues that prevent independent skin inspection. Denial is a powerful force, and many individuals may have skin issues that require attention but have been ignored.

A study by Schoonhoven et al. (2002) found length of surgery to be the only reliable risk indicator for pressure ulcer development. Becuase the length of surgery can only be predicted, not determined, the focus of pressure ulcer prevention should concentrate on decreasing pressure and shearing forces applied during surgery. Heels are the most often

---

EXHIBIT 14.1 Preoperative Risk Factors for Pressure Ulcers During Surgery

- General physical condition
- Altered mental status
- Type and length of surgery
- Hydration
- Nutritional status
- Age > 65
- Moisture on the skin
- Infection
- Immobility

- Incontinence
- Use of body preparation solution (chlorhexidine)
- History of diabetes, peripheral vascular disease
- Previous pressure damage
- Hypotension
- Body habitus

- Hemoglobin < 10
- Comorbidities (American Society of Anesthesiologists 3 or greater)
- Low serum albumin < 3.5
- Pressure
- Shear
- Friction
- Extremes of weight

EXHIBIT 14.2 **Intraoperative Factors for Pressure Ulcer Risk**

- Duration of surgery
- Surgical position
- Type of mattress
- Positioning devices
- Warming devices
- Epidural anesthesia/analgesia
- Anesthetic agents
- Type of surgery
- Extracorporeal circulation
- Inappropriate manual handling
- Hypotension

cited areas for pressure ulcers. The use of pressure-reducing mattresses and pressure-reducing positions when placing the patient on the OR table can reduce the incidence of pressure ulcers.

In order to decrease pressure to heels during the perioperative period, the Agency for Health Care Policy and Research advises that heels be kept off the OR table. By placing a pillow under the length of the lower leg, the leg is supported while leaving the heel free. Heel protectors may help reduce pressure in instances where pressure to the heels occurs over long periods as a result of the lower leg not being able to be elevated. Other nursing interventions include placement of transparent dressings over bony prominences to prevent friction and shearing, protection of pressure-sensitive areas during positioning, and correct use of positioning aids such as stirrups for lithotomy position (Exhibit 14.3).

During the postoperative period, constant vigilance is necessary. Schoonhoven et al. (2002) noted that most stage 1 pressure ulcers are not identified postoperatively. Instead, atypical lesions are noted but not considered pressure ulcers as they do not fit the pressure ulcer staging definitions.

Pressure ulcer development is assessed during the immediate postoperative period to determine the effects of immobility, direct pressure to bony prominences, shear forces, and friction. Shearing forces and friction occur from improper handling of patients, poor positioning, poor lifting techniques, and moisture from perspiration, urine, or skin preparation

EXHIBIT 14.3 **Nursing Interventions to Prevent Intraoperative Pressure Ulcers**

- Transparent dressings over bony prominences
- Elevation of heels
- Maintain proper body alignment
- Correct positioning
- Cushion pressure-sensitive areas when positioning
- Minimize skin exposure to moisture
- Avoid pooling of solutions
- Proper handling, moving, and transferring
- Appropriate use of positioning aids
- Alleviate pressure on nerves to avoid nerve injury
- Prevent leaning on patient by surgical team
- Dry wrinkle-free linen surface

solutions. These ulcers do not heal easily and take longer to heal than the surgical wound. In the event that a pressure ulcer heals, the risk of recurrence is high due to poor tensile strength and revascularization.

Postoperatively, prevention of pressure ulcers requires vigilance and a multidisciplinary approach. Frequent turning, moving, and ambulation can reduce the risk of postoperative pressure ulcer development. Keeping patients clean and dry and the skin well hydrated with emollients can keep skin supple and less prone to shearing. Special padding for mattresses and chairs helps to reduce pressure as does proper positioning. Adequate nutrition is essential for prevention and treatment of pressure ulcers. Physical therapy, nursing, nutritionists, and the primary provider must work together to ensure the best possible care and outcomes for gerioperative surgical patients. In the event a pressure ulcer develops, early referral to wound care is imperative.

Healing pressure ulcers is a long, expensive, and debilitating patient experience. The cost of pressure ulcer treatment can vary from $14,000 to $40,000. The hospital length of stay can increase as much as 7 days. Preventing pressure ulcers is a preferred alternative to attempting to heal pressure ulcers. The list of negative outcomes from pressure ulcers is long: pain, depression, anxiety, low self-esteem, multiple surgeries, disfigurement, increased length of stay, loss of income, and increased cost of care. Gerioperative patients are at increased risk of morbidity and mortality from pressure ulcers. More research is necessary to identify risk factors for surgical patients and methods to prevent pressure ulcers in the perioperative period.

> *Pain sensations are diminished, so pain may not alert the patient that there is a problem.*

SURGICAL SITE INFECTIONS

Surgical site infections (SSIs) can increase morbidity and mortality in the gerioperative patient. Eleven percent of nosocomial infections in the elderly are surgical wound infections. Several studies have shown that SSIs in elderly patients can reduce physical and social functioning, increase mortality, double the rehospitalization risk, increase the length of stay up to 2 weeks, and can increase health care costs by 300%.

The most common organism responsible for SSI in the gerioperative patient appears to be methicillin-resistant *Staphylococcus aureus* (MRSA). The prevalence of MRSA has increased 20%. Routine surgical antibiotic prophylaxis protocols do not cover MRSA. Chen et al. (2010) identified that the risk of SSI was highest among elders that lacked independence in three or more activities of daily living, specifically a lack of independence with bathing and/or dressing. Interestingly, these patients were not from long-term care facilities. Screening all gerioperative patients for MRSA may be of benefit in preventing MRSA wound infections. The correlation between increased MRSA infection and age requires additional study.

Wound infections and infections in general present differently in the elderly, leading to delays in diagnosis. Gerioperative patients exhibit lower body temperatures rather than fever, with few outward signs of infection. Pain sensations are diminished, so pain may not alert the patient that there is a problem. Eyesight in the elderly is altered and, along with a lack of mobility, the gerioperative patient may not be able to see changes or recognize the lack of healing. The usual signs of purulent exudate or redness may not be apparent.

The first sign of infection in the elderly may be confusion and falling. These signs are often overlooked or misinterpreted as stroke- or age-related dementia. When gerioperative patients present with confusion or falls, it is essential for nurses and caregivers to adequately assess elderly individuals for any infectious processes. In the postoperative period, common sites of infection are the wound and the respiratory and urinary tracts.

INTERVENTIONS

Nurses can provide elders and their caregivers with information to improve skin care. Frequent bathing or showering in the elderly washes away natural oils that moisturize and protect the skin. Less frequent bathing or bathing without the use of harsh soaps allows body oils to keep the skin more supple. Mild cleansers with moisturizers are preferred. Using warm rather than hot water prevents drying of the skin. The use of rough washcloths when bathing or showering damages thin skin. Wash cloths and towels should be soft and nonabrasive.

After bathing or showering, application of a skin moisturizer before drying the skin is recommended. Emollients should be applied liberally and in the direction of hair growth. If skin must be dried, patting rather than rubbing the skin dry is recommend. Rashes to inguinal and skin fold areas can be prevented by daily washing and drying completely by patting with a highly absorbent soft towel. Small amounts of powder applied to thoroughly dried areas can prevent moisture. Only small amounts of powder should be applied to prevent balling up of the excess powder that may rub and irritate the skin.

Surgical wounds will not heal if nutrition and hydration are inadequate.

If a rash is noted, patients should be instructed to consult a provider and use an antifungal powder rather than talcum or cornstarch. Patients with diabetes are prone to *Candida* rashes in the genital areas and under breasts. These are made worse with cornstarch powders, as yeast feeds on the cornstarch.

Gerioperative foot care is important as elders are more prone to corns, calluses, dry skin, fungal infection, blisters, bunions, and thick, rough toenails. Regular podiatry appointments for routine foot care and trimming of the nails are recommended. Patient education regarding foot care should include wearing comfortable shoes at all times, even in the house. The feet should be washed and dried daily, especially between the toes. The patient should be instructed to thoroughly rub moisturizer into the feet, except between the toes.

Good nutrition and hydration are imperative to promote healthy skin and wound healing. The patient should be educated throughout the perioperative period about proper nutrition and hydration. Adequate protein, vitamins, and minerals enhance the skin's ability to maintain and repair itself. Sufficient hydration keeps skin moist to promote wound healing. If the patient has a low albumin level or appears malnourished or dehydrated, a nutritional consult should be ordered. Surgical wounds will not heal if nutrition and hydration are inadequate.

PATIENT REPORT: Mr. Kilty

Mr. Kilty's hip replacement surgery takes 3 hours. In the OR, he is positioned on his left side and is supported by positional aids. No areas of pressure were noted before surgery began. During hip replacement, the surgeon frequently pulled on the leg to manipulate the joint, causing the patient's body to shift. At the end of surgery, the nurse anesthetist notices a reddened area on the left bicep, where the Kraus arm rest applied pressure. Mr. Kilty's blood pressure was stable during surgery, but at times, it dipped below 100 systolic. In the postanesthesia care unit, he complains of burning in his arm. The postanesthesia care unit nurse notes a darkened area on the left bicep and notifies the surgeon. A consult is entered for the wound service. Mr. Kilty has multiple risk factors for a perioperative pressure ulcer. His risk factors include pre-diabetes, age, smoking history, and possible protein deficiency due to alcohol ingestion. Intraoperative repositioning, length of surgery, and blood pressure contributed to his risk. Despite attention to positioning and padding, the patient can shift during surgical manipulation. Gerioperative care requires careful assessment throughout the perioperative course and immediate intervention.

SUMMARY

Although rarely fatal, changes in the skin are responsible for significant morbidity and impacts elders' quality of life. Emotional, psychological, and physical responses may accompany changes in skin conditions before, during, and after surgery. The nurse must be aware of age-related changes to elders' skin and how these changes affect the patient emotionally, physically, and spiritually, and should implement interventions to prevent complications. In the event that complications occur, the nurse must immediately implement interventions to decrease the risk of more severe complications.

KEY POINTS

- The skin plays a very important role in human socialization. Because of this, many elders may be sensitive about their appearance.
- The skin is a window into the body. The nurse can identify many health issues, such as smoking and sun exposure, by examining the gerioperative patient's skin.
- The decreased number of nerve endings in the skin can predispose the elderly to injury.
- When age-related changes are combined with disease processes, healing can be delayed or compromised.
- The best opportunity for the promotion of wound healing in the gerioperative patient is to identify and understand the risk factors that can interfere with healing and provide adequate intervention.
- Prevention of pressure ulcer development during surgery is focused on assessment and intervention.
- Wound infections and infections in general present differently in the elderly.
- Good nutrition and hydration are imperative to healthy skin and wound healing.

FIFTEEN

Gastrointestinal

Susan J. Fetzer, Jennifer V. Long, and Raelene V. Shippee-Rice

PATIENT REPORT: Ms. Stine

Ms. Stine is an 81-year-old active widowed senior admitted for a small bowel obstruction. She is generally healthy and takes no prescription medication. She attributes her healthy state to a positive attitude, regular use of vitamin C and D, and calcium. She is 64 inches and weighs 130 lbs. She denies any recent weight loss. She prepares her own meals and does her own shopping using a van service for older adults. She takes omeprazole as needed and admits to a history of peptic ulcers when she was 55. She is concerned about the surgery because of her age. She feels well generally but states "I'm not as young as I used to be." She feels there is a difference in the way she responds to "things" that started about 4 months ago. "I just don't have the same energy."

During surgery, a carcinoid tumor of the ileum with metastasis to the liver was identified, and a palliative approach was determined as the best choice for Ms. Stine's quality of life. Within the first 36 hours after returning to the surgical floor, Ms. Stine develops an ileus with bloating and significant abdominal discomfort.

The gastrointestinal system processes food; absorbs nutrients, minerals, vitamins, and water; excretes byproducts; and manufactures hormones, vitamins, and substances needed for organ function. The gastrointestinal system shown in Figure 15.1 includes the functional system of the mouth, esophagus, stomach, intestines, and rectum, as well as the endocrine organs of the pancreas, liver, and gallbladder.

Gastrointestinal Considerations

The salivary glands, teeth, and tongue, along with muscles of mastication prepare the food bolus for digestion. Over 1 L of saliva is secreted by three sets of salivary glands each day: parotid, submaxillary, and sublingular. Secretion is controlled by the autonomic nervous system in response to smell, thought, or sight of food, as well as any food or irritating substance in the mouth. Saliva is composed of primarily of water (95%), mucous, electrolytes, enzymes,

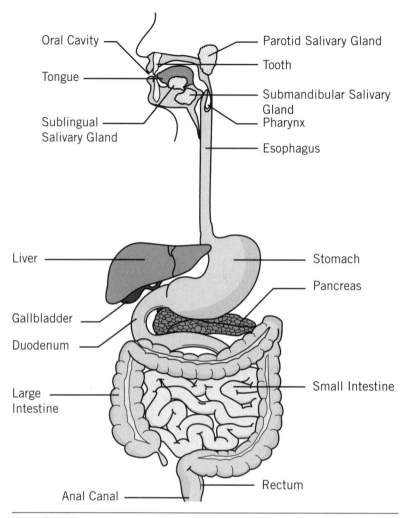

FIGURE 15.1
Gastrointestinal System

and water. Three important enzymes in saliva are amalyse to begin the breakdown of starches, lipase to begin the breakdown of fats, and lysozyme, which lyses bacteria and prevents the overgrowth of oral microbes. The mucous offers a protective barrier and lubricating function. Mucous turns the chewed food into a slippery bolus that can easily slide down the esophagus. Electrolytes result in a slightly acidic salivary pH at rest between 6.3 and 6.8.

A tooth is composed of two minerals: the enamel that covers the crown and the dentine that comprises the inner core and root of the tooth (see Figure 15.2A). The dentin is produced by the underlying pulp. The pulp is rich with blood vessels and nerve fibers. Enamel can withstand pH changes in the mouth as low as 5.5 without becoming demineralized. Dentin has a critical pH of 6.0. When oral bacteria come in contact with refined carbohydrates (sugar), acids are produced as a byproduct of metabolism. These acids can drop the pH below 5.5 and begin demineralizing tooth enamel. The presence of saliva acts as a defense mechanism by neutralizing the demineralizing acid. The enamel can be remineralized after an acid attack, but saliva is required. However, the production of saliva is virtually stopped when sleeping.

The muscular tongue functions to move food around where it can be best broken down by the teeth. When fully chewed, the tongue propels the food bolus to the back of the oral cavity for swallowing. In addition to being required for speech, the tongue also is the organ of taste. Small structures on the upper side of the tongue called papillae contain taste receptor cells for sweet, salty, bitter, sour, and savory substances. The receptor information is sent to the gustatory areas of the brain via the cranial nerves. The substance must be dissolved in saliva for the receptor cells to perceive a taste.

Four muscles of mastication connect the mandibular bone to the skull. These muscles act to open and close the jaw, provide side to side movement, and protrude or retrude the chin. The mandibular nerve is a branch of the trigeminal nerve.

Age-Related Changes

The composition of the salivary glands changes with age. The secretary cells are replaced with fatty and fibrous tissue. However, under normal conditions the glands are able to maintain salivary flow because of their vast reserve capacity.

Xerostomia or dry mouth is a common complaint of older adults and is reported in nearly 15% of all elders and 45% of institutionalized elders. Side effects of more than 500 over-the-counter and prescription drugs are the most common cause of dry mouth, in addition to poor hydration. Xerostomia results in difficulty chewing, tasting, and swallowing food. Speech can also be impaired by a dry mouth.

Taste receptors do not change with age, yet elders often report a diminished sense of taste and a less intense stimulation. With age, the ability to differentiate between taste qualities decreases, particularly with salty, bitter, and sour tastes. The decline in salivation, due to polypharmacy, results in an increased taste threshold for sodium (11 times normal), bitter (7 times normal), and sour (4 times normal). As a result, it is not uncommon for elders to oversalt their food or select foods that are overbitter or oversour.

DENTURES

While advances in dental care and prevention of disease have resulted in greater tooth retention among elders, over 60% of elders are edentulous among some populations. Over a quarter of patients aged 65 to 74 are without teeth, with the number nearly doubling for those over 75 years of age. Ninety percent of edentulous individuals wear dentures. However, dentures are not fitted for life. As the boney structure and muscle structure of the oral cavity changes, dentures can become ill fitting. It is estimated that 30% of elders have oral lesions from poorly fitting dentures. Chewing efficiency is nearly 75% lower in denture wearers.

Poorly fitting dentures cause oral lesions in 30% of elders.

Taste buds normally reproduce every 10 days in healthy adults. With aging, the renewal is slower. Decreases in zinc and body protein can prolong taste bud regeneration. Loss of sensation on the lateral tongue and floor of the mouth with aging may be related to the prolongation of the oral phase of swallowing in healthy elderly people. Smell is just as important as taste in influencing food preferences. As the number of nerve receptors in the roof of the nasal cavity declines with age, olfactory acuity declines. Older adults have less discriminatory ability of food odors. Aging affects the sense of smell greater than the sense of taste (see Chapter 11).

Chewing efficiency is nearly 75% lower in denture wearers.

With age, the soft tissue of the gums recedes, exposing the tooth root and dentine (Figure 15.2B). Enamel is worn with time allowing the underlying yellowish dentine to show through. Teeth tend to darken with age. Dental caries occur during the first three decades and periodontal disease occurs through the fifth decade; in elders, tooth decay again becomes the major reason for dental loss. The decay occurs at the edges of previously restored cavities or crowns and on the surfaces of the tooth exposed by the receding gums.

As the volume of dental pulp decreases with age, the nerves within the pulp decrease in size and number. Elders have a decreased sensitivity to dental pain and temperature. Damage has already occurred when elders seek help, usually from food that sticks between receding gums or a fractured tooth that lacerates the tongue. Elders may have advanced caries with drainage, swelling, fever, and swallowing discomfort and may not be able to relate their symptoms to dental problems. The decrease in dental pulp also makes the teeth more brittle and at risk for fractures.

Gingival recession contributes to elders' caries at the base of the tooth where enamel does not cover the dentin, leading to increased sensitivity. More than 85% of people over 65 have

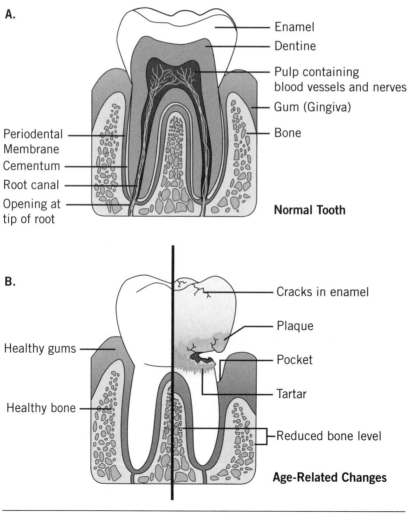

FIGURE 15.2
Age-Related Changes in Teeth, Bone, and Gums

moderate to severe gum recession. The unprotected roots are prone to caries. Gaps at the base of the teeth form when the gum recedes, trapping food particles. Caries in these areas are common among elders. Xerostomia further contributes to caries production as saliva is not available to neutralize bacterial acids. Finally, the ability to perform self-oral hygiene declines with age. As the gum changes, it is more difficult to clean some areas, creating a greater risk for caries. It has been estimated that a quarter of all elders have root caries; the estimate jumps to 80% in institutionalized elders.

Aging reduces the muscle mass of the muscles of mastication, which is even more pronounced among edentulous elders. Contractions of the muscles are less precise and less efficient. Combined with the loss of teeth and decline in salivation, the food bolus contains coarser particles prior to swallowing. In response, elders develop preferences for smooth, moist, and slippery textured foods rather than hard, crunchy, or fibrous substances. With few teeth, diets become low in fruit and vegetables and higher in fat. Food preparation changes as elders prefer cooked processed vegetables to raw items. Changes in the oral cavity with age can affect quality of life as well as nutrition.

SWALLOWING

Once food has undergone physical and chemical changes, the tongue squeezes against the palate and generates a wave that propels the bolus to the pharynx. The muscular upper esophageal sphincter (UES) opens, the larynx is sealed off with the epiglottis, and the slippery food bolus enters the esophagus. The smooth muscles of the UES contract behind the bolus, and the peristaltic wave of contractions moves the contents toward the stomach. The primary wave takes 5 to 8 seconds. If the food bolus is large or sticky and not passed by the primary wave, the distended esophagus stimulates salivation for more lubrication and initiates a second more forceful peristaltic wave. The lower esophageal sphincter (LES) reflexively relaxes and allows food to pass to the stomach.

Age-Related Changes

The duration of the swallowing sequence increases with age. The time required to chew and the number of chewing strokes needed to achieve the same level of food maceration increase with age. As the number of teeth decline, the number of strokes increases. The age-related loss of muscle function, chewing inefficiency, and reduced salivation results in a drier food bolus. In addition, the food bolus is not propelled to the pharynx with as much force.

Dysphagia, or difficulty swallowing, occurs in an estimated 15% of community-dwelling elders and up to 40% of institutional elders. However, dysphagia is not a result of normal age-related change. Swallowing difficulties in the elderly occur as a result of age-associated diseases such as stroke, Parkinson's disease, and myasthenia gravis. Up to two-thirds of elders have a decreased UES pressure, but it is usually not symptomatic. The UES of elders has a longer relaxation phase after swallowing, potentially exposing the pulmonary tree to aspiration. There also appears to be a positive relationship between impaired chewing ability and the frequency of aspiration.

Esophageal peristalsis decreases in both amplitude and duration with age. Secondary peristalsis to clear substances from the esophagus is also diminished. Diabetes further increases the likelihood of abnormal motility. The delayed esophageal transit is of concern for elders taking oral medications. Medications can become "stuck," dissolve in place, and result in mucosal damage. Capsules have a slower transit time than tablets. Particularly damaging are potassium supplements, tetracycline, doxycycline, quinidine, aspirin, nonsteroidal anti-inflammatory drugs, and ferrous sulfate.

The incidence of a hiatal hernia increases with age from less than 10% under age 40 to 40% under age 70 and as much as 70% after age 70. The hernia results in a less competent LES, which predisposes elders to gastroesophageal reflux disease (GERD). When GERD is diagnosed in elders it is usually more severe, though symptoms are milder. It appears that esophageal sensitivity to acid declines with age. Therefore, acid reflux may not result in heartburn. Nausea, vague chest discomfort, and regurgitation are more prevalent symptoms along with chronic cough and hoarseness. Proton pump inhibitors are just as effective for elders in treating the symptoms of GERD.

Acid reflux causes vague chest discomfort, chronic cough, and hoarseness.

STOMACH

The stomach serves as the short-term holding area for swallowed food boluses. Once the food bolus enters the stomach, enzymatic digestion of proteins is initiated. The muscular folds of the stomach mix and grind the boluses with the gastric secretions, resulting in a liquid called chyme. The chyme is slowly release into the duodenum of the small intestine through the pyloric valve. Secretory epithelial cells cover the surface of the stomach. Mucous cells protect the stomach lining against shear stress and acid by secreting an alkaline mucus.

Parietal cells secrete hydrochloric acid, killing most bacteria from the food bolus and activating pepsinogen. The secreted acid has a pH of 0.8. Secretion, however, requires active transport of ions in the form of a "proton pump." Administering proton pump inhibitors blocks acid secretion by parietal cells. Parietal cell secretion is stimulated by several substances including the hormone gastrin and histamine. The parietal cell receptor for histamine is the H2 type. Administering H2 blockers will decrease stimulation of parietal cell secretion of acid. The parietal cells also secrete intrinsic factor, a protein necessary for the absorption of vitamin B_{12} in the intestine. Chief cells secrete pepsinogen, the precursor of pepsin, the enzyme that breaks down proteins. The gastric cells also secrete hormones into the blood, most importantly gastrin. Gastrin stimulates acid secretion by the parietal cells and stimulates mucosal cell development.

The pH of gastric acid in healthy adults is usually below a pH of 4, an environment that kills enteric organisms and renders the stomach sterile. At a ph from 4 to 5, salivary bacteria survive in the stomach, and a pH over 5 allows viral, protozoan, and bacterial pathogens to exist. Drugs used to decrease acid production or neutralize acid such as H2 blockers, antacids, and proton pump inhibitors create an environment conducive to the growth of microflora. Overgrowth of microflora contributes to diarrhea. An example is the use of H2 blockers as a risk factor for *Clostridium difficile* infection.

The volume and composition of gastric contents determine the rate at which the stomach empties. After a solid meal, the stomach actively mixes and digests for 20 to 30 minutes, emptying then occurs with 50% of the stomach contents being passed to the intestine over the next 3 hours. On average, there is total emptying of the stomach in 4 to 5 hours. Clear liquids, such as water, immediately begin to empty out of the stomach. The larger the volume, the faster the stomach empties. If the fluid is hypertonic or acidic and contains protein (such as milk), the rate of stomach emptying is slower. Strong peristaltic waves move the chyme toward the pylorus, creating a pressure that forces liquids through the pylorus in spurts.

When larger solids are propelled toward the pylorus, they are refluxed back until they are reduce to a diameter of less than 1 to 2 mm and able to pass through to the duodenum of the small intestine.

Vomiting occurs when gastric contents are propelled back through the esophagus and out of the mouth. A highly coordinated series of events are in place during the act of emesis. First, the glottis closes, and the larynx is raised to open the UES. Simultaneously, the soft palate rises to close off the opening to the nares. The diaphragm contracts, creating a negative thoracic pressure. The negative pressure serves to open the LES to the esophagus. With the diaphragm contracted, the abdominal muscles vigorously contract applying external pressure to the stomach. The stomach is squeezed, elevating pressure inside the stomach, which is higher than the open esophagus, and the contents are expelled.

Vomiting is controlled external to the stomach in two areas of the brain. The vomiting center of the medulla receives afferent signals from at least four major sources. Afferent impulses from the vagus and sympathetic nerve inform the brain of gastrointestinal distention and mucosal irritation from toxic substances such a blood. Distention is a potent stimulus for vomiting. Outside the stomach, impulses from the bile duct (as in gallbladder disease), the peritoneum (as in appendicitis), the heart (as in vomiting during a coronary event), and other organs send signals to the brain. Signals from within the brain can trigger vomiting. Psychic stimuli such as fear, odors, vestibular disturbances (motion sickness), and cerebral trauma can send signals to the vomiting center. Finally, a significant influence on the vomiting center comes from the chemoreceptor trigger zone (CTZ). The CTZ, located in the brainstem under the fourth ventricle, is sensitive to emetic drugs and substances in the blood such as uremia, hypoxia, and high blood sugars. When stimulated, the CTZ sends a powerful message to the vomiting center to initiate retrograde stomach emptying. Antiemetic drugs such as dexamethasone, which act at the level of the CTZ, are effective in reducing the risk of vomiting.

Age-Related Changes

Aging affects the ability of all smooth muscle to contract effectively, and the stomach is a smooth muscle. Age is associated with alterations in both the secretory and motor activities of the stomach.

Gastric acid production, both at rest and with eating, declines. Achlorhydria occurs in up to 20% of elders over 60 years. Aging also increases the stomach's vulnerability to mucosal damage. Decreased mucosal blood flow and mucous production impair the barrier function of the stomach lining. Elders' stomachs are more vulnerable to gastric ulcers despite the decline in gastric acid.

Gastritis occurs when the mucosal layer of the stomach becomes inflamed. Cell injury occurs with submucosal hemorrhage and edema followed by regeneration. Infection with the organism *Heliobacter pylori* is responsible for most cases. The organism attaches to the mucous-producing cells of the stomach and alters cells' structure, creating an inflammatory response and ultimately cell death. As the secretory glands are destroyed, they are replaced with atrophic mucosa cells with impaired secretory activity. Atrophic gastritis results in a decrease in acid production, low gastrin levels, lower levels of intrinsic factor, which can lead to anemia, and an increase in stomach pH. Iron and calcium require the acidifying effects of gastric acid to be kept soluble and absorbable. Thus, atrophic gastritis can result in lower levels of these key nutrients. Up to a quarter of all elders have atrophic gastritis, which can be asymptomatic.

Infection with *H. pylori* has been strongly linked to peptic ulcer and gastric cancer. The prevalence of *H. pylori* increases with advancing age. The increase in the infection duration of *H. pylori* and long-term use of medications that can injure the mucosal lining, particularly nonsteroidal anti-inflammatory drugs, thus contributing to the higher incidence of ulcers among elders. The classic peptic ulcer symptom of burning epigastric pain are muted or absent in older adults. One-third of elders hospitalized for peptic ulcers will deny pain. As a result, bleeding and perforation are more frequent, yielding a higher mortality rate in patients over age 65.

Healthy aging is associated with a slowing of gastric emptying of solids and nutritional liquids. The stomach is slower to distend with meals, leading to earlier sensation of fullness, or satiation. Delayed emptying leads to nausea and bloating, thus decreasing appetite and intake. Gastric distention is longer and the expulsion of chyme through the pylorus takes more time.

Among elders, blood pressure can drop significantly after meals as a result of blood flow shunting to the splenic circulation to promote nutrient absorption. Postprandial hypotension can lead to syncope and falls.

SMALL INTESTINE

The three segments of the small intestine, the duodenum, jejunum, and ileum, are responsible for the final stages of enzymatic digestion, liberating nutrients small enough to be absorbed. The vast absorptive surface area of the small intestine, approximately 250 m^2, is made possible by circular mucosal folds, projections of villi into the lumen, and microvilli on the endothelial surface of the villi. The endothelial surface is the site of absorption and secretion.

Motility of the small intestine is an important defense mechanism against pathogens and harmful substances. Motility is managed by migrating myoelectric complexes that stimulate peristalsis. Alternating periods of rest with bursts of intense contractions propel the intestinal contents while removing the mucous layer, which is continuously being replaced. When the migrating myoelectric complex is abolished by drugs such as morphine, peristalsis ceases and bacterial overgrowth will occur within 6 to 15 hours.

Age-Related Changes

Only minor changes occur in the small intestine during aging, partly due to its large reserve capacity. Motility, transit, and absorption maintain their ability to provide the body with most of the nutrients, water, and electrolyte balance. However, even in healthy elders, calcium absorption declines with age. Healthy women over 75 years have over a 25% decrease in calcium absorption. When older adults are given a low-calcium diet, they are less able to adapt by increasing calcium absorption. Vitamin D absorption is impaired as well as the absorption of zinc. Vitamin B$_{12}$ deficiency, found in 10% to 15% of elders, occurs due to the lack of intrinsic factor, a substance that is unable to be secreted by atrophic stomach mucosa.

With age, specific enzymes secreted by the intestinal villa decline. Lactase, the enzyme that breaks down lactose into glucose, is reduced resulting in lactose intolerance. While healthy elders have no difficulty digesting protein or fat, they cannot tolerate massive intakes of either substance as well as younger adults.

Proton pump inhibitors promote overgrowth of bacteria.

Among elders, *H. pylori* is most likely to result in peptic ulcers; however, duodenal ulcers can also be prevalent. Treatment for *H. pylori* and gastritis can alter the environment of the intestine. In healthy elders, the small intestine is normally sterile. However, bacterial overgrowth is common due to acid-base alterations secondary to coexisting illness and diabetes. Acid-reducing drugs such as proton pump inhibitors also alter the intestinal environment. The bacterial overgrowth results in poor absorption, pain, bloating, diarrhea, and eventually malnutrition with weight loss.

LARGE INTESTINE

The large intestine includes the appendix, colon, and rectum. The colon continues the work of water and electrolyte reabsorption, though 90% of the water has been removed by the small intestine. While the stomach and small intestine are typically sterile, the colon harbors over 500 species of anaerobic bacteria adhering to the mucosa. Adherence to the colonic mucosa avoids eviction during evacuation and prohibits new organisms from gaining occupancy. Enzymatic activity by the bacteria allows for the digestion of carbohydrates not completed by the small intestine. As the human body does not have cellulase, an enzyme to break down cellulose, bacterial action accomplishes this task. The major byproducts of bacterial action on carbohydrates and cellulose are methane, hydrogen, and carbon dioxide, all components of intestinal flatus. A critical product of colon bacteria is the synthesis of vitamin K. The breakdown of bilirubin by colonic bacteria gives feces its brown color.

Overgrowth of bacteria promotes C. difficile diarrhea and synthesis of vitamin K.

Large intestine motility is compromised of segmental contractions, antiperistaltic waves forcing the contents back toward the ileum for additional digestion and absorption to occur, and mass movements. Mass movements are intense, sustained peristaltic movements that clear an area of colon.

Rectal smooth muscle near the anus forms the internal sphincter, which is contracted at rest. When fecal matter enters the rectum, the internal sphincter relaxes. The consistency and volume of the fecal matter and the condition of the rectum triggers an awareness of the need to defecate. The external sphincter, composed of skeletal muscle, does not relax until the message is sent to the cerebral cortex and the individual adopts a sitting or squatting position. This position straightens the anorectal angle and promotes effective propulsion. For defecation to occur, the rectal muscles must contract with the internal and external sphincters relaxing.

Age-Related Changes

Absorption and secretion of the large intestine is maintained in the healthy elder. Age has a slight effect on the large intestine by slowing transit time through the colon. The species of bacteria in the large intestine changes with age. There is an increase in species diversity with fewer bifodobacteria, also referred to as probiotics. Probiotic bacteria may be responsible for limiting the growth of *C. difficile* bacteria. These microflora changes may contribute to constipation, a common complaint among elders.

Elasticity of the rectal wall declines with age. The internal sphincter becomes thicker, while the external sphincter thins. There is an increase in the pressure threshold to produce the sensation of rectal filling. A large volume is required to stimulate the urge to defecate. As rectal tone declines, the ability to generate squeeze pressure declines with age. The result is fecal incontinence, which occurs in up to 20% of community elders over age 65 and over 50% of institutionalized elders.

Constipation is not a natural part of aging, yet over two-thirds of elders will report an increase in constipation with age. Constipation is defined as less than three bowel movements per week. In practice, straining, hard stools, pain, and incomplete evacuation are also referred to as constipation. Physiologic decline in elders' smooth muscle and neural function can contribute to constipation. However, constipation is also a side effect of a number of drugs administered to elders, including opiods, diuretics, antidepressants, and antihistamines. Up to one-third of community-dwelling elders admit to using laxatives on a weekly basis, the number doubling in institutionalized elders. Women report more laxative use than men. Changes in pelvic floor function secondary to childbirth make constipation twice as common in women. Fecal impaction has been identified in up to 42% of frail elders admitted to geriatric facilities.

If solid waste stays in the colon too long, the buildup exerts pressure on the intestinal wall. Aging results in declining tensile strength in smooth muscle, and under chronic pressure, the wall weakens and pouches, or diverticula, develop. Two-thirds of elders will have diverticula by age 80. Trapped undigested food in the diverticula, called diverticulosis, can result in inflammation, or diverticulitis. It is estimated that half of older adults will develop diverticulosis, with 25% of those experiencing diverticulitis. A lifetime diet rich in refined foods and low in fiber is associated with diverticulosis risk. Diverticulitis can be more difficult to identify in geriatric patients as they can lose sensitivity and are often unaware of abdominal cramping or bloating.

Age changes in the colonic flora coupled with antibiotic usage are risk factors for acquisition of *C. difficile*. Normal intestinal flora resists *C. difficile* colonies, but when antibiotics suppress normal flora, *C. difficile* is opportunistic. Elders become contaminated with spores carried on health care workers' hands and objects in the environment. *C. difficile* produces toxins that lead to an inflamed colon. *C. difficile*–associated diarrhea has a 25% mortality rate among the frail elderly. Antibiotic usage may also reduce the production of vitamin K by healthy bacteria. The decrease in vitamin K can have hematologic consequences.

LIVER

The liver is the largest gland in the body, weighing 2 kg in the average adult. It is a very vascular organ, receiving 30% of the cardiac output. Seventy-five percent of the blood flow through the liver is from the portal vein, which drains the small and large intestines and is high in nutrients with the remaining blood from the hepatic artery. The liver has numerous functions including the formation of lymph; controlling synthesis; utilization of carbohydrates, lipids, and proteins; removing dead cells and byproducts of metabolism; and synthesis and secretion of bile.

Age-Related Changes

There is a progressive decrease in liver size with age. By 80 years old, the liver mass has declined by 40% compared to the young adult. A decline in hepatic blood flow parallels the decline in liver mass. Blood flow through the liver decreases from 0.3 to 1.5% per year. The change in blood flow and liver mass explains elders' sensitivity to medications, slower metabolism of medications, and reduced elimination. When the aged liver becomes diseased, difficulty with drug metabolism is usually more severe.

Despite the change in mass, liver enzymes are unchanged. Routine liver enzyme tests do not show age-related changes. The activity of drug-metabolizing enzymes in the liver does not appear to decline with age. While protein synthesis and albumin synthesis by the liver are reduced in the elderly, the reduced synthesis is independent of protein intake.

GALLBLADDER

The liver cells, hepatocytes, secrete bile into the collecting ducts, which pass into the hepatic duct. The hepatic duct merges with the cystic duct to form the common bile duct. Bile is concentrated and stored in the gallbladder until a food bolus stimulates the gallbladder to contract and send bile down the common bile duct through the sphincter of Oddi to the duodenum. Bile contains water, electrolytes, bile acids, cholesterol, phospholipids, and bilirubin. The average person produces 400 to 800 mL of bile each day, with the gallbladder concentrating bile by a factor of five.

Cholecystokinin is a hormone secreted into the blood by the duodenal mucosa in response to fat entering the intestine. An increase in cholecystokinin stimulates gallbladder contraction and relaxes the sphincter of Oddi. Bile acids are critical for the intestinal digestion and absorption of fats and fat-soluble vitamins. Their chemical properties break down fat globules much like a detergent. The emulsification increases the surface area of the fat droplets making them available to digestive lipases.

Age-Related Changes
Bile flow and the amount of bile acid produced by the liver are reduced by about 50% with age. These findings suggest an impairment of the energy-requiring transport processes. Concurrently, there is an increased liver secretion of cholesterol. As a result, the bile becomes supersaturated with cholesterol. The major effect of aging on the biliary system is the increased risk of cholesterol gallstones; by age 70, gallstones will be found in 35% of women and 20% of men. Despite the common bile duct increasing in diameter with age, stones in the common bile duct are more common in the elderly, with nearly triple the incidence of younger adults with cholecystitis.

Open laparotomies for cholecystitis are more common among elders.

Despite the increasing incidence of gallstones with age, most elders never experience complications. Symptoms of cholecystitis in the elderly can be nonspecific; pain may be dull, absent, or poorly localized. More than half of elders are afebrile. Delirium and septic shock can be the only presenting sign of cholecystitis in elders. The difficulty in diagnosing cholecystitis results in more complications for older adults. Laparoscopic surgeries turn into open laparotomies more often among elders than for younger adults. Obstructing gallstones account for most cases of pancreatitis in elders.

Elders have higher blood levels of fasting and stimulated cholecystokinin. However, the emptying volume and the rate of emptying do not change, so that with age, there is a reduced sensitivity to cholecystokinin.

NUTRITION AND AGING

The large reserve capacity allows gastrointestinal functions to remain intact with aging. Health promotion, disease prevention, and chronic disease management relies on nutrition. Poor nutrition is not a natural response to aging. A variety of age-related changes place elders at high risk for poor nutritional status. With aging, there is a decrease in total body protein, total body water, bone density loss, and a redistribution of body fat with decreased fat stores. Four factors influence elders' nutritional status: food acquisition, food ingestion, digestion and absorption, and tissue requirements. Poverty, immobility, or inadequate cooking facilities contribute to elders' difficulty obtaining or maintaining adequate food and nutrients. Food choices may be limited by dietary traditions or availability. Protein can cause early satiety, prompting elders to ingest more carbohydrates. Protein deficiency is common among elders. Vegetables can be gas-producing and may be avoided altogether, resulting in vitamin and mineral deficiencies. Many elders resort to canned soup as it is cheap, easy to prepare, and does not make them feel as full. However, the salt content in canned foods can precipitate heart failure, which is a risk factor in surgery.

Nurses and health care providers should coach gerioperative patients and family members about the need for changes to diet along with the importance of good nutrition and hydration. A multivitamin should be taken daily to compensate for decreased food, vitamin, and mineral intake. Dental and oral health may present ingestions problems as well as dysphagia. Problems with digestion and absorption are usually created by coexisting illnesses. Finally, nutrition utilization depends on physical activity, stress of disease, and pharmacological requirements. Over 50% of elders are malnourished or at risk for malnutrition, with the number increasing to 85% among institutionalized elders. The impact of malnutrition on gerioperative patients are numerous and contribute to postoperative mortality and morbidity (Exhibit 15.1).

ENERGY

The decrease in body mass with aging decreases the total energy expenditure. Between ages 30 and 80, energy requirements decrease by 30%, primarily due to decreased activity. While basal metabolic rate (BMR) does not change with age, a negative energy balance is common during increased times of stress when energy expenditure increases. Elder's metabolic rate can increase 20 to 40% during the immediate postoperative period. During this time, the calorie requirements increase 1.2 to 2 times the BMR. The decline in BMR means that elders have difficulty generating heat to maintain normothermia. The decline in BMR is related to the change in body mass composition as adipose tissue requires less energy to maintain.

Energy needs determine calorie intake. Elders have a 30% reduction in calorie consumption. However, elders have the same requirements for all other nutrients except for carbohydrates. Thus, less food means that nutritional deficiencies can occur. With age, hunger

EXHIBIT15.1 Impact of Malnutrition in Gerioperative Patients

- Decreased immune system
- Increased risk of surgical site infections
- Decreased respiratory function
- Increased risk of pneumonia
- Increased muscle weakness and fatigue
- Altered skin integrity
- Changes in neurological status and cognitive function
- Increased morbidity and mortality
- Increased recovery time
- Increased hospital length of stay
- Altered fluid and electrolyte balance
- Changes in drug absorption and interaction
- Decreased sensory function

decreases, and as a result, elders eat less, consume smaller meals slower, eat fewer snacks, and become satiated rapidly after eating. It has been noted that elders consume a less varied, more monotonous diet. Flavor of food is derived from taste, smell, texture, and temperature, all of which are altered with age.

BODY MASS INDEX

By age 70, men and women will lose up to 5% of their peak height. The vertebral disc compression results in a decrease of approximately 1 cm per decade after age 20. Body mass increases up to advanced ages over 70, when weight declines.

Lean body mass is defined as the difference between total body mass and adipose tissue mass. Throughout their lifetime, men have greater lean body mass than women. As both genders enter adulthood, lean body mass declines yearly, 0.3% for men and 0.2% for women. Simultaneously, the percentage of body fat increases with age. The body fat of young adult males averages 18%, while at age 70, body fat is 26%. In young women, body fat accounts for 24% compared to 36% in women over 70 years. The adipose or fat tissue is redistributed with aging, moving from subcutaneous toward the abdominal viscera. The increase in fat accentuates an elder's ability to store lipid-soluble drugs. Storage of these drugs leads to slow and prolonged release with a longer elimination time.

After age 65, a body mass index (BMI) between 24 and 29 is recommended. A BMI below 22 indicates the elder is underweight and is cause for concern. A BMI below 18.5 kg/m^2 suggests nutritional compromise, while a BMI over 29 defines obesity. Older adults who have unintentionally lost 10 or more pounds in 6 months are at risk of malnutrition.

PROTEIN

Forty-five percent of body weight in young adults is protein; only half of this amount is found in the very old. There is a decrease in protein synthesis and protein breakdown. The protein molecules are exposed to gradual damage. A decreased secretion in growth hormone, produced by the anterior pituitary gland, is responsible. The reduction in growth hormone, which usually spares the use of protein for energy, results in the decreased use of fat. The protein decline is manifested as a decrease in skeletal muscle mass. Particular losses are noted in the small muscles of the hand and face. The muscles for mastication can be affected. Protein malnutrition is also evident in dry, flaking skin; dull-appearing hair; and peripheral edema. The availability of protein is a major factor in wound healing.

FAT

The ability to use fat or triglycerides as a source of fuel does not change with age. Triglycerides and cholesterol, insoluble in body fluids, are carried by lipoprotein molecules. Low-density lipoproteins have been implicated in heart disease, while high-density lipoproteins are cardioprotective. With aging, men increase low-density lipoproteins to age 50 and women to age 70.

CARBOHYDRATES

Sugars are a valuable source of energy and are available as intrinsic or extrinsic according to their metabolic availability. Food cell structure contains intrinsic sugar. Extrinsic sugars include milk, fruit juices, and refined sugars. Elders consume approximately 18% of their food energy in extrinsic sugars, which has been correlated with dental root caries. The consumption of extrinsic sugars threatens elders' nutrition.

VITAMINS AND MINERALS

With age, there is clear evidence of deficiency in B_1, B_{12}, C, and D vitamins (Table 15.1). B_1 (thiamin) is found in fortified cereals and breads. Confusion among postoperative patients has been attributed to low thiamin intake. Half of older adults have vitamin and mineral intakes less than the recommended daily allowance.

While the ingestion of vitamin B_{12} is adequate, 5 to 20% of elders have insufficient levels, over half of which are due to absorption defects. The use of histamine blockers and proton pump inhibitor treatment for gastritis further decreases vitamin B_{12} absorption. Specific to vitamin B_{12} is the presence of intrinsic factor secreted by the gastric mucosa. Atrophic gastritis, or bacterial overgrowth, can impair secretion and result in low levels of vitamin B_{12}. Deficiency is manifested as pernicious anemia. Low vitamin B_{12} is associated with increased levels of homocysteine, an amino acid responsible for cardiovascular disease.

Vitamin C is needed for protein synthesis during wound healing. However, foods high in vitamin C usually require preparation and chewing. When these foods are exposed to prolonged heating to increase palatability for elders with oral problems, the vitamin is oxidized. Up to 40% of institutionalized elders have vitamin C deficiency.

Vitamin D acts to promote small intestinal absorption of calcium and phosphate. It is synthesized in the skin by exposure to sunlight and converted to the active form by the liver. At age 80, vitamin D production in the skin in response to sun exposure is half that at age 18. Vitamin D is obtained in lesser amounts by ingesting eggs, margarine, and oily fish (e.g., tuna fish). Limited skin exposure makes dietary supplements more important, especially during the northern winter months. Over 30% of institutionalized elders will present with a vitamin D deficiency.

With a vitamin D deficiency, calcium absorption declines with age. In addition, milk consumption falls with age, further adding to a calcium deficiency. The reduced bone density can impair mobility and increase the rate of falls. Hypocalcaemia can lead to cardiac arrhythmias and neuromuscular dysfunction.

Zinc plays an important role in cell development, protein synthesis, and a sense of smell and taste. Zinc deficiency can result in poor wound healing and make patients more susceptible to infections. Zinc is used to epithelialize the wound and add strength.

TABLE 15.1
Sources of Important Vitamins and Minerals

Vitamin/Mineral	Deficiency	Sources
C	Scurvy	Citrus fruits, raw leafy vegetables, tomatoes, broccoli, peppers
B_{12}	Anemia	Liver, cereal, salmon, beef, yogurt
D	Decreased bone density	Sunlight, eggs, margarine, oily fish
B_1	Confusion	Fortified cereals and breads
Zinc	Poor wound healing	Beef, pork, cereals, baked beans

The body's need for every nutrient except carbohydrates does not change with age. Nutrition impacts surgical recovery. Protein-calorie, iron, vitamin, and mineral deficiencies impact the ability of any patient to tolerate surgery with the elderly even more vulnerable. Malnutrition leads

> *Daily multivitamins compensate for vitamin and mineral loss.*

to an impaired immune system with poor wound healing. Malnourished patients are more prone to infection and multisystem organ failure complications of surgery and death.

Gerioperative Care

PREOPERATIVE CONSIDERATIONS

History

In addition to obtaining information about prior gastrointestinal diseases, a nutritional assessment includes the risk factors associated with malnutrition: history of weight loss, vomiting, diarrhea, and change in appetite. Identify the regular meal schedule and intake as well as use of vitamin and mineral supplements. Awareness of bowel movement frequency, schedule, and any aids to defecation are important for postoperative care. As the quantity of food intake decreases with age, the quality of the food ingested becomes more important. Note any recent dietary changes. Not eating food for a week before surgery is worse than eating a limited regular diet for a long period.

Surgery on malnourished elders should be postponed if possible. A recent weight loss greater than 10% of lean body mass increases wound complications.

Physical Assessment

Assess the oral cavity for hydration, overall oral health, and problems with dysphagia. If the elder uses dentures, note if they fit properly. An accurate height and weight is important for BMI calculation. If malnutrition is suspected from an analysis of the BMI or physical findings, laboratory analysis should include a complete blood count to evaluate anemia, serum albumin, and cholesterol. Elders are predisposed to malnutrition. Malnutrition is often misdiagnosed or underdiagnosed in the gerioperative population. It is important to remember that obese patients can also be malnourished. Nutritional assessment is essential to evaluate patients at risk for perioperative complications secondary to nutritional compromise. A quick assessment of daily intake can give an idea of calorie count and protein intake. The nurse should ask about fast food and preprepared foods. Soups and frozen dinners can have high sodium and fat content with little nutritional value. This information combined with laboratory values and visual assessment can help determine which gerioperative patients may be at risk for poor outcomes secondary to malnutrition. Albumin is an excellent measure of protein status, changing very little with healthy aging. The albumin level reflects nutritional status over the previous 1 to 2 months and is considered the best predictor of postoperative complications. Healthy elderly have an albumin level over 4 g/dL, while surgical complications double in patients with an albumin less than 3.0. An albumin less than 3.5 is considered protein calorie malnutrition

Interventions

Severely malnourished elders may require nutritional support to prepare them for the increased energy demands caused by the stress of surgery and anesthesia. Over-the-counter, high-protein oral supplements can be suggested during the preoperative interview for otherwise healthy elders. Rapid replenishment of depleted nutrients is effective, and a few days of parenteral nutrition can restore an elder.

Preoperative and postoperative oral care in the gerioperative patient is essential. Normal age-related changes, medications, and disease processes predispose the elderly to dry mucous membranes. Mouth care should be performed by the patient, the caregiver, the assistant, or the nurse several times each day and as necessary. The mouth should be assessed for any trauma or lesions daily. Oral care is easily accomplished with a soft toothbrush. The teeth and tongue should be brushed with a fluoride toothpaste, and the mouth should be rinsed. Flossing should also be encouraged. Commercial mouthwashes containing alcohol are drying to mucous membranes and should be avoided. Chlorhexidine rinse may be effective to decrease oral bacteria contributing to postoperative pneumonia.

Frequent mouth care increases patients' well-being and protects against infection.

Frequent mouth care accomplishes several objectives including increased patient sense of well-being, decreased oral colonization, and moisturization of mucous membranes. Exhibit 15.2 presents a serious consequence of poor oral hygiene that was not identified until the patient went to the operating room.

Moisturized mucous membranes facilitate chewing, swallowing, medication intake, and decreased risk of infection due to traumatized membranes. Frequent mouth care is even more important postoperatively secondary to changes in hydration and nutrition caused by nothing-by-mouth status. Also, many gerioperative patients may be less able to perform mouth care after surgery or not feel it is important. The nurse is responsible for ensuring mouth care is completed either by encouraging the elder to engage in self-care or by actively performing the oral care for patients not able to care for themselves.

Many elders have dentures. Prior to surgery or anesthesia induction, the dentures are often removed. It is part of nursing care to ensure that patients have dentures in place prior to oral intake. It is also the nurse's responsibility to determine if the dentures are cleaned frequently, whether the nurse, patient, or caregiver cleans them.

POSTOPERATIVE CONSIDERATIONS

In response to nothing-by-mouth status and the stress of surgery, elders are less hungry than their younger counterparts. Postoperative nursing responsibility includes coaching family and patients about nutrition and nutritional monitoring in order to prevent postoperative complications. Small frequent meals throughout the day are well tolerated by gerioperative patients. Protein is important for healing and should be encouraged unless contraindicated.

EXHIBIT 15.2. Clinical Implications of Oral Care

An 85-year-old woman, Mrs. Marcy, was brought to the operating room for evaluation of dysphagia and a "mass" in oropharynx. Patient was anesthetized and intubated for endoscopy by endotracheal tube. The "mass" was found to be a mucous plug in the oropharynx with extremely dry and cracked mucous membranes. Poor oral care and lack of hydration led to dry mucous membranes, mucous plug formation, and dysphagia as well as the risk of unnecessary anesthesia delivered to a frail gerioperative patient.

High nutrition drinks can be made into milkshakes for an easy tasty snack that promotes healing. Consulting with a dietician can be useful in determining which product may be most cost-effective given an individual patient's financial and clinical situation. If nutritional monitoring shows that intake is not adequate, a nutritional consult must be obtained. Enteral and parenteral sources of nutrition may need to be considered.

Opiates administered before, during, or after surgery stimulate the release of inhibitory neurochemicals, increasing the occurrence of nonpropagating contractions in the distal gut. Excessive use of opioid medication can cause constipation. Postoperative constipation is a common complaint in the gerioperative population. The nurse should coach patients and families regarding adequate fluid intake and stool softeners, especially for those discharged on pain medications. Adequate fluid intake and stool softeners can maintain bowel motility. Bran mixtures of bran cereal, applesauce, and prunes provide fiber and stimulate defecation. However, physical activity, within the limits set by the surgeon, is most effective in promoting gastric motility. In the event that bowel movements are decreased, laxatives and enemas may be added to stimulate defecation. The nurse should assess bowel sounds and palpate the abdomen for distension. Pertinent questions to ask include frequency of preoperative and postoperative bowel movements, fluid intake, medication changes, amount of activity, and time of normal bowel movement, as coaching can then be focused. Routine orders for stool softeners and bulk laxatives should be implemented prophylactically.

One of the major complications experienced in the postanesthesia period, nausea and vomiting, is uncommon among elderly patients. Changes in the vomiting center and diminished sensory input reduce the occurrence of postoperative nausea and vomiting. However, the occurrence of dysphagia and dyspepsia increase elders' risk of aspiration. As soon as possible, the head of the bed should be elevated

Sitting at 90 degrees when taking fluids, foods, or medications decreases aspiration risk.

at least 30 degrees to avoid regurgitation of stomach acids. When administering any oral medications, provide water before and after the medications. Drugs should be swallowed upright with a full glass of water. Sitting the patient in high Fowler's position facilitates the swallowing process and prevents swallowing complications.

PATIENT REPORT: Ms. Stine

Ms. Stine does not like to complain. She waited to tell the nurse about her abdominal distention and discomfort until she could no longer tolerate it. The nurse had been encouraging her to take more walks, but Ms. Stine felt she could not even get out of bed she was so uncomfortable. She also had been told she could start liquids the first morning after surgery but she had not done so because the medication made her feel "queasy." She was eating little, not drinking, and spending most of her time in bed. She was using her patient-controlled analgesia pump with morphine as often as the pump allowed. One the evening of the second day after surgery, the gerioperative care facilitator spent some time explaining the problem to Ms. Stine. The nurse told the patient that one of the contributing factors to her ileus was the amount of morphine she was using. In other words, although the morphine helped decrease some of her pain, it was contributing to her bloating by slowing down her bowel function. Ms. Stine was almost in tears. She was so uncomfortable, and the very medicine that should make her feel better was actually making her feel worse. She had lost her appetite. The nurse was very positive and told her there were several things they could work on that might help. The first was to get her started on intravenous fluid as a precautionary measure. The nurse would then start Ms. Stine on gum chewing. This astounded Ms. Stine, gum chewing to make her stomach bloat go away did not make much sense, but she was willing to give anything a try. The nurses suggested that Ms. Stine try to decrease her morphine use with nonpharmacological pain relief methods. The nurse would get an order for nonopioid medication to help with pain relief. Combining nonopioid mediation with nonpharmacological pain methods could help to decrease the need for the patient-controlled analgesia opioid, an important step in getting her gastrointestinal function back. Moving around and walking would help prevent pneumonia. Ms. Stine really needed to get up and move even if only for a few minutes several times a day.

The nurse told Ms. Stine that the bowel would probably start working by itself and the interventions they could work on together would move the process along a bit faster. Ms. Stine agreed. She was willing to try anything. Within 2 days, Ms. Stine reported that she thought she had passed some gas. The nurse administered a bisacodyl suppository, ordered as needed, to increase lower colon motility. Ms. Stine started on clear liquids, and by that evening she tolerated a vanilla milkshake her family had brought. She continued on frequent small nutritious drinks. Bowel function returned, and Ms. Stine continued to recover without any additional challenges.

SUMMARY

While age has little effect on the gastrointestinal system due to its large functional reserve, the rate of cell growth declines, making tissues more vulnerable to damage. A decrease in smooth muscle slows contraction along the gastrointestinal tract. While the prevalence of gastrointestinal disorders increase with age, age-related malnutrition is of most concern.

KEY POINTS

- The duration of the swallowing sequence increases with age.
- The age-related loss of muscle function, chewing inefficiency, and reduced salivation results in a drier food bolus.
- When GERD is diagnosed in elders, it is usually more severe, though symptoms are milder.
- A significant influence on the vomiting center comes from the chemoreceptor trigger zone (CTZ). The CTZ, located in the brainstem under the fourth ventricle, is sensitive to emetic drugs and substances in the blood such as uremia, hypoxia, and high blood sugars.
- Atrophic gastritis results in a decrease in acid production, low gastrin levels, lower levels of intrinsic factor that can lead to anemia, and an increase in stomach pH.
- Up to a quarter of all elders have atrophic gastritis.
- One-third of elders hospitalized for peptic ulcers will deny pain.
- Postprandial hypotension can lead to syncope and falls.
- Vitamin B_{12} deficiency, found in 10 to 15% of elders, occurs due to the lack of intrinsic factor secreted by atrophic stomach mucosa.
- A critical product of colon bacteria is the synthesis of vitamin K.
- Fecal incontinence occurs in up to 20 % of community elders over 65 and over 50% of institutionalized elders.
- *C. difficile*–associated diarrhea has a 25% mortality rate among the frail elderly.
- The change in blood flow and liver mass explains elders' sensitivity to medications, slower metabolism of medications, and reduced elimination.

- Symptoms of cholecystitis in the elderly can be nonspecific and pain may be dull or absent. Pain is poorly localized and over half of patients are afebrile.
- Poverty, immobility, or inadequate cooking facilities contribute to elders' difficulty in acquiring adequate food and nutrients.
- Over 50% of elders are malnourished or at risk for malnutrition with the number increasing to 85% among institutionalized elders.
- The decline in BMR means that elders have difficulty generating heat to maintain normothermia.
- The increase in fat accentuates an elder's ability to store lipid soluble drugs. Storage of these drugs leads to slow and prolonged release with a longer elimination time.
- With age there is clear evidence of deficiency in B1, B12, C, and D vitamins.
- Forty percent of institutionalized elders have reported vitamin C deficiency.
- Over 30% of institutionalized elders will present with a vitamin D deficiency.
- Drugs should be swallowed upright with a full glass of water. Sitting the patient up facilitates the swallowing process and prevents swallowing complications.
- Reduced salivation due to polypharmacy results in an increased taste threshold for sodium (11 times normal), bitter (7 times normal), and sour (4 times normal).

SIXTEEN

Hematology

Susan J. Fetzer, Jennifer V. Long, and Raelene V. Shippee-Rice

PATIENT REPORT: Mrs. Nagele

Mrs. Nagele is admitted for an abdominal hysterectomy. She is 68 years old and has a history of angina, varicose vein ligation, and right carotid endarterectomy. She is a nonsmoker, having quit 5 years ago when she developed angina. She is taking metoprolol 25 mg daily and an aspirin 81 mg daily. She has not required sublingual nitroglycerin for 6 months, when she started a cardiac rehabilitation program. She exercises 3 days a week. During the preoperative interview, she expresses concern that her "blood" is low as she has experienced vaginal spotting for the past 3 months. A preoperative complete blood count (CBC) revealed hemoglobin of 12. 2 g/dL, hematocrit of 36%, white blood cell (WBC) count of 8,000 and a platelet count of 110,000. Mrs. Nagele is fitted for knee-high compression stockings. While applying the stockings, the nurse instructs Mrs. Nagele in the proper technique for applying and wearing the stockings, as well as their purpose.

The cavities of the long bones contain bone marrow, the source of all blood cells. Within the bone marrow are stem cells, which are cells that have the ability to regenerate and differentiate throughout life. In the bone marrow, stem cells are capable of producing eight different types of mature blood cells. However, only a few stem cells replicate and differentiate at a time, allowing the cells ample time to rest and regenerate.

Blood Components

PLATELETS

Stem cells can differentiate into megakaryocytes, which fragment to become thrombocytes or platelets. One trillion platelets (10×10^{11}) are produced each day to maintain a normal blood level range of 150 to 400×10^9 platelets per liter. Platelets are clear cell fragments without a nucleus that have a lifespan of 5 to 9 days. The role of platelets is to initiate hemostasis and release growth factors. Hemostasis is begun when endothelial damage exposes collagen to the blood vessel. When platelets make contact with collagen, they are activated and aggregate or clump together. Growth factors signal cells to differentiate thereby promoting tissue healing. A reserve of platelets is stored in the spleen and released by sympathetic stimulation.

RED BLOOD CELLS

Red blood cells (RBCs) or erythrocytes are disks that are concave on both sides. From the stem cell, the RBCs enter the blood stream as reticulocytes or immature cells. At any one time, approximately 1% of RBCs in the blood are immature. Within a day, they have matured into erythrocytes. By the time they enter the bloodstream, reticulocytes have lost their nuclei, but can still live for up to 120 days. The RBC contains a large iron-containing protein molecule that is capable of binding to oxygen. The iron protein, or hemoglobin, transports the bound oxygen to the cells for metabolism. The shape of the RBC enables them to squeeze through the narrow capillaries. The production of the hemoglobin molecule inside the RBC requires a nutrient source of iron.

A normal 70-kg adult has a circulating RBC mass of 2000 mL or 300×10^9 RBCs per kg. RBCs live for 100 to 120 days, which means that 1% of the cells die each day, about 20 mL. The stimulus of a hemorrhage or hypoxia can increase RBC production by 300% within 5 to 7 days. An elevated reticulocyte count is an index of the bone marrow's ability to produce new cells.

The development of RBCs in the bone marrow, or erythropoiesis, is controlled by feedback mechanisms. The number of RBCs is determined by the amount of oxygen delivered to body tissues. If the tissues become hypoxic, particularly the sensitive cells of the kidney, the hormone erythropoietin is released by the peritubular renal cells. Once released, erythropoietin is bound to circulating RBCs. If there are inadequate cells to bind the erythropoietin, unbound erythropoietin acts on the bone marrow to stimulate erythropoiesis. Once additional RBCs are produced, the level of unbound erythropoietin decreases. Inflammation can interfere with the action of erythropoietin. A limiting factor of erythropoietin's effectiveness in increasing the RBC volume is the availability of iron for hemoglobin molecule production. A lack of iron will render erythropoietin's action to increase RBC volume ineffective.

WHITE BLOOD CELLS

The WBCs, or leukocytes, originating from the bone marrow stem cells include the neutrophils, macrophages, eosinophils, basophils, and B- and T-lymphocytes. Each is involved in different aspects of immunity from infection. The normal adult WBC count ranges from 3,900 to 10,000 mm³, with neutrophils comprising up to 70% of the cells. Approximately 10% of the WBCs are replaced by the bone marrow each day. The cells of immunity are discussed in Chapter 17.

Age-Related Changes

Platelets produced by older megakaryocytes have shown hyperactivity or an increased susceptibility to aggregation. Hyperactive aggregation creates a risk for clots to develop in smaller blood vessels, leading to cerebral or myocardial thrombosis, stroke, and myocardial infarction. Most elders are prescribed medications, such as aspirin or clopidogrel, which irreversibly disrupts platelet function. Aspirin and other anticoagulation medications work by inhibiting the chemical that encourages platelets to stick together. Even a small amount (81 mg or "baby" aspirin) taken daily can permanently affect the stickiness of platelets emerging from the bone marrow. However, the short life span of platelets means the effect of the aspirin on platelet function is 5 to 9 days.

Aspirin's platelet effect lasts for 5 to 9 days.

Aging changes the bone marrow. Up to age 16 the bone marrow appears red, with 80 to 100% of the marrow composed of hematopoietic cells actively producing blood cells. With age, the active marrow is gradually replaced by connective tissue and fat. By age 65, only 50% of the marrow is hematopoietic. By age 75, there is a further decline to 30% as more of the red marrow transitions to yellow. These age-related changes explain why bone marrow donated by older donors is more likely to fail when transplanted.

Bone marrow donated by older donors is more likely to fail when transplanted.

The reduction in the number of active stem cells with age is offset as the number of remaining stem cells involved in replicating and dividing increases. Despite the changes in the bone marrow, there is only a very slight decrease in the number of RBCs with age. Basal parameters are not affected. The lifespan of an RBC does not change, with hemoglobin concentration only decreasing slightly after age 65.

As the spleen shrinks with age, it becomes less efficient at removing old or damaged RBCs from the circulation. While it allows RBCs to remain in the circulation longer, the cells are older and less effective oxygen carriers.

ANEMIA

Anemia, or low level of serum hemoglobin, was once thought to be a normal condition of aging. However, there is no evidence that the bone marrow cannot supply an adequate number of RBCs to elders. While stems cells do lose their proliferative capacity with age, there is a limited reserve to meet the normal requirements. Age-related changes make elders more sensitive to anemia-producing events and less able to respond quickly.

Age-related changes make elders more sensitive to anemia producing events and less able to respond quickly.

The World Health Organization defines anemia as less than 12 g/dL in women and 13 g/dL in men. The prevalence in elders ranges from 4 to 48%, with a higher frequency in men especially after age 85. Elderly Black men have the highest prevalence of anemia. While anemia occurs in up to 12% of community-dwelling elders, the rate increases 400% in institutionalized elders. Anemia has been diagnosed in about 13% of older Americans, with a higher number not tested.

A lack of cellular oxygen tissues as a result of anemia produces a wide range of symptoms (see Exhibit 16.1). The degree of anemia, rapidity of onset, underlying cause, comorbid illness, and medications often make the symptoms of anemia difficult to assess. Acute anemia often causes tachycardia and hypoxemia, whereas chronic anemia rarely exhibits any symptoms as the body compensates for hypoxemia over time. In chronic anemia, symptoms rarely develop unless the hemoglobin falls below 7 g/dL.

Age-Related Changes

Acute anemia can be readily diagnosed in young adults. Typical signs and symptoms of anemia such as tachycardia, shortness of breath, pallor, and dizziness are often difficult to identify in the elderly due to comorbid conditions and medications. The tachycardia or anemia

EXHIBIT 16.1 Symptoms of Anemia

- Fatigue
- Syncope
- Postural hypotension
- Falls
- Apathy
- Irritability
- Muscle weakness

- Shortness of breath
- Exertional dyspnea
- Tachycardia
- Pale skin and mucous membranes
- Cognitive impairment
- Confusion

causes myocardial oxygen consumption to increase, which can produce cardiac complications. However, many gerioperative patients are on medications such as beta blockers that prevent tachycardia. Many elderly are often pale, so pallor is less recognizable. Dizziness can be caused by narcotics and anesthetic agents, further diminishing the ability to diagnose anemia after surgery. Maintaining an index of suspicion and close monitoring can identify anemia early in order to intervene and prevent complications.

Elders with anemia have difficulty responding to stressful situations and require additional oxygen. Anemia results in decreased wound healing. In the face of anemia, elders with comorbid pulmonary or cardiovascular disease can not compensate for the decrease in oxygen delivery to the cells.

Anemia is the result of nutrient deficiencies, hemolysis due to comorbid diseases, or idiopathic causes. Older adults are at high risk for nutritional deficiency of iron, vitamin B_{12}, and folic acid, which are associated with anemia. Up to 20% of elders over 70 have some sort of nutritional deficit. Iron deficiency anemia is related to poor dietary intake (see Exhibit 16.2) or chronic blood loss. Vitamin B_{12} deficiency is related to lack of intrinsic factor produced by gastric parietal cells. Atrophy of the parietal cells is prevalent in elders (see Chapter 15). Folic acid deficiency is related to alcoholism and intestinal malabsorption. Comorbid diseases, such as gastrointestinal bleeding, malignancy, rheumatoid arthritis, chronic kidney disease, and infection, contribute to anemia in older adults. Idiopathic anemia is found in up to one-third of elders.

Though anemia is not an age-related disease, it is associated with increased mortality and hospitalization. In addition to decreasing muscle strength, which presents a risk factor for postoperative pulmonary complications, anemia results in delayed wound healing. Anemia is associated with frailty in the elderly.

The total number of leukocytes in older adults decreases slightly. There is little effect of age on the number of neutrophils and macrophages. There is a decline in T-cell function with an increase in B-cells (see Chapter 17). The ability of eosinophils to react to a foreign antigen

EXHIBIT 16.2 Foods Rich in Iron

- Beans (kidney, navy, soy, lentil)
- Fortified cereals
- Spinach
- Prune juice
- Raisins

- Clams, oysters, scallops, tuna
- Liver
- Turkey (dark meat)
- Beef

declines with age. Overall, stem cells in healthy elders will continue to produce WBCs under normal conditions. However, in the presence of chronic inflammation or stress, the leukocytes are less able to be mobilized, leaving the elder vulnerable to devastating infections.

Gerioperative Care

PREOPERATIVE CONSIDERATIONS

The preoperative history evaluates the gerioperative patient for bleeding problems and infections. A history of requiring blood transfusions outside of surgery prompts the need for focused questioning. A list of current medications is vital as many elders are taking prescription or herbals that interfere with coagulation. Antiplatelet drugs interfere with surgical coagulation and may be stopped up to a week before elective surgery (see Exhibit 16.3), especially prior to cardiac, neurologic and plastic surgery. Symptoms of anemia prompt the need for laboratory tests.

Gerioperative patients scheduled for surgery that is high risk for bleeding, such as cardiac, vascular, plastic, or orthopedic procedures, should have CBC with platelet count. If the platelet count is below 50 ($\times$ 10^9/L), abnormal bleeding will occur. Regional anesthesia is avoided if the number of platelets is below 100 ($\times$ 10^9/L) due to the risk of an epidural hematoma, which could result in spinal cord compression.

A test of bleeding time has been advocated for patients taking aspirin or other antiplatelet drugs to determine platelet deficits. However, the poor reliability of the test due to operator technique has decreased it use. Ask the patient or family members the last time an aspirin or antiplatelet drug was ingested.

The high rate of anemia among otherwise healthy elders suggests the need to evaluate hemoglobin preoperatively. For elective surgery, obtaining serum hemoglobin 30 days prior to surgery allows timely evaluation and intervention if anemia is detected. Iron supplements, B_{12} and erythropoietin administration, or red cell transfusion may be indicated. Even mild anemia among elders has shown a significant increase in 30-day postoperative mortality.

> *Even mild anemia in older adults has shown a significant increase in 30-day postoperative mortality.*

The hemoglobin is compared to the hematocrit, or percentage of RBCs to blood volume. The hemoglobin/hematocrit ratio is approximately one to three in normovolemic patients. When hemoglobin is more than three times the hematocrit, the patient is hypvolemic or dehydrated. When the hemoglobin is less than three times the hematocrit, the patient is fluid overloaded.

EXHIBIT 16.3 **Medications and Herbals With Antiplatelet Actions**

- Aspirin
- Nonsteroidal anti-inflammatory drugs
- Dipyriadamole
- Caffeine
- Aminophylline
- Clopidogrel
- Monoclonal antibodies
- Abciximab
- Ginkgo biloba
- Ginseng
- Garlic
- Ginger
- Vitamin E

INTRAOPERATIVE CONSIDERATIONS

Blood loss is a natural consequence of most surgeries. The decision to transfuse packed RBCs is dependent on the vital signs, symptoms of hypoxemia, and rate of blood loss. There is no evidence that hemoglobin trigger for transfusion improve outcomes. The American Society of Anesthesiologists stratifies anemic patients into three groups according to risk. Age places elders in the moderate- or high-risk strata. For elders with stable cardiac disease who have adequately compensated for anemia, transfusion is recommended if the hemoglobin is less than 8g/dL. High-risk patients who are older than 55 years and cannot compensate for anemia should be transfused to keep the hemoglobin over 10g/dL. The group includes those at risk for a myocardial event.

Preoperative autologous blood donation has been successful in older adults who are screened for anemia. Autologous blood can be used for orthopedic, cardiac, vascular, and other high-risk surgeries. Transfusion to bring the hemoglobin over 30 has shown to reduce 30-day short-term postoperative mortality in older adults.

Blood transfusion in the elderly must be done slowly to avoid circulatory overload. The hypertonic infusion of blood products can draw considerable cellular and interstitial fluid into the vascular system. The adage "start low and go slow" applies to blood administration as well as medication administration for elders. Units of packed RBCs can be split in half by the blood bank to increase the duration of infusion from 4 hours per unit to 4 hours for each split unit. Administering furosemide prior, during, or after the infusion can minimize volume overload. If a blood transfusion is ordered for an older adult, preoperatively or postoperatively, the nurse should ask the health care provider if furosemide should be administered.

> *The adage "start low and go slow" applies to blood administration as well as medication administration for elders.*

POSTOPERATIVE CONSIDERATIONS

During the immediate postoperative period, gerioperative patients must be carefully assessed for bleeding. Drains and drainage tubes must be carefully monitored for excessive bleeding. Procedures such as lithotripsy that involve trauma require frequent assessment for the presence of hematomas. Procedures on highly vascular organs or tissues such as the bladder or prostate may require continuous irrigations systems to avoid drainage obstruction by clots.

Estimated perioperative blood loss, communicated during the intraoperative-postoperative handoff, should be considered when evaluating for signs and symptoms of anemia. The perioperative transfusion of any blood products should also be communicated with the transition of care. The nurse should ask whether any furosemide was administered with the blood products during surgery. If not, the nurse should monitor the patient closely for signs of fluid overload. If the patient develops signs of fluid overload, the nurse should contact the surgeon or anesthesia provider to determine if the patient needs a diuretic.

HEMOSTASIS

Hemostasis, the changing of blood from a liquid to solid clot, is a complex process involving numerous proteins and particles. Hemostasis is triggered by injury to the vascular endothelium, exposing proteins that attract clotting factors and platelets. Tissue damage initiates the clotting cascade. Thrombin is produced by the cascade and acts to convert fibrinogen to fibrin.

The fibrin protein strands form a mesh with the platelets that resembles a "plug." Plasminogen from the liver is converted into plasmin, which begins the process of breaking down the clot, or fibrinolysis. The breakdown of fibrin results in circulating fibrin degradation or split products.

Age-Related Changes

Age-related changes occur at several levels of hemostasis. Several coagulation factors increase with age. Fibrinogen, the precursor to fibrin, increases 10 mg/dL per decade. Thus fibrin, the major circulating protein that acts to inhibit fibrinolysis, is increased with age. Platelet activity accelerates with age as platelets become more responsive to collagen exposure of the vascular endothelium. Changes in the vascular epithelium involve increase in collagen and calcium of the vessel wall. Stiffness and inelasticity contribute to endothelial dysfunction. The sum of these age-related changes is a greater likelihood of thrombosis.

In addition to physiologic changes related to hemostasis, several environmental factors contribute to risk of thrombosis. Diets rich in polyunsaturated fats, a diet not seen in nutritionally deficient elders, can reduce thrombotic tendency. Smoking increases fibrinogen levels. Lack of physical activity increases inflammation and the propensity to clot.

The consequence of age-related and environmental influences on hemostasis is a higher incidence of thromboembolic disorders in the elderly. The hypercoagulable state represents body proteins that are out of balance.

Hypercoagulability is one of the three arms of Virchow's triad, or risk factors for venous thromboembolism. Decreased blood flow and trauma to the vessel are the other arms of the triad. The gerioperative patient is positive for all three of Virchow's risk factors. Decreased blood flow, or stasis, occurs as a result of venous pooling due to supine positioning and the effects of anesthesia. Trauma to the intima of the vessel is the result of excessive vasodilation and constriction caused by vasoactive amines and anesthetic medications. In addition to age, additional risk factors for deep venous thromboembolism, or DVT, have been identified that are commonly identified in gerioperative patients (see Exhibit 16.4). Elders at particular high risk for DVT include hip or leg fracture/replacement, major general surgery, major trauma, or spinal cord injury.

GERIOPERATIVE CARE

The risks of DVT are considerable for older adults. Prophylaxis begins preoperatively with the application of knee-high compression stockings to support venous return. Stockings must be properly sized to fit snugly and work effectively. Intraoperative interventions include application of intermittent pneumatic compression stockings (PCS), which will be transferred to the postoperative unit. The PCS stockings are used until the elder is ambulatory. It is recommended that, while

The risks of DVT are considerable for older adults.

EXHIBIT 16.4 Risk Factors for Deep Vein Thromboembolism

- Age > 50 years
- History of varicose veins
- History of myocardial infarction
- History of cancer
- History of atrial fibrillation
- History of ischemic stroke
- History of diabetes mellitus

in bed or sitting in a chair, the stockings remain on. Depending on the surgery and ambulation potential, thromboprophylaxis with heparin, low-molecular-weight heparin, warfarin, or other anticoagulants are indicated. For better absorption, all heparin products ordered subcutaneously should be administered in the tissue of the abdomen below the umbilicus.

PATIENT REPORT: Mrs. Nagele

The preoperative nurse informs the anesthesia provider of Mrs. Nagele's laboratory values. A type and cross of blood products is ordered, just in case blood would need to be administered. Once admitted to the operating room, the circulating nurse applies PCS over Mrs. Nagele's compression stockings. Mrs. Nagele loses 350 mL of blood during her 2-hour surgery. In the postanesthesia care unit, laboratory work includes a hemoglobin and hematocrit. Mrs. Nagele is transferred to the surgical floor. The laboratory reports hemoglobin as 9.8 g/dL and hematocrit as 33g/dL. Intravenous fluids are decreased from 100 mL/hr to 75 mL/hr because the hemoglobin/hematocrit ratio is greater than one to three. After consulting with the surgeon, Mrs. Nagele will have a CBC drawn in the morning. Her compression stockings and PCS remain on while she is on bed rest.

SUMMARY

The bone marrow of elder adults is capable of supporting the hematological needs under baseline conditions. Like other systems, the reserve capacity and prompt response of the stem cells to produce platelets, RBCs, and WBCs is diminished. When faced with the stress of surgery in the presence of comorbid illnesses responsible for anemia or chronic inflammatory response, the hemopoeitic system is slow to respond. Without adequate oxygen provided by hemoglobin molecules, wounds are slow to heal and risk of cardiac complications increases. Without sufficient WBCs, the risk of infection is great. The hypercoagulabity of aging challenges health care providers to promote venous return and reduce DVT, so compression devices are necessary to reduce the risk of DVT. Chemical prophylaxis by heparin or low-molecular-weight heparin may also be used along with compression devices to reduce the incidence of DVT.

KEY POINTS

- Anemia is not an age-related disease but occurs more frequently in the elderly.
- Anemia results in decreased wound healing, increased mortality, and hospitalization.
- Older adults are at high risk for deep vein thrombosis.
- Prevention, assessment, and early intervention of hematologic complications after surgery are critical to promoting recovery in the gerioperative patient.

SEVENTEEN

Immunity

Kathleen M. Gilkey, Jennifer V. Long, and Susan J. Fetzer

PATIENT REPORT: Mr. Cheney

Mr. Cheney, a 68-year-old attorney, underwent a hernia repair with mesh under general anesthesia. This is his second surgery to repair this hernia. He has an extensive medical history including a liver transplant 4 years ago. He is a nondrinker, nonsmoker and still works part-time in his law office. His medication regime includes cyclosporine and prednisone. He reports regular dental checkups, pays careful attention to his diet including washing fresh fruits and vegetables, and follows up on his blood work at regular intervals. The preoperative nurse recognizes that Mr. Cheney is at high risk for postoperative surgical site infection because of his immunosuppression and communicates this finding to the perioperative team.

The immune system, an integral part of the lymphatic system, is a complex network of chemicals, cells, organs, and tissues that protects the body against illness and infection. The immune system and lymphatic system work closely together to protect the body from harmful external microorganisms and toxins as well as internal neoplastic cells. The lymphatic system works closely with other body systems to aid in immunity by removing excess fluid, waste, debris, pathogens, cancer cells, and toxins. It also supports lymphocytic activity while preventing an imbalance of fluids in the internal environment. Fluid imbalance is prevented by returning interstitial fluid to the vascular system via the lymphatic system.

This chapter reviews the lymphatic and immune systems with attention to age-related changes. Nursing implications for preoperative, intraoperative, and postoperative care of the gerioperative patient with altered immunity are presented.

IMMUNE AND LYMPHATIC CONSIDERATIONS

LYMPHATIC SYSTEM

When blood flow slows in the capillary beds, interstitial fluid seeps out of the capillary walls through the capillary pores into the tissues and becomes interstitial fluid. Interstitial fluid bathes and surrounds cells of the body, delivering nutrients to cells, removing metabolic waste, and providing intercellular communication. Interstitial fluid contains amino acids, sugars, fatty acids, hormones, neurotransmitters, salts, coenzymes, and waste products from the cell. It is the primary component of extracellular fluid.

Interstitial fluid normally returns to the blood by venous absorption. However, not all interstitial fluid is able to return to the blood. Capillary outflow exceeds the venous reabsorption rate by approximately 3 L a day. Excess interstitial fluid enters the lymphatic system and is described as lymph.

Lymph is similar to blood plasma but has less protein. Lymph also contains various foreign substances such as bacterial cells and viruses that have been removed from the cell and entered the interstitial fluid. The lymph must eventually return to the bloodstream in order to maintain sufficient blood volume in the vascular space. The lymph system prevents loss of interstitial fluid from the blood circulation that would result in decreased circulatory volume.

LYMPHATIC VESSELS

The lymphatic vessels begin as microscopic, closed-ended capillaries that extend into the interstitial spaces. The vessels join together to form a mesh-like network of tubes that run parallel to the blood capillaries. These lymphatic capillaries merge together to form the afferent lymphatic vessels.

The afferent lymphatic vessels lead to lymph nodes where the lymph is filtered. The vessels leave the lymph nodes and become the efferent lymphatic vessels. The efferent vessels merge to form the lymphatic trunks and are named for the region of the body that they serve. For example, the intestinal lymphatic trunks drain fluid from the abdominal viscera. The trunks join into two large ducts: the right lymphatic duct or left thoracic duct.

Lymph collected by the right lymphatic duct from the right side of the head, neck, thorax, and right arm returns to the right subclavian vein. The thoracic lymph duct drains lymph from the rest of the body into the left subclavian vein near the internal jugular vein. Damage to the left lymphatic duct during procedures involving the left subclavian vein can affect lymph drainage. Such damage results in edema to the abdomen, gastrointestinal tract, pelvis, left side of the thorax, left arm, and lower extremities due to the inability of the lymph to drain into the venous circulatory system.

Valves similar to those in veins keep the lymph flowing in a one-way direction toward the heart. Surgical removal of lymph nodes and other changes to lymph drainage hinders movement of lymph. Disruption in the lymphatic flow results in fluid accumulation in the interstitial spaces causing edema.

Lymph is carried through the lymphatic system by contraction of skeletal muscles and by the muscular walls of the lymphatic vessels. As skeletal muscles and the muscular walls of the lymphatic vessels contract, they compress the lymphatic vessels causing the lymph to move toward lymphatic ducts. Change in thoracic and abdominal pressures during respiration forces the lymph into the lymphatic system and toward the lymphatic ducts.

LYMPH NODES

The human body contains between 600 and 700 lymph nodes, which are bean-shaped structures located at intervals along the lymphatic system. The major lymph node locations are the cervical region, axillary region, thoracic cavity, abdominal cavity, inguinal region, and the pelvic cavity.

Lymph nodes contain large numbers of lymphocytes and macrophages to defend against invading pathogens. As lymph passes through the honeycomb of lymph node connective tissue, the lymphocytes and macrophages destroy and filter potentially harmful foreign particles before they reach the bloodstream.

Lymph nodes enlarge when an infection is present due to enhanced activity and increased division of lymphocytes. The increased activity leads to increased fluid and noticeable swelling of the lymph node. The failure of the lymphatic system due to trauma, disease, or genetic factors can lead to lymphedema. Lymphedema is localized lymph fluid retention and swelling. There are two types of lymphedema: primary and secondary. Primary lymphedema is a congenital defect causing dilated lymphatic capillaries and subsequent swelling. Secondary lymphedema occurs after removal of lymph nodes, damage to the lymphatic vessels, or a functional deficiency. Some causes of secondary lymphedema are surgical removal of nodes, trauma, cancer, inflammation, and infection.

Age-Related Changes

Age-related changes to the lymphatic system decrease the ability of the lymph vessels to collect fluid from the interstitial space and transport the lymph back to the blood. Pressure- and flow-dependent regulatory mechanisms are impaired secondary to decreased muscle mass, strength, and decreased muscle contractility. The result is a general slowing of lymph flow into and through the lymph vessels. These changes can lead to the back up of lymph and lymphedema. Elders are more prone to inflammation, infections, and cancers that lead to lymphedema.

IMMUNE DEFENSE

The human body has multiple strategies to defend against invading organisms. The first defense is that of a surface or barrier defense. The physical barrier of the skin, mucous membranes, and conjunctiva are protective. Bacteria are removed mechanically by tears, sloughing of skin cells, ciliary action, coughing, sneezing, vomiting, urinating, and defecating. Chemical barrier defenses include gastric acid, lactic acid, fatty acids, and bile salts.

The second defense is known as nonspecific resistance factors. These factors include fever, lysozymes, C-reactive proteins, alpha-1-trypsin, and interferon. Interferon is a group of proteins produced by cells in response to the presence of viruses that interfere with the reproduction of viruses in other cells.

The third type of defense against an invading pathogen is a tissue response, known as the inflammatory response. Inflammation occurs within seconds of an invading pathogen and includes localized redness, swelling, heat, and pain. Inflammation is an attempt to remove injurious stimuli in order to initiate the healing process. The process of inflammation begins when blood vessels dilate in response to an invading pathogen or injury. Capillary permeability increases and tissues become red, swollen, warm, and painful. White blood cells (leukocytes) invade the region and pus may form as these cells, along with bacterial cells and cellular debris accumulate. Body fluids then seep into the area, causing swelling. A clot containing threads of fibrin may form if there is a vascular injury. Fibroblasts appear, forming a connective tissue sac around the injured area. During this defensive response, plasma and leukocytes move from the blood to the injured tissue. Leukocytes accumulate at the injured site and help control the invading pathogen by phagocytosis. The leukocytic phagocytes include circulating neutrophils, eosinophils, monocytes, and macrophages. Phagocytes remove dead cells and debris, allowing cells to reproduce and replace the injured cells. Neutrophils and macrophages engulf and destroy the foreign particles and cells.

The inflammatory response occurs in response to tissue injury, tissue repair, infection, allergic reactions such as allergic rhinitis, and other injuries. The inflammatory response

TABLE 17.1

Functions of Specific Lymphocytes

Immune Response	Lymphocyte	Function
Inflammation	Neutrophil	Nonspecific ingestion and phagocytosis of antigens
	Macrophage	Nonspecific recognition of antigens; ingestion andphagocytosis of antigens
	Eosinophil	Weak phagocytosis
	Basophils	Releases histamine in areas of tissue damage
Antibody-mediated immunity	B lymphocyte	Becomes sensitized to antigens
	Plasma cell	Secretes immunoglobulins in response to the presence of antigen
	Memory cell	Remains sensitized to a specific antigen that B-cell had previously encountered; secretes large amount of antibodies specific to that antigen
Cell-mediated immunity	T-lymphocyte Helper T-cells	Enhances immune activity through secretion of cytokines and lymphokines
	Cytotoxic T-cells	Selectively attacks and destroys nonself cells, including viruses, grafts, transplanted tissues
	Natural killer	Nonselectively attacks nonself cells, especially cells that undergone mutations and have become malignant, also attacks transplanted tissues

occurs in response to an antigen without the presence of an active infection. A mediator of the response to inflammation is the cytokines, proteins produced by white blood cells that act as messengers. When white blood cells have been activated, cytokines alert the brain that a disturbance requiring an immune response has occurred. Fever develops in response to the cytokines and additional defenses are initiated. The final type of defense is the immune response, the most complicated and yet comprehensive response.

The immune response occurs slower than the inflammatory response and targets its response to provide long-term protection against very specific microorganisms. A number of immune mechanisms are involved in which select cells recognize the presence of particular foreign substances and then act to eliminate them. The immune-specific cells are lymphocytes, polymorphonuclear cells, natural killer (NK) cells, and macrophages. Two specific response mechanisms are the humoral response (B-cell, plasma cells, and immunoglobulins [Ig]) and the cell-mediated response (T-cells, lymphokines). Table 17.1 lists functions of the different lymphocytes.

CELLS OF IMMUNITY

Macrophages

Wound healing is regulated by macrophages, which are impaired in the older adult.

Macrophages are white blood cell phagocytes that engulf and digest (phagocytosis) cellular debris and pathogens. The macrophage processes the antigen and presents the antigen fragments to the T-cell, which results in the formation of an antibody. In addition to phagocytosis, macrophages produce cytokines, signaling proteins that alert the brain and other white blood cells to inflammation. Wound healing is regulated by macrophages.

Age-Related Changes

Macrophages in the elderly show decreased ability for phagocytosis and decreased cytokine production. There is a general decrease in infiltration and antigen presentation. Macrophages have an impaired ability to kill invading tumor cells. The decline in macrophage function impairs wound healing. The consequence is longer healing times with greater risk of infection.

POLYMORPHONUCLEAR LEUKOCYTES

Polymorphonuclear (PMN) cells, also known as neutrophils, are the most abundant phagocytes and the first line of defense. The PMN cells are one of the first cells recruited to tissue sites in response to inflammation and infection. Once a PMN cell engulfs a virus or bacteria, they die and undergo phagocytosis by macrophages. The debris composed of foreign cells, PMN cells, and macrophages appears as pus. PMN cells also stimulate monocytes and macrophages, causing an increase in phagocytosis.

Age-Related Changes

While there is no apparent difference in the number of PMN cells in the elderly, PMN cells are slower to respond to inflammation and infection. The presence of chronic diseases also affects the ability of PMN cells to respond. In elders with cardiovascular disease or poorly controlled diabetes, PMN cells show further deterioration in their response and function, which increases the risk of infection and delayed wound healing.

IMMUNOCYTES

The primary immunocyte is the lymphoid stem cell, which originates in the bone marrow of an adult. The undifferentiated lymphoid stem cell is a precursor to one of three types of lymphocytes: NK cells, B-cells, or T-cells. Figure 17.1 shows the process of immunocyte formation from bone marrow to the periphery.

NATURAL KILLER CELLS

Natural killer (NK) cells, not to be confused with killer T-cells, kill tumors and cells infected by viruses by releasing a protein that causes the tumor or virus cell to die by apoptosis or programmed cell death. Because NK cells do not express an antigen receptor or surface marker for the development of antibodies, they must receive an activating signal by a cytokine. The NK cells contain the viral infection while the adaptive immune response is generating antigen lymphocytes that can remove the antigen.

Age-Related Changes

With age, the NK cells become less responsive to activation by cytokine due to a decrease in activating receptors. However, the impact is minimized by an increase in the actual number of NK cells available in the blood. Thus, NK cells continue to provide the same protection in the elderly as in the younger population.

T-CELLS (CELL-MEDIATED IMMUNITY)

Lymphoid stem cells that leave the bone marrow and migrate to the thymus are described as T-cells. Once in the thymus, the cells undergo cell division to generate a large population

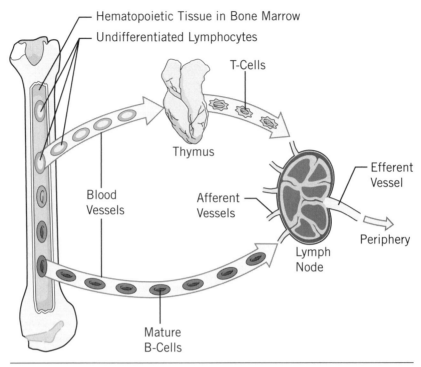

FIGURE 17.1

Lymphocyte Formation

Undifferentiated lymphocytes are released into the bloodstream and are processed in the thymus gland to become T-cells. Others mature to become B-cells
while in the marrow and then are released into the bloodstream. B-cells and
T-cells are transported to the lymphatic organs by the blood where they remain
until needed.

*Immune system cells are considered
naïve when they have not yet been
exposed to an antigen.*

of immature cells. The immature cells move into the inner
cortex of the thymus where they mature and differentiate.
The cells are then known as naïve T-cells until they are
exposed to an antigen. T-cells act directly against bacteria
and viruses with no need to form antibodies. The T-cell
response is referred to as a cell-mediated response. T-cells
are mobilized when the macrophage has ingested an antigen and is displaying antigen fragments bound to its molecules. The complex activates the T-cell receptors and the T-cells
secrete cytokines necessary for T-cells to mature. Cytokines promote the growth and differentiation of T-cells.

When the T-cell encounters an antigen, five subtypes of cells are produced with each
having its own immune response. Lymphokine-producing T-cells secrete proteins that activate other T-cells, stimulate the production of leukocytes in bone marrow, cause the growth
and maturation of B-cells, and activate macrophages. Cytotoxic T-cells attack antigens
directly and destroy cells that contain foreign antigens. These cells, known as killer T-cells,
are capable of causing the direct death of infected tissue or tumor cells. Killer T-cells act on
viruses or cells that are otherwise damaged or dysfunctional. When transplanted tissue is
rejected, cytotoxic killer T-cells are involved.

Memory T-cells induce the secondary immune response and are antigen-specific cells that persist long after an infection has resolved. Memory T-cells quickly proliferate to very large numbers when reexposed to the initial antigen. Helper T-cells assist other lymphocytes in the immunologic process and activate cytotoxic T-cells and macrophages. Helper T-cells participate in the maturation of B-cells and secrete cytokines to facilitate the immune response. Suppressor T-cells are known as regulatory T-cells and act to suppress the immune response of other cells. The process by which the immune system does not attack an antigen, immunologic tolerance, is mediated by the suppressor T-cells. Lack of suppressor T-cells contribute to autoimmune disease.

> *The inability of the aging thymus to regenerate naïve T-cells results in immunosuppression.*

Age-Related Changes

Age-related changes of the thymus lead to decreased production of naïve T-cells. The decrease in production is dramatic with advanced age and results in an overall reduction in the T-cell pool. T-cell reduction leads to an increase in severity of infections, inflammation, and decreased protectiveness of vaccines. The decrease in thymocyte production leads to decreased T-cell diversity and function. When exposed to a new or reoccurring antigen, there is impaired activation and proliferation of T-cells. The naïve T-cells that survive to old age are less functional and less responsive to antigens. Memory T-cells proliferate and become overabundant, restricting the few naïve T-cells from migrating out of the thymus to respond to new antigens. The memory cell proliferation leads to a chronic antigen load and is responsible for the chronic inflammatory status of the elderly. Figure 17.2 shows age-related changes in production of T-cells and B-cells.

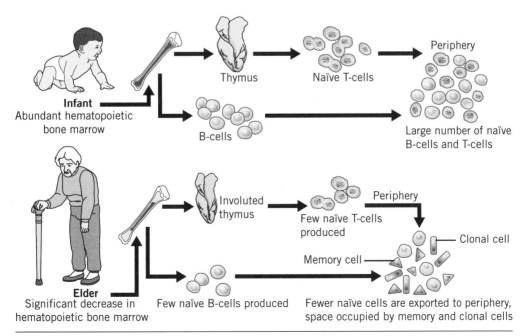

FIGURE 17.2

Age-Related Changes' Impact on T-cell and B-cell Formation

The decline in helper T-cells impairs B-cell to T-cell interaction. Unable to be presented with antigens by missing helper T-cells, B-cells do not form an antibody. The inability of the aging thymus to regenerate naïve T-cells results in immunocompetence in an older adult.

B-CELLS (HUMORAL RESPONSE)

Lymphoid stem cells that remain in the bone marrow until maturity are known as B-cells. Once released into the blood, they travel to the spleen where they undergo differentiation. B-cells are described as naïve when they have never come into contact with an antigen.

Age-related fat deposits in the bone marrow decrease naïve B-cells.

It is only when B-cells encounter an antigen that they are activated and engulf and digest the antigen. After ingestion, the cell displays antigen fragments on the cell surface, attracting the help of a mature, helper, or suppressor T-cells. The T-cells secrete cytokines, which enables B-cell maturity and enables them to produce and secrete Ig, or antibodies, when activated. Antibodies act directly against the antigen. Once released into the blood, antibodies lock onto matching antigens and begin to eradicate the antigens. B-cells reproduce and form memory cells capable of recognizing the same antigen for a faster, more efficient, and more powerful response in future antigen encounters.

Age-Related Changes

B-cells are produced in the vertebrae, ribs, sternum, flat bones of the pelvis, cranium, and the ends of long bones. As fat deposits accumulate in the bone marrow with age, there is a decrease in bone marrow producing cells resulting in a decline in naïve B-cells. Aged bone marrow also has a reduced ability to support B-cell proliferation once the person has been exposed to an antigen.

The decrease in naïve B-cells is accompanied with an increase in B-cells that have already been exposed to antigens: memory B-cells. The increase in memory B-cells further depresses the production of naïve B-cells, rendering those that are produced with less of a chance to respond to new antigens. The new B-cells also are unable to migrate to the secondary lymphoid structures because of the presence of memory B-cells. This further reduces the chance that an antigen will come in contact with its antigen-specific B-cell. Age-related changes to the B-cells make the immune system of the gerioperative patient less effective.

ANTIBODIES

The immune system uses antibodies or Ig to identify and neutralize bacteria and viruses. Each antibody is capable of recognizing one individual antigen. There are five known classes of Ig, with each having a specific function: IgA, IgD, IgE, IgG, and IgM. Table 17.2 describes the function of each class of Ig.

IgA, the most abundant antibody, protects the surfaces that are directly exposed to external substances and is commonly found in mucosal tissue as well as milk, tears, nasal fluid, gastric juices, intestinal juices, bile, and urine. IgA prevents pathogen colonization. IgD is found on the surface of some B-lymphocytes. It functions mainly as an antigen receptor on the B-cell that has not been exposed to an antigen. IgD also signals B cells to become activated.

IgE is the least abundant antibody and responsible for binding to allergens and triggering a histamine reaction. Upon the first exposure to an antigen, the antibody becomes

TABLE 17.2

Specific Functions of Immunoglobulin Classes

IgA	Prevents pathogen colonization
	Protects the surfaces that are directly exposed to external substances
IgD	Antigen receptor on the B-cell that has not been exposed to an antigen
	Signals B-cells to be activated
IgE	Responsible for binding to allergens and triggering a histamine reaction
IgG	Provides immunity against infections of bacteria, viruses, and all other toxins
IgM	First to be produced in response to an infection
	Interacts with blood cell type A and B antigens

sensitized. When reexposure occurs, the antigen binding to the antibody IgE initiates the release of chemical mediators, including histamine. The mediators produce a symptom complex known as anaphylaxis, which includes bronchospasm, upper airway edema, urticaria, and increased capillary permeability. The increase in capillary permeability combined with histamine results in vasodilatation, hypotension, and eventually leads to shock. IgE is found in very high concentrations in persons with allergies.

IgG is found primarily in plasma providing immunity against infections of bacteria, viruses, and all other toxins. IgM, the largest of the antibodies, is the first to be produced in response to an infection. IgM also interacts with blood cell type A and B antigens.

Antibodies act directly by combining with an antigen and causing agglutination (clumping) or precipitation (formation of a soluble substance). Antibodies can also block or neutralize the action of the pathogen's toxin or cause the invading pathogen's cell membrane to rupture. Antibodies act indirectly through the complement pathway. Antibodies combine with antigens to cause enzyme activation. The enzymes produce a variety of reactions including chemotaxis, inflammation, lysis, opsonization, and alterations of the virus' molecular structure. Chemotaxis is the attraction of macrophages and neutrophils while inflammation promotes local tissue changes that help prevent the spread of the antigen. Lysis ruptures the cell membrane while opsonization alters the membranes making it susceptible to phagocytosis.

Age-Related Changes

With age, there is a decline in circulating antibodies and a decrease in antibody secretion. However, with age there is an increase in the production of nonspecific Ig antibodies with a low affinity for antigens. The decrease in specificity and efficacy leads to a diminished primary and secondary response, especially to vaccines. Elders who receive vaccines respond with a lower antibody titer and less affinity of the vaccine for an antigen. The production of aberrant antibodies has been implicated in the development of autoimmune diseases.

SPLEEN

The spleen, located in the left upper quadrant of the abdomen, is the largest of the lymphatic organs and serves as a reservoir for blood. The blood that is stored in the spleen can be returned to the circulation during times of anemia, hypoxia, or hemorrhage. As a lymphatic organ, the spleen stores lymphocytes, monocytes, and macrophages.

Elders' decreased immunity is directly related to the decline in thymus gland function.

Structurally, the spleen consists of two distinct areas: red pulp and white pulp. The red pulp is a mechanical filtration system for red blood cells and storage site for half of the monocytes. The white pulp houses lymphocytes and macrophages that remove antibody-coated bacteria. The lymphocytes and macrophages are essential in defending against infection. The macrophages engulf and destroy foreign material such as bacteria that may be carried in the blood. Lymphocytes mount immune responses to foreign invaders.

Age-Related Changes

A decrease in the elastin fibers of the spleen with age contributes to a decrease in splenic mass. Functionally, there are few changes in the spleen, despite a decrease in the number of circulating lymphocytes.

THYMUS

Located in the mediastinum, behind the sternum, the thymus gland is a soft structure that is composed of two identical lobes: medulla and cortex. The two lobes contain a large number of lymphocytes that have developed from precursor cells originating in the bone marrow. The function of the thymus is to further develop and differentiate the T-cells. As a gland, the thymus secretes thymosin, a hormone that stimulates T-cell growth. The thymus contains a lifetime supply of T-cells by age 16.

Age-Related Changes

With age, the thymus undergoes a significant decrease in size, composition, and function. Having reached a maximum size of up to 37 grams shortly after puberty, by age 75 the thymus is scarcely visible at 6 grams. As thymus size and weight decreases, cells in the cortex and medulla are replaced with fat and connective tissue. The decline in the thymus gland activity with aging is reflected in the decrease in immunity experienced by elders. With the decline in thymus function, elders become more susceptible to bacterial invasion, immune-related diseases such as arthritis and cancer, and are less likely to respond to antigens and allergens.

IMMUNITY

Immunity is the resistance to specific foreign antigens that invade the body and the actions the body undergoes to combat these antigens. An antigen is a foreign protein that is capable of inducing a specific immune response. Antigens can be infectious, such as viruses, fungi, bacteria, and parasites, or noninfectious, such as pollen, foods, bee venom, drugs, vaccines, transfusions, and transplanted tissues.

There are two types of immunity: natural immunity and acquired immunity. Natural immunity is native or innate immunity and does not require prior exposure or sensitization to an antigen. The skin, lymphocytes, macrophages, PMN cells, NK cells, stomach acid, and chemicals in the bloodstream are all present at birth and provide natural immunity. Natural immunity represents a primary defense system responsible for spontaneous killing of select tumor cells and viruses. Acquired immunity is gained after birth as a result of the immune response. There are two types of acquired immunity: passive and active. Passive immunity occurs during short-term exposure to a specific antigen or disease. A comprehensive immune response does not occur, but specific lymphocytes are transferred to the recipient. A trauma patient who receives tetanus immune globulin obtains passive immunity.

Active immunity occurs after natural exposure to an antigen or by immunization. There are three responses involved in the active immune response: primary, secondary, and tertiary. The primary response is the initial exposure to an antigen followed by a latent phase and finally the formation of antibodies. The primary response primes the body to recognize the specific antigen whenever a second exposure occurs. The secondary response occurs when memory cells are present after the primary response. During this response, there is a quicker formation of antibodies and faster reaction to the antigen. The tertiary phase is long-term immunization when the antigen is made less infectious or is altered so that it may cause a primary response but will not cause illness.

Age-Related Changes

Immunosenescence is the dramatic reduction in responsiveness as well as a functional regulation of the aging immune system. A complex process, immunosenescence causes alterations in immune reactions. Elders are less able to generate an immune response to invading pathogens than their younger counterparts. The decline leads to an increase in infection rates, cancer, autoimmune diseases, and a subsequent decrease in the quality of life. Death from infection is a much greater risk in the elderly.

Chronic illnesses, common among the elderly, increase the risk of infection. Chronic low-grade inflammation and an increase in inflammatory cytokines are associated with increased risk of physical disability, cardiovascular disease, upper and lower respiratory infections, and urinary tract infections. Chronic low-grade inflammation masks inflammation caused by more serious pathogens, explaining why the elderly are much sicker and may develop sepsis before the body exhibits any outward signs or symptoms of infection.

Decreased cytokine production with age leads to a decrease in the ability of the skin to mount an inflammatory response. The decreased inflammatory response leads to impaired wound healing with greater risk for infection. Depression and physical and psychological stressors enhance the production of inflammatory cytokines. The stress response triggers the release of cortisol and catecholamines, which in turn cause a decrease in cytokine function. Stress further limits the body's ability to produce an acute inflammatory response.

Malnutrition is associated with significant impairment in immunity. Poor dentition, medication anorexia, restrictive diets, gastrointestinal disorders, and metabolic disorders, such as diabetes and renal insufficiency, all cause a reduction in nutrient intake that can increase the risk of infection. Infections in turn increase the nutrient requirements that, if not corrected, will lead to further vulnerability and increased episodes of worsening infections. Obesity is associated with several immunological disorders as well as an overall increased risk of infection. Hormonal changes during menopause and adrenopause decrease cellular responses to infections.

Elders must be considered an immunocompromised population.

The diminished function of the immune system results in a weaker antibody response to vaccinations. Vaccine-induced antibody responses wane rapidly in the elderly. The long-term effects of vaccines administered to elders cannot be taken for granted. As the response to vaccines becomes weaker, minimal protection is provided against deadly illnesses such as pneumonia and influenza. The diminished immune system results in the recommendations to administer the pneumonia vaccine to elders every 5 years and the influenza vaccine every year.

There are two types of influenza vaccine. The flu shot is an intramuscular injection of nonviable influenza that is not contagious or infectious. The Flumist (MedImmune, Inc.) nasal spray contains attenuated live influenza virus that usually does not cause infection. If influenza infection occurs, the virus and the symptoms it produces are much weaker and illness is far less severe than the influenza. Elders should not receive Flumist as it contains the live influenza virus that can actually inoculate elders with influenza. In the geriatric population, the resulting illness can be much worse than in younger individuals and can progress to pneumonia.

Elders must be considered an immunocompromised population. Health care providers should receive the flu shot because the live nasal vaccine virus can produce mild flu symptoms. Viral load can be shed from nasal drainage of the mild symptoms, potentially infecting others for up to 3 days. Because many patients cared for by health care providers are elderly and immunocompromised, the Flumist vaccine can indirectly infect elders with influenza.

AUTOIMMUNITY

Immune responses are usually directed toward foreign molecules but sometimes the tolerance to self is lost or decreased enough to make the immune response turn towards an individual's own cells. The attack on self is known as autoimmunity. Autoimmune diseases such as Grave's disease, lupus erythematosus, Hashimoto's thyroiditis, diabetes mellitus type I, and rheumatoid arthritis can attack specific organs or be systemic. A small amount of autoimmunity may be beneficial in aiding the recognition of neoplastic, precancer cells before they are able to proliferate, but overactive autoimmune responses can be detrimental.

Age-Related Changes
With the aging of the immune system and the decline in T- and B-cell function, there is a loss of ability to distinguish between foreign antigens and the "self." Thus, autoimmune diseases come more common in the elder population.

Gerioperative Care

PREOPERATIVE CONSIDERATIONS

Preoperative assessment focuses on identifying additional risk factors for postoperative infection in the immunocompromised elder and identifying risk factors for allergic reactions. Risk factors for postoperative infection include preoperative medication regimens, underlying undiagnosed infections, and malnutrition. Risk factors for allergic reactions include environmental exposure to foreign substances, anesthetic drugs, and latex.

Chronic disease medications such as prednisone, antirheumatics, beta blockers, nonsteroidals, and antihistamines suppress a febrile reaction to invading pathogens. The decline in immune responsiveness makes diagnosing an infection in an elder difficult. There is a lack of typical symptoms such as fever or rash. An unexplained alteration of behavior, sudden confusion, agitation, lethargy, urinary incontinence, or loss of appetite is often the only sign of infection in an older adult. The onset of infections is often missed among the elderly population.

It is imperative that nurses complete a thorough preoperative evaluation and adequately assess for possible infections. This includes exploring any unusual behaviors with patients or their families if the patient is unable to answer questions.

Autoimmune diseases are more common among older adults than younger adults.

The white blood count may not be elevated during an untreated infection in an elder adult.

An allergy history includes drug, food, and environmental allergens. Elders often misunderstand an adverse reaction for an allergic response. An allergic reaction accounts for less than 10% of all adverse reactions. Allergic reactions rarely occur after a week of drug therapy and symptoms do not resemble the drug's intended action.

Patients may be prescribed antibiotics preoperatively. During the preoperative assessment, inquire as to recent or current antibiotic use, the purpose of the antibiotic, and the duration of treatment. Confirm that the symptoms of the infection were relieved by the preoperative antibiotic. Elders have a decreased affinity for antibiotics and the antibiotic may not have been effective.

The skin is inspected and open wounds assessed for signs and symptoms of infection. Wounds that are not healing may not demonstrate the typical signs of infection such as redness, drainage, or odor. All nonhealing wounds should be brought to the attention of the surgeon. Open areas should be covered with an occlusive dressing before surgery to avoid "shedding" of bacteria or viruses. Additional focused areas of assessment include urinary and respiratory systems, which are high risk for infection among elders.

Preoperative laboratory testing can include a complete blood count with differential if an undiagnosed, untreated infection is being considered. However, an elevated white blood cell count, leukocytosis, may not be present due to elders' weakened immune system. Serum creatinine and liver enzymes may be needed to detect organ damage related to inappropriate antibiotic dosing. Many facilities require that elders habituating in long-term care facilities be screened for methycillin-resistant *Staphylococcus aureus*. In additional to nasal swabbing, open wounds should also be cultured.

If an infection is suspected or the surgery is high risk for poor outcomes if the surgical site becomes infected (total joint replacement), a urinalysis should be obtained. If the urinalysis or dip stick urine results show nitrates and leukocyte esterase, a clinically significant urinary tract infection is present, even if the patient does not exhibit signs or symptoms of an infection. The surgeon must be notified if the leukocyte esterase and nitrates are positive.

Antibiotics given within 1 hour of surgical incision have been shown to decrease the incidence of postoperative would infections. The preoperative nurse must coordinate the administration of the antibiotic with the anesthesia provider to ensure that the ordered antibiotic is available and infused within the 1 hour timeframe.

INTRAOPERATIVE CONSIDERATIONS

The greatest perioperative concern related to immune function is anaphylactic reactions. The large number of drugs given rapidly during induction of anesthesia can stress the weakened immune system of elders. Several commonly identified agents that induce allergic reaction are listed in Exhibit 17.1. Of the medications listed, muscle relaxants and antibiotics are the biggest offenders.

Hypotension is common in the elderly surgical patient secondary to anesthesia. However, if a patient is experiencing hypotension that is refractory to fluids and vasoconstrictors, anaphylaxis should be considered and treated appropriately. Initial treatment includes administering 100% oxygen, discontinuing anesthetic drugs if possible, providing volume expansion, and administering epinephrine or vasopressin.

POSTOPERATIVE CONSIDERATIONS

Health care workers are inundated with hand washing information and techniques and consequences of poor hand washing. However, in the care of the gerioperative patient, excellent hand washing techniques and practices are necessary to prevent infection.

EXHIBIT 17.1 Perioperative Agents Known to Trigger Anaphylaxis

Anesthetics
    Induction agents: propofol, etomidate, barbiturates
    Local anesthetics
    Muscle relaxants: succinylcholine, vecuronium, mivacurium
    Opioids: meperidine, morphine, fentanyl

Perioperative medications
    Antibiotics: cephalosporins, penicillin, sulfonamides, vancomycin
    Cyclosporine
    Furosemide
    Nonsteroidal anti-inflammatory drugs
    Protamine
    Radiocontrast dye
    Colloid volume expanders: dextran, albumin, hydroxyethyl starch

Perioperative materials
    Bone cement
    Latex

A lack of clinical symptoms at the onset of infection often delays diagnosis and treatment. If wound healing is delayed, so frequent inspection of postsurgical sites is needed. Antibiotic therapy may be necessary to combat an infection and should be started early. Changes to the immune system in surgically stressed gerioperative patients can delay a response to infection. Nurses must be vigilant to prevent infection and provide early intervention in the event an infection begins.

Postoperative pulmonary toileting is necessary as elderly have decreased ciliary action, decreased gag reflexes, and decreased cough reflexes, which predisposes them to pulmonary infections. Even after immunization with the pneumonia vaccine, the risk of infection is still greater in elders than in younger patients.

Patients and caregivers should receive information that changes in behavior may signal the onset of an infection. A health care provider should be notified immediately if the older adult demonstrates sudden or evolving behavioral or cognitive changes. Hand washing to prevent infection is mandatory, and nurse coaching surrounding proper hand washing and the use of alcohol hand sanitizers for family members is essential.

PATIENT REPORT: Mr. Cheney

Preoperatively, Mr. Cheney's intravenous line was started by the anesthesia provider using strict sterile technique in the operating room. The perioperative nurse conducted a thorough skin preparation of the area, and reminded the team members during the perioperative "time out" that Mr. Cheney was a transplant recipient. A large sterile transparent dressing was placed on the surgical site postoperatively and was covered with a snug abdominal binder. The circulating nurses discussed Mr. Cheney's preoperative drug regimen with the postanesthesia care unit nurse to ensure as little disruption as possible. After recovering from his anesthesia, Mr. Cheney is able to drink liquids and sit in a lounge chair in the phase 2 postanesthesia care unit. He takes his antirejection medication on time and does not require any pain medication. Prior to discharge, he is able to "talk back" the procedure for wound care and symptoms of infection he should report immediately. He is discharged home accompanied by his sister.

SUMMARY

Elders' immune systems and lymphatic systems are compromised by age-related changes. The gerioperative patient is at increased risk of infection due to these age-related changes, in addition to malnutrition, surgical stress, and altered tissue integrity after surgery. The nurse and health care providers should be vigilant to prevent surgery-related infections, and in the event that an infection occurs, initiate rapid appropriate intervention critical to achieving positive outcomes.

KEY POINTS

- Age-related changes in the skin and mucous membranes reduce the effectiveness of the first line of defense.
- Swollen glands during an infection result from increased activity of B-cells and T-cells in lymph nodes.
- Lymph circulation is diminished in elderly secondary to decreased overall movement and muscle tone.
- Thymus gland function is so reduced in elders that it is unable to supply enough new T-cells to combat invading antigens.
- Immunosenescence occurs with aging as a dramatic reduction in overall function of the immune system.
- Malnutrition is associated with significant impairment of the immune system.
- The elderly may not exhibit normal signs and symptoms of infection. The only indication of infection may be a sudden change in behavior or level of consciousness.
- Thorough assessment and early intervention are essential to prevent, identify, and treat infections in the gerioperative patient.

EIGHTEEN

Endocrine

Susan J. Fetzer, Jennifer V. Long, and Raelene V. Shippee-Rice

PATIENT REPORT: Ms. Wagaman

Ms. Wagaman is a single 72-year-old former waitress who lives with her widowed 65-year-old brother in a country farmhouse. She is attending the clinic for a scheduled preoperative evaluation by the nurse practitioner. A right breast biopsy with lumpectomy is scheduled for Ms. Wagaman in a week. Ms. Wagaman is 66 inches and weighs 210 pounds, for a body mass index of 33.9, which is reflective of obesity. She is a nonsmoker with no previous surgical history. Five years ago, she was diagnosed with type 2 diabetes, which is well controlled with diet and exercise. Recently, she has curtailed her daily walks with her brother complaining of shortness of breath and fatigue. She sees her primary care provider every 6 months and she takes rosiglitazone 4 mg every morning before breakfast. She reports that she has lost 5 pounds in 3 months. Ms. Wagaman is also taking levothyroxine 75 mcg every morning.

All organs and body cells are influenced by the effect of hormones throughout life. Multiple hormones engage in similar responsibilities, providing negative and positive feedback controls. Hormonal effects depend on blood and extracellular concentrations. Control is needed to avoid diseases created by high or low concentrations. Concentration is dependent on the rate of production, rate of delivery, and rate of elimination of each hormone.

> *Throughout life, all organs and body cells are influenced by hormones.*

Control over the endocrine system lies in the interactions among the hypothalamus gland, the pituitary gland, and the adrenal gland, also referred to as the HPA axis. Hormones from the HPA axis provide feedback and regulatory influences of the body's endocrine organs (Figure 18.1).

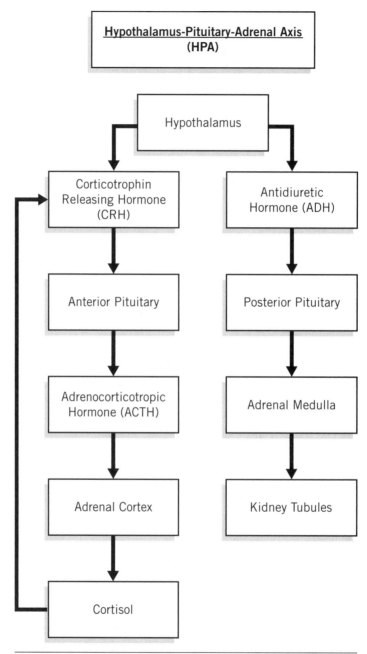

FIGURE 18.1

Hypothalamus-Pituitary-Adrenal Axis

Endocrine Considerations

HYPOTHALAMUS-PITUITARY-ADRENAL AXIS

The hypothalamus synthesizes and secretes vasopressin and corticotropin-releasing hormone (CRH). Vasopressin or the antidiuretic hormone (ADH) travels to the posterior pituitary where it is stored until osmoreceptors sense dehydration or pressure receptors sense lowered blood pressure. In addition to influencing kidney tubule reabsorption (see Chapter 10), ADH is a potent vasoconstrictor.

In response to stress CRH is released from the hypothalamus and stimulates the anterior pituitary to secrete adrenocorticotropic hormone (ACTH). ACTH acts directly on the adrenal cortex to release the glucocorticoid cortisol. Cortisol secretion results in negative feedback by turning off the production of CRH. Thus, the three components of the HPA axis are interdependent.

While the HPA axis controls hormone secretion, most hormones are secreted in "pulses" with a limited life span or half-life. For example, ACTH has a half-life of 10 minutes. Cortisol is secreted upon wakening and peaks in 30 to 45 minutes, declines throughout the day, and increases in late afternoon. These changes define the circadian rhythm dictated by the pineal gland and the hormone melatonin.

Twenty-five percent of bone loss from onset of menopause to age 60 is due to estrogen loss.

The pineal gland, the size of a piece of rice, and located deep in the brain between the hemispheres, secretes the hormone melatonin. Photosensitive cells in the retina of the eye send stimulating impulses to the pineal gland when light is absent, which results in melatonin secretion. Secretion is inhibited during daylight. The duration of melatonin secretion is related to the length of the night. Melatonin communicates information about environmental lighting to various parts of the body. Melatonin regulates circadian rhythms and aids in inducing sleep. It is also a powerful antioxidant that can easily cross cell membranes and the blood-brain barrier.

Age-Related Changes

The HPA axis is generally untouched in healthy aging. There is some evidence that CRH secretion is increased under basal conditions; however, the brain also has reduced sensitivity to the negative feedback of cortisol. The amount and duration of melatonin secretion decreases beginning with early childhood and continuing with age. The decline in melatonin may be responsible for elders' complaints of insomnia. Falling levels of melatonin are thought to increase oxidative damage to cell structure, which supports the findings that melatonin supplements have had a positive effect on reducing delirium and improving Alzheimer's disease symptoms.

SEX AND GROWTH HORMONES

The hypothalamus releases gonadotropin-releasing hormone, which works on the anterior pituitary to release luteinizing hormone (LH) and follicle-stimulating hormone. In men, LH stimulates the testes to synthesize and secrete testosterone. In women, LH stimulates the ovaries to produce estrogen. In addition to mediating sexual characteristics and behavior, testosterone and estrogen act to increase metabolism, decrease body fat, and increases bone mineral density (Figure 18.2).

The hypothalamus stimulates the anterior pituitary to synthesize and secrete growth hormone (GH) at 3- to 5-hour intervals with the largest secretion occurring after the onset of sleep. GH, an anabolic steroid, plays a role in numerous metabolic processes (Exhibit 18.1), which are all designed to promote body growth by stimulating muscle mass and bone growth. GH acts directly on fat cells by stimulating them to break down triglycerides and blocks the uptake of circulating lipids. GH assists in the conversions of the thyroid hormone T4 to the more active hormone T3. Indirectly, GH acts on the liver to secrete insulin-like growth factor (IGF-I). IGF-I stimulates bone growth by increasing cartilage cells, stimulates muscle growth by increasing muscle cell numbers and differentiation, and encourages protein synthesis by encouraging cellular amino acid uptake.

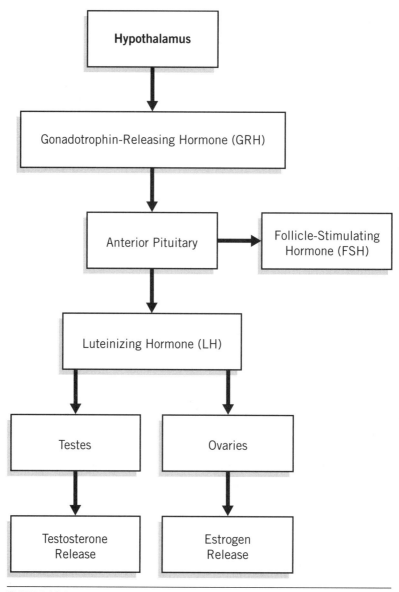

FIGURE 18.2
Effect of Growth Hormones

Age-Related Changes

Estrogen ceases to be released when a woman has completed menopause usually by her mid-50s. Thus one-third of a woman's life is spent without this important hormone. Women lose an average of 25% of their bone mass from the time of menopause to age 60, due in part to the loss of estrogen. Twice as many elder women have osteopenia and osteoporosis compared to their age-matched male counterparts. The presence of estrogen has been associated with managing blood cholesterol and after menopause a woman's risk of coronary artery disease increases. Loss of estrogen has also been implicated in bladder dysfunction, decreased elasticity in the skin, decrease muscle tone, vision deterioration, and weight gain. Low estrogen levels have also been associated with a risk of Alzheimer's disease.

EXHIBIT 18.1 **Metabolic Process Promoted by Growth Hormone**

- Increase calcium retention by bone
- Increase muscle mass
- Promote lipolysis for energy
- Increase protein synthesis
- Decrease liver uptake of glucose
- Promote liver gluconeogenesis
- Stimulate the immune system

A steady decline in testosterone levels occurs in males as they age. By age 70, one-quarter of males meet the criteria for testosterone deficiency. The extent of decline depends on health. Healthy males show less decline than their matched counterparts with comorbid illnesses. Evidence suggests that this decline may be at least partially responsible for a variety of physical and mental changes associated with the aging process. For instance, abnormally low levels of androgens can lead to profound changes in bone density, body composition, as well as sexual and cognitive function. Low testosterone or andropause is manifested as low libido, decreased stamina and energy, increased irritability, loss of muscle mass with increased abdominal fat, gynecomastia, osteopenia, and osteoporosis. Between the ages of 40 and 70, the average man loses up to 20 pounds of muscle, 15% of his bone mass, and up to 2 inches in height. Testosterone decline has also been associated with cognitive impairment.

Aging is associated with a steady decline of the production and secretion of GH. Half of adults over 60 have reduced GH levels. Serum IGF-I levels also decline with age. Aging is associated with catabolism: a decrease in lean muscle mass, an increase in fat mass, and a decrease in bone density. Decreased GH secretion is a contributory cause to these body composition changes, which occur with advancing age. Undernutrition is accelerated when GH is low. In addition, GH deficiency immobilizes the immune system. The decline in T4 to T3 conversion promotes hypothyroidism and a state of limited energy production. The decline in GH and T3 results in an undernourished and hypoenerergic organism with decreased serum glucose for nervous system metabolism, an ultimately cognitive decline. Numerous investigators have sought to supplement GH to reverse aging catabolism with little success.

ADRENAL GLANDS

The adrenal glands, located anterior to the kidneys, are composed of two functionally different endocrine organs: the cortex and the medulla. The cortex secretes steroid hormones while the medulla releases epinephrine and norepinephrine (Figure 18.3).

CORTEX

Over two dozen different steroid hormones are produced by the adrenal cortex; however, the three main regulatory hormones are the mineral corticoids (aldosterone), the glucocorticoids (cortisol), and the androgens (testosterone and estrogen). The mineral corticoids are responsible for sodium, potassium, and water homeostasis and exert effect on the kidney (see Chapter 10).

Cortisol, also known as hydrocortisone, is under direct control of ACTH secretion from the anterior pituitary. The anterior pituitary receives signals from the hypothalamus in the form of CRH. Any type of stress, physical or mental, actual or perceived, results in an

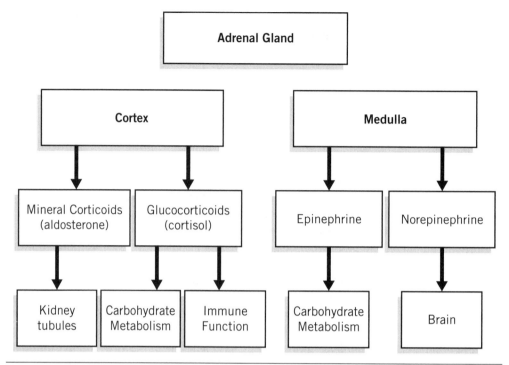

FIGURE 18.3

Influence of Adrenal Gland Hormones

elevation of serum cortisol. Cortisol serum concentration exerts a negative feedback on CRH release, which turns off adrenal cortex secretion. The feedback is cyclical, resulting in a circadian rhythm of cortisol secretion that is higher during the day, with a peak from 4:00 p.m. to 8:00 p.m., and lower at night with a trough from 2:00 a.m. to 4:00 a.m.

Normal cortisol secretion is approximately 5 mg/m^2 or 20 mg per day. The maximal output of the adrenal cortex is 150 to 300 mg per day. As would be anticipated, the stress of surgery activates the HPA axis. ACTH increases at the time of surgical incision and peaks with extubation in the immediate postoperative period. As a result, cortisol levels increase within 30 minutes of anesthesia induction. Cortisol production during minor surgical procedures can exceed 50 mg/m^2 and up to 150 mg per day during major surgical procedures. Surgery stimulates an immediate rise in glucocorticoid levels, peaking in the immediate postoperative period. Levels remain elevated for 24 to 48 hours. The circadian rhythm of cortisol is lost after surgery, severe illness, or trauma.

Two weeks of prednisone 5 mg or hydrocortisone will depress the HPA axis, and it will remain suppressed for up to 1 year.

Cortisol receptors are found throughout the body. Two important effects are the hormone's impact on carbohydrate metabolism and immune function. The goal of carbohydrate processes is to maintain or increase glucose availability for stressed cellular functions (Exhibit 18.2).

Cortisol has potent anti-inflammatory and immunosuppressive properties. Cortisol promotes lysosome integrity. Lysosomes within the cell engulf bacteria and viruses with their digestive enzymes. Capillaries are also supported as cortisol reduces the ability of white blood cells to adhere to the endothelium and reduce their response to local irritation.

EXHIBIT 18.2 Effects of Cortisol Secretion on Carbohydrate Metabolism

- Increase blood sugar by stimulating gluconeogenesis in the liver
- Mobilize amino acids for gluconeogenesis
- Stimulate fat breakdown for gluconeogenesis
- Decrease glucose uptake by muscle and fat tissue to conserve glucose

---

Adequate adrenal function is critical to mediate the stress of surgery by cortisol. When 90% of the cortex is destroyed, adrenal insufficiency occurs. The etiology can be within the adrenal gland or anterior pituitary ACTH deficiency. Primary adrenal dysfunction (Addison's disease) is usually the result of autoimmune mechanisms. Tuberculosis is the second most common cause of primary adrenal insufficiency.

Many patients require exogenous glucocorticoid therapy, including those with chronic asthma, organ transplants, or depressed immune systems. Two weeks of 5 mg of prednisone or 20 mg of hydrocortisone will depress the HPA axis. The cortisol response to stress controlled by the HPA axis can be suppressed for up to a year after the last dose of steroids.

MEDULLA

Epinephrine is the main catecholamine comprising 80% of the hormone secretion of the adrenal medulla, the remainder being norepinephrine. Once released into the blood, epinephrine binds to adrenergic receptors and creates effects that mimic sympathetic nervous stimulation. However, the effect of epinephrine lasts longer than stimulation by the sympathetic nervous stimulation.

Different organs have different classes of adrenergic receptors, with alpha 1, alpha 2, beta 1, and beta 2 receptors all responsive to epinephrine stimulation. The goal of the epinephrine response (Exhibit 18.3) is to increase blood glucose and fatty acids to provide quick energy sources for cell activity. The goal of norepinephrine secretion is to modulate

---

EXHIBIT 18.3 Effect of Adrenal Medulla Hormones

Epinephrine	Norepinephrine
• Smooth muscle relaxation in airways for bronchiole dilation	• Increase peripheral vasoconstriction to increase blood pressure
• Arteriole smooth muscle constriction	• Increase attention span of brain
• Inhibit insulin secretion	
• Stimulate liver glycogenolysis	
• Stimulate muscle glycolysis	
• Stimulate glucagon secretion	
• Increase adrenocorticotropic hormone secretion by pituitary gland	
• Increase heart rate	
• Increase strength of myocardial contraction	
• Increase lipolysis of fat tissue	
• Inhibits gastrointestinal secretion and motility	

EXHIBIT 18.4 Illnesses Associated With Steroid Use

- Rheumatoid arthritis
- Inflammatory bowel disease
- Degenerative joint disease
- Chronic obstructive pulmonary disease
- Organ and tissue transplants
- Skin disease

stress responses in the brain by increasing attentiveness and attention. Norepinephrine has a powerful effect on peripheral blood flow throughout the body by causing vasoconstriction.

Age-Related Changes

The rate of cortisol secretion declines with age, reduced by as much as 30%. However, serum cortisol remains unaffected because of decline in the ability of the liver and kidneys to clear the hormone. Under stress, serum cortisol increases and lasts longer in the elderly than their younger counterparts. The response can promote immediate adaptation; however, the long-term effects may be deleterious.

The most common cause of elevated cortisol levels in the elderly is the administration of exogenous glucocorticoids, usually in the form of prednisone. Many elders are prescribed steroids for a variety of ailments (Exhibit 18.4) either episodically or on a routine basis.

The output of medullary norepinephrine increases with age. Epinephrine secretion is markedly reduced with age; however, there is also reduced plasma clearance. Thus, the change in secretion is not reflected in plasma concentrations. Adrenergic receptors to the catecholamines become less responsive with age, particularly in the heart.

Gerioperative Care

PREOPERATIVE CONSIDERATIONS

Surgery and anesthesia stimulate the HPA axis and the endocrine stress response. The extent of the adrenal response is related to the duration of surgery, extent of surgery, and the patient's ability to produce cortisol. The type of anesthesia also modulates the stress response. Cortisol production during surgery of the lower abdomen and lower extremities is reduced under regional anesthesia. Thus, regional anesthesia requires less response by the HPA axis, which benefits older adults.

Careful assessment of adrenal sufficiency is required preoperatively. During the preoperative interview, symptoms of adrenal insufficiency should be further investigated (Exhibit 18.5). Any history of exogenous steroid use must be documented. Administration can be oral, inhaled, topical, or epidural. While topical or inhaled steroids are less likely to produce adrenal suppression, frequent use or high doses can require perioperative supplementation during times of stress. A history of oral steroid use in the past year, including elders who have received steroid joint injections or epidural steroids within the past 3 months, suggests the need for steroid supplementation.

Steroid supplementation should be considered with steroid joint injections or epidural steroids within the past 3 months.

Patients taking over 5 mg of prednisone per day should receive their usual dose of steroid preoperatively, either by mouth or intravenously, and a supplement. The dose of additional hydrocortisone is based on the degree of surgical stress.

The optimal dosage for steroid supplementation to combat surgical stress is controversial. One method classifies the surgery as exposing the body to minor, moderate, or major

EXHIBIT 18.5 **Symptoms of Adrenal Insufficiency**

- Lethargy
- Diarrhea
- Weakness
- Anorexia

- Hyperpigmentation
- Hyponatremia
- Fasting hypoglycemia

stressors. Minor stress is experienced during surgeries such as hernia repair, colonoscopy, or laparoscopic diagnostic procedures. For minor procedures, an additional 25 mg of hydrocortisone is administered. Patients return to their usual regimen the following day. Other regimens supplement the patient's usual dose taken the day of surgery with an equivalent supplement.

Moderate stress is encountered during procedures such as bowel resection, peripheral revascularization, joint replacement, or open cholycystectomy. The equivalent of 50 to 75 mg/day of hydrocortisone administered for 1 to 2 days is suggested. Surgeries producing major stress include aortic surgery, coronary artery surgery requiring bypass, esophagostomy, or pancreaticoduodenostomy. For these involved and longer surgeries, 100 to 150 mg/day of hydrocortisone for 2 to 3 days is suggested.

Another regimen uses the maximum stress dose of hydrocortisone as 10 times the maintenance dose up to 300 mg per day. The first dose of 100 mg is administered intravenously at least 1 hour before anesthesia induction and then every 8 hours for at least 24 hours. Once the acute stress is passed, the patient is weaned back to a maintenance dose over several days. However, there is no conclusive research supporting supraphysiologic doses of supplemental steroids.

Steroids can be administered orally, intravenously, or intramuscularly. The provider must be careful to prescribe the appropriate potency of steroid (Table 18.1).

INTRAOPERATIVE CONSIDERATIONS

Unexplained hypotension unresponsive to fluid replacement and vasopressors suggests an Addisonian crisis, which is a severe deficiency of cortisol under stress. Immediate administration of dexamethasone 8 mg intravenously, along with fluids and glucose, can be life-saving.

POSTOPERATIVE CONSIDERATIONS

Following surgery, the stress response continues. Steroid replacements must be administered on schedule. As steroid affects glucose metabolism, blood sugars must be assessed and treated while the patient is receiving supplemental steroids.

TABLE 18.1

Steroid Types

Medication	Potency Compared to Cortisol
Hydrocortisone	1x
Prednisone	4x
Methlyprednisolone	5x
Dexamethasone	30x

THYROID

A highly vascular gland, the thyroid gland is one of the largest in the body, storing enough of its own hormones for a 100-day supply. The gland is under the control of the hypothalamus and anterior pituitary. Thyroid-releasing hormone (TRH) from the hypothalamus stimulates the anterior pituitary to release thyroid-stimulating hormone (TSH). TSH triggers the thyroid gland to secrete T3 and T4 hormones. In addition, 75% of the circulating T3 results from the conversion of T4. The presence of T3 and T4 hormones create a negative feedback on the hypothalamus. Similarly, a decline in circulating thyroid hormones will trigger the hypothalamus to release additional TRH. Exercise, stress, malnutrition, and hypoglycemia also trigger TRH release.

Synthesis of thyroid hormones depend on the availability of dietary iodine, which is absorbed by the small intestine. After synthesis, the hormones rely on plasma proteins for delivery to the target organs. In the periphery, T4 is converted to T3. When in the blood, 99% of T3 and T4 hormones are bound to proteins. Once the hormones are unbound the free T3 and T4 bind to receptors for transport into the cell.

Thyroid hormones affect every cell and organ of the body. Once inside the cell, fat is mobilized for energy, leading to more circulating fatty acids. Carbohydrate metabolism is enhanced with increased gluconeogenesis and glycogenolysis to generate free glucose. These effects on metabolism increase the basal metabolic rate and increase heat production.

Age-Related Changes

With age, there is a decline in hormone production as the thyroid gland becomes smaller. The atrophy and fibrosis of the gland makes assessment through palpation difficult. There is a blunted response to TRH and less conversion of T4 to T3. However, the decline in production is balanced by a decline in metabolic clearance, resulting in unchanged serum levels. T4 in the elderly is within the normal range with T3 in the low normal range. In adults over 80 years, the half-life of T4 is prolonged, with less production of T4, compounded by a decline in TSH. Hypothyroidism is more common in elders than hyperthyroidism.

Hypothyroidism is primarily a disease of adults aged 50 to 70 years old. Over 70% of newly diagnosed patients with hypothyroidism will be over 50 years old. The level of T4 and TSH will be below normal. Symptomatic or clinical hypothyroidism affects nearly 1% of adults, with women six more times likely to be hypothyroid than men. Over 10% of elder women over age 65 and 15% over 75 experience hypothyroidism. Subclinical hypothyroidism is asymptomatic and is diagnosed based on laboratory findings. Thyroid antibodies can develop with age, with the resulting thyroiditis responsible for producing low levels of thyroid hormones. Autoimmune disease has been implicated, but hypothyroidism can occur spontaneously in more than 5% of women.

Subclinical hypothyroidism increases with age and is reflected in normal T3 and T4 levels but increased TSH levels. It occurs in up to 18% of elders in the general population, with a higher prevalence in women. The diagnosis is difficult because subclinical hypothyroidism is asymptomatic. Yet, the impact of subclinical hypothyroidism on elders can be significant. It has been associated with cognitive dysfunction when other contributing factors are controlled. Subclinical hypothyroidism is an independent risk factor for atherosclerosis, acute coronary syndrome, and left ventricular diastolic dysfunction leading to heart failure.

The development of hypothyroidism is insidious, often over a period of years. In elders, the signs are subtle. Elders commonly report fatigue and weakness as symptoms of hypothyroidism. Additionally, there may be other findings of low T3 and T4 (see Exhibit 18.6). Thyroid disease in the elderly is difficult to diagnose as some of the symptoms of thyroid

EXHIBIT 18.6 Signs and Symptoms of Hypothyroidism

- Fatigue, lethargy, weakness
- Thick, course, drying skin
- Brittle and coarse hair
- Alopecia
- Fluid retention with weight gain
- Hypoactive reflexes
- Sensitivity to cold

- Hypothermia
- Facial puffiness
- Goiter
- Trouble breathing or swallowing
- Hoarseness
- Constipation
- Ataxia
- Depression

- Memory loss
- Irritability
- Bradycardia, atrial fibrillation
- Hypertension
- Anorexia
- High low-density lipoproteins, low high-density lipoproteins

disorders are common to illnesses prevalent among elders. An index of suspicion is needed when the signs and symptoms of hypothyroidism are identified. For example, dementia screening should always include thyroid testing.

The decline in thyroid hormones has major cardiovascular, neurological, and metabolic effects. In hypothyroidism, the heart is less responsive to epinephrine and exhibits a blunted response to adrenergic stimulation. The result is a decrease in cardiac output and blood pressure. Combined with the decrease in metabolism, these changes result in cold intolerance. Neurologically, the central nervous system becomes depressed in hypothyroidism with a slowing of thought, memory, and speech. These changes can result in somnolence and lethargy. Hypothyroidism decreases insulin metabolism resulting in higher serum insulin and resulting hypoglycemia.

The hypometabolic state created by hypothyroidism can develop into myxedema. Skin changes and pleural and pericardial effusions result from mucoploysaccharide production. The appearance of nonpitting edema around the eyes, feet, and hands; a thickened tongue; and pharyngeal and laryngeal edema can result in thick, slurred speech. An altered mental status is one of the hallmarks of myxedema along with significant hypothermia. Myxedema is more common in adults over 70 years old. It can be precipitated in stress situations that also require surgery such as trauma and burns. Administering hypnotics to elders with myxedema will result in a coma in half of all patients.

Agitation and confusion in hyperthyroidism can mimic dementia.

Hyperthyroidism affects one of five older adults, yet only 75% will be symptomatic. The term masked or apathetic thyrotoxicosis refers to elders' hyperthyroidism. Undiagnosed hyperthyroidism may manifest as heart failure, angina, or stroke. Weight loss, anorexia, and constipation are classic signs but are found in only 15% of elders with hyperthyroidism. The agitation and confusion associated with hyperthyroidism can mimic dementia. The heart's sensitivity to elevated thyroid hormone can result in unexplained atrial fibrillation in up to 20% of elders.

Medications treating unrelated illnesses can mask the symptoms of hyperthyroidism in elders. Beta blockers can decrease the heart rate, blood pressure, and hand tremors associated with elevated thyroid hormones. Similar to hypothyroidism, a level of suspicion is needed when unexplained signs and symptoms appear such as mood changes, weakness, fatigue, or atrial fibrillation.

Gerioperative Care

PREOPERATIVE CONSIDERATIONS

Primary care screening for thyroid disorders is recommended every 5 years after age 35. Screening includes TSH, free T3, and T4. During the preoperative history, the patient should be routinely asked about thyroid screening. If any of the signs and symptoms of hypothyroidism are identified, thyroid testing is indicated. Patients receiving thyroid replacements for hypothyroidism should have yearly thyroid testing. As elders lose weight, supplemental thyroid replacement dosage must be monitored to avoid hyperthyroidism. The decrease in metabolic clearance of the thyroid hormones with age means that older adults require lower replacement doses than younger adults with the same deficit. Supplementation with synthetic thyroxine must begin slowly to minimize the stress to the heart and central nervous system.

Thyroid storm mimics signs of malignant hyperthermia.

INTRAOPERATIVE CONSIDERATIONS

When possible, surgery should be postponed in hypo- or hyperthyroid elders until a euthyroid state is achieved. Patients who are hypothyroid have a decreased rate of metabolism of administered drugs. Careful dosing is required to reduce the risk of toxicity.

The hypermetabolic state created by undiagnosed hyperthyroidism is exacerbated by the stress of surgery and anesthesia. The signs of a thyroid storm, an excessive secretion of thyroid hormones, include hyperthermia, hypertension, life-threatening tachycardias, and cardiovascular collapse due to high output cardiac failure. These life-threatening symptoms require immediate interventions including adrenergic blockers, beta blockers, and iodine to reduce the effects of the circulating hormones and block further hormone release. Glucocorticoids can lower T3 levels and provide adrenal support in the face of high metabolic demand. The symptoms of thyroid storm can mimic malignant hyperthermia (see Chapter 8).

POSTOPERATIVE CONSIDERATIONS

Surgery and anesthesia results in a decrease in T3 levels within 24 hours of nonthyroid procedures. Prolonged surgery and stress can precipitate a fall in T4 levels. Surgery requiring heart-lung bypass will result in up to a 75% decline in T3 levels up to 4 postoperative days.

Surgery and anesthesia cause a decrease in T3 levels within 24 hours of surgery.

Elders who require synthetic thyroid or thyroid-suppressing drugs must be returned to their preoperative regiment as soon as possible. Thyroxine can be administered crushed via a nasogastric tube if needed.

PARATHYROID

The parathyroid hormone (PTH) regulates calcium and phosphorous by targeting processes in the bone and kidney. The parathyroid gland's secretion of PTH inhibits the reabsorption of bicarbonate and phosphate in the proximal tubules of the kidney. PTH stimulates calcium reabsorption in the kidney distal tubules. In addition to regulating absorption, PTH stimulates the kidney to activate vitamin D. With vitamin D, intestinal absorption of calcium is enhanced. PTH also stimulates bone cells to release calcium. By excreting phosphate, retaining calcium, and releasing bone calcium, serum calcium levels are maintained. With adequate serum calcium, bone calcium can be preserved (Figure 18.4).

Age-Related Changes

There is an increase in PTH secretion with age. One-third of patients with hyperparathyroidism are over 60 years. Postmenopausal women are three times more likely to have hyperparathyroidism than men of the same age. The incidence of hyperparathyroidism in the elderly is double that of younger adults.

Serum calcium concentration begins to decline after 50 years. Decreases in intestinal absorption and increases in urinary calcium secretion contribute to hypocalcemia. The low serum calcium triggers a parathyroid response. The increase in PTH increases the serum calcium at the expense of osteopenia and calcium deposits in the kidney. The renal deposits result in elevated creatinine levels. Symptoms of hyperparathyroidism are often overlooked or explained by aging: bone demineralization, weakness, and joint complaints. Postmenopausal women with forearm fractures and low bone density should be evaluated for hyperparathyroidism.

INTRAOPERATIVE CONSIDERATIONS

Hypercalcemia impacts cardiac conduction. Changes in the electrocardiogram include prolonged PR, widened QRS, and shortened QT intervals. Continuous segment monitoring when hyperparathyroidism is suspected is imperative. Digitalis toxicity is enhanced by hypercalcemia. Elevations in serum calcium can be manifested as skeletal muscle weakness. Adjustments in muscle relaxants may be required.

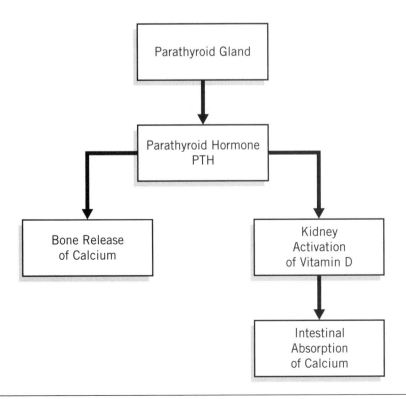

FIGURE 18.4
Influence of Parathyroid Hormones

PANCREAS

Three major hormones are excreted by the pancreas: delta cells secrete somatostatin, alpha cells secrete glucagon, and beta cells produce insulin. Somatastatin is an inhibitory hormone that decreases the release of insulin and glucagon in addition to several other hormones such as GH, cholycystokin, and gastrin in the gut. An elevated serum level of glucose stimulates insulin release from the beta cell and promotes additional insulin production within the cell. When glucose levels fall, glucagon is secreted from the alpha cells and travels to the liver where it triggers the liver to break down stored glycogen into glucose as well as produce glucose from amino acids (gluconeogenesis) (Figure 18.5).

Diabetes is the most common endocrine disease among surgical patients. Most diabetics will require surgery or procedures related to the consequences of diabetes during their lifetime. Diabetes is not a risk factor for surgical mortality or morbidity. However, the organ damage and hormonal disruptions caused by uncontrolled diabetes contribute to intraoperative and postoperataive complications.

Type 1 diabetes is an early-onset, abrupt disease with low or absent levels of insulin production. Glucose balance requires insulin administration with its difficulties of tight control of glycemia. End organ complications occur earlier in life. Type 2 diabetes is adult-onset, occurs gradually, and reflects both a decrease in insulin production and an increase in insulin resistance. Insulin resistance reflects the inability of the target cells to use the secreted insulin. Insulin resistance occurs as a result of the decrease in physical activity and the increase in fat tissue with age. Insulin resistance usually precedes the development of type 2 diabetes.

Age-Related Changes

While the pancreas undergoes atrophy, fat infiltration and fibrotic changes with aging, there is little functional change due to the large reserve capacity of the organ. Basal somatostatin is increased in elders, but the effect of this change is not understood.

With age, insulin levels decrease, though basal insulin is not affected. The stimulus for serum glucose is the sympathetic nervous system, which detects hypoglycemic stress in the brain. The brain requires a continuous supply of glucose for functioning. The decline in insulin is believed to be a protective measure of the aging brain to guarantee an adequate glucose supply.

More than half of all diabetics are over 65 years old. Twenty percent of elders between 65 and 74 suffer from type 2 diabetes. The number of elders with diabetes continues to increase as diagnosis improves and the number of elders at risk grows. Diabetes develops in elders due to insulin resistance and a decrease in insulin production. Metabolic syndrome (MS) is a cluster of findings used for adaptation of the aging body: central obesity, abnormal fasting glucose, lipidemia, and hypertension. The development of MS has been associated with diabetes and cardiovascular disease. The prevalence of MS increases with age; however, elders who are physically fit rarely show insulin resistance.

Hypoglycemia and electrolyte balance is poorly tolerated by elders.

The treatment of diabetes in the elderly is difficult. Hypoglycemia is poorly tolerated by elders, and they are less able to maintain fluid and electrolyte balance brought on by a low blood sugar. While lower serum glucose levels can improve cognitive function, elders can appear confused with hypoglycemia.

Aging appears to accelerate the negative effects of diabetes. Morbidity and mortality increase when elders experience hyperglycemia. Contributing to the hyperglycemia is the severity of the causative event, decreased insulin reserve, and diminished physiological reserve. Hyperglycemia of elders is usually associated with infection and pancreatitis. The

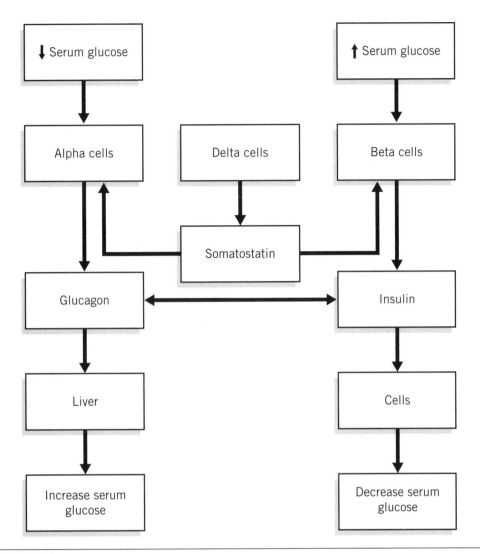

FIGURE 18.5
Hormones of the Pancreas

hyperglycemia leads to cognitive dysfunction. Elders with diabetes have slower reflexes than age-matched healthy elders.

The importance of recognizing diabetes in elders is the impact of diabetes combined with age-related change to increase elders' vulnerability and the creation of an added layer of surgical risk.

Gerioperative Care

PREOPERATIVE CONSIDERATIONS

Anxiety and the stress of surgery trigger the HPA axis to secrete ACTH, which in turn stimulates cortisol release from the adrenal gland. The function of the stress response is to increase the amount of energy available to the cell in the form of glucose. Even an individual without impaired insulin production and receptivity can experience hyperglycemia. In older adults with diabetes, the hyperglycemia is magnified. Anesthesia and surgery metabolically destabilize gerioperative patients who have little tolerance of stress.

Because the onset of type 2 diabetes is insidious, many elders may fail to seek treatment. Careful preoperative assessment can identify changes suggesting blood sugar abnormalities. Obese elders with a family history of diabetes should be questioned about polyphagia, polyuria, and polydipsia, although these signs and symptoms are easily masked by other age-related or disease-related changes in organ function. Elder women with a history of gestational diabetes require careful screening. Changes in vision, frequent infections, or evidence of cardiovascular compromise suggests type 2 diabetes. A routine fasting blood sugar performed preoperatively may reveal abnormalities requiring further evaluation prior to surgery.

For known elder diabetics, preoperative assessment focuses on determining any end-organ complications of diabetes. A 10-year or more history of diabetes is associated with an increase risk of end-organ disease. Atherosclerosis is more prevalent in diabetics with manifestations of acute coronary syndrome, peripheral vascular disease, renovascular disease, and cerebral vascular disease. The patient with long-standing diabetes has an increased risk of postoperative stroke, myocardial infarction, and renal failure. Diabetic neuropathy increases risk for pressure ulcer development, intraoperative hypothermia, and delayed gastric emptying.

Diabetes increases risk of pressure ulcers, hypothermia, deep vein thromboembolism, and delayed gastric emptying.

The goal of diabetes management during the perioperative period is optimal control of blood sugar and prevention of significant hyperglycemia. Preoperative fasting creates catabolism, a response of the body to breakdown glycogen, amino acids, and fats to serve as the source of glucose. For a type 1 diabetic, the result is an accumulation of ketones from fat metabolism. Surgery scheduled early in the day limits the duration of nothing-by-mouth status, missed medications, and blood sugar fluctuations.

A detailed record of the patient's current diabetic medications with administration time is crucial. Long-acting insulins taken the evening before surgery can impact perioperative blood sugars.

Laboratory Assessment

Glycosolated hemoglobin is an essential blood test to determine blood glucose control.

During the preoperative visit, laboratory testing should include glycosylated hemoglobin (HbA1C) to reflect the fluctuations in blood sugars over the past 3 months. Also indicated are tests of potential end-organ damage from poorly controlled blood sugars: electrocardiogram, electrolyte panel, blood urea nitrogen/creatinine, and urinalysis. On the day of surgery, a finger stick blood sugar should be obtained upon arrival in the preoperative holding area. Blood sugars outside the 80 to 130 mg/dL range must be reported to the anesthesia provider for additional intervention.

Interventions

Elders with type 1 diabetes require insulin before, during, and after surgery. Even if the patient is on nothing-by-mouth status, insulin is still required. Patients with an insulin pump are allowed to maintain their pump settings on a basal infusion rate. One-half of the intermediate acting insulin dose is administered preoperatively.

Elders with type 2 diabetes are more prevalent and most will not require insulin therapy perioperatively. Patients on a short-acting oral hypoglycemic can have the medication held on the day of surgery, while patients on a longer-acting oral hypoglycemic should take their medication per routine on the day of surgery.

Depending on the blood sugar control, patients with diabetes may be dehydrated preoperatively. An intravenous line of normal saline is initiated while waiting for surgery. Lactated Ringer's solution is avoided as the lactate is converted to glucose and exacerbate the hyperglycemia.

INTRAOPERATIVE CONSIDERATIONS

Patients with diabetes may require insulin administration during surgery. A source of glucose is required to prevent catabolism. A standard dose of glucose during surgery is 5 to 10 g/hr, which is equivalent to a continuous infusion of 5% dextrose at 100 mL/hr. The 5% dextrose solution in water is administered separately so that if vigorous fluid replacement is needed, normal saline can be administered. A blood sugar is obtained after induction and hourly to provide tight control over hyperglycemia. Supplemental short-action insulin using a sliding scale is administered to maintain the blood sugar below 200 mg/dL; close to 110 mg/dL is optimum.

POSTOPERATIVE CONSIDERATIONS

A postoperative blood sugar is obtained immediately upon admission to the postanesthesia care unit and then upon discharge if insulin has been required. Once the blood sugar has returned to the tight control range of 80 to 120 mg/dL, blood sugars are obtained every 6 hours if the patient is on nothing-by-mouth status, or before meals and at bedtime if the patient has resumed a normal diet. Encourage the patient to resume their normal diet as soon as possible. Once the diet is resumed, medication schedules can be resumed.

PATIENT REPORT: Ms. Wagaman

Preoperatively, Ms. Wagaman's electrocardiogram, T4, and TSH were within normal limits indicating a euthyroid state. The glycosolated hemoglobin was 8.5, with a fasting blood sugar of 150. The nurse completed a neurovascular assessment and documented diminished pedal pulses and sensation. The nursing assistant reported that Ms. Wagaman's finger stick blood sugar upon admission was 190. She had not taken her rosiglitazone that morning. The nurse communicated and documented her finding to the nurse anesthetist. An intravenous line of normal saline is started. Surgery and anesthesia are unremarkable. After arriving in the postanesthesia care unit, Ms. Wagaman's finger stick blood sugar is 162. She recovers from her anesthesia and is transferred to phase 2 postanesthesia care unit.

Postoperatively, Ms. Wagaman was instructed in how to care for her wound dressing and drain. She was to resume her levothyroxine in the morning as well as her rosiglitazone. She tolerates fluids and crackers before discharge. The discharge nurse makes a referral to the outpatient diabetic educator for diet teaching and exercise regimen.

SUMMARY

With aging, changes occur in the production, effectiveness, and breakdown of hormones. Hormone receptors show decreased function as well as the response of the end organ to hormone stimulation. The decline in function with age becomes overt when the endocrine system becomes stressed as in the perioperative period. The endocrine system modifies life span by enhancing body adaptation to the aging process as well as accelerating the aging process. The decline in endocrine function becomes obvious during periods of stress, when the hormonal reserves are expended and recovery is slow. The hallmark of aging is difficulty coping with stress.

KEY POINTS

- Aging is associated with catabolism: a decrease in lean muscle mass, an increase in fat mass, and a decrease in bone density.
- The most common cause of elevated cortisol levels in the elderly is the administration of exogenous glucocorticoids, usually in the form of prednisone.
- A history of oral steroid use in the past year, including elders who have received steroid joint injections or epidural steroids within the past 3 months, may indicate the need for steroid supplementation.
- Thyroid disease in the elderly is difficult to diagnose as some of the symptoms of thyroid disorders are common to illnesses prevalent among elders. An index of suspicion is needed when the signs and symptoms of hypothyroidism are identified. Dementia screening should always include thyroid testing.
- As elders lose weight, dosage must be monitored to avoid hyperthyroidism.
- Symptoms of hyperparathyroidism are often overlooked or explained by aging: bone demineralization, weakness, and joint complaints.
- The importance of recognizing diabetes in elders is the impact of diabetes combined with age-related changes, which increases vulnerability and creates an added layer of surgical risk.

NINETEEN

Frailty and Reserve Capacity

Raelene V. Shippee–Rice, Susan J. Fetzer, and Jennifer V. Long,

PATIENT REPORT: Mr. Ditmer

Mr. Ditmer is scheduled for a knee arthroscopy. He is 78 years old, plays golf three times a week, and works part-time as a Walmart greeter because he enjoys interacting with people. He twisted his knee playing golf with resulting moderate to severe pain. Mobility has been diminished for 3 weeks due to the pain. He is taking hydrocodone on an as-needed basis. Over the past few weeks, he has been inactive, spending much of his time watching television and showing evidence of mild cognitive changes. He has lost 10 pounds over the past 3 weeks due to pain, immobility, uncomfortable abdomen, and mild nausea. He comes to a same-day surgical center for his arthroscopy.

Frailty is a geriatric condition characterized by deterioration in physiologic systems and is associated with alterations in psychosocial functions and systems. Frail older adults have higher rates of postoperative complications, longer hospital stays, more discharged to nursing home or assisted living facilities, and more hospital readmissions than nonfrail gerioperative patients (Dasgupta, Rolfson, Stolee, Barrie & Speechley, 2009; Kristjansson et al., 2010; Makary et al., 2010).

Surgery challenges the ability to maintain homeostasis in multiple physiological, cognitive, and psychological systems. The interactive and simultaneous nature of the challenge creates a trauma to overall integrity that is greater than the sum of trauma to each individual organ or system. In frail older adults, the complex homeostatic responses needed to maintain physiological and psychological integrity are diminished, increasing vulnerability to adverse surgical outcomes.

Interdisciplinary assessment and prevention can improve surgical outcomes. Recognizing early onset disruption in homeostasis and responding with rapid, accurate interventions can prevent escalation of adverse events. This chapter describes frailty and the concept of reserve capacity in relation to the gerioperative patient. An overview of the perioperative care needs of frail older adults with suggested interventions is offered.

The number of research articles and commentaries on the subject of frailty has increased dramatically over the past 30 years. Despite the increase in clinical interest and research, no single best definition of frailty has emerged. There is a consensus in the geriatric community that frailty is marked by loss of reserve capacity or resilience. This loss results in decreased resistance to stressors and increased vulnerability to adverse events.

Models of Frailty

Definitions of frailty vary depending on the model of frailty. The biological model and the dynamic model are two predominant models of frailty. The biological model provides a unidimensional perspective focusing on the physiological dimensions of frailty. The dynamic model is a biopsychosocial model incorporating psychological, social, and physiological dimensions.

BIOLOGICAL MODEL

Biological or physiological models of frailty incorporate core elements involving loss of physiologic reserve capacity, involvement of multiple organ systems, and inability to maintain homeostasis in the face of severe physiologic threat. Frailty is a physiologic state resulting from the interaction of aging, disease, disuse, and diminished physiological reserve. Vulnerability to adverse effects is a hallmark of frailty (Buchner & Wagner, 1992; Fried et al. 2001). Kingsnorth and Majid (2006) describe frailty specific to the gerioperative patient as an impaired physiological reserve leading to an inability to adapt to the stress of anesthesia, surgery, and postoperative demands.

DYNAMIC MODEL

The dynamic model extends frailty beyond physiological systems to psychological and social systems. Frailty occurs in the absence of disease. Rockwood and colleagues (1994) proposed a dynamic model of frailty that considers biological, psychological, and social elements as assets or deficits. In this model, when the assets in each of area outweigh the deficits, the older adult is fit; when the deficits outweigh the assets, the older adult is considered frail; when the assets and deficits are in a state of balance that can be easily tipped toward deficits, the older adult is prefrail or intermediate frail. The dynamics of the model suggest that a deficit in any one area can initiate an interaction that can decrease the stability in any other area, causing the balance to be upended and result in frailty.

Reserve Capacity and Resilience

Frailty creates a self-perpetuating decline.

Reserve capacity and resilience are fundamental precepts that refer to an organism's ability to maintain or regain equilibrium in the face of adverse events or challenges. The term reserve capacity is more commonly used in the physiological literature, while resilience is commonly used in the psychosocial literature.

In the physiological literature, reserve capacity refers to the ability of a system to maintain homeostasis when under severe physiological threat. Most systems require at least 30% of total available capacity to maintain normal function, suggesting there is a reserve capacity of 70%. When stressors beyond normal function are placed on the system, such as strenuous exercise, emotional intensity, medication, disease, trauma, or other events, reserve capacity provides the physiologic resources to meet the added challenge and return the system to homeostasis.

In the psychosocial literature, resilience refers to the capacity of the individual to successfully cope with life events and adversity. Resilience serves as a buffer (reserve) that enables the individual to regain equilibrium (homeostasis) when challenged. Challenges for the older adult encompass chronic illness, pain, and loss of significant others, independence, or physical abilities.

Pathophysiology

Age-related changes diminish physiologic reserve. Chronic and acute disease processes further deplete physiologic reserve. Frailty results when body systems can no longer integrate and regulate functions that maintain homeostasis. Physiologic frailty rests in the lack of system synthesis and integration rather than in any single organ or system. The increasing inability to regulate and integrate systems is *homeostenosis*.

The risk of frailty is increased when the system is placed under greater stress, such as acute illness, medications, hospitalization, or surgery.

The effects of dysregulation across multiple systems are seen most readily in impaired muscle strength, mobility, balance, and endurance. Frailty occurs in response to early disease in multiple systems with disruption in neuroendocrine and inflammatory processing systems.

Inflammatory pathways associated with frailty relate to skeletal muscle homeostasis (Ershler, 2007). When the inflammatory pathways become dysfunctional, the resulting changes in muscle structure predispose to diminished muscle strength. Elevated levels of interlukin-6 and C-reactive protein have been found in frail older adults, lending credence to the association between inflammatory process, dysregulation, and frailty.

Activity levels and mobility depend on functional skeletal muscle. Impairment in skeletal muscle inhibits muscle strength, mobility, and endurance contributing to loss of physiological reserve. Diminished activity causes a physiological stress response that triggers psychological disruption as well as loss of physical function. The cumulative effect compounds the cycle further, disrupting neuroendocrine and inflammatory processes. Thus, frailty creates a self-perpetuating decline.

The frailty trajectory is not predetermined or absolute and can therefore be interrupted. The trajectory is a continuum from nonfrail to very frail, incorporating static and dynamic elements. Static frailty is capacity measured at a single point in time, indicating that at a single point a person can be categorized as nonfrail, intermediately frail, or frail. It provides a snapshot that serves as a predictor of actual and potential risk for adverse events.

Levels of frailty are categorized along a continuum from nonfrail to intermediate or pre-frail to frail. Nonfrailty or being fit implies sufficient reserves to manage stress demands. When an older adult who appears fit is on the borderline of diminished reserve capacity, there is no way to measure or evaluate frailty directly. Older adults who have intermediate frailty show evidence of frailty but are able to maintain stability between physiologic demands and physiologic capacity. The system may have sufficient reserve to maintain homeostasis but only in the face of minor stressors. The risk of frailty is increased when the system is placed

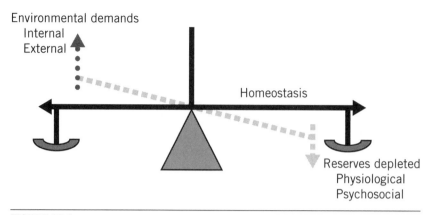

FIGURE 19.1

Tipping Point for Frailty

Frailty occurs when environmental demands become of sufficient intensity to create a tipping point. Reserve capacity is diminished to a point that disrupts the demand–reserve balance and homeostasis cannot be maintained.

under greater stress, such as acute illness, medications, hospitalization, or surgery. An elder with intermittent frailty quickly depletes any reserve capacity. Frailty results when there is minimal reserve and even small demands become tipping points, pushing the older patient into acute distress, as shown in Figure 19.1.

The trend for older adults predisposed to physiological frailty is a trajectory progressing from nonfrail to frail. The speed and complexity of the trajectory depends on the frequency and severity of internal and external challenges. When frailty is associated with chronic illness, disuse, or inactivity, timely and accurate interventions can help to diminish indicators of frailty. If frailty is due to age-related changes or the reserves are depleted beyond recovery, no interventions will be able to restore the system, and frailty becomes a precursor to death. Figure 19.2 compares a slow decline in reserve capacity compared with acute depletion that can occur with sudden acute illness, accidental trauma, or surgery.

CHARACTERISTICS OF BIOLOGIC FRAILTY

Characteristics of frailty depend on the model of frailty. Fried and colleagues (2001) developed a "phenotype" that refers to a set of characteristics used to operationalize and measure the presence of frailty. The five characteristics are shrinking, weakness, poor endurance or exhaustion, slowness, and low activity. The presence of three or more characteristics is needed for an older adult to be considered frail. One or two characteristics establish a state of prefrail or intermediate frailty. An older individual is considered robust when no characteristic of the phenotype is present. The phenotype serves as a predictive measure for adverse outcomes such as falls and disability (Fried et al., 2001).

Dynamic models of frailty incorporate physiologic and psychosocial characteristics. The Edmonton Frailty Scale (EFS) is multidimensional, incorporating functional, physical, pharmacological, and psychosocial factors (Rolfson, Majumdar, Tsuyuki, Tahir, & Rockwood, 2006). Cognition, mood, functional independence, medication use, social support, nutrition, general health status, functional performance determined by balance and gait, and continence are the measurement elements used to evaluate level of frailty. These elements are akin to the components that are included in a comprehensive geriatric assessment, a standard model for providing and improving health care in older adults.

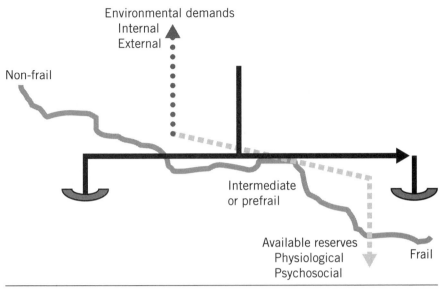

FIGURE 19.2

Frailty Trajectory

Frailty can be a slow trajectory with chronic illness and advancing age depleting reserves. Nonfrail reserves meet environmental demands to maintain homeostasis. In the intermediate or prefrail individual, environmental demands begin to increase and available reserves diminish but are not depleted. As the trajectory continues, available reserves become depleted and frailty ensues. Surgery, sudden trauma, or acute illness causes rapid depletion. Rapid depletion also occurs in apparently healthy aging adults with subclinical illness.

MULTIDIMENSIONAL FRAILTY

The prevalence of frailty is difficult to evaluate. Prevalence varies depending on definition, model, measurement criteria, and study population characteristics. Between 3% to 7% of older adults aged 65 to 75 meet criteria for frailty (Fried et al., 2005). In those over age 90, 32% were found to be frail (Walston et al., 2002). A longitudinal study of 2049 Mexican Americans reports that 58% of those over 65 years of age were assessed as frail (Ottenbacher et al., 2009). In hospital-based populations, between 60% and 63% of older adults are frail. Not all frail older adults have multiple chronic diseases. Fried and colleagues report that 7% of the frail older adults in their analysis of over 5000 older adults had no major chronic illness defined as hypertension, diabetes, arthritis, cancer, or cardiovascular disease, and 25% had just one. Frailty can exist in older adults without evidence of comorbid disease.

Few studies have evaluated frailty in older adults undergoing surgery. Makary and colleagues (2010) reported a frailty rate of 10.4% in a population of 594 older adults attending a pre-evaluation clinic. Results indicated that 31% met the criteria for intermediately frail, and 58% were nonfrail. Sundermann and colleagues (2011) tested a new frailty measurement tool in 400 patients over 75 years of age undergoing cardiac surgery. Study results revealed severe frailty in 7.7%, with 42.5% moderately frail and almost 50% considered robust or not frail.

> *Frailty can exist in older adults without evidence of comorbid disease.*

Gerioperative Care

Recognizing early-onset disruption in homeostasis and responding with rapid, accurate interventions can prevent escalation of adverse events.

Frail older adults have a narrow reserve capacity. The reality of diminished reserve means that providers must be hypervigilant to prevent perioperative adverse events. Careful preplanning is needed to ensure there is a rapid response process available if physiological or cognitive changes indicate impending complications. The therapeutic window of opportunity is small before reserve capacity is depleted and multisystem failure ensures.

Figure 19.3 depicts a frailty cascade beginning with predisposing triggers leading to a loss of reserve, increasing frailty, and finally to negative surgical outcomes. What is not shown here is how prehabilitation and preventative postoperative care may be able to interrupt the trajectory at any point in the process. Prevention and diligent observation shape the frailty surgical trajectory in the direction of successful outcomes.

PREOPERATIVE CONSIDERATIONS

Assessment

Ask the patient to describe past and current illnesses, especially onset of new illness situations. Using a standardized assessment form adapted for persons with vision impairment is

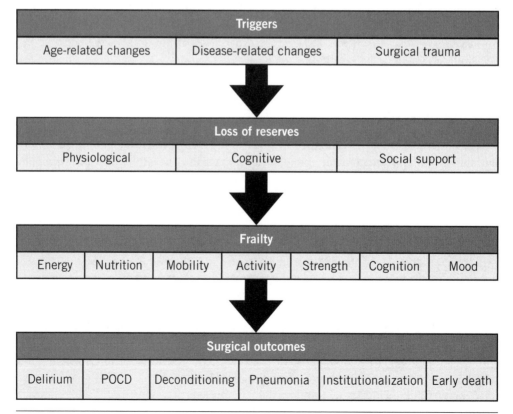

FIGURE 19.3
Frailty Cascade for Gerioperative Patients

useful for eliciting this information. Older adults can have difficulty completing self-administered questionnaires accurately and efficiently, especially in potentially or actual stressful situations. Preoperative interviews can be potentially stressful. Reviewing any self-administered document item by item is important to ensure that the information written by the patient is what is intended. The number of chronic illnesses has been identified as a potential measure of frailty. The greater the number of comorbid diseases, the greater the risk of frailty. However, the relationship is not deterministic; it provides a measure for concern about the presence of frailty.

Limiting the evaluation to number and severity of comorbid conditions does not consider type of conditions or the combined effect of diseases depending on organ systems involved. Evaluating the interactions of disease processes, physiologic pathways, and age-related changes contributes to an understanding of the dynamic of frailty. Understanding the dynamic contributes to determining effective interventions.

Questions about activity levels, feelings of exhaustion, weight changes, cognitive changes, and mood are used to evaluate the presence of frailty. Assessment tools used to evaluate frailty in older adults undergoing surgery include the Cardiovascular Health Study Index (Makary et al., 2010), Comprehensive Geriatric Assessment (CGA; Kristjansson et al., 2010), and the EFS (Rolfson, Majumdar, Tsuyuki, Tahir, & Rockwood, 2006).

The Cardiovascular Health Study Index (Fried et al., 2001) measures five biological variables to assess frailty in older adults. Frailty variables include shrinking, exhaustion, weakness, slowness, and low activity. Two of the items, shrinking and weakness, include performance measures: weight to measure shrinking and grip to measure weakness.

The EFS and CGA reflect a biopsychosocial model of frailty. The CGA is comprehensive covering major geriatric care problems. The items on the CGA are not standardized as clinicians include different items based on the patient's health and social situation. The items cover the major geriatric syndromes with the ability to add items depending on presenting data. Kristjannson and colleagues (2010) used the following assessment parameters in a study evaluating frailty in an aging surgical population: depression, cognition, activities of daily living, instrumental activities of daily living, polypharmacy, nutrition, and comorbid disease. Each assessment area relied on a standardized assessment tool for evaluation criteria to determine frailty. An important consideration in conducting a CGA is the energy level of the older adult. If the purpose is to measure frailty and a characteristic of frailty is low energy, conducting a multi-item CGA may be counter to the best interests of the older adult. Data obtained when the older adult is fatigued or stressed by multisensory inputs over long periods of time may introduce bias into the results. The EFS provides an alternate approach. Table 19.1 compares the EFS items with items included in a basic comprehensive geriatric assessment.

The EFS is a 10-item frailty assessment tool based on comprehensive geriatric assessment items. Each item in the EFS is weighted with a quantitative score between 0 and 2 points for a total of 17 points. Eight items are assessed through observation or patient questioning. Two items, a clock face drawing test and a get up and go test, are performance measures. The test is easy to use in a clinical setting. Social support is included in the EFS. Although availability of social support is an important variable in discussions of frailty, it is not always included in frailty scales.

In all three scales, poor nutritional status is measured by weight loss of greater than 10 pounds. Some studies have noted that older adults can be obese and meet the criteria for frailty. Hubbard and colleagues (2009) found a U-shaped correlation between body mass index and frailty in a secondary analysis of 3055 community-dwelling older adults over age 65.

TABLE 19.1

Comparison of Edmonton Frail Scale and Comprehensive Geriatric Assessment

Edmonton Frailty Scale	Comprehensive Geriatric Assessment
Cognition	Dementia
General health status	Comorbid conditions
Functional independence	Functional capacity
Social support	Social support
Medication use	Polypharmacy
Nutrition	Malnutrition
Mood	Depression
Continence	Urinary incontinence
Functional performance	Mobility

Active listening develops trust that leads to patient sharing of concerns and values.

Asking the older adult for a diet history presents a challenge due to poor patient recall. Family members can assist in collecting data on nutritional status. Asking the older adult about the type of foods preferred and commonly eaten, grocery shopping frequency, how groceries are obtained, and meal preparation information provides an overview of nutritional access. Asking about type and frequency of vitamin supplements, snack bars, and fast foods provides additional data about nutrition adequacy.

Stress is a risk factor that can be a tipping point in prefrail or intermediately frail older adults. Presence of depressive symptoms, anxiety, and heightened stress must be evaluated. Depression screening can be done through inclusion of two key questions during the assessment process. The two question test and follow-up questions are described in detail in Chapter 20.

Frail older adults are often ambivalent about surgery. Concerns about cost of care, benefits of care, feelings of family members, and fears of death and dying are not uncommon in this population. Active listening is important to get an accurate insight into the patient's own concerns and values rather than the concerns and values expressed by the patient but based on what others think. Asking about expectations for surgery and what the older person hopes the surgery will achieve along with assessing anxiety levels can help determine if the patient is making an informed decision.

Assessing social support and availability of caregivers and potential for caregiver burnout can be key factors in determining postdischarge plans of care. Evaluating the social support situation preoperatively provides time to make plans for discharge to sites other than home if needed. If not needed and the patient is expected to receive postsurgical care at home, exploring the level of skills, knowledge, and resources must begin during the preoperative period in order to evaluate the education and coaching needs that need to be implemented throughout the care continuum.

It is important to discuss advanced directives and proxy decision-making with frail adults. Surgery in this vulnerable population increases risk of surgical and postsurgical morbidity and mortality. The informed consent process provides the opportunity for such a discussion. Providing decisional support about surgery and treatment in the event of complications requires awareness of the patient's values and beliefs about health care and life goals.

Discussions can guide patient and provider decision-making across the perioperative continuum. The preoperative interviewer has the responsibility to raise the issue with the patient, provide decisional support, and honor the patient's decisions.

Physical Assessment

The screening physical assessment includes all elements customary in a standard assessment process with attention to problem areas identified in the history. Performance measures specific to frailty are grip and gait speed. Gait speed has been found to be highly relevant in estimating morbidity and complication risk (Makary et al., 2010). Grip is measured using a standard dynameters based on parameters suggested by Fried and colleagues (2001). Gait speed is measured by a get up and go test that asks the patient to stand from a chair walk, turn around, and return to the chair.

Preoperative Testing

Serum albumin and prealbumin are significant markers for nutritional status and availability of protein. Older adults at risk for frailty have poor nutritional intake and generally are in an anabolic state. Serum albumin less than 3.75 g/dL in surgical patients is associated with delayed wound healing and increased wound dehiscence. Albumin level is associated with muscle strength, an important variable in activity and mobility after surgery. Physiological stress and hydration levels can interfere with albumin results. Prealbumin is a more stable measure and should be evaluated as well. Additional preoperative tests suggested in frail elders are hematocrit and hemoglobin, C-reactive protein, and vitamin D.

The interdisciplinary care team should discuss abnormal test results. Although preoperative test results rarely lead to preoperative intervention, in the frail older adult test results can be a harbinger of intraoperative and postoperative problems. Low hemoglobin and hematocrit are linked to postoperative delirium, as is low serum albumin. Albumin and nutritional status are concerns in the gerioperative patient with even greater significance in frail gerioperative patients. Poor nutrition is often ignored too long. Evidence on the benefits of preoperative nutrition intervention is limited and with mixed results. However, vitamin supplements, high nutrition drinks, and frequent small meals of high nutritional value may prove beneficial. More research is sorely needed on both the potential benefits of preoperative nutrition intervention and the most effective intervention methods.

PREHABILITATION

The preoperative fitness of the older adults influences intraoperative and postoperative outcomes. Older adults, even frail older adults, are tough. They have lived long lives and mounted many hurdles. With advice and counsel from the interdisciplinary team, frail elders can better prepare themselves for surgery.

Four major areas of prehabilitation with the frail older adult center on increasing fitness and conditioning, increasing nutrition, optimizing clinical conditions, and improving cognition and mood. Other interventions center on strengthening psychological well-being and ensuring commitment by available social support systems. Emergent surgery limits opportunities for prehabilitation. Nevertheless, prehabilitation should be initiated in the time available between the decision to undergo surgery and the scheduled date of surgery. Preoperative improvement in any dimension of physical, psychological, or social support system preparation for the gerioperative patient can have a positive influence on surgical outcomes and postoperative recovery.

Using a multidisciplinary model of care, interventions are targeted to the individual's assessment, focusing on areas of greatest need and most amenable to intervention. The interdisciplinary team should develop an overall plan of care, including problem identification, best outcomes, interventions, discipline responsible for implementing intervention, and timing and methods of evaluation. In an ideal situation, the team meets regularly to review progress and revise the plan as needed. In many preoperative settings, a nurse or other provider is responsible for coordinating the plan of care, collecting information on patient progress, and ensuring revisions are made as needed. A gerioperative care coordinator can be highly effective in managing the prehabilitation program while also providing support and motivation to the older adult and support system.

Fitness and Conditioning

A prehabilitation exercise program includes resistance, aerobic, flexibility, and balance activities. The exercise plan must be tailored to the level of frailty and functional capacity of the older adult. Activities begin slowly, alternating different activities on different days, gradually increasing in number of days, repetition, and intensity in response to the patient's progress and conditioning (Hamann & Minaker, 2009). Motivation, encouragement, and attention to the psychological resiliency are important to ensure the older adult continues with the exercise recommendations. Assist family members and companion-coaches in becoming coaches to the older adults in order to improve adherence to the exercise plan.

Nutrition

Improving nutrition in the preoperative frail gerioperative patient can be challenging and difficult. Frailty is marked by low energy and weakness, two factors that interfere with appetite. Breaking the downward spiral of poor appetite and inadequate nutrition causing low energy and weakness contributing to poor appetite demands the combined thinking and collaboration of the interdisciplinary geriatric nutritional support team. Motivational interviewing and health coaching, as described in Chapter 6, is a useful strategy to help those who are frail to make changes in nutritional intake. The gerioperative care facilitator and companion-coach provide continuity and familiarity necessary to promote and support changes in behavior. An important contribution of the companion-coach is being a meal companion. Eating alone can be isolating. Evidence shows that older adults are more likely to eat better when they have someone with whom they can share a meal than when eating alone.

The exercise plan must be tailored to the level of frailty and functional capacity of the older adult.

Nutritional supplements are a mainstay of preoperative nutritional support. Nutritional supplements include high-nutrition liquid foods. Homemade smoothies, milkshakes, and other liquefied foods contribute to improved nutrition. The latter offers important substitutes if the patient refuses other types of high-energy liquid foods.

Small, frequent, nutrient-dense snacks and meals, high-energy protein bars, and vitamin supplements contribute needed calories, protein, and carbohydrates. Timing is a problem for improving nutritional status preoperatively. Improvements in nutritional states from oral intake typically take 6 to 8 weeks. However, benefit can be derived from even short-term improvement. Nutritional guidelines recommend giving a high-carbohydrate drink up to 2 hours before surgery. The high-carbohydrate drink helps to reduce anxiety, prevent dehydration, minimize surgical stress response, and reduce insulin resistance.

Studies on perioperative parenteral nutrition have produced mixed results. Few studies have documented the benefit of preoperative parenteral nutritional support except in the severely undernourished patient. For severely malnourished older adults, parenteral and enteral nutrition given for 7 to 10 days has been found to improve the patient's condition. Frail older adults are vulnerable to infection from parenteral nutrition. The risks and benefits of implementing parenteral and enteral support in frail older adults must be evaluated carefully.

Optimizing Clinical Conditions

Optimal management of all preexisting medical illnesses is a priority in the preoperative care of the frail older adult management, including medication review and revision.

Ensuring older adults are receiving an optimum medication regimen that maximizes benefit and minimizes risk is a preoperative target goal in frail older adults. Frailty is a risk factor for increased adverse medication events due to changes in pharmacodynamics and pharmocokinetics resulting from sarcopenia and weight loss. A medication review evaluates potential for drug-drug and drug-disease interactions. A key question in medication use in frail adults is, "Is this medication necessary?" Attention to dose and interval of administration is required.

Maximizing Cognition and Mood

Engaging in games, conversations, puzzles, and other activities that require concentration and attention can increase alertness and attention span. Participating in leisure activities with friends or family members helps to decrease feelings of isolation and depression. Cognitive behavioral therapy is a formal strategy for treating depression. Exercise, nutrition, and adequate sleep also decrease depression and enhance overall well-being. Many frail elders reside in assisted living centers or nursing homes. Staff or family members serve as partners in motivating and encouraging the older adult to be active.

INTRAOPERATIVE CONSIDERATIONS

Frail older adults have higher risks for intraoperative adverse events. Instituting preventive actions can improve surgical outcomes. Recognizing the potential effects of surgery and anesthesia on the frail older adults enables providers to monitor the older adult for possible adverse events. Intraoperative factors that increase the risk for adverse postoperative events in frail gerioperative patients include length of surgery and anesthesia, amount of blood loss, number of blood transfusions, and depth of anesthesia.

Hypothermia

The loss of physiologic reserves in frail older adults makes them highly vulnerable to hypothermia and the resulting adverse events. Minimizing intraoperative hypothermia requires constant body temperature monitoring, use of warming blankets and warming fluids, and maintaining a warm ambient temperature. Frail older adults undergoing abdominal surgery are at highest risk of hypothermia due to loss of body heat through the open abdomen. An even greater degree of vigilance is needed to maintain normothermia in this highly vulnerable population. For more extended discussion of hypothermia in the gerioperative patient, see Chapter 8.

Frailty predisposes the postoperative older adult to higher risk of postoperative complications.

POSTOPERATIVE CONSIDERATIONS

Postoperative considerations for frail older adults do not vary significantly from postoperative considerations for all older adults. However, attention to the timeliness of early detection and the immediacy and adequacy of a therapeutic response is crucial.

The focus of care with frail gerioperative patients must be based on sensitivity to the lack of reserve and critical attention to minimal levels of stress acting as a tipping point. Once the tipping point is reached, postoperative complications easily occur, and recovery is difficult. Although "prevention, prevention, and prevention" is the byword in care of all gerioperative patients, in the frail older adult, the value of the old adage "an ounce of prevention is worth a pound of cure" must be taken seriously.

Frailty predisposes the postoperative older adult to higher risk of postoperative complications. Table 19.2 shows postoperative complications rates in three populations of frail older adults. Complication rates ranged from 43to 76%. Many of these complications are preventable by involving the interdisciplinary geriatric care team preoperatively. Identifying the underlying strengths of frail gerioperative patients is critical in helping them to meet the challenge of surgery. Old people have lived long enough to be old by overcoming hardships, illness, and a lifetime of challenges. Harnessing previous coping abilities while supporting available physiological reserve by decreasing stress and preserving energy promotes faster rehabilitation and recovery.

Taking immediate preventive actions as soon as possible after surgery remains the key to positive patient outcomes. Postoperative care is outlined in Table 19.3. Frail older adults are at highest risk for falls, pressure ulcers, infection, thromboembolism, cognitive changes, and medication-related adverse events. Consistent, systematic monitoring to detect earliest signs and symptoms of impending complications is a high priority. Maintaining alertness to atypical signs and symptoms contributes to early detection of emerging problems. Cognitive or behavioral changes may be the first sign of impending complications. The interdisciplinary health care team must initiate rapid, intensive evaluation and response.

Reviewing the preoperative assessment, perioperative plan of care, prehabilitation outcomes, and intraoperative events assists in detecting and evaluating changes in the clinical status of the frail older adults. Postoperative care providers need to review the medical record to determine how long the gerioperative patient required anesthesia, amount of blood loss and number of transfusions, if any, and core temperature reading during and after surgery. Medical record review highlights risk factors and assists in targeted prevention and

TABLE 19.2

Percent of Frail Older Adults Experiencing Postoperative Complications

	Scale	Number	Percent Fit	Percent Intermediate Frail	Percent Frail	Percent Frail with Complications
Krisjansson et al. (2010)	CGA	178	12%	46%	43%	76%
Makary et al. (2010)	Fried phenotype (five variables)	346	58%	31%	10%	43% (major surgery) 11% minor surgery
Dasgupta et al. (2009)	EFS*	125	40%	48%	12%	56%

CGA, Comprehensive Geriatric Assessment; EFS, Edmonton Frailty Scale.

TABLE 19.3

Selected Prehabilitation and Recovery Targets, Intervention, and Care Team Involvement for Frail Older Adults

Stage	Target	Intervention	Interdisciplinary Involvement
Preoperative	Mobility and exercise	Exercises to improve: Balance Aerobic capacity Flexibility	MD PT OT Physiotherapist Self Family GFC CC
	Nutrition and fluid	Small nutrient dense meals Sip nutrition between meals Vitamin supplements Vitamin D	MD Nutritionist Self/family
	Optimize physical, mood, cognitive, social well-being	Maximum control of preexisting illness and disease Assess and treat depression, anxiety Cognitive stimulation Identify, support, and coach social support system	MD Geropsychiatrist ARNP SW Self/family
	Medication	Medication review and adjustment as needed	MD Pharmacist Self/family
	Smoking cessation	Smoking cessation program Implement coaching program on smoking cessation	MD Respiratory therapist Anesthesia provider Self CC GFC
	Pulmonary prehabilitation	Increase chest flexibility Improve lung expansion Practice controlled breathing	Pulmonogist Respiratory therapist Self/family
	Information support	Coach on benefits of: Correct use of spirometer Effective coughing Minimizing pain when moving Nutrition	RN
	Decrease anxiety	Share information about surgery from preoperative prehabilitation through discharge planning	RN SW Family CC GFC

(continued)

TABLE 19.3
Selected Prehabilitation and Recovery Targets, Intervention, and Care Team Involvement
for Frail Older Adults *(continued)*

Stage	Target	Intervention	Interdisciplinary Involvement
	Perioperative plan of care	Identify patient alerts Anticipate problems Share information across care continuum Inform next step providers Review last step events	RN Anesthesia provider Surgeon
	Evaluation postdischarge plan of care and follow-up	Review preoperative discharge options Explore patient preferences Assess discharge environment Anticipate health and social support needs Evaluating strengths and resources	RN SW Surgeon PT OT Self/family Long-term support Counselor GFC CC
	Informed consent	Assessing cognitive capacity Reviewing options Exploring patient values and beliefs Exploring advance directives and proxy decision-making	MD RN Self Family
Intraoperative	Anxiety	Medication Therapeutic communication	RN Anesthesia provider
	Normothermia	Warming blankets Ambient temperatures	RN
	Pain control	Monitoring pain Administering analgesia	Anesthesia provider
	Depth anesthesia		Anesthesia provider
	Positioning	Ensuring comfort Supporting joints Padding joints	RN Anesthesia provider Surgeon
	Pressure points	Avoiding pressure points Padding superficial nerves and blood supply	RN
	Fluid management	Intravenous fluids Monitoring fluid balance	Anesthesia provider Surgeon
Postoperative care: PACU, immediate and postdischarge	Pain relief	Analgesic medication Nonpharmacological methods Routes of administration	RN MD Self/family

(continued)

TABLE 19.3

Selected Prehabilitation and Recovery Targets, Intervention, and Care Team Involvement for Frail Older Adults *(continued)*

Stage	Target	Intervention	Interdisciplinary Involvement
	Systematic monitoring Standardized tools when appropriate		RN Self/family
	DVT prevention		MD RN Self/family
	Pneumonia protocol including oral care		RN MD Respiratory therapist Self/family
	Fluid maintenance		RN MD surgeon Nutritionist/dietician Self/family
	Nutrition		Surgeon Nutritionist/dietician RN Self/family
	Ambulation/ activity		RN Physiotherapist PT OT Surgeon MD Self/family
	Geriatric care units (ACE, HELP)		Full IDT
Follow-up	Appointment		MD ARNP Self/family SW
		Recovery activities and log	RN SW OT

ACE, acute care for elders; ARNP, advanced registered nurse practitioner; CC, companion-coach; DVT, deep vein thrombosis; GFC, gerioperative care facilitator; HELP, Healthcare and Elder Law Programs Corporation; IDT, interdisciplinary care team; MD, medical doctor; OT, occupational therapist; PACU, postanesthesia care unit; PT, physical therapist; RN, registered nurse; SW, social worker.

intervention strategies. Medication reviews must be completed as soon as possible after surgery to determine medications that need to be restarted immediately and medications that create risk factors for delirium and other adverse events.

Conserving energy and promoting recovery can appear to be contradictory goals. Recovery activities require significant levels of energy to complete. Frail older adults have preexisting low energy levels and poor endurance. Surgery and anesthesia further deplete the frail patient's limited energy reserves. Conserving remaining energy is important if frail older adults are to conduct recovery activities. A third element important to conserving sufficient energy to meet recovery demands is adequate nutrition. Interventions targeting improvement in nutrition increase energy stores and availability. In the postoperative older adult, activities, uninterrupted rest periods, and nutritional interventions must be carefully planned and coordinated among all members of the health care team.

Nutrition involves multiple small meals coordinated with recovery and rest periods. Meals should be offered at a time that does not interfere with rest periods or immediately before or after energy depleting activities such as walking, toileting, or deep breathing and incentive spirometry. A functional schedule follows a rest, activity, rest, meal, rest, and activity pattern throughout the day. Frail patients need time to consume even small meals. Having family members or the companion-coach present during meals can help improve intake. Ensuring good oral hygiene between meals encourages intake.

Pain is a major barrier to activity and nutritional intake. Providing adequate pain relief improves activity participation and general comfort that can improve appetite. However, medications, including pain medications, contribute to nausea. Taking multiple medications at a single point in time can deplete energy and interfere with appetite. Giving medications can be used as a nutrient-inclusive activity depending on the medication. Administering fewer medications at a time and giving medications with food or high-nutrient drinks contribute to caloric and nutrient intake. An important consideration in medication management, especially polypharmacy, is avoidance of a pharmacological cascade, giving a medication that causes side effects to relieve side effects of another medication.

Mobility

Movement is one of the most significant activities in preventing complications and promoting recovery. Movement decreases risk of pulmonary complications, venous thrombosis, delirium, and pressure ulcers. Increasing activity improves wound healing, cognition, appetite, and sleep. In-bed exercises, such as passive and active range of motion, can be used for severely frail older individuals or those whose clinical condition requires bed rest. Sitting with the head of the bed elevated improves ventilation and cardiac function and prevents aspiration. Chair exercises rely on similar activities. Elastic bands are used to increase resistance. Slumping positions must be avoided and shearing pressures carefully monitored to prevent pressure ulcer development when sitting in an upright or partially position. Standing and ambulating with assistance increases lower leg muscle strength, improves balance, and decreases fall risk.

Guidelines and standards have not been established for postoperative activity levels in frail older adults. General guidelines for postoperative exercise, mobility, and activity may not be relevant or appropriate. Interventions must be targeted to the individual patient's clinical condition and functional capacity identified through interdisciplinary team assessment and must be consistent with overall treatment goals. Providing emotional and structural support helps the patient gain confidence in performing postoperative activities and establishing a pattern that can be continued postdischarge. Activity can be increased as function improves. Unless a comorbid clinical condition limits activity, the frail older adult should be encouraged to engage in range of motion or an exercise group on a daily basis.

DISCHARGE CONSIDERATIONS

Frailty is associated with increased risk for discharge to assisted living or nursing home. However, many frail older adults can be discharged to the home if there is adequate social support and support services available and the patient expresses the desire to return home. To be ready for discharge home, the patient must be in maximum presurgical condition. Family education, coaching, teaching, and support contribute to prehabilitaton adherence. The local adult and disability services center can be contacted regarding home discharge and obtaining long-term support services for frail older adults who need assistance postdischarge. Initiating contact with the aging and disability center before surgery provides times for the agency and long-term coordinator to ensure that needed services will be available and in place at time of discharge. Preoperative discharge plans for frail older adults are subject to revision due to postoperative clinical events that alter hospital length of stay and postdischarge placement. However, preplanning can facilitate the potential for discharge home when services needed are identified in a timely fashion.

PATIENT REPORT: Mr. Ditmer

Mr. Ditmer is discharged home after his day surgery. Three days later, the family brings him to the emergency room. He shows no evidence of any identifiable pathological process or diagnosis. The conclusion is possible delirium due to preexisting pain, medication, changes in nutrition, and stress of surgery and anesthesia. The surgery was a tipping point. Although apparently healthy prior to his knee injury, Mr. Ditmer had osteoarthritis that was very painful but minimally acknowledged. His change from active older adult to a perceived label of "old man" caused by his inability to "get around" led to a mild depression that was not evaluated prior to surgery but put him at risk for delirium.

SUMMARY

The number of frail older adults undergoing surgery is increasing as a result of improved surgical techniques and anesthetic approaches. Frailty is associated with decreased physiological and psychological reserve capacity. Frail older adults are less able and have less capacity to meet the demands of surgery, making them more vulnerable to intraoperative and postoperative complications. However, intensive prehabilitation and diligent attention to postoperative prevention programs may be able to preserve whatever reserve capacity the frail gerioperative patient possesses, and surgery can result in successful patient outcomes.

KEY POINTS

- Surgery is a stressor that can increase frailty by overstressing physiologic and psychological reserve. The goal is to minimize the stress of surgery at all stages.
- Older adults identified as frail are 2.5 times more likely than nonfrail adults to have adverse outcomes and 20 times more likely to be admitted to a nursing home after hospital discharge.
- The high preponderance of frail older adults in the acute care setting can create a normative expectation among professional care providers that aging and frailty are synonymous.
- Only through diligence and meticulous attention to gerioperative care can providers assist frail adults to remain at their maximum level of health, well-being, and functional ability.

PART III

Gerioperative Considerations

TWENTY

Depression and Dementia

Raelene V. Shippee–Rice, Susan J. Fetzer, and Jennifer V. Long

PATIENT REPORT: Mrs. Rosner

Mrs. Rosner emigrated from the Czech Republic 15 years ago at age 55. She lives with her daughter and son-in-law. She was found 2 days ago passed out on the floor of the kitchen when her daughter came home from work. Very little of her medical history is known by her daughter. However, her son-in-law has noticed that Mrs. Rosner has seemed withdrawn lately, not wanting to go out of the house, and seldom finishes her meals. She wakes early in the morning and takes frequent naps during the day. She has refused to attend church services for the last month.

After treatment in the emergency room with a temporary pacemaker for sick sinus syndrome, she undergoes surgery for an 80% occlusion of her right carotid artery. The vascular surgeon and anesthesia provider agree on a regional anesthetic, and Mrs. Rosner has an uncomplicated surgery. In the postanesthesia care unit, she is pleasant but quiet, and is able to follow commands during the neurological assessment. She has an uneventful recovery from her anesthesia and is transferred back to the surgical unit. Her daughter greets her upon her return to her room.

Depression and dementia are not normal consequences of growing old. However, there is evidence that age-related changes increase vulnerability to depression and dementia. Older adults with preoperative depression or dementia are highly vulnerable to the physiological and psychological stress induced by surgery and anesthesia. The vulnerability contributes to postoperative complications in the gerioperative patient. Detection of depression and dementia allows for treatment and supportive interventions that can improve perioperative outcomes. Understanding depression and dementia in the gerioperative patient leads to interventions that protect the integrity of the older adult, prevents postoperative events that exacerbate depression and dementia, and prevents risk of complications induced by physiological changes associated with depression and dementia. This chapter compares and contrasts early- and late-onset depression, depression and dementia, and depression and dementia in relation to delirium and postoperative cognitive dysfunction.

Depression and dementia are not part of normal aging.

Postoperative depression and dementia can exist prior to surgery or occur in response to surgical, anesthesia, pain, and postoperative recovery demands. Depression and dementia create risks to client safety, recovery, and well-being after surgery. Detection of depression and dementia before surgery allows for prehabilitation that can help minimize preoperative anxiety associated with depression and dementia, contribute to an intraoperative and postoperative plan to decrease risk of complications, and establish an alert system for systematic monitoring and early detection of new symptoms that signal a new onset of depression or dementia. The signs and symptoms associated with dementia and depression in the older adult are similar, making a differential diagnosis difficult. Further, the symptoms are common to diseases associated with aging. The presence of coexisting dementia and depression in older adults with comorbid diseases compounds the problems of assessment and intervention. The right treatment for the right problem at the right time to prevent surgical complications or to initiate early intervention becomes a major challenge for nurses and other providers facing complex depression, dementia, and disease interactions.

Depression

Depression is defined as an alteration in mood marked by diminished interest or pleasure in regular activities and feelings of sadness. It is characterized by changes in a person's affect, behavior, cognition, and soma. Depression results from a complex interaction of physiological, psychosocial, generic, cognitive, psychodynamic, and health-related factors. Physiological processes involve neuroendocrine and neurotransmitter alterations. Three major mechanisms are neurotransmitter depletion, diasthesis-stress, and hypothalamic-pituitary-adrenal (HPA) axis disruption.

The neurotransmitter deficiency theory posits that disrupted regulation of neurotransmitters in the central nervous system results in mood alterations and depression. Serotonin is the primary neurotransmitter of interest along with the norepinephrine and dopamine. The neurotransmitters are major influences on mood and emotional responses including feelings of well-being, pleasure, pain, anxiety, and arousal.

Neurotransmitter concentration and the number of receptor sites available that can bind the neurotransmitter regulate the availability of neurotransmitter in the central nervous system. When neurotransmitter production is reduced or fewer receptor sites are present, nerve signals are not conducted. Depression occurs with low concentration of or loss of receptor sites for serotonin, norepinephrine, or dopamine. One of the most convincing arguments supporting the neurotransmitter theory is the beneficial effect of drug therapy in decreasing or increasing neurotransmitter activity. However, medications used to treat depression are not effective for every patient, suggesting that additional explanations contribute to the etiology of depression.

The diathesis-stress hypothesis argues that elevated stress levels trigger depression in individuals who have a genetic or biologic predisposition or diathesis. The level of stress needed to evoke a depressive episode depends on the degree of predisposition, which is highly variable across individuals. In the absence of a family history suggesting a genetic diathesis, there is no way to predict vulnerability to stress-related depression. Not all persons with predisposition to depression will experience a depressive episode. It is only when the intensity of stress becomes overwhelming that the vulnerability becomes evident and depression ensues.

The HPA axis has also been implicated in depression. Dysfunction in the HPA causes changes in neurotransmitter receptor sites. High levels of stress trigger the hypothalamus to release corticotropin-releasing factor (CRF). CRF activates the release of adrenocorticotropic

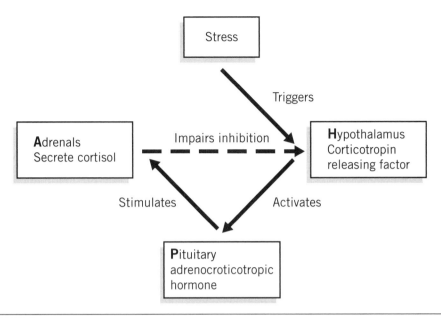

FIGURE 20.1
Hypothalamus-Pituitary-Adrenal Axis Model of Depression

hormone from the pituitary. Adrenocorticotropic hormone triggers cortisol secretion from the adrenal glands. Due to negative feedback, increased cortisol secretion triggers receptors in the central nervous system to decrease corticotropin releasing factor activation. Figure 20.1 presents the HPA-elevated cortisol model. Depression occurs when, because of changes in feedback receptors, CRF is not inhibited due to changes in feedback receptors. Lack of CRF inhibition causes brain cortisol levels to remain elevated. There is a positive association between elevated cortisol, decreased serotonin receptor function, and the onset of depression.

The physiological processes explaining depression result in symptoms identified by the *Diagnostic and Statistical Manual of Mental Disorders, 4th edition (DSM-IV)*, as criteria for diagnosis. Criteria are divided into four symptom categories: affective, behavioral, cognitive, and somatic symptoms. The patient's symptoms must be present almost every day for most of the day for at least 2 weeks to be considered for diagnosis. The presence of at least one of two cardinal symptoms, depressed mood and anhedonia (loss of pleasure), is needed for a diagnosis. Demonstrated mood changes must show a difference from the person's normal mood to one that interferes with social, occupational, or educational function. A depressed mood cannot be the result of drugs, alcohol, medications, or a comorbid medical condition. In addition to the two cardinal symptoms, at least four of the following symptoms are needed: significant weight change, insomnia or hypersomnia, psychomotor agitation or retardation, excessive fatigue or loss of energy, feelings of worthlessness or excessive guilt, difficulty concentrating, or recurrent thoughts of death or suicide.

Late-Onset Depression

Depression that occurs for the first time after age 65, referred to as late-onset depression, is different than depression found in younger adults. Late-onset depression is the most common mood alteration in older adults. The reported

Depressive symptoms can be atypical in older adults.

prevalence for late-onset depression in the United States is highly variable because of the difficulty distinguishing among the multiple classifications of depression. Depression is classified into five categories of special relevance to the older adult. Categories include major depressive disorder, depressive symptoms, mood changes due to general medical conditions, vascular depression, or depression of Alzheimer's disease (AD). Onset of depression in any classification occurring in elders over 65 is termed late-onset depression.

The reported prevalence of major depression is estimated at 5%, with a 15% prevalence of depressive symptoms in community-based elders. The percentage increases to 42% in older adults living in nursing homes. Older adults in hospitals have rates of depression up to 50%. Depression is closely linked with disease in older adults. The number of comorbid conditions, including persistent pain, is highly correlated with the number or severity of depressive symptoms.

Older adults with cardiovascular disease are a subpopulation with higher rates of depression. Depression is associated with increased platelet reactivity and markers for inflammation. These changes lead to cardiovascular disease. Approximately 20% of older adults undergoing cardiac bypass graft report five or more depressive symptoms (Sorenson & Wang, 2010). Among older adults having major, noncardiac surgery, 15% showed evidence of depressive symptoms during preoperative screening (Bass, Attix, Phillips-Bute, & Monk, 2008).

PATHOPHYSIOLOGY

The physiology of late-onset depression involves the interaction of predisposing and precipitating biological, psychological, and psychosocial factors represented in Figure 20.2. Predisposing biological factors include cognitive predisposition and age-related neurobiological changes. Chronic disease conditions, particularly cardiovascular, neurological, and persistent pain, serve as precipitating factors along with medication effects.

Aging is associated with reduced central nervous system neurotransmitters and loss of postsynaptic receptor sites. Decreased levels of serotonin, norepinephrine, and dopamine, an alteration in their distribution, and changes in the synaptic gap increase the vulnerability

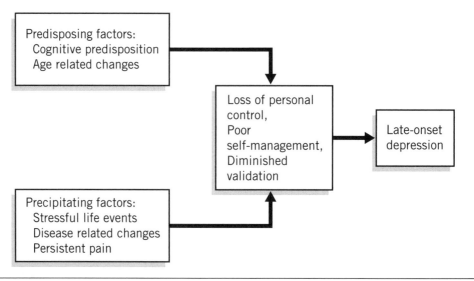

FIGURE 20.2
Predisposing and Precipitating Factors for Late-Onset Depression

of older adults to depression. Elevated stress levels from multiple biological, psychological, and social events stimulate the HPA axis, triggering depressive symptoms. Depression risk is increased in older women as a result of decreased estrogen and increased in older men with low testosterone levels.

As older adults age, they lose many of their friend networks and support systems. Family members often live at a distance or are busy with work, children, or other responsibilities. Although family members are the major source of support for older adults, many elders experience burden worry, the fear of becoming a burden to their families. As functional capacity diminishes in response to aging and disease-related changes, increasing concerns about their families' ability to continue supporting them, fear of nursing home admission, decreased financial resources, and ability to maintain self-care become increasingly stressful. In vulnerable older adults, the increase in psychosocial stress can precipitate a late-onset depression.

Older adults with depression are often misdiagnosed, underdiagnosed, and undertreated. One of the major reasons for undertreatment is the difference in symptoms in older adults. Many older adults exhibit signs and symptoms of a depressed mood without meeting all the criteria for major depression or major depressive episode. Subthreshold or minor depression exists when a patient exhibits fewer than the five symptoms listed in the *DSM-IV* criteria but significant clinical evidence of depressive mood still exists. Subthreshold depression is an important consideration in the care of older adults. Ignoring subthreshold depression in the perioperative care of the older adult creates a risk for inadequate treatment of depression and adverse effects of perioperative depression.

DETECTING DEPRESSION

Detection of depression is critical for patient safety and well-being throughout the perioperative continuum. The lack of a preoperative diagnosis prevents older adults from receiving treatment before surgery. Inadequate treatment increases the potential for adverse events in the immediate postoperative period or after discharge from the hospital or ambulatory care center. Adverse events include an increase in pain severity, less effective analgesia outcomes, impaired wound healing, diminished ability to participate in recovery activities, impaired ambulation, increased deconditioning, inadequate nutrition and hydration, sleep disturbance, increased fatigue, and impaired coagulation.

Detecting depression and distinguishing depression from other conditions that result in behavioral and cognitive changes is challenging. Late-onset depression presents differently in older adults than depression in younger age groups. Depression symptoms are confounded by symptoms associated with chronic disease, pain, and postoperative effects of surgery and anesthesia.

Table 20.1 displays differences in signs and symptoms in older adults with late-onset depression and depression in younger adults. Older adults show less evidence of depressed mood or feelings of guilt. Somatic complaints are often the most common presenting symptom. Common somatic concerns are fatigue, sleep disturbance, appetite loss, psychomotor retardation, and complaints of headache, gastrointestinal discomfort, shortness of breath, back and joint pain or muscle aching, and paresthesias. They are more likely to be irritable or upset about money, health, or how they will get along in the future.

Depression can occur after surgery independent of preexisting depression. The onset of postoperative depression leads to impaired recovery, poor adherence to medication regimens postdischarge, increased rate of hospital readmission, prolonged length of stay, impaired cognition, and loss of the ability to perform self-care.

TABLE 20.1

Comparison of Symptoms of Late-Onset Depression and Early-Onset Depression

Category	Older Adults (Late-Onset)	Younger Adults (Early-Onset)
Affective	Loss of feelings of pleasure Lack of interest in daily activities	Depressed mood Feelings of worthlessness and guilt Lack of feelings of pleasure
Behavioral	Irritability Apathy Psychomotor retardation	Withdrawal Agitation
Cognitive	Reduced cognitive processing Poor memory Inability to concentrate Memory loss Impaired executive function	Difficulty with concentration Inability to make decisions
Somatic	Sleep disturbance Gastrointestinal disturbances Palpitations Weight loss Back or joint pain Muscle aching Incontinence	Insomnia or hypersomnia Decreased or increased appetite

Symptoms of postoperative depression can be misinterpreted as pain, resistance to treatment, postanesthesia effects, or exacerbation of comorbid illness. Factors contributing to immediate postoperative depression include fatigue, pain, inability to sleep, feelings of weakness, and concerns about recovery. Postsurgical depression may not become evident until after discharge from the hospital. Postdischarge depression can result from prolonged recovery.

Physical symptoms caused by depression are hard to distinguish from symptoms caused by physical disease or exacerbation of comorbid illness. Symptoms are often treated with medication independently of a more comprehensive assessment. Careful observation, history taking, and physical examination can help to detect evidence of depression. Not making assumptions that symptoms are a normal part of aging or normal responses to surgery can help providers remain alert to evidence of depressive mood. Screening tools can help distinguish depression from other causes of symptoms.

Comorbidity is associated with higher rates and severity of depressive symptoms. Altered cognitive function, decreased vision and hearing, changes in executive function, and slowed processing time are common confounding variables. Loss of independence particularly after surgery, concerns about future health and well-being, as well as worries over financial resources, housing, and ability to maintain functional capacity exacerbates presurgical factors.

Medications contribute to depression by acting on the central and autonomic nervous systems, regulating cortisol excretion, or disrupting inflammatory pathways. Some medications interfere with neurotransmitter availability or the stability of the HPA axis. Betablockers, benzodiazepines, corticosteroids, narcotics, and statins are the most common medications used in the surgical setting that can cause depressive symptoms among gerioperative patients.

Pain is a major contributor to depression. Older adults with preexisting pain have higher levels of depression. Unrelieved postoperative pain can lead to feelings of depression.

The onset of surgical related physiological, psychological, and social stressors heightens stress, exacerbating preexisting depression or depressed mood or triggering new-onset post-surgical depression.

Depression and Dementia

There is a strong positive correlation between depression and dementia. Older adults with depression have an increased risk of developing dementia, particularly of the AD type. In a longitudinal study of 949 participants, findings indicated that 21.6% of those who were depressed at study baseline developed AD compared with 16% of those who did not have depression. Those with depression had a 50% increase in risk for dementia (Saczynski, Beiser, Seshadri, Auerbach, Wolf, & Au, 2010). A study of older adults with late-onset depression and cognitive impairment revealed that 40% subsequently were diagnosed with AD (Fiske, Wetherell, & Gatz, 2009). In the reverse, patients with dementia are at risk for late-onset depression due to the increase in stress from cognitive, behavioral, and psychosocial changes accompanying the disease and to the uncertainty about the future and concerns for self and family. There is a potential for either disease to mask the other due to the similarity of signs and symptoms and presence of comorbidity. Gerioperative patients presenting with either depression or dementia must be carefully screened for both conditions using standardized tools, observation, active listening, and clinical judgment.

Dementia

Dementia is a general term describing brain pathology. In dementia, there is a loss of memory and cognitive deficits with an overall decline in language and executive function that leads to motor retardation, increasing functional incapacity, and changes in mood and behavior.

Dementia is not a single disease; there are over 40 forms of dementia. The most common forms are AD, vascular dementia (VaD), and mixed dementia. Mild cognitive impairment (MCI) is an intermediate stage between typical age-related cognitive changes and early clinical signs of dementia. Patients with MCI experience a decline in memory, language, thinking, and judgment. Between 50% and 70% of older adults with MCI will progress to a diagnosis of AD.

DSM-IV criteria for AD and VaD are outlined in Table 20.2. There are no defined criteria for mixed dementia.

ALZHEIMER'S DISEASE

AD, a progressive, degenerative disease, is the most common cause of dementia. AD is characterized by the development of amyloid plaques, neurofibrillary tangles, neuronal loss, and alterations in neurotransmitter availability and function. Although similar changes occur in the brain of older adults without dementia, the severity of physiologic change and effect on function is much greater in AD.

In the early onset of AD, physiologic changes occur in the hippocampus with the primary effect on memory. Over time, there is progressive involvement of the cerebral cortex, leading to loss of executive function and long-term memory. Cerebral cortex changes also

TABLE 20.2

Comparison of Signs and Symptoms of Alzheimer's Type Dementia and Vascular Dementia

Alzheimer's Type Dementia	Vascular Dementia
• Memory impairment	• Memory impairment

• Cognitive disturbance manifested by
  • Aphasia
  • Apraxia
  • Agnosia
  • Impaired executive function
	• Cognitive disturbance manifested by
	  • Aphasia
	  • Apraxia
	  • Agnosia
	  • Impaired executive function

• Memory and cognitive changes lead to impaired social or occupational function	• Memory and cognitive changes lead to impaired social or occupational function
• Gradual onset and continuing decline	• Intermittent periods of stabilization
	• Step down progression

lead to alterations in mood and personality. Eventually, beginning in the moderate disease stage, motor function degenerates. In late-stage AD, neuronal loss encompasses the entire cerebral cortex including the ventricles affecting speech, motor function, sensory processing, and conscious thought. With the loss of neurons, there is depletion of acetylcholine, serotonin, and norepinephrine neurotransmitters important to cognitive function. Brain atrophy results from the loss of neurons. Figure 20.3 makes the extent of brain atrophy in late-stage disease evident and explains the extensive loss of function that occurs in older adults with AD.

The degenerative process is gradual and progressive beginning long before signs and symptoms appear. The progressive atrophy and alterations in neurotransmitter function result in few signals getting transmitted in the cerebral cortex where thought, mood, and personality reside, leaving little of the unique personhood of the individual. The loss of brain integrity in both structure and function is critical to understanding the behavior and needs of the older adult with AD. The only parts of the brain left relatively intact are those that control basic body function and responses to external stimuli with little voluntary control.

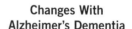

Normal Brain   **Changes With
                            Alzheimer's Dementia**

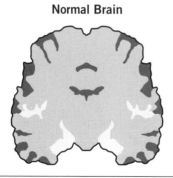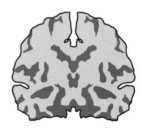

FIGURE 20.3

Transition From Normal Adult Brain to Brain Atrophy From Alzheimer's Disease

The brain of an older adult with Alzheimer's disease is atrophied with large ventricles. There is very littlef functioning cortical matter to manage cognition, emotions, and behavior.

The older adult is at the mercy of a progressive, degenerative process. The loss of personhood is a seamless downward spiral. The lack of interruption in disease progression is one factor distinguishing Alzheimer's type dementia from VaD. In VaD, disease progression makes a step-down pattern with intermittent periods of stabilization.

VASCULAR DEMENTIA

VaD, or multi-infarct dementia, is caused by atherosclerosis in the blood vessels supplying nutrients to the cerebral cortex. In the 1960s, the diagnoses of arteriosclerotic brain disease or chronic obstructive brain disease were commonly used for older adults who demonstrated cognitive deficits, personality and mood changes, and memory loss. The changes in cognition were believed to be due to atherosclerosis or hardening of the arteries in the brain.

The process of atherosclerotic plaques in VaD interferes with cerebral blood flow, causing a loss of tissue oxygenation similar to that seen in a myocardial infarction. The location of the ischemia determines symptoms. The process is the same as that seen in stroke and myocardial infarction. In VaD, microemboli occur causing "mini" strokes or silent strokes. Symptoms appear as step-wise changes in the patient's condition and functional ability as new "infarcts" occur.

Risk factors for VaD are similar to those of cardiovascular disease: smoking, hypertension, hypercholesterolemia, heart disease, diabetes, or other conditions that control vascular integrity. Older adults with VaD have motor and cognitive changes as well as mood and behavior changes depending on the area of the brain affected by infarcts or plaques. Patients with VaD often show disorientation or confusion similar to that seen in cerebral vascular accidents or transient ischemic attacks.

MIXED DEMENTIA

Mixed dementia occurs when there is a coexistence of documented VaD and AD. Up to 50% of older adults with dementia show brain lesions consistent with both AD and VaD. The impairment in cognitive function may be greater when there the physiological changes of AD and VaD are combined than with either disease alone.

The overall prevalence of dementia in elders is estimated at 14%. The prevalence ranges from 5% in 71- to 79-year-olds to almost 38% in adults over age 90. AD accounts for approximately 70% of the reported dementia, followed by VaD at nearly 18%. Parkinson's disease and other forms of dementia account for the remaining 12%. As age increases, AD accounts for a greater proportion of the reported dementia. Approximately 22% of adults over age 75 present have mild cognitive impairment. In older adults with MCI and late-onset depression, the risk of developing an Alzheimer's type dementia is twice that of older adults with MCI without an accompanying depression.

Gerioperative Care

As the population of older adults increases, the number of gerioperative patients with depression, mild cognitive impairment, and dementia will increase. Understanding the special needs of older adults with cognitive impairment regardless of etiology enables providers to anticipate potential problems and initiate preventive actions to ensure patient safety, prevent complications, initiate early interventions, and achieve positive surgical outcomes.

PREOPERATIVE CONSIDERATIONS

Identifying the presence and severity of depression and dementia influences the type of pre-habilitation program and coaching strategies that can be used to prepare the older adult for surgery. Care providers can plan care that centers on safety and unique needs of older adults with depression and cognitive impairment. Care includes primary intervention to prevent delirium, delayed wound healing, impaired mobility, poor nutrition, and extended recovery period prevalent in gerioperative patients with a history of depression or dementia. Communication needs are a high priority. Depression and dementia can interfere with reception of information and with expressing needs and concerns.

Many older adults may have undiagnosed or undetected signs and symptoms of depression or dementia that can be identified through the preoperative assessment. Up to 25% of older adults will not self-report symptoms of depression or dementia. Fears of being labeled, treated differently, or losing independence all interfere with self-acknowledgement of symptoms or sharing symptoms and concerns with others. Conducting depression and dementia assessment requires sensitivity to the concerns of the older adult. Exhibit 20.1 outlines general guidelines for depression and dementia screening. Table 20.3 identifies assessments to be completed.

HISTORY

Chronic Disease

Depression is strongly associated with duration, severity, and number of comorbid disease. Ask the patient about current medical history and duration of each condition. Assess symptom severity and the effect of symptoms on patient function.

EXHIBIT 20.1 Guidelines for Preoperative Depression and Dementia Screening

- Maintain a high index of suspicion for the presence of depression, mild cognitive impairment, or dementia in the gerioperative patient.
- Be aware that older adults with depression often present with atypical signs and symptoms.
- Depression and dementia have a high degree of comorbidity and present with overlapping symptoms.
- Gerioperative patients should be screened for depression, mild cognitive impairment, and dementia using standardized screening tools.
- Gerioperative patients with questionable or positive scores on screening tests should be referred for further evaluation by a primary care provider, geriatrician, or interdisciplinary care team before surgery.
- A patient safety alert must be attached to the medical record of all older adults with diagnoses of depression or dementia.
- A plan for prehabilitation, intraoperative, postoperative, and postdischarge care directed to ensure patient safety, prevent complications, and implement systematic monitoring and early intervention should be developed prior to surgery, implemented across the perioperative continuum, and revised as necessary based on the patient's clinical condition.
- A patient safety alert should be posted for older adults taking antidepressants and other mood-altering medications due to potential interactions with anesthesia and postoperative analgesia.

TABLE 20.3
Dementia and Depression Screening Components

	Component
History	

Mental status and mood changes	• Signs and symptoms
	  • Cognitive changes
	  • Somatic symptoms
	  • Affect
	  • Behavior change
	  • Functional changes
	• Onset
	• Duration
	• Severity
	• Effect on function

Comorbid conditions	For each condition: • Symptoms • Onset • Duration • Severity • Effect on function

Drugs	• General medication history
	• Special attention to:
	  • Benzodiazipines
	  • Hypnotics
	  • Antianxiety
	  • Opioids
	  • Sterioids
	  • Hypertensivies
	  • Betablockers
	• Alcohol
	• Over-the-counter medications
	• Herbal and culture-related home remedies

Special problems	• Sleep patterns • Appetite and nutrition • Disruptive behaviors • Apathy • Motor retardation • Activity impairment
Social support systems	• Living arrangements • Caregiver availability and commitment • Financial resources • Social and health services availability

Physical examination	• Observe
	  • General appearance, grooming
	  • Behavior
	  • Thought processes
	  • Verbal fluency
	  • Functional capacity
	• Cardiovascular function
	• Motor function and gait
	• Somatic symptoms
	• Geriatric Depression Scale-Short Form
	• Mini-Cog

Laboratory testing	• Complete blood count • Renal function • Electrolytes

---

EXHIBIT 20.2 **Chronic Health Conditions Associated With High Rates of Depression in Older Adults**

- Cardiovascular disease
- Cancer
- Rheumatoid arthritis
- Skin disorders
- Osteoarthritis
- Spinal stenosis
- Polymyalgia rheumatica
- Dementia
- Parkinson's disease
- Stroke
- Anemia

- Vitamin deficiencies
- Hematologic disorders
- Dehydration
- Hypoxia
- Azotemia
- Diabetes mellitus
- Hyperthyroidism, hypothyroidism
- Cushing's disease
- Addison's disease
- Infections
- Chronic obstructive pulmonary disease

Exhibit 20.2 lists common diseases associated with increased rates of depression. Older adults with a history of cardiovascular disease are a high-risk population for late-onset depression and are at risk for VaD. The duration, severity, and number of recent and past illnesses are important considerations in determining risk for depression. The American Heart Association recommends that any older adult with a history of cardiac disease be screened for depression. Depression can trigger myocardial infarction in older adults with history of cardiac disease, a significant concern in the gerioperative patient.

Persistent Pain

Persistent pain is a major cause of depression in older adults. Asking about pain severity and duration of pain provides clues to the need for more extensive questioning about medication use and depression symptomatology. Medications used to treat persistent pain can also trigger late-onset depression. Initial screening can detect depression in older adults with a history of persistent pain.

Medication

Alcohol use and medications can increase the risk of depression and can exacerbate cognitive decline in older adults with dementia. The patient should be asked about alcohol use during an assessment of medication history.

Benzodiazepines, sedatives, antianxiety agents, and hypnotics are commonly prescribed for older adults with undetected depressive symptoms. Most of these drugs are not recommended for use in older adults due to severe side effects and potential for drug-drug interactions. These medications, also prescribed for older adults with dementia, present similar concerns for patient safety and potential adverse effects. Steroids, betablockers, antihypertensives, immunosuppressive agents, and opioids can trigger depression in older adults. In addition, older adults with dementia are more sensitive and vulnerable to the depressive side effects of medications. Preoperatively, elders should be asked about the use of herbal and culture-specific remedies. Of special concern in the gerioperative patient is the use of St. John's wort due to the potential interaction with anesthetics.

Patients with depression or cognitive impairment have difficulty taking their medications as prescribed and are at risk for overmedication or undermedication. Obtaining a clear medication history often depends on the availability of a family member or friend familiar with the patient's medication regimen. However, family members are often unaware of or do not want to acknowledge the older person's depression or level of cognitive impairment if it is undiagnosed. As a result, they ignore evidence of the person's difficulty managing day-to-day functions, even medication use. Inability of the patient to recall names, dose, and scheduling of medications is a warning signal for over- or undermedication.

Over-the-counter medications used for sleep, anxiety, incontinence, and constipation often have anticholinergic properties that increase risk of depressive episodes and cognitive dysfunction. Home remedies are a concern. St. John's wort, a common home remedy for depression, can cause hypertension and hyperpyrexia in the presence of certain anesthetics. A patient alert should be posted on the medical record for any older adult taking St. John's wort, benzodiazepines, antipsychotics, or monoamine oxidase inhibitors.

Special Concerns

Altered sleep patterns and appetite changes are common in older adults with depression and dementia. Changes in sleep or appetite can be symptoms of onset of illness or the result of depression or dementia. Assess duration of symptoms and steps the patient has taken to address them, especially the use of herbal products or home remedies.

To assess sleep, ask about sleep patterns, daytime napping, feelings of being rested, fatigue levels, and energy. In patients reporting sleep problems, ask specific questions about bed times, preparation for sleep, number of times the patient wakes at night, and time of morning awakening. Patients with depression and dementia have disrupted sleep patterns with multiple nighttime sleep interruptions and early morning awakening.

Assessment of appetite changes includes not only quantity of food, but types of food, changes in meal patterns such as time of day, and foods eaten at different times. Identifying who prepares meals is important. Older adults with poor intake due to the need to self-prepare food presents a different picture from older adults who have meals prepared for them.

Social Support

Preoperatively, evaluating the patient's social support system prompts planning for prehabilitation activities and promotes support during hospitalization and postdischarge recovery. Older adults with depression or dementia feel more secure and experience less anxiety when in familiar environments. Hospitals are unfamiliar environments. Finding ways to include support systems in the ongoing care of the older adult across the perioperative continuum contributes to feelings of security and safety offered by the presence of familiar faces. Family members and friends will be important in providing care needed after discharge. Involving them during the preoperative discussions of postoperative care needs contributes to more realistic planning and promotes their awareness of patient's ongoing needs after discharge.

DEPRESSION AND DEMENTIA SCREENING

Changes in Affect and Cognition

Ask the patient to describe any changes in memory, attention span, ability to concentrate, and decision-making that can indicate the presence of depression or dementia. If changes are identified, a more focused assessment based on screening tools is conducted. However, some older adults may find these questions threatening to their self-esteem or fear confirmation of their own concerns about mental ability and changes in mood. Reassuring patients that

Preoperative screening for depression and cognition must become routine screening with older adults.

the questions are directed at ensuring their safety and well-being throughout the surgical process can help to allay fears that the questions are directed at their personhood or personal integrity. Maintaining a calm, matter-of-fact, caring interaction also can relieve anxiety associated with questions about cognitive function and mood.

Ask the patient to describe experiences with inattention, apathy, irritability, aggressiveness, or feelings of anxiety, fears, getting lost, or other unusual or disturbing behaviors or sensations. Panic is a common symptom in older adults with dementia. Surgery creates high psychological stress that can trigger feelings of panic. Assessing the type of situations where the patient experiences panic is critical in preventing gerioperative-related panic. The stress induced by panic behaviors, fear, and anxiety escalates physiological and psychological responses before and after surgery and anesthesia. Alerting members of the interdisciplinary team about these behaviors, fears, and concerns allows for ongoing support and prevention of depression or increases in severity of dementia.

SUICIDE IDEATION

Suicide ideation is always a concern in older adults with depression or cognitive impairment. It is of special concern in men over the age of 85. Gerioperative patients who demonstrate depressive symptoms or cognitive impairment with depressive mood should be questioned about suicide. Older adults with severe persistent pain, cancer, or who have multiple or severe chronic illness should also be asked. Patients can view surgery as a treatment that will improve their quality of life. Surgery can also be viewed as trauma or source of increased pain and discomfort. For older adults who are depressed or who have undetected depression or underreported symptoms, surgery may be an overwhelming physical, psychological, or financial hurdle.

Surgery can be a precipitating factor for depression.

Providers are often hesitant to ask about suicide. One reason is a concern that raising the subject of suicide will inhibit or disrupt a comfortable, caring interaction or offend the older adult. Another is the discomfort of the provider. Asking the patient about the decision to go ahead with surgery allows for a discussion about the patient's life goals and preferences and values about surgery. It provides an opportunity for assessing patient concerns, questions, and fears about the procedure or process as well as assessing effectiveness of the patient's coping mechanisms. Using the patient's response as a guide, providers can direct questions to patient concerns about dying, becoming a burden, and to consideration of suicide. Opening the door to a conversation about the patient's feelings and concerns demonstrates concern, willingness to listen, and availability to the older adult in a profound and caring way.

DEPRESSION SCREENING

Two initial open-ended questions useful in assessing depression are: "Over the past 2 weeks, have you felt down, depressed, or hopeless?" and "Over the past 2 weeks, have you felt little interest or pleasure in doing things?" If the patient responds yes to either question or reports two or more of the following symptoms, a more extensive depression screening is needed: change in appetite or sleep patterns, excess fatigue or lack of energy, inability to concentrate, or memory impairment.

Though not diagnostic, the Geriatric Depression Scale-Short Form (GDS-SF) and the Patient Health Questionnaire (PHQ-9) are recognized tools used to screen for depression in older adults. Both tests are easy to use in the clinical environment, take 5 minutes or less to complete, and are easy to score. The GDS-SF and PHQ-9 are in the public domain, making them freely accessible for use. Older adults with scores suggesting presence of depression should have a follow-up evaluation by a primary care provider, geriatrician, or interdisciplinary team prior to surgery.

The GDS-SF consists of 15 yes or no questions (see Appendix II). The tool can be self-administered or completed by a family member or companion-coach in the event of cognitive impairment, visual impairment, or low literacy. The answers indicating depressive symptoms are bolded. The bolded scores are summed for a score. A score greater than 5 suggests possible depression; a score greater than 10 is strongly suggestive of depression.

The PHQ-9 is a 9-item Likert-type scale with options ranging from not at all, several days, more than half the days, and most every day. A 10th question asks the person taking the test to determine if any of the answers checked create difficulty in carrying out daily activities and functions. The test is designed to be self-administered. However, for older adults who have low literacy or visual impairment, the questions can be read. A family member or companion-coach familiar with the patient can complete the questionnaire if cognitive impairment interferes with patient self-administration. The responses are not as standardized as in a self-administered questionnaire but can be useful for screening. The PHQ-9 is translated into more than 50 languages. The English version of the PHQ-9 and directions for use are available in Appendix II.

DEMENTIA SCREENING

Dementia screening tools used in the clinical environment are the Folstein Mini-Mental State Examination (MMSE) (Folstein, Folstein, & McHugh, 1975) and the Mini-Cog (Borson, Scanlan, Brush, Vitallano, & Dokmak, 2000). The MMSE is a series of 11 questions that assess memory, orientation, attention and calculation, recall, and language. Results of the MMSE are influenced by age, education, and literacy. The Mini-Cog is less time-consuming, easier to use, and as accurate as the MMSE without the potential bias created by age, education, or literacy. An additional advantage is that the Mini-Cog is in the public domain, which makes it easily available and accessible for use without the need for permission. The Mini-Cog is a three-item word learning and recall activity combined with a clock drawing task to be completed between the word learning and the recall.

PHYSICAL ASSESSMENT

During the preoperative interview, pay particular attention to general appearance and behavior. Hygiene provides clues to mood and cognitive function, especially for older adults who manage their own personal hygiene and dressing. Often, family members help older patients maintain appropriate dress, bathing, and general presentation. Asking the patient if anyone helps with dressing or hygiene helps distinguish whether appearance is due to self-care or care by others.

Observing behavior can affirm data obtained through the history or elicits the need for further evaluation or clarification. Behaviors to observe include affect, ability to sustain attention and interaction, language use, eye contact, and thought processes. Vision and hearing evaluation is important especially for older adults with dementia. Misinterpretation of visual or verbal stimuli can increase anxiety and provoke aggressive self-protective reactions detrimental to the safety of the patient and caregivers. Screening for dementia, cognitive impairment, and depression preoperatively is needed to establish a baseline for determining changes in mood and cognitive function after surgery. Screening assists in the development of a patient safety plan of care including systematic monitoring, prevention of complications and adverse events, and early intervention when there are changes in the clinical condition.

PREOPERATIVE TESTING

There are no specific diagnostic tests routinely conducted for preoperative evaluation of depression or dementia. Reviewing preoperative testing to detect abnormalities prevents unnecessary complications that can increase dementia or depression severity. Monitoring renal function is important for medication safety in gerioperative patients with increased sensitivity to medications. Abnormal hemoglobin, hematocrit, and electrolyte reports are associated with delirium risk, a condition highly correlated with depression and dementia.

Prehabilitation

Depression and dementia are high-risk preoperative conditions strongly correlated with development of postoperative complications. Coaching encourages and motivates the older adult and support systems to initiate and maintain treatment that optimizes health and well-being prior to surgery. Being clear about the goals and the benefits in decreasing surgery-related problems helps older adults understand the importance and value of actively participating in prehabilitation activities.

Improving cardiac and pulmonary status, physical function, psychological comfort, sleep patterns, and nutritional status can stabilize and improve mood, decrease anxiety, and maximize cognitive function. Multivitamins can improve nutrition along with feelings of depression. Giving the older adult and caregiver a sleep protocol can help improve sleep patterns. Ensuring the older patient receives sufficient rest and sleep to maintain energy levels to carry out prehabilitation activities is critical to the success of the program. Recommending small highly nutritious meals and snack foods, and high-nutrition drinks improves nutritional intake often depleted in older adults with depression or dementia.

The interaction of depression, dementia, and cardiovascular disease demands that risk factors such as hypertension be under maximal control. Pulmonary function is important to ensure optimal oxygenation for cerebral function. Physical activity and exercise is well documented in improving depression and depressive symptoms as well as cardiovascular function. Physical activity such as walking increases brain gray matter and improves cognition in older adults with early-stage dementia.

Ensuring availability of social support, reducing social isolation, and reviewing environmental safety can reduce anxiety and fear generated by the disease condition as well as impending surgery. Encourage participation in education and support groups targeted to the older adult's clinical condition: depression, dementia, or comorbid illness. Encouraging a caregiver, family member, or friend who will serve as a gerioperative support system or companion-coach while the patient undergoes surgery to accompany the older adult to support and education groups can benefit both the patient and the family member or friend. Identifying the level of caregiver commitment and the potential for caregiver "burnout" is an important element in considering postoperative discharge planning. Social support for caregivers should be considered as important as a direct treatment intervention in care of the older adult with depression or dementia.

Initiating cognitive behavioral or behavioral activation therapy before surgery can improve mood and decrease anxiety. Therapies are more effective in patients with mild to moderate depressive mood or depression.

Older adults often are averse to hearing the term *psychotherapy* or *mental health*. Focusing the purpose on improving surgical outcomes can help the older patient be more accepting of the intervention. Directing attention to preventing complications and enhancing recovery and not on mental health needs can relieve some of the stigma older patients often associate with the word psychotherapy.

Older adults with depression or dementia are highly vulnerable to medication side effects. A medication review is critical to evaluate risks and benefits of each medication, correct dosing and scheduling, drug interactions and side effects, and presence of potentially inappropriate medications. In addition to concerns about polypharmacy and overmedication, an equal concern with an older patient who is depressed or cognitively impaired is ensuring the patient is taking medications important to controlling comorbid conditions, particularly cardiovascular disease and diabetes. Individuals who are depressed or have cognitive impairment may not understand medication instructions or have the cognitive capacity to manage multiple medication regimens. This is a critical area of medication assessment in this vulnerable population.

Of special importance in the care of the gerioperative patient with depression or dementia is managing antidepressant, benzodiazepine, hypnotic, and psychotropic medications across the perioperative continuum. Benzodiazepines have been linked with an exaggerated response to neuromuscular blocking agents. Opioids should be avoided in older adults taking monoamine oxidase inhibitors. Although rarely used in older adults, monoamine oxidase inhibitors are important in older adults with major depression when other antidepressant medications are ineffective. Acetylcholinesterase inhibitors used in treatment of dementia can trigger atypical responses in older adults receiving the anesthetic propofol.

The patient or caregiver assisting the older adult with medications must receive written instructions on the medications that should be taken or omitted the day of surgery. Equally important is information on medications that should continue to be taken up until surgery. Clearly written instructions should indicate medications to be tapered and how to taper them, as well as when other medications are to be discontinued. Have the patient and family or companion-coach make note of the medications to be continued after surgery. Providing coaching on asking providers about restarting medications helps patients and families to be more effective advocates. Emphasizing that benzodiazepine use is to be continued prior to surgery is critical information for patients who have been taking the medication for a prolonged period. Benzodiazepines are prescribed regularly with older adults who have anxiety due to undetected depression or early-onset undiagnosed cognitive impairment. Abrupt discontinuation can cause withdrawal symptoms.

The nurse conducting the preoperative interview is responsible for confirming that the older adult, support person, or care facility receive written instructions about medication use and that the patient and caregiver have adequate understanding to carry out the regimen successfully. The written instructions must be reviewed with the patient before the end of the preoperative interview. The preoperative provider asks the older adult and support person to state in their own words how medications are to be managed in the weeks before surgery and on the morning of surgery. A review of instructions continues until the patient or caregiver provides evidence of a client-centered plan to manage medications before surgery.

Intraoperative Considerations

Many of the intraoperative prevention and intervention actions addressing risk factors for older adults with dementia or depression are decided by the anesthesia provider during the surgical procedure. An important consideration by the nurse in the operating suite is the use of perianesthesia medications. Providing a calm, reassuring presence can decrease anxiety and the potential for panic in patients with dementia, minimizing the need for medication. Alerting postoperative providers about intraoperative medication use during the handoff is critical to preventing or detecting postoperative delirium. Postoperative delirium is the most common complication caused by preoperative and intraoperative medications in older adults with dementia or depression.

Postoperative Considerations

Depression and dementia are risk factors for a multitude of postoperative complications. New onset of depression or dementia as a result of surgery is a postoperative complication in itself as well as a trigger for other adverse events.

Altered physiology is important in the development of postsurgical complications in older adults with preoperative dementia or depression. It is not unusual for professional providers to focus on the psychosocial and behavioral element of depression and dementia at the risk of ignoring the underlying physiological changes. Recognizing the impact of physiological changes on development of postoperative complications adds additional import to prevention and intervention.

There is a positive relationship between depression and dementia and each of the following postoperative complications: delirium, postoperative cognitive dysfunction, impaired wound healing, increased pain severity, and deconditioning. Neurobiology and neuropsychology continue to demonstrate that physiologic factors both contribute to and derive from age- and disease-related neuronal loss and dysfunction in neurotransmitter regulation. Pain perception is affected by changes that occur in the brain secondary to dementia and depression, while cognitive function is influenced by pain severity and duration. Elevated stress levels seen in dementia and depression disrupt endocrine and immune systems important to wound healing. Disruptions in neurotransmitter availability evident in depression and dementia contribute to onset of delirium.

POSTOPERATIVE ONSET DEPRESSION

Older adults often exhibit depressive symptoms after surgery. Symptoms may be due to preexisting depression or from a new-onset depression. Postsurgical depression can occur in the immediate postoperative period or several months later. Older adults who have had cardiac- or cancer-related surgeries are particularly vulnerable to immediate and long-term postsurgical depression. Anesthesia has been identified as a precipitant of postoperative depression. Additional causes of depression include awareness of one's vulnerability or frailty, recognition of the shortness of life and time to complete life tasks, postcrisis let down, and worries about pain and the ability to function independently. Pain and discomfort can stimulate the stress cycle, initiating or exacerbating a preexisting depression. Opioids, commonly used to manage pain in older adults, can trigger depressive symptoms.

Providers must remain alert to the fact that depression can mask onset of postoperative complications and that pain and discomfort can mask depression. The similarity in symptoms between hypoactive delirium, depression, dementia, and postoperative cognitive dysfunction create a challenge to early detection and targeted intervention. Table 20.4 distinguishes signs and symptoms between depression and dementia. Table 21.5 differentiates signs and symptoms across the four Ds: depression, dementia, delirium, and postoperative cognitive dysfunction. Older adults demonstrating any change in affect, mood, or behavior must be evaluated as soon as symptoms appear.

Patients on antidepressant medications before surgery should continue to take their medication throughout the perioperative period. There are few pharmacologic options for older adults who are on nothing-by-mouth status or are unable to take oral medications. Closely monitoring patients for evidence of adverse effects, seeking alternative medications, and providing strong, consistent psychoemotional support can help protect the patient until medications can be resumed. The use of nonpharmacologic therapies such as massage, music therapy, heat and cold, the presence of familiar and comforting items, and caring touch can be effective in managing depression. These interventions are equally useful in the care of the older adult with dementia.

POSTOPERATIVE ONSET DEMENTIA

Cognitive impairment is common after surgery alone or in conjunction with depression. Cognitive impairment may be a continuation of preoperative impairment or of new onset. The changes in cognition may be short-term, lasting only a few days, or more extensive lasting more than a year after surgery. Chapter 21 presents a more extensive review of cognitive changes due to onset of postoperative cognitive dysfunction and delirium. Being alert to changes in cognition is important to ensure quality care, prevention of further cognitive decline, decreased patient anxiety, and detection of acute onset of other postoperative complications.

Surgery and anesthesia can exacerbate preexisting dementia or precipitate previously unrecognized dementia, especially in older adults with preexisting condition, mild cognitive impairment (MCI). Having results of preoperative dementia screening available can help to determine if the dementia reflects a new onset of dementia. Hypoactive delirium can mimic dementia. It is critical that postoperative nurses routinely assess cognitive status. Assessments using both the Mini-Cog for dementia and either the Confusion Assessment Method or Neelon and Champagne Confusion Scale (NEECHAM) for delirium help differentiate the two conditions. The NEECHAM tool can be found in Appendix II.

Interventions for care of older adults with dementia depend on the level of cognitive impairment and presence of depression or other comorbid conditions. Preventing cognitive deterioration after surgery requires awareness of the underlying physiology and its effects on patient behavior and needs. Patience, caring, and attention to elder-sensitive care are essential.

POSTOPERATIVE INTERVENTIONS

An interdisciplinary care team is important in coordinating treatments and interventions for depression and dementia. A social worker, geriatric psychiatrist, physical and occupational therapists, nutritionist, nurses, and geriatricians are needed to coordinate a treatment plan that will decrease the negative effects of depression and dementia, prevent postoperative complications, and promote a rapid recovery.

TABLE 20.4

Differences Among Normal Age Changes, Depression, and Dementia

	Normal Age Changes	Depression	Dementia
Definition	Minimal to moderate decline in: Processing speed Attention Memory	Feelings of sadness that affect sleep, appetite, energy, and confidence that are out of the ordinary for the individual and most of the time on most days for at least 2 weeks	A gradual and progressive decline in cognition and mental processing ability affecting short-term memory, communication, language, judgment, reasoning, and abstract thinking
Onset	Gradual over years	Unexplained flattening of affect or mood that persists for 2 weeks or more. May coincide with changes in life event	Changes occur over months or years
Course	Changes over years	Gradual onset over days or weeks Usually reversible with treatment Often worse in morning	Slow, chronic progression or step-wise progression over months to years
Early presentation	Word loss Processing speed	Reduced memory, concentration, low self-esteem Slowed response Apathy, low energy Sleep disturbance	Impaired short-term memory Impaired judgment, language ability Progressive decline in cognition
Sensorium	No change	No change	Delusions Hallucinations
Mood	Normal	Depressed mood Flat affect Changes in appetitive Possible suicidal ideation Hopelessness	Depends on stage of disease Depressed in early stages Apathy Angry outbursts
Behavior	Normal	Withdrawn, apathy, decreased motivation May be agitated	Agitated or withdrawn Aimless/nonpurposeful activity
Consciousness level	Clear	Clear	Clear until late stages
Screening tools	Trail Making Test Digital Symbol Substitution Test	Geriatric Depression Scale	Mini-Mental Status Exam Clock Drawing Test Mini-Cog Dementia Screen
Response/action/ intervention	None needed	Notify attending physician Refer for geriatric mental health consult	Notify attending physician and inter-disciplinary care team Refer for geriatric mental health consult

Older adults with dementia or depression require additional time to process information, initiate activity, and respond to verbal instructions. Taking time to demonstrate expected activities and providing consistent cueing and coaching decreases anxiety and facilitates active participation. Ensuring a low-stress environment by managing noise, light, clutter, and the number of unfamiliar personnel further contributes to maintaining patient safety and security. Continuity of providers is highly significant in the care of older adults with dementia. Familiarity decreases stress and is a cornerstone of care in patients with cognitive impairment. Maintaining a consistent, caring, unhurried approach improves patient participating in rehabilitation and recovery. Attending to patient psychological comfort is as important in this vulnerable population as is attention to physical comfort.

Ambulation, hydration, nutrition, and intermittent rest periods are core ingredients to a successful postoperative recovery in the hospital, the rehabilitation center, and in the home. Providing encouragement and support through calm, caring interactions increases older patients' ability to attend to postoperative recovery activities.

Promote self-efficacy as much as possible by obtaining the patient's attention prior to initiating an activity, coaching the patient through the activity, providing time for the patient to carry out the activity, and providing supporting supervision. These interventions enhance personal integrity, safety, and security.

Initiating protocols to be used by all providers for addressing specific care concerns ensures care consistency and promotes familiarity. Specific protocols that must be implemented for the gerioperative patient with dementia or depression are the systematic monitoring for changes in cognition and detection of early onset of deconditioning, attention to fall prevention, promoting sleep, relieving pain, and preventing delirium and pressure ulcer development. Medication reconciliation after surgery is a must to ensure continuation of all needed medications and elimination of those that are no longer needed.

PATIENT REPORT: Mrs. Rosner

After her return to the surgical unit, Mrs. Rosner remains quiet. She drinks and eats little and is reluctant to participate in postoperative care routines. She responds positively when asked about pain and is given medication that is effective in minimizing her pain. She is pleasant but does not want to get out of bed or eat. She plucks at the bed linens several times throughout the day on the second postoperative day but remains quiet. The nurse notices she does not sleep during the night and is awake very early in the morning. The nurse asks her daughter about her behavior and if this is typical. The daughter tells the nurse that her mother is a quiet woman, but that she seems almost withdrawn which is unlike her. The nurse decides to conduct a depression screening. The daughter is shocked at the idea her mother might be depressed. The nurse explains that older adults with heart disease are at a high risk for delirium. The results of the screening indicate that Mrs. Rosner has depressive symptoms. The nurse goes on to conduct a delirium assessment based on the knowledge that hypoactive delirium and depression have overlapping symptoms. The delirium screen is negative. The nurse notifies the surgeon and requests a consult with the geriatric interdisciplinary team. The care plan involves extensive psychoemotional support and coaching, with time to engage Mrs. Rosner in postoperative recovery activities. Her daughter is coached in how best to help her mother in the hospital and after discharge. Mrs. Rosner responds positively to the intervention by participating in mobility activities. Her appetite remains poor. Mrs. Rosner reassures the nurse she will be fine as soon as she can get home.

SUMMARY

Depression and dementia are preexisting conditions that are identified risk factors for postoperative complications. Surgery, anesthesia, and postoperative demands can exacerbate preexisting conditions or result in new onset of depression or dementia. Late-onset depression differs from depression in younger populations. Depression and dementia result from alterations in physiological functioning. Depression is undetected, undiagnosed, and undertreated in older adults due to atypical presentation of late-onset depression. Benzodiazepines, sedative, hypnotics, and antianxiety agents, medications are contraindicated in most older adults, and causes of drug-anesthesia interactions are often prescribed to treat anxiety symptoms. Dementia severity ranges from mild cognitive impairment to incapacity to total dependency. Assessing suicidal ideation is fundamental to the care of the gerioperative patient with depression. Depression and dementia screening are highly recommended for all older adults undergoing surgery. Providing care to gerioperative patients with depression or cognitive dysfunction must be done with sensitivity to the changes in memory, thinking, information processing, and altered ability to understand and follow directions. Providers must be on the alert for any changes in cognition that herald the onset of delirium or other postoperative complications including new-onset depression and dementia.

KEY POINTS

- Depression and dementia are major risk factors for delirium, postoperative cognitive dysfunction, and other postoperative complications.
- Depression and dementia result from pathophysiological processes.
- Depression is underdiagnosed and undertreated in vulnerable older adults.
- Cardiac disease is highly correlated with depression.
- All older adults with a history of heart disease should have depression screening prior to surgery.
- Suicide ideation should be evaluated in older adults with a history of depression or dementia.
- Postoperative care must be sensitive to the heightened vulnerability of older adults with dementia or depression to adverse events.

TWENTY-ONE

Delirium and Postoperative Cognitive Dysfunction

Raelene V. Shippee-Rice, Susan J. Fetzer, and Jennifer V. Long

PATIENT REPORT: Mrs. Postemsky

Mrs. Postemsky is an 85-year-old widowed housewife who emigrated from Poland 60 years ago. While she speaks English, her comprehension is limited, having never attended high school. While tending her flower garden, she twisted and fell, fracturing her hip. She arrives in the preoperative holding area in her bed with 20 pounds of Buck's traction. There is an intravenous infusion in her right forearm of lactated Ringer's solution at 125 ml. A Foley catheter is in place and draining clear yellow urine. She has no allergies and is on no medications. Her last pain level was a 3/10, and her last dose of acetaminophen 500 mg was 6 hours ago. She is alert and cooperative as she discusses the anesthesia plan for a spinal anesthetic. This is her first hospitalization. Preoperatively, the primary nurse for Mrs. Postemsky discusses the risk of postoperative delirium with the patient and her six children. The nurse identifies that the patient enjoys gardening, looking at magazines, and watching the history channel on television. The family is encouraged to bring her favorite magazines for postoperative cognitive stimulation. In addition, the family arranges to have a member available to stay with Mrs. Postemsky after surgery.

The mind is the repository of a person's history and sense of self. The mind holds the memories, knowledge, and beliefs of the past and builds the bridges to the future. "Losing my mind" is one of the most feared events in the lives of older adults. "As long as I don't lose my mind" is an adage of aging.

Half of all surgeries performed in the United States are in adults 65 years and older, with approximately 50 million surgeries a year on older adults worldwide. The incidence of postoperative cognitive impairment ranges between 10% and 60%, or 5 million to 30 million patients per year. Postoperative delirium (POD) and postoperative cognitive dysfunction (POCD) are two of the most common forms of postoperative cognitive impairment. The onset of these adverse events faced by gerioperative patients, their families, and their providers is unexpected.

POD and POCD remain undetected, misdiagnosed, and undertreated postoperative complications in gerioperative patients.

While they are not routinely mentioned in the preoperative informed consent discussion, their impact on the older adult is profound, leading to physiological, emotional, and spiritual distress; increased days of hospitalization; delayed healing and rehabilitation; increased health care costs; deterioration in quality of life; and even early death.

This chapter provides an overview of POD and POCD including incidence, outcomes, pathophysiology, risk factors, and perioperative considerations.

Delirium

Delirium is a syndrome, or group of symptoms, that reflect acute malfunction in the brain secondary to trauma, disease, metabolic changes, or toxicity in other areas of the body. The American Psychiatric Association *Diagnostic and Statistical Manual of Mental Disorders, 4th edition (DSM-IV)* (2000), uses the following criteria as diagnostic for delirium: acute onset with fluctuating course and inattention combined with either altered level of consciousness or disorganized thinking manifested by disturbances in orientation, memory, thought, or behavior. Commonly, POD is defined as an acute change or fluctuation in mental status manifesting as disordered cognition and characterized by cognitive, emotional, and behavioral disturbances. Table 21.1 outlines the *DSM-IV* diagnostic criteria.

POD is characterized by acute onset of fluctuating consciousness with intermittent periods of lucidity; disorientation to person, place, or time; and difficulty maintaining attention. The sleep-wake cycle is often disrupted. Signs and symptoms vary from patient to patient and within the same patient at different times. Delirium can present as a hyperactive, hypoactive, or mixed state. Presentation varies depending on whether the delirium is hypoactive, hyperactive, or mixed. Changes are seen in cognitive, emotional, behavioral, and sensory domains, as identified in Table 21.2.

Hyperactive delirium is associated with restlessness, agitation, and an overreactive response to stimuli. Patients often experience hallucinations or illusions. Conversely,

TABLE 21.1

DSM-IV Criteria for Delirium

Criterion	Description
Consciousness	• Disturbances of consciousness (i.e., reduced clarity of awareness of the environment) • Reduced ability to focus, sustain, or shift attention
Cognition	• Changes in cognition (e.g., memory deficit, disorientation, language disturbance, perceptual disturbance) that are not accounted for by a preexisting, established, or evolving cognitive impairment
Timeframe	• Disturbance develops over a short timeframe (usually hours to days) • Fluctuations occur during the course of the day
Etiology	• Cognitive/mental status changes are caused by a physiologic consequence of a medical or surgical condition, intoxicating substance, medication use, or more than one cause

From American Psychiatric Association (2000).

TABLE 21.2

Cognitive, Emotional, Behavioral, and Sensory Changes in Delirium

Cognitive Changes	Emotional Changes	Behavioral Changes	Sensory Changes
• Altered consciousness • Inattention • Disorganized thinking • Disorientation • Thought disturbances • Loss of comprehensive ability	• Anxiety • Anger • Fear • Irritability • Affective ability	• Agitation • Restlessness • Lethargy • Sleep disturbances • Motor retardation • Hyperactive responses	• Visuospatial alterations • Perceptual disturbances

hypoactive delirium is characterized by reduced psychomotor response lethargy, apathy, sleepiness, or withdrawn behaviors. Mixed delirium is characterized by unpredictable demonstration of hyperactive and hypoactive behaviors vacillating at different points in time.

Hypoactive delirium is difficult to distinguish and therefore less likely to be diagnosed. Patients are quiet, and their behavior is subdued. Older adults with hypoactive delirium are most likely to be misdiagnosed with dementia or depression. Older adults with hypothyroidism show symptoms similar to those seen in hypoactive delirium. Distinguishing hypothyroidism and hypoactive delirium requires critical analysis and acute observation. Hypoactive symptoms are often ignored because the patient is quiet, not complaining, and considered by others to be comfortable. Detecting hypoactive delirium early is important as over half of the patients will go on to develop a hyperactive state.

EPIDEMIOLOGY

Delirium is one of the most common causes of acute cognitive impairment in hospitalized older adults. Annually, over 2.5 million older adults exhibit some degree of delirium during hospitalization. Up to 20% of older adults meet the diagnostic criteria for delirium at the time of hospital admission, with another 25 to 60% meeting diagnostic criteria during hospitalization. The early onset of delirium is often overlooked due to the emergent nature of the older adult's diagnosis and clinical status. Older adults in intensive care units have the highest rates of delirium.

Statistics on surgically related delirium are highly variable because of differences in definition, assessment methods, type of surgery, and sample. Various reports indicate postoperative delirium rates in older adults range from 15 to 67%. Rates are highest for older adults undergoing orthopedic, cardiac, and emergency surgery. Table 21.3 lists reported rates of delirium by type of surgery. However, reported rates do not capture the extent of the problem, as POD is unrecognized in 30 to 60% of older adults. After age 65, the probability of an episode of POD can increase by as much as 2% per year.

Over 2.5 million older adults exhibit some degree of delirium during hospitalization.

PATHOPHYSIOLOGY

Until recently, health care providers commonly referred to delirium as "confusion," a common condition in hospitalized older adults. As a normative response, health care providers became concerned only if the patient demonstrated behaviors that were disruptive, interfered

TABLE 21.3

Delirium Rates by Type of Surgery

Type of Surgery	Reported Rates
Orthopedic surgery	25–65%
Joint replacement	25–41%
Hip fracture	4–54%
Cardiac surgery	25–67%
Coronary artery bypass grafting	25–32%
Cardiotomy	50–67%
Cataract surgery	4–7%
General surgery	20–33%
Vascular surgery	29–42%
Emergency surgery	59%

with patient care, or posed a safety risk. Treatment consisted of physical restraints and medication. There was little concern about the etiology of the condition. Engel and Romano (2004) first described delirium as a syndrome of cerebral insufficiency caused by a derangement in functional metabolism.

While the pathophysiology of delirium has received greater attention in recent years, delirium is still not well understood. There is consensus that delirium arises from and causes a disruption in brain metabolism and neurotransmission, but the pathophysiology remains unclear. Current hypotheses center on acetylcholine neurotransmitter dysfunction, oxygen deprivation, neuronal aging and cellular signaling changes, inflammation, and physiological stress. Maldanado (2008) suggested that presence of multiple hypotheses does not create competing arguments but rather complementary ones in that delirium may well be an interaction of two or more mechanisms or pathways. He further suggested that different types of delirium may be a result of different pathways or combinations of pathways.

NEUROTRANSMITTER HYPOTHESIS

Interruption and interference in neurotransmitter function is the most common hypothesis explaining delirium. The major neurotransmitters involved in delirium are acetylcholine, dopamine, serotonin, and norepinephrine. Delirium is related to a disturbance in acetylcholine synthesis with alterations in other neurotransmitters acting as contributing agents. Loss of cholinergic neurons as a consequence of aging reduces the availability of acetylcholine. Disruption in neurotransmission also arises from changes in neuronal structure and intracellular signaling. The signal disruption increases vulnerability to delirium. Alterations in synthesis and function of dopamine or serotonin may contribute to the behavioral, emotional, and cognitive changes seen in delirium.

Age-Related Changes

Normal aging is associated with a decrease in brain size, mass, and weight. Increased ventricular dilatation and lesions in the basal ganglia have also been reported in the aging brain. Although these structural changes may not be a direct cause of delirium, they have the potential to increase the brain's vulnerability to delirium. Such age-related physical changes may increase elders' vulnerability to changes in neurotransmitter levels during surgery and anesthesia, surgical hypoxia, hypoglycemia, and surgical stress.

INFLAMMATORY PROCESSES

Surgically related hypoxia and hypoglycemia inhibits neurotransmitter synthesis, especially acetylcholine. The physiologic stress of surgery increases anti-inflammatory cytokine production. The increase of inflammation alters perfusion and brain oxygenation, which contributes to further loss and dysfunction of neurotransmitters.

Neurological imaging studies of patients with delirium have shown a decrease in cerebral blood flow. In a study of 22 older adults, Fong, Sands, and Leung (2006) found frontal or parietal cerebral perfusion abnormalities during delirium in half of the study population. It is unclear whether there is a direct relationship between the decrease in blood flow and delirium or if blood flow changes indirectly alter biochemical function.

POD is most likely a cortical dysfunction resulting in incorrect or misinterpretation of sensory input, causing poor integration of incoming stimuli. The inability of the older adult to correctly interpret stimuli leads to behavioral responses inconsistent with the data and the environment, and the person becomes labeled as confused. Although confusion correctly describes the older person's experience, the term carries connotations that inhibit a therapeutic response. Understanding the etiology of delirium and its devastating consequences can prompt providers to take delirium seriously, respond quickly, and interfere therapeutically.

RISK FACTORS

Multiple predisposing and precipitating factors are identified as creating a risk for delirium. Many risk factors are modifiable through primary prevention. Delirium is preventable in an estimated 30 to 40% of older adults. The severity of delirium also can be decreased or limited through early detection and secondary intervention.

There is significant heterogeneity in the literature on delirium-related risk factors. Differences in risk assessment, populations at risk, type of surgeries, methods of measurement, and timing of assessment account for the variety of risk factors described across studies. However, several risk factors consistently emerge with an interaction effect involving predisposing and precipitating factors.

Predisposing or preexisting factors are present prior to surgery or hospital admission. Age-related physiological changes, preoperative cognitive function, preoperative mood, medication, and severity of comorbid disease are most often cited. Precipitating factors are incidents or events that can trigger delirium onset. Type and length of surgery, anesthesia, blood loss, and development of hypothermia are cited intraoperative precipitating factors. Inadequate pain relief, sleep deprivation, immobility, and unfamiliar, disruptive environments are listed most often as postoperative precipitating events. Delirium can result from a single event but is most often the result of an interaction between and among predisposing and precipitating factors.

Predisposing and precipitating risk factors can be further categorized as modifiable or not modifiable. Table 21.4 categorizes common predisposing and precipitating risk factors. An important caveat is that some risk factors are easily modifiable while others are minimally modifiable. For example, a preexisting or comorbid disease may be modifiable or only minimally modifiable depending on the severity of the condition and the older adult's ability to attend to and manage chronic illness. Knowing the modifiability of predisposing and

TABLE 21.4

Modifiability of Predisposing and Precipitating Risk Factors in Postoperative Delirium

Predisposing Factors	Modifiable (H, M, S, N)*
Cognitive impairment	S
Age > 65	N
Depression or psychopathology	M
Medical comorbidities or severe illness	S

Medications
  Antipsychotics
  Hypnotics, sedatives
  Anticholingergics
  Multiple drugs (more than five)
	M

Nutrition and/or dehydration	M
Impaired functional status	S
Sensory impairment	S
Abnormal laboratory values: albumin, hematocrit, electrolyte	M
Precipitating Factors	

Medications
  Opiates
  Hypnotics
  Addition of four or more in one day
	M

Surgical delay	M
Surgical blood loss > 800 mL	S
Long or complex surgical procedures	S

Environmental factors
  Hospitalization
  Increased noise levels
  Multiple diagnostic procedures
  Multiple staff changes
  Multiple room/setting changes
	H

Hypoxia, fever, infection	S
Abnormal laboratory values: albumin, hematocrit, electrolyte	S
Poorly managed pain	H
Sleep deprivation	H

*H, highly modifiable; M, modifiable; S, somewhat modifiable; N, not modifiable.

precipitating factors allows providers to focus on prevention strategies, the most important delirium intervention.

Timing and severity of events are important aspects of precipitating factors. Noimark (2009) suggests a delirium risk factor typology based on the rapidity of the insult to the patient and the severity of the insult. For example, rates of POD are higher in older patients who have emergency surgery and for elders who require intensive care unit stay for acute postoperative surgical reactions or illnesses. Sudden trauma or severe insult can be a single precipitating event in an older adult with or without predisposing risk factors.

The list of risk factors is extensive, covering a span of physiological and psychological elements. A systematic review of POD risk factors in patients having noncardiac surgery concluded that cognitive impairment and preoperative use of psychotropic drugs were the most robust predictors of POD (Dasgupta & Dumbrell, 2006). Several authors have developed clinical prediction rules and scoring systems to determine the weight of risk factors for POD (Freter, Dunbar, Macleod, Morrison, MacKnight, & Rockwood, 2005; Marcantonio et al., 1994; Weed, Lutman, Young, & Schuller, 1995). Although not all factors are included in all prediction rules and checklists, a number of predisposing factors are consistently identified: cognitive status, substance abuse, age, functional status, sensory impairment, and low serum albumin and hematocrit. The factors are confounding in that some conditions are linked with each other as well as associated with delirium. The question then becomes which factor is the cause. For example, functional status is closely associated with age- and disease-related changes. Considering functional status as a predictor of delirium may actually reflect severity of chronic illness. Providers must be cognizant that delirium is not "confusion" nor is it a normative response to illness and hospitalization. It is a complex, multifactorial, devastating condition easily triggered in vulnerable gerioperative patients.

A key factor that must be considered in the care of the gerioperative patient is increasing age as an independent factor regardless of other variables. Other variables increase the risk, but nurses and other providers must be attentive to the potential effect of patient age on susceptibility to delirium.

Attention to modifiable risk factors and using a preventative paradigm is fundamental to decreasing the incidence of delirium in the gerioperative patient. Delirium is triggered more easily in an older adult with several predisposing factors. Being aware of the gerioperative patient's risk factors allows for targeted prevention and intervention strategies.

Early detection and prompt intervention can limit the duration and severity of delirium. Treatment is most effective when delivered in context of all predisposing and precipitating factors and not limited to a single precipitating event.

COGNITIVE RESERVE

The concept of reserve, applied to aging and disease, affects all body systems (see Chapter 19). Reserve is the ability of a physiological system to maintain integrity when challenged by aging, disease, or surgery. Reserve helps to explain clinical variations seen in individuals with similar age-related changes or diseases.

When applied to the brain, cognitive or neurocognitive reserve is the capacity of the brain to maintain functional capacity when challenged by neurological insult, disease, or injury. Cognitive reserve fills the gap in cognitive function that neurological aging, disease, or injury depletes. The concept of cognitive reserve, or what is "left over" after working capacity is lost, is used to explain clinical variations in cognitive deficits seen in elders with similar levels of brain function. Delirium occurs when cognitive reserve is depleted and function can no longer be maintained. The point at which cognitive reserve is depleted is unique to the individual and cannot be predetermined. What can be predetermined is the type of stress generated by predisposing and precipitating factors. Exhibit 21.1 shows relationships among cognitive reserve, insult, and outcome.

The level of cognitive reserve depends on both passive and active reserve capacity. Passive reserve capacity refers to brain size and neural capacity, whereas active reserve capacity is the ability of the brain to use compensatory processes (Stern & Jayasekara, 2009). Larger brains have more neurons. As a result, larger brains may have more "reserve" neurons that are not needed for day-to-day functions but are available for use under

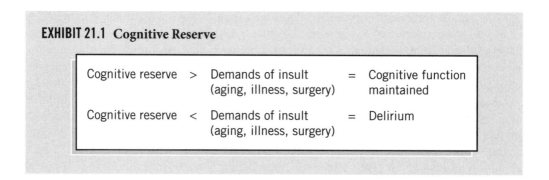

EXHIBIT 21.1 **Cognitive Reserve**

Cognitive reserve	>	Demands of insult (aging, illness, surgery)	=	Cognitive function maintained
Cognitive reserve	<	Demands of insult (aging, illness, surgery)	=	Delirium

conditions of stress or injury. The reserve neurons can substitute for damaged neurons. A larger brain can sustain greater damage and loss of neurons before the effect on cognitive function becomes evident.

Age-related physiological changes create demands on the brain, forcing the use of cognitive reserve. Figure 21.1 shows the combined effects of age, disease, and surgery on cognitive reserve.

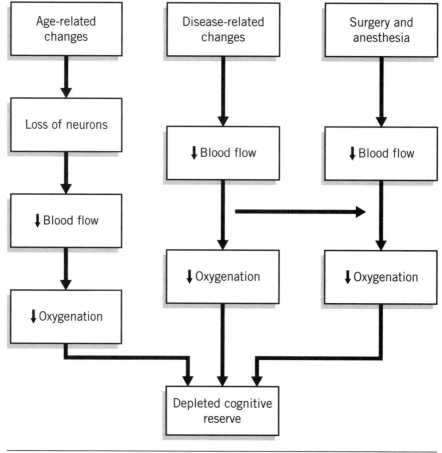

FIGURE 21.1
Effect of Age, Disease, and Surgery on Cognitive Research

Active reserve is the capacity of the brain to actively use available neurons and neural networks effectively. By using available neural networks and systems in new ways or establishing new networks, the brain maintains cognitive function. Similar to passive reserve, there is great individual variation in core capacity before active reserve capacity is needed. There is also individual variation in the level or amount of active reserve. Depletion of active reserve occurs with aging as available networks are altered in function due to changes in neuron and neurotransmitter availability.

Preoperatively, active and passive reserve may be sufficient to compensate for loss of brain reserve due to age-related changes. However, surgery, anesthesia, and postoperative complications create severe and often overwhelming physical, psychosocial, physiological, and environmental stress. The resulting stress-inflammatory response further depletes brain reserve. When clinical stressors become overwhelming, reserve can be temporarily or permanently depleted. Figure 21.2 shows a schematic of cognitive reserve depletion in the geri-operative patient with the shaded areas representing reserve. In adults, there is an unknown cognitive reserve capacity. Aging decreases the level of reserve. Chronic illness continues to deplete reserve capacity, and the stress of surgery further causes depletion. Reserve levels may be restored depending on causation and degree of pathology but not to the level of original capacity.

While passive reserve can be evaluated using brain imaging studies, there is no measure for active reserve. The level of passive reserve does not equate to total cognitive reserve capacity. Older adults with low passive reserve levels can show little evidence of cognitive changes while others with greater passive reserve have obvious cognitive impairment. Providers must be alert for early signs indicating that cognitive reserve is approaching a level where even apparently small stressors can become tipping points for delirium.

Normal Cognitive Reserve

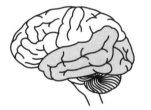

Cognitive Reserve With Aging

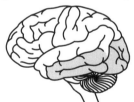

Cognitive Reserve With Aging
After Surgery

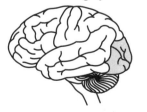

Cognitive Reserve With Aging
After Surgery and Delirium

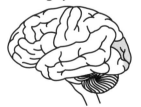

FIGURE 21.2

Schematic of Cognitive Reserve Capacity

Shaded areas represent cognitive reserve capacity. Reserve capacity diminishes in response to normal age-related changes. It is further threatened by surgery and disease. Each added stressor further depletes reserve.

DELIRIUM TRAJECTORY

The typical clinical course of acute POD begins with a period of lucidity during the immediate postanesthesia period. The onset of POD occurs within 1 to 3 days after surgery but can develop as late as 5 to 7 days postoperatively. Delirium manifested as a transient single episode is the most common form of POD. Other forms of delirium include persistent and subsyndromal delirium. Persistent delirium extends beyond the time of hospital discharge. Patients with subsyndromal delirium show a few signs of delirium but do not fully meet the delirium criteria. Conceptually, delirium can be placed on a continuum from subsyndromal to episodic to persistent. However, subsyndromal and persistent delirium may represent separate entities with different etiologies, pathophysiology, treatment needs, and outcomes. Further research is needed.

Acute onset POD, while described as a short-term syndrome, may evolve into a prolonged persistent delirium. Delirium is a medical emergency. It is often the earliest sign of an acute change in the patient's condition.

DELIRIUM OUTCOMES

If treated promptly, delirium can resolve with little negative effect. However, most providers do not address delirium as a medical emergency and delay intervention. When untreated or with delayed treatment, delirium causes short- and long-term negative outcomes.

Delirium is frightening with episodes of panic and anger.

Delirium was described by Balas (2005) as "one of the most frequent, dangerous, and costly complications" encountered by hospitalized older adults (p. 1). POD predisposes the patient to iatrogenic falls, incontinence, pressure ulcers, adverse medication events, and prolonged hospital stay. Patients asked to describe their delirium experience call it frightening with episodes of panic and anger. Long-term outcomes can include prolonged cognitive and functional loss, dementia, and likelihood of postdischarge nursing home placement, decreased quality of life, and early death. Mortality rates associated with delirium range from 20 to 70% with 35 to 40% mortality within 1 year after surgery (Fearing & Inouye, 2009).

Gerioperative Care

Historically, care providers considered delirium a normal aging response to disease and hospitalization. Up to 60% of hospital-based delirium is misdiagnosed or never detected. Prevention, early detection, and intervention can improve patient outcomes. Considering mental status as a sixth vital sign and using standardized assessment tools provides needed systematic monitoring if delirium is to be detected early.

Diligent and vigilant provider care is critical to prevent onset, progression, and negative outcomes of acute cognitive changes.

More recent research points to delirium as a complex multimodal syndrome. Diligent and vigilant provider care is critical in preventing the onset and decreasing the severity, duration, and negative outcomes associated with POD. McNicoll and Besdine (2007) argue that prevention and early detection as a standard part of geriatric care will occur only when providers recognize that delirium is predominately iatrogenic and preventable. Figure 21.3 outlines risk factors with prevention and intervention guidelines applied across the gerioperative care continuum.

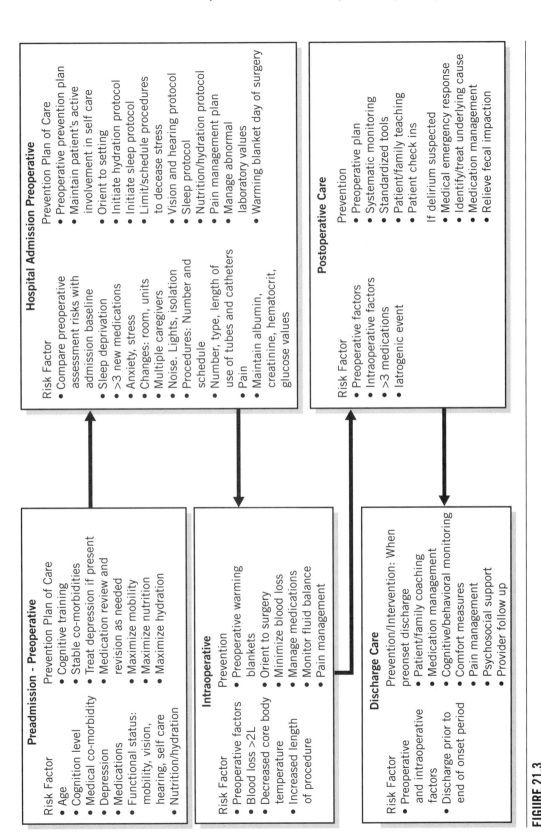

Preadmission - Preoperative

Risk Factor
- Age
- Cognition level
- Medical co-morbidity
- Depression
- Medications
- Functional status: mobility, vision, hearing, self care
- Nutrition/hydration

Prevention Plan of Care
- Cognitive training
- Stable co-morbidities
- Treat depression if present
- Medication review and revision as needed
- Maximize mobility
- Maximize nutrition
- Maximize hydration

Hospital Admission Preoperative

Risk Factor
- Compare preoperative assessment risks with admission baseline
- Sleep deprivation
- >3 new medications
- Anxiety, stress
- Changes: room, units
- Multiple caregivers
- Noise. Lights, isolation
- Procedures: Number and schedule
- Number, type, length of use of tubes and catheters
- Pain
- Maintain albumin, creatinine, hematocrit, glucose values

Prevention Plan of Care
- Preoperative prevention plan
- Maintain patient's active involvement in self care
- Orient to setting
- Initiate hydration protocol
- Initiate sleep protocol
- Limit/schedule procedures to decease stress
- Vision and hearing protocol
- Sleep protocol
- Nutrition/hydration protocol
- Pain management plan
- Manage abnormal laboratory values
- Warming blanket day of surgery

Intraoperative

Risk Factor
- Preoperative factors
- Blood loss >2L
- Decreased core body temperature
- Increased length of procedure

Prevention
- Preoperative warming blankets
- Orient to surgery
- Minimize blood loss
- Manage medications
- Monitor fluid balance
- Pain management

Postoperative Care

Risk Factor
- Preoperative factors
- Intraoperative factors
- >3 medications
- Iatrogenic event

Prevention
- Preoperative plan
- Systematic monitoring
- Standardized tools
- Patient/family teaching
- Patient check ins

If delirium suspected
- Medical emergency response
- Identify/treat underlying cause
- Medication management
- Relieve fecal impaction

Discharge Care

Risk Factor
- Preoperative and intraoperative factors
- Discharge prior to end of onset period

Prevention/Intervention: When preonset discharge
- Patient/family coaching
- Medication management
- Cognitive/behavioral monitoring
- Comfort measures
- Pain management
- Psychosocial support
- Provider follow up

FIGURE 21.3
Delirium Risk Factors With Prevention and Intervention Guidelines

Preoperative Considerations

ASSESSMENT

The preoperative interview involves standard preoperative assessment with special attention given to predisposing risk factors previously identified. Identifying POD risk factors before surgery is needed to develop targeted primary interventions. Patient alerts inform intraoperative and postoperative providers to maintain prevention and to establish systems for delirium detection and rapid response. The presence of two or more risk factors requires further evaluation by other members of the interdisciplinary care team.

Age

Increasing age is an independent risk factor for POD. As one ages, cognitive, mental, emotional, physical, and physiologic reserve diminishes in even the healthiest of older adults. System integrity becomes strained when trying to meet demands from multiple internal and external sources. When the system is overloaded, delirium is a common outcome. Marcantonio and colleagues (1994) and Litaker and colleagues (2001) identified greater than 70 years as a risk factor for delirium. Freter and colleagues (2005) identified age 80. When age is the only risk factor, older adults are at lower risk for POD than those of the same age with additional risk factors. However, older adults with no risk factors are at greater risk than their younger counterparts.

Cognitive Status

Preexisting cognitive impairment is consistently identified as a major risk factor for POD in older adults. The risk of POD in older adults with cognitive impairment is highest in those with dementia, possibly due to the inflammatory process that characterizes dementia. There is an inverse relationship between cognitive level and delirium severity and duration. Mild cognitive impairment becomes a risk factor when other risk factors are present in addition to severe physiological, psychological, or environmental stress.

Cognitive impairment is not limited to a diagnosis of dementia. Cognitive changes begin as early as the early 40s. Older adults begin to be aware of the effects of cognitive changes around age 70. Changes in information processing speed, attention, and memory are the most common cognitive changes. In healthy older adults, these changes rarely have a significant impact on function. Under conditions of high stress or in patients with limited cognitive reserve, the cognitive changes become more noticeable. Even mild changes in cognition, especially in the area of executive function, increase the risk for delirium. Mild cognitive impairment often goes undetected unless evaluated using standardized screening tools.

The Mini-Mental Status Exam (MMSE) (Folstein, Folstein & McHugh, 1975) is used most often to screen for cognitive impairment. A score equal to or greater than 25 out of a possible 30 points is considered intact cognitive function. Lower scores indicate severe (≤ 9 points), moderate (10 to 20 points), or mild (21 to 24 points) impairment. The MMSE has been translated into several languages.

The MMSE tests global cognitive function. It is not an effective tool for evaluating executive function, the cognitive ability to organize thoughts and activities, problem solve, and make decisions. The Trail Making Test and clock drawing test are common screening tools to evaluate executive function. See Chapter 20 for a more complete discussion of cognitive screening.

Depression

The relationship between preoperative depression and POD remains unclear. Although a number of clinical rules or checklists do not include depression as a risk factor, studies have identified preoperative depression as an important contributor to POD onset (Greene, Attix, Weldon, Smith, McDonagh, & Monk, 2009; Leung, Sands, Mullen, Wang, & Vaurio, 2005). Approximately 30% of elders and 70% of elders with chronic illness exhibit some form of depression. Due to misdiagnosis and lack of systematic screening, the 30% rate may underestimate the overall incidence of depression. Older adults admitted with depression who go on to develop a delirium while in the hospital are at even higher risk for poor outcomes, including death.

Depression can be easily confused with dementia. The presenting symptoms are similar: lack of concentration, disorganized thinking, limited attention span, and slowed response to stimuli. One distinguishing feature is the ability of people with depression to describe their symptoms and articulate their memory problems. Older adults with dementia often are unaware they have a cognitive impairment or tend to downplay its severity or interference with function. A more complete discussion of depression and dementia can be found in Chapter 20.

Multiple studies have investigated depression as a risk factor for delirium in geriatric surgical patients. Results indicate a positive association between depression and delirium. The number of depressive symptoms reported preoperatively is positively related to delirium duration.

Overlap syndrome is the presence of preoperative depression and hospital-based delirium. Older adults with overlap syndrome have "five times greater odds of nursing home placement or death at 1 year and three times greater odds of 1-month functional decline than patients with neither depression nor delirium and three times greater odds of 1-month functional decline than patients with neither depression nor delirium" (Givens, Jones, & Inouye, 2008, p. 1350). While no studies on overlap syndrome in geriatric surgical patients have been reported to date, similar effects would be expected. The evidence indicating preoperative depression is a risk factor for POD is extensive and consistent.

The potential for poor surgical outcomes is high in older adults with depression and in those with delirium. The potential is even greater when depression and delirium are combined. Despite the available evidence, depression screening is rarely included in standard preoperative assessment protocols. Chapter 20 discusses depression and preoperative screening in greater detail. Preoperatively, a two-item screening tool is recommended followed by additional screening if the answer to either of the two questions is affirmative. The two questions are: "During the past two weeks, have you often been bothered by feeling down, depressed, or hopeless?" and "During the past two weeks, have you often been bothered by little interest or pleasure in doing things?" An affirmative response to either question indicates a need for additional screening.

Preexisting Disease

The health history provides insight into the number and duration of chronic diseases, a predictor of POD. Conditions most frequently correlated with delirium are diabetes, stroke, cardiac disease, hypertension, and chronic obstructive pulmonary disease. Cardiovascular disease is highly correlated with POD. Older adults with alterations in thyroid function should be carefully evaluated for control to protect against delirium.

Medication

Medication assessment is a standard element of a preoperative assessment. Medications are a contributing factor for delirium in up to 40% of older adults admitted to medical services.

EXHIBIT 21.2 **Prescription and Over-the-Counter Drug Classifications Associated With Delirium**

Gastrointestinal and urinary antispasmodics
Antiemetics
Antihistamines
Muscle relaxants
Antidepressants
Antiarrhythmics
Antihypertensives
Analgesics
Anxiolytics
Benzodiazepines
Antiparkinsons
Anticoagulants
Glucocorticoids
Alcohol use

Older adults do not tolerate polypharmacy well. Delirium results from medication toxicity, drug-drug interactions, and drug-disease interactions. The risk of delirium increases as the number of medications increases.

Exhibit 21.2 identifies drug classifications that should be evaluated as risk factors. Older adults experiencing a stress response from surgery and anesthesia are at high risk for medication-induced delirium due to the effects of age-related changes in pharmacokinetics and pharmacodynamics. Psychoactive and psychotropic drugs have been linked with delirium onset in older adults undergoing cardiac, hip fracture, arthroplasty, vascular, and general surgery. Anticholinergic medications and narcotics have been positively associated with POD. Medications with anticholinergic activity commonly prescribed in patients undergoing surgery include antispasmodics, analgesic, bronchodilators, benzodiazepines, antidysrthymics, and analgesics. Other drugs with potential anticholinergic effects include warfarin, ranitidine, codeine, and nifedipine. Diuretics, antibiotics, anticonvulsants, anti-inflammatory agents, antiparkison medications, and oral hypoglycemic agents have also been associated with POD.

Many over-the-counter medications and herbs contain anticholinergic properties. During the preoperative assessment, the patient should be asked to list all the over-the-counter medications and any herbs, herbal medication, or herbal teas taken during the last month. It is helpful to offer specific suggestions such as: Any antihistamines? Antispasmodics for diarrhea or incontinence? Antacids or medications for stomach upset? Offering ideas as to type of medications prompts patients to remember specific incidents when over-the-counter medications were used.

More than three medications, the addition of three or more medications on any one day, psychotropic drug use, and the existence of three or more medical conditions should place the nurse on alert for instituting delirium prevention and systematic monitoring for evidence of early symptoms.

Visual and Hearing Impairment

Normal age-related changes contribute to varying degrees of vision and hearing loss among older adults. These sensory changes, creating the potential for decreased communication and social isolation, are significant predisposing factors for the onset of POD. Impaired hearing contributes to misunderstanding information, which leads to increased stress. Health care providers spend less time and communicate less frequently with hearing impaired older adults. Poor vision hinders elders' ability to perceive nonverbal cues and interpret environmental stimuli. Visual impairment contributes to misidentification of people, misinterpretation of visual messages, and misperception of environmental cues. The result of vision and hearing loss and subsequent effect on communication and comfort diminishes social interaction, increases withdrawal and social isolation, and increases functional impairment.

Older adults often state it is "tiring" to try and attend to events due to vision or hearing changes. In the hospital environment, noise levels and unfamiliar environments compound hearing and vision difficulties. Illness and environmental stress places additional demands on the older adult's ability to comprehend what is happening in the environment and consider appropriate responses, creating further stress. The inability to process and attend to environmental stimuli and the resulting sensory overload overwhelms coping mechanisms and overwhelms cognitive reserve. Professional care providers often label the older adult as "confused" when older adults who are hearing or vision impaired do not respond to verbal stimuli or respond out of context.

Preoperatively, vision can be assessed using a standard Snellen chart. Hearing is easily assessed using the "whisper test." Standing behind the older adult, whisper a word, and ask the older adult to repeat it. Vision and hearing assessment should be conducted with and without assistive devices. Testing without an assistive device provides a measure of what the patient can see or hear before and after surgery if assistive devices are not readily available. If loss is severe, a patient alert should be posted in the medical record so staff caring for the patient during and after surgery can ensure effective communication processes. Patient understanding of information must continually be assessed using talk back to prevent misunderstanding that can exacerbate the potential for delirium.

Nutrition and Dehydration

Functional impairment negatively affects nutritional status and hydration. Community-dwelling adults, especially those who live alone or who are caregivers, are at risk for poor nutrition. Inadequate transportation, limited resources, energy depletion, and anxiety contribute to the onset of malnutrition and dehydration.

Increased frailty (see Chapter 19) is closely linked with poor nutritional and hydration status and weight loss. Brain metabolism depends on quality nutrition and adequate hydration. Inouye and Charpentier (1996) identified malnutrition as one of the five factors included in a predictive model for delirium in hospitalized older adults on medical units. Dehydration inhibits kidney function, contributing to the potential for electrolyte imbalance, a major precipitating factor in POD.

No screening battery test has been shown to have good sensitivity and specificity for identifying persons at risk for delirium secondary to nutrition or dehydration. Nutritional assessment must rely on the patient or companion-coach. Asking for a history of intake of foods and fluids for several days prior to surgery provides data for determining risk of inadequate nutrition and dehydration. A history of 10% or more weight loss accompanied by loss of muscle strength and function indicates that the patient is moving toward frailty. Body measurements are used to assess physiological stamina and function.

The laboratory assessment of malnutrition generally includes a complete blood cell count and albumin level. Albumin levels of less than 3.2 g/dL in hospitalized elders are highly predictive of subsequent mortality.

Rapidity of Insult

Rapidity of surgical insult causes excessive stress that can trigger POD. Sudden excessive stress can overwhelm available cognitive reserve, triggering delirium.

Emergency surgery has a high correlation with delirium onset. Hip fractures are common emergency surgeries in older adults and a well-established risk factor for delirium. The factors that predispose older adults to hip fractures also predispose the older adults to delirium: cognitive impairment, sensory impairment, comorbidity, and medications. Delay in surgical intervention after hip fracture also has been associated with delirium. The need to stabilize the patient prior to surgery suggests that the patient's poor preoperative physiologic status may contribute to delirium risk rather than the surgical delay. Pain levels and microemboli formation that accrue from postponements may contribute to the higher incidence of delirium in postfracture patients. More research is needed to determine the relationship between surgical delay following acute or traumatic events and confounding factors.

Patients requiring surgery for accidental trauma do not have time to be prepared physically, physiologically, or emotionally for the rigors of surgery. The stress response is high before the addition of the surgical stress and can overwhelm the patient's cognitive reserve. Ansaloni and colleagues (2010) reported that of 47 older adults with POD (sample = 357), 37 (78.7%) had emergency surgery. None of the emergency surgeries involved hip fracture. Nearly 20% of those with emergency surgery developed POD, three times the incidence of older adults having elective surgery.

INTERVENTION

The goal of prehabilitation programs, based on preoperative assessment data, is to improve overall function, clinical status, and well-being of the older adult prior to surgery. However, there has been little investigation on the effect of preoperative physical exercise or cognitive activity in preventing POD or POCD.

Improving nutrition, exercise, and functional capacity; optimizing treatment of chronic illness; reducing high-risk medications; and improving sleep patterns are well-established interventions to improve overall health. Interventions targeted to reduce delirium risk focus on optimizing cognition and overall health as well as decreasing onset or severity of postoperative cognitive impairment. For example, music therapy is effective in decreasing preoperative anxiety. Exercise improves depression. Smoking cessation improves cardiorespiratory function. Thus, any documented preoperative intervention that targets predisposing, modifiable risk factors has the potential to decrease onset or severity of POD. In addition, ensuring the older patient has hearing and vision aids that are based on recent vision and hearing assessments available optimizes sensory functioning and reduces delirium risk.

Once risk factors are identified, an interdisciplinary prehabilitation treatment plan can be designed in collaboration with the older adult and the participation of companion-coach or family. Preferably, prehabilitation should be initiated at least 8 weeks before surgery. However, even minimal levels of exercise, smoking cessation, or reduction in high-risk medications have beneficial effects.

Intraoperative Considerations

The type of surgery is a consistent risk factor associated with POD. Patients undergoing orthopedic or cardiac surgery have the highest incidence of POD. The most frequently cited intraoperative factors associated with POD are complex surgeries, blood loss, transfusion greater than 1 L, and low body temperature. Chang, Tsai, Lin, Chen, and Liu (2008) noted a low body temperature of 25° C, while Detroyer and colleagues (2008) indicated temperatures of 32.8° C or lower as precipitating events. Blood loss and transfusions ranged from two units (Chang, Tsai, Lin, Chen, & Liu, 2008) to more than five units (Katzelson et al., 2009). Fluid balance, glycemic control, hypoxia, and management of hypotension are additional areas of risk for POD.

Anesthesia and intraoperative medications are precipitating factors for delirium in gerioperative patients. Medications used during surgery include muscle relaxants, analgesics, cardiac medications, antihypertensives, and anticholinergics. Chapter 8 presents a more extensive overview of intraoperative medications.

PRIMARY INTERVENTION

Surgical complexity, blood loss, and number of transfusions are minimally modifiable variables. Hypothermia is a modifiable risk factor. The use of warming blankets, ensuring the patient is adequately covered during transfer and throughout surgery, and maintaining room temperature at approximately 24° C help maintain body temperature.

Consideration of intraoperative medications and delirium risk is a risk-benefit ratio. Many of the drugs associated with delirium are important in maintaining hemodynamic stability and homeostasis during surgery or in relieving pain. Postoperative care providers must review the intraoperative medication record to assess the type and amount of risk medications the older patient received. Analysis of the intraoperative medications provides an estimate of delirium risk.

Postoperative Considerations

Preoperative interventions impact predisposing risk of delirium, but the risk continues after surgery. Precipitating intraoperative and postoperative factors are additive. Postoperative prevention of delirium begins immediately in the postanesthesia care unit by initiating interventions to address modifiable precipitating factors.

Medications, oxygenation, blood transfusions, fluid and electrolyte imbalance, and hypothermia are sources of precipitating events. Although delirium onset typically occurs 24 hours after surgery and gerioperative patients are typically lucid in the postanesthesia care unit, taking preventive actions to prevent later onset is critical. Adequate oxygenation, monitoring glucose levels, warming blankets, comforting presence, pain relief, minimizing medication use, and use of nonpharmacological interventions for comfort contribute to delirium prevention.

ASSESSING POSTOPERATIVE DELIRIUM

Delirium is underassessed, underdiagnosed, misdiagnosed, and undertreated in older adults. Few health providers are adequately prepared to recognize the signs and symptoms of hyper- and hypodelirium, or to conduct systematic delirium assessments with the gerioperative patient. Less than 20% of surgical facilities report a protocol for assessing postoperative delirium in older adults (Neumann, Speck, Karlawish, Schwartz, & Shea, 2010).

One reason for missed diagnosis is the widespread assumption that confusion is a normal response in older adults who are hospitalized and acutely ill. Such an assumption is one of the most dangerous safety risks to older adults in the acute care setting. The presence of cognitive, attention, or behavioral changes in an older adult without a prior diagnosis of cognitive impairment, depression, or psychiatric illness is a medical emergency requiring an immediate response. Obtaining information from someone who knows the patient well and is familiar with the patient's preoperative behaviors and activities assists in differentiating in-hospital behaviors from prehospital behaviors, an important criterion when making the diagnosis of delirium.

The documentation of vague descriptors such as "confused" with no supporting data is inappropriate. Standardized delirium assessment tools provide systematic data for detecting delirium onset. Standardized tools assist in making informed, knowledgeable judgments about the degree and type of changes in an older adult's behavior, cognitive ability, and environmental awareness. Standardized tools, based on a common language, promote understanding across caregivers in describing the cognitive and behavioral status of the older adult.

The Confusion Assessment Method (CAM), Neelon and Champagne Confusion Scale (NEECHAM), and Delirium Index (DI) are commonly used. The NEECHAM scale is a public domain document available in Appendix II. The assessment tools are short, reliable, and have been tested for use in assessing POD in older adults. Although each of the tools is described as easy to use, providers require information and training on their use, the interpretation of results, and integrating results with clinical judgment. The most commonly used tool is the CAM. The CAM is cited in a number of protocols for delirium care and as a tool in numerous research studies on delirium. The DI is one of the few available tools that measure delirium severity. A delirium assessment protocol can be found in Appendix I. Best practice guidelines for assessing delirium in older adults are listed in Exhibit 21.3. Figure 21.4 presents a flow chart for delirium assessment.

EXHIBIT 21.3 Best Practice Guidelines: Assessing Delirium in Older Adults

- Establish and document baseline assessment data
- Conduct systematic assessment of at-risk patients using standardized assessment tools and compare with baseline
- Screen patients whenever symptoms of changes in cognitive function or mental status present or whenever family or friend expresses concern about patient behaviors
- Select assessment tools in consideration of patient's sensory, physical, and physiological status
- Document assessment data and nursing evaluation
- Be cognizant of overlapping symptoms in patients with dementia or depression and influences of overlap on delirium assessment
- When probable delirium determined, immediately initiate therapeutic, safety, and preventive interventions
- Initiate an immediate medical referral or rapid response when screening indicates probable delirium

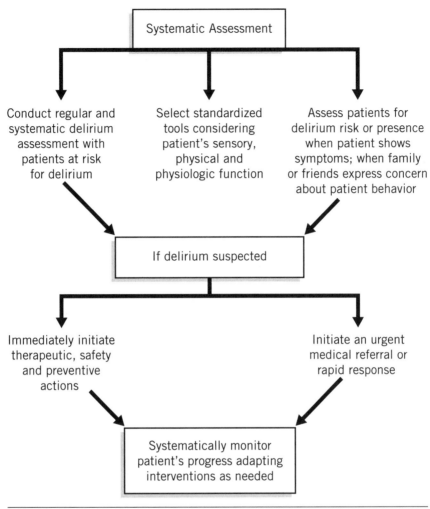

FIGURE 21.4
Delirium Assessment Guidelines

However, regular assessment should not be limited to older adults identified as high risk for POD. Delirium has been reported in 3 to 9% of patients who had no risk factors for delirium and up to 23% of older adults identified as having an intermediate risk of only one or two factors. Providers must recognize that the POD risk continuum in postoperative older adults does not range from "no risk to high risk" but from "risk to higher risk."

INTERVENTION

Interventions should be patient-centered and matched to the identified actual and potential risk factors, clinical situation, and unique preferences, values, and needs of the individual patient. Maintaining rigorous and continued attention on prevention strategies strengthens remaining cognitive and physiologic reserve, an important element in minimizing delirium severity and duration.

Delirium Package of Care

Effective prevention and intervention strategies depend on basic care issues and Maslow's hierarchy of needs: oxygenation, nutrition, hydration, sleep and rest, bowel and bladder regimens, activity and exercise, pain relief, environmental comfort, social support, cognitive stimulation, and avoidance of adverse medication effects. Prevention and intervention effectiveness may be achieved through a comprehensive "package of care," which is not a policy and procedures manual or a written set of protocols but a way of thinking holistically about postoperative care of the older adult and prevention of delirium. Protocols are useful, but attending only to protocols without a framework for carrying out the protocol limits their effectiveness. A set of protocols is available in Appendix I-1 that address many of the care issues important in delirium prevention and assessment. However, critical thinking, clinical judgment, and a practice framework must guide their use. The gerioperative care model that integrates comfort, relationship-centered care, and best practice across the perioperative continuum guides the care of gerioperative patients at risk for delirium.

The package of care relies on prevention as the primary mode of care. However, delirium may not always be preventable. Being on the alert and using systematic assessment based on standardized tools and clinical judgment during observation for changes in behavior is critical. The fluctuating nature and the potential for onset of a mixed type delirium suggests that relying only on standardized assessments at regulated intervals will miss early onset. Every patient interaction is an opportunity to detect changes in behavior that may signal early onset of delirium. Older adults who show any atypical behavior must have further evaluation with intense investigation into the underlying cause.

Family caregivers and care providers in rehabilitation settings or nursing homes can use the package of care concept after discharge to improve recovery and decrease postoperative readmission. A gerioperative care facilitator or other member of the care team coaches the patient, family, companion-coach, and other providers on the package of care as a tool for thinking and planning for postdischarge care with the older adult.

Oxygenation and Glucose

The brain consumes a large percentage of the body's need for oxygen and glucose. Physiological and psychological stress increases the brain's demand for these nutrients. Ensuring adequate oxygenation, fluid, and glucose are basic elements in preventing postoperative delirium.

Preventing Postoperative Complications

The excessive physiological and psychological stress caused by postoperative complications is a major contributor to delirium onset. Many of the prevention and intervention strategies targeting delirium contribute to preventing other postoperative complications. Prevention of pneumonia, wound infection, urinary tract infection, hemodynamic instability, dehydration, malnutrition, and adverse medication events all contribute to prevention of delirium.

Therapeutic interventions can increase risk for delirium. Examples include bed rest and medications. Finding alternative strategies to mitigate these situations and doing a risk-ratio analysis helps to determine if such treatments are necessary or can be modified in ways to decrease delirium risk. Clinical judgment, knowledge of the patient, and clinical status must be considered before making treatment decisions.

COGNITIVE ENGAGEMENT

Surgery, anesthesia, and medications generate additional physiological and psychological stressors that exacerbate preexisting cognitive dysfunction. Undetected preoperative changes in cognition become evident as the level of cognitive reserve continues to be depleted due to the stress of surgery and postoperative recovery demands. As recovery progresses, cognitive strength and function can return to presurgical levels. Continuing to engage older adults in cognitively stimulating activities at the individual's functional level helps to maintain and regain cognitive function. Interaction with friends and family avoids social isolation, which is strongly associated with altered cognition. The companion-coach can be extremely beneficial in providing activities, encouragement, and cognitive challenges important to for functional abilities.

Vision, Hearing, and Environment

Minimizing negative effects of vision and hearing impairment can be a challenge in the hospital environment. Environmental noise, lights, communication styles, the rapid pace of change in providers, numerous activities, and speed with which care is conducted exacerbate the misinterpretation that occurs when vision and hearing are impaired. The majority of older adults have some degree of vision and hearing changes that influence sensory acuity and sensory perception. Providers are responsible for adapting the pace of care and treatment to meet the needs of the older adult. Older adults with hearing impairment experience less interaction with care providers and less communication interaction when care occurs. Sensory isolation can occur and induce delirium from the lack of sensory stimulation.

Pain Relief

Pain and pain relief are priority concerns in gerioperative care. An increased pain level is strongly correlated with higher rates of delirium. Patients with severe pain are nine times more likely to experience POD. Pain interferes with attention, coping, and problem solving. The lack of attention and problem solving can impede effective pain assessment that can result in over or under medication and ineffective pain relief.

Inadequate pain relief confounds the ability to determine the best route for pain management. Older adults receiving parenteral opioids have higher levels of delirium than those receiving oral doses. Patients appear to have an increased use of patient-controlled anesthesia in the 24 hours preceding POD. Additional research is needed to identify low-risk opioid administration delivery methods.

Inadequate pain relief and its relationship to delirium is an ethical care issue. There is no reason to undertreat pain. Pain relief does not rely solely on medication administration. Multimodal pain relief methods using the World Health Organization stepladder approach to pain management are effective in relieving acute, severe pain in most situations. When traditional methods fail, regional anesthesia and other interventions can be initiated in collaboration with the interdisciplinary care team. Providers must be vigilant in assessing pain, not only severity but pain quality and effect on function. A holistic approach to pain relief calls for clinical judgment that attends to vigilant and sensitive pain assessment, collaborative decision-making on pain intervention, and evaluation of intervention effectiveness.

Nutrition and Hydration

Dehydration is a concern in the postoperative older adult. Changes in thirst mechanisms, renal changes, comorbid disease, diuretic use, self-care practices, and preparation for surgery contribute to postoperative dehydration. Dehydration contributes to altered kidney function, hemodynamic instability, and electrolyte disturbances that contribute to postoperative delirium. Monitoring fluid balance can be accomplished by checking intake and output at scheduled intervals and through handoff reports. Keeping fluids within easy reach, hydrating before and after ambulation or out-of-bed activities, and providing time during oral medication administration for the patient to drink a glass of fluid contributes to maintaining fluid balance in the older adult.

Low serum albumin is both a predisposing and a precipitating risk factor for delirium. Surgery increases catabolism and interferes with nutritional intake secondary to postoperative pain and fatigue. Older adults with low albumin, of no more than 3.5 g/dL, should receive a nutritional consult. A common intervention is providing small, high-nutrition snacks at regular intervals along with high-nutrition fluids that increase both nutrition and fluid intake. Foods and fluids that act as "comfort foods" can help stimulate intake.

Successful intervention depends on early detection through systematic assessment and rapid response. Rapid response is the prompt identification of underlying cause and targeted treatment. Health care providers must be reminded that older adults present with atypical symptoms, making diagnosis of the underlying cause of delirium difficult. Careful listening to the older adult's verbal description of symptoms, observation of nonverbal cues, and careful review of previous interventions including medications, procedures, tubes, drains, or assistive devices provide evidence into the nature of the precipitating problem. Interventions are targeted to the immediate problem.

Delirium and Postoperative Cognitive Dysfunction

Cognitive impairment can last up to 1 year and many patients never recover.

The exact nature of the relationship between delirium and POCD is unclear, although there is no doubt that there is a relationship. Some researchers suggest there is a continuum of cognitive disorders ranging from mild cognitive impairment to dementia. Delirium and POCD may be points along the continuum with similar and overlapping pathways or may be separate and distinct entities with different pathophysiologies. Evidence suggests that delirium is a risk factor for POCD and that preventing delirium may help prevent POCD. However, not all older adults who have delirium complain of POCD. The reverse is also true; not all patients with POCD have a history of POD. Ongoing research is needed to determine the nature of the two entities and to identify effective prevention and treatment interventions.

Postoperative Cognitive Dysfunction

POCD is a decline in cognitive ability detected after surgery. While the condition can occur in any age group, in younger adults, the condition is temporary and lasts a few hours or days. Older adults are particularly vulnerable to the onset of postoperative cognitive changes and long-lasting effects. In the gerioperative patient, the recovery from POCD is prolonged; in some cases cognitive deficits persist up to a year, and many patients never recover.

Bedford (1955) conducted one of the first retrospective reviews on postoperative cognitive changes in older adults. As an anesthesiologist, he was interested in the role of anesthesia in what was considered at the time as postanesthesia dementia of older adults. He reported that 10% of the sample of 1169 elders evidenced cognitive changes. He concluded that no patient over the age of 60 should undergo surgery unless absolutely necessary. Surgical care of the older adults has advanced since Bedford's admonition. Anesthesia techniques are improved, and geriatric surgery is common but more complex. Despite advanced knowledge, research, and technology in anesthesia, surgical techniques, geriatrics, and gerontology, POCD remains a common, serious, and devastating postoperative complication for the older adult.

The incidence of POCD in patients undergoing cardiac and orthopedic surgery is as high as 80%, with 60% having continued dysfunction after 3 months. In major noncardiac surgery, the incidence of POCD is nearly 30% with half reporting symptoms after 3 months. In older adults undergoing repair of hip fracture, POCD occurs in over one-third of patients. In older adults undergoing elective noncardiac, nonthoracic surgery, figures have shown a 20 to 50% incidence of POCD with nearly a third experiencing decline after 3 months.

Currently, 50% of the 50 million of surgeries worldwide involve adults over age 60. This number is expected to increase dramatically as the world population continues to age. By extrapolating POCD rates similar to those provided by Bedford, approximately 5 million older adults will suffer from POCD. Most will recover; however, even with a rate of unresolved POCD, there will be 3 million people with diminished cognitive function; most of whom will rely on family caregivers for emotional and functional support for an undefined period of time after surgery.

DEFINITION

While POCD lacks a consistent, standardized definition, it is typically described as a mild to severe decline in memory, verbal abilities, perception, attention, executive functions, and abstract thinking. The lack of a standardized definition impairs comparison of research results and clinical recommendations. In addition, clinical details related to assessment criteria, etiology, pathophysiological mechanisms, prevention, and treatment are not well defined.

Avidan and colleagues (2009) challenged previous research findings that surgery is a causative factor in the onset of POCD. In a retrospective cohort study, the researchers investigated the effects of noncardiac surgery, illness, or neither illness or surgery on long-term cognitive decline. The authors concluded there was no evidence of a "long term effect on cognition independently attributable to surgery or major illness" (p. 968).

ASSESSING POSTOPERATVE COGNTIVE DYSFUNCTION

There is no *DSM-IV* code, nursing diagnosis, or International Classification of Diseases that specifically addresses the syndrome of POCD. The *DSM-IV* criterion most closely related to POCD is the mild cognitive disorder listed under the section entitled "cognitive dysfunction not otherwise specified." The mild cognitive disorder is described as a cognitive impairment evidenced by neuropsychological testing (NPT) or clinical assessment that is accompanied by a systemic general medical condition or central nervous system dysfunction. POCD is not characterized as a systemic general medical condition or a result of central nervous system dysfunction. While the signs and symptoms reflect a disturbance in central nervous system function, the cause may not be in the central nervous system.

POCD symptoms are vague, usually characterized as difficulty with memory, attention, and slowed thinking processes. Subjective indicators of POCD are patient complaints of "fuzzy thinking," "not being the same since surgery," and "not feeling all there." Behavioral manifestations are not easily recognizable. Patient complaints or family concerns about the older adult's thinking, memory, problem solving, or attention should be carefully reviewed and evaluated. Alterations in cognitive function can herald adverse medication effects or deterioration in physiological function. A thorough evaluation of the patient's status should be conducted immediately in any older adult who demonstrates or complains of changes in cognition.

> *A rapid response interdisciplinary team evaluation is required when gerioperative patients demonstrate changes in cognition or behavior.*

Subjective indicators are poorly correlated with results of NPT. While NPT is the gold standard for identifying POCD, there are no standards to guide decisions on a determination of POCD, the most effective tests for POCD, or the best timing for POCD testing. A major issue in NPT is deciding which tests to use, as different tests measure different cognitive abilities. As POCD evokes a spectrum of impairments, researchers and clinicians can use different tests to measure different types of impairments. Seventy different tests and composites batteries have been used in POCD evaluation.

A standard neuropsychological assessment covering most cognitive domains takes approximately 2.5 hours to complete. Testing with older adults recovering from surgery could easily take longer. During the postoperative period, older adults have limited capacity to respond to multiple testing procedures. Pain, stress, anxiety, fatigue, dehydration, and sleep disturbance interfere with cognition. Conducting NPT in the early postoperative period may capture cognitive dysfunction due to normal postsurgical events or postoperative recovery interventions rather than true cognitive decline. A diagnosis of POCD should only be determined after comprehensive NPT to ensure accuracy of diagnosis.

POCD can be misinterpreted as hypoactive delirium, depression, or dementia. An evaluation must be conducted to determine cognitive changes reflecting onset of delirium or POCD. Key differences differentiating delirium and POCD are listed in Table 21.5 along with distinguishing differences with dementia, depression, and normal age-related changes.

Delirium usually occurs within 24 to 72 hours after surgery but has been seen as long as 5 to 7 days later. There is often a period of lucidity between anesthesia withdrawal and onset of delirium symptoms. Delirium onset is characterized as a rapidly developing fluctuating course with changes in level of consciousness and an inability to sustain attention. There is often a precipitating cause. Older adults with delirium demonstrate changes in behavior that reflect hyperactivity, hypoactivity, or unpredictable swings from restlessness and agitation to apathy and withdrawal. Hallucinations or illusions are not uncommon in delirium. In comparison, POCD has a slow insidious onset occurring over several days or weeks, and lasting for a prolonged period of several weeks, months, or years. Yet, POCD has been reported as early as day 1 and day 2 postsurgery.

POSTOPERATIVE COGNITIVE DYSFUNCTION TRAJECTORY

POCD is divided into three phases. The early phase occurs after the first week of surgery, the intermediate stage lasts 3 to 12 months, and long-term POCD lasts 1 to 2 years. A greater

TABLE 21.5
Distinguishing Features of Normal Age Changes, Delirium, Postoperative Cognitive Dysfunction, Depression, and Dementia

	Normal Age Changes	Delirium	Postoperative Cognitive Dysfunction	Depression	Dementia
Definition	Minimal to moderate decline in: Processing speed Attention Memory	A medical emergency characterized by an acute fluctuating onset of confusion, disturbances in attention, and disorganized thinking; may have decline in level of consciousness	A mild to severe decline in memory, verbal abilities, perception, attention, executive functions, and abstract thinking	Feelings of sadness that affect sleep, appetite, energy, and confidence that are out of the ordinary for the individual and most of the time on most days for at least 2 weeks	A gradual and progressive decline in cognition and mental processing ability affecting short-term memory, communication, language, judgment, reasoning, and abstract thinking
Onset	Gradual over years	Acute, fluctuating Occurs in hours, 1 to 6 days after surgery	Typically occurs 1 week after surgery	Unexplained flattening of affect or mood that persists for at 2 weeks or more; may coincide with changes in life event	Changes occur over months or years
Course	Changes over years	Rapid onset, Fluctuates over 24 hours; amenable to treatment; may be worse at night	May resolve over 3 months; known to last up to 1 year; may never resolve	Gradual onset over days, weeks; usually reversible with treatment; often worse in morning	Slow, chronic progression, or step-wise progression over months to years
Early presentation	Word loss; Processing speed	Increase or decrease in reactivity, response to stimuli Fluctuations in alertness, cognition, judgment, thinking; fails to understand tasks	Subjective symptoms of not remembering clearly; symptoms vague; general loss of cognitive acuity; symptoms need a baseline for comparison	Reduced memory, concentration, self-esteem; slowed response; Apathy, low energy; sleep disturbance	Impaired short-term memory; Impaired judgment, language ability Progressive decline

(continued)

TABLE 21.5

Distinguishing Features of Normal Age Changes, Delirium, Postoperative Cognitive Dysfunction, Depression, and Dementia *(continued)*

	Normal Age Changes	Delirium	Postoperative Cognitive Dysfunction	Depression	Dementia
Sensorium changes	None	Misperceptions; Hallucinations; Illusions	None	None	Delusions Hallucinations
Mood	Normal	Fluctuating emotions; Apathy, outbursts, anger, fear		Depressed mood Flat affect Changes in appetitive Possible suicidal ideation Hopelessness	Depends on stage of disease Depressed in early stages Apathy Angry outbursts
Behavior	Normal	Hyperactive delirium: agitated, restless, fidgeting, increased arousal Hypoactive delirium: apathy, lethargy, low arousal		Withdrawn, apathy, decreased motivation- May be agitated.	Agitated or withdrawn Aimless/nonpurposeful activity
Consciousness level	Clear	Often impaired; fluctuating	Clear	Clear	Clear until late stages
Screening tools	Trail Making Test Digital Symbol Substitution Test	Confusion Assessment Method (CAM) Delirium Observation Screening Scale (DOS) Neelon-Champagne Confusion Scale (NEECHAM)	Common screening tools Mini-Mental Status Exam CLOX test Trail Making Test: Parts A and B	Geriatric Depression Scale	Mini-Mental Status Exam Clock Drawing Test Mini-Cog Dementia Screen
Response/ action/ intervention	None needed	Notify medical or rapid response team; Immediate referral to geriatric consult or interdisciplinary team	Refer to interdisciplinary care team Consult geriatric psychiatrist	Notify attending physician Refer for geriatric mental health consult	Notify attending physician and interdisciplinary care team; Refer for geriatric mental health consult

percentage of older adults have early onset POCD occurring within the first week after surgery. Symptoms typically diminish or resolve within 3 months in the absence of dementia. Patients who have intermediate POCD have an increased mortality in the first year following surgery.

ETIOLOGY

The etiology of POCD is not well understood. Pathophysiological mechanisms reflect those found in other clinical syndromes associated with cognitive dysfunction. Mechanisms center on heightened neuroinflammatory response, altered neurotransmitter function, diminished cognitive reserve, and hyperactive neuroendocrine stress response. Cardiac disease is strongly associated with elevated levels of inflammatory markers and alterations in cognitive function.

The neurotransmitter acetylcholine has been linked to cognitive function. Older adults are highly sensitive to changes in levels of acetylcholine. Opioid administration decreases acetylcholine, which may be one explanation for the occurrence of POCD after major surgery requiring opioid anesthesia.

Hospitalization and environmental factors have long been identified as risk factors for changes in cognitive function in older adults. Cognitive dysfunction increases in the presence of heightened anxiety. Hospitalization increases anxiety as a result of alteration in normal routines, disrupted sleep patterns, decreased environmental familiarity especially in relation to toileting, and uncertainty about disease prognosis and outcomes. The added stress of surgery and postoperative pain, presence of tubes such as catheters and intravenous lines, dehydration, and low nutritional intake may deplete cognitive reserves. In older adults with significant age-related changes or mild cognitive impairment not detected preoperatively, cognitive reserves may be insufficient to cope with the added stress of hospitalization.

RISK FACTORS

Predisposing factors directly associated with POCD are age and minimal preoperative cognitive reserve. Low educational level has been used as a proxy for minimal cognitive reserve. However, the relationship between education and cognitive reserve is insufficiently demonstrated for education to be used as a clinical reference. The lack of cognitive reserve may predispose older patients by decreasing the capacity for withstanding the severe stresses imposed by surgery and anesthesia.

Precipitating factors of POCD are type and length of surgery. Older adults undergoing cardiac or orthopedic procedures, surgeries usually requiring over 2 hours, are at highest risk. Anesthesia has not been identified as a risk factor for POCD. Severity and duration of postoperative delirium severity, opioid use, history of stroke, postoperative infections, and pain have been associated with POCD. However, the relationship between proposed risk factors and the mechanisms of POCD remain unknown.

Gerioperative Care

PREOPERATIVE ASSESSMENT

Older patients and family members should be asked if the patient has experienced changes in the ability to manage daily living situations, problem solve, or ability to complete tasks previously done with ease. Family members can identify changes in ability to carry out daily and instrumental activities of daily living or changes in participation in activities previously found enjoyable. Assessment should focus on: What can the patient no longer do that he or she used to do? What are some of the reasons? Other factors such as impaired mobility, energy, and fatigue are commonly associated with changes in activity.

Providers are often hesitant to ask about changes in cognition for fear of upsetting the patient and causing potential harm. Often, older adults are "protected" by families and friends who avoid discussing changes in behavior that may signal cognitive decline. Asking the patient about any changes offers an opportunity for discussion and additional follow-up.

Current recommendations suggest that the MMSE be administered to older adults having major surgery to evaluate overall cognitive function. Although the MMSE does not evaluate executive function, it provides the foundation for further follow-up of executive function. Patients with scores below 24 on the MMSE should have a follow-up neurological evaluation. A patient alert should be placed on the medical record to prompt postoperative providers to monitor for evidence of POCD.

INTERVENTION

Getting the older patient prepared for surgery involves attending to the patient's agenda, providing information as needed, decreasing anxiety, and improving overall health and well-being. The goal of primary intervention for POCD centers on prehabilitation activities designed to improve cognitive function, managing depression, and maximizing overall health and functional status. Interventions are similar to those for prevention of delirium.

Intraoperative Considerations

Intraoperative interventions focus on the prevention of POCD. While there is little correlation between intraoperative interventions such as prevention of hypothermia, positioning, preoperative anxiety, anesthesia, or pain for POCD, these are important interventions in the overall care of the older adult. Providing an adequate level of oxygenation and perfusion, fluid and electrolyte maintenance, and pain control may prevent cognitive harm in older adults with preexisting cognitive vulnerability. The correlation between delirium and POCD suggests that interventions targeted to minimizing onset, severity, and duration of delirium may be effective in decreasing onset, severity, and duration of POCD.

Postoperative Considerations

An awareness of the onset of POCD increases safety and security of older adults. Although there is minimal literature addressing safety in older adults with POCD, there is extensive evidence that cognitive decline is associated with higher rates of falls and adverse events. Older adults with impaired cognition are less effective in managing postoperative recovery activities unless they have consistent and supportive coaching. POCD is associated with a greater risk of respiratory complications, suggesting that older adults are not engaging in postoperative respiratory activities. Health care providers must be more diligent in supervising respiratory activities in older adults who are cognitively impaired. There is an urgent need for focused research on postoperative primary and secondary interventions in the treatment of older adults vulnerable to POCD and its effects.

Detecting early onset of POCD is a challenge in hospitalized older adults due to the timeline of onset of symptoms. The average length of stay for older adults after surgery is about five days. With the onset of POCD ranging from 2 to 10 days after surgery, the majority of older adults will not have signs or symptoms of POCD until after hospital discharge. Thus, POCD will go undetected. Informing and coaching family members and companion-coaches and educating community health nurses about the importance of monitoring patient statements and behaviors that may indicate cognitive decline is needed to maximize the potential for detection.

Older adults having day or ambulatory surgery are less vulnerable to the onset of POCD. The reasons for the difference are not well documented. However, POCD can occur in older adults who have had same day surgery. Older adults, who may not show evidence of cognitive changes until 7 to 10 days after being released from surgery, are at high risk for having the changes in cognition ignored or if acknowledged, untreated. "Feeling fuzzy" or "not quite right" are not symptoms that prompt older adults to seek medical attention. Explaining POCD, the timeline for symptoms, and the need to contact providers will assist in follow-up care for this potentially life-altering condition.

Prevention and intervention for treatment of delirium may benefit older adults at risk for POCD. Attention to care issues including nutrition, hydration, environmental and interpersonal support for vision and hearing impairment, early ambulation and range-of-motion exercises, and medication review may impact the onset of POCD. Areas of particular importance include increased use of multimodal pain relief methods to decrease opioid dose, adherence to sleep protocols including minimal use of opioid analgesia, and avoidance of noise, light, and environmental factors. Activity scheduling that prevents sleep disturbance and supplemental oxygenation the first 24 to 48 hours after surgery may be helpful.

DISCHARGE CONSIDERATIONS

Cognitive changes are distressing and highly stressful to patients and family members. Concerns center on how long the changes will last, the meaning of the changes, and if they represent the beginning of dementia. POCD typically occurs a week after surgery, meaning that patients are already discharged to home, a rehabilitation center, or long-term care facility. Supporting and preparing the family for possible onset of cognitive dysfunction is crucial. Coach patients and families on the benefits of self-care including activity and exercise, nutrition, pain relief, hydration, and sleep along with correct use of medication. Providing a calm, secure environment that minimizes psychological stress, involves the patient in enjoyable activities, and provides a sense of safety, security, and control may help prevent POCD.

Explaining the signs and symptom the patient may experience, what to do if signs and symptoms become evident, and giving resource contact numbers increases feelings of control and competence. Encourage older adults and their families to seek a provider if symptoms occur. It is important to note that symptoms can range from mild

Supporting and preparing families for potential changes in cognition is crucial.

to more severe. There is a possibility that POCD may interfere with the patient's ability to manage instrumental or basic activities of daily living. Coaching family members on the value and important of providing maximum support and resources for the older patient, ensuring mental stimulation and social interaction, adequate rest and exercise, and encouragement in context with the patient's preferences, health status, and living situation cannot be underestimated.

PATIENT REPORT: Mrs. Postemsky

Mrs. Postemsky has several risk factors for POD in addition to age. On the morning of the second postoperative day, she becomes quiet and responds to her family member with simple answers. She continually picks at her intravenous line site dressing and the hip dressing, as well as tries to remove the incisional drain. The primary nurse suspects early onset hypoactive delirium. A plan is developed with the help of her family to stimulate Mrs. Postemsky with her favorite music, television shows, and magazines. Nonsteroidal anti-inflammatory drugs are ordered on a fixed schedule. The next morning, Mrs. Postemsky shows no evidence of hypoactive delirium, and she is discharged to the rehabilitation unit. The primary nurse provides a complete report to the rehabilitation nurse about the patient's symptoms of delirium and the prevention plan.

SUMMARY

Threats to cognition and losing one's mind are among the greatest fears in older adults. Delirium is a serious, devastating, and often unrecognized postoperative complication affecting cognitive function in older adults. The incidence of delirium ranges from a low of 4% to a high of 67% depending on type of surgery. In the past, providers have not viewed delirium as a serious complication but a normative consequence of being old and sick in the hospital. Recent studies have identified the complex nature of delirium in the gerioperative patient and its deleterious consequences. Most important is the recognition that delirium can be prevented or minimized through diligent, targeted prevention and treatment interventions. POCD, although identified more than 60 years ago, remains an enigma in clinical practice. The use of astute clinical judgment, accurate observation, and critical attention to basic principles of perioperative care is essential to protecting and preserving cognitive function in the older adult.

KEY POINTS

- POD and POCD remain undetected, misdiagnosed, and undertreated postoperative complications in gerioperative patients.
- Delirium is one of the most common causes of cognitive impairment in hospitalized older adults.
- Delirium occurs when cognitive reserve is depleted and function can no longer be maintained. The threshold or critical level below which cognitive impairment begins to emerge is unique to the individual.
- Prevention and early detection as a standard part of geriatric care will occur only when providers recognize that delirium is predominately iatrogenic and preventable.
- Although there are many unanswered questions about causes and treatment of cognitive changes, providing the patient and family with available information will increase understanding and decrease fear of the unknown.

TWENTY-TWO

Gerioperative Pain Relief

Raelene V. Shippee–Rice, Jennifer V. Long, and Susan J. Fetzer

PATIENT REPORT: Mrs. Oakley

Mrs. Oakley is a 75-year-old woman admitted after surgery for a hip fracture. Mrs. Oakley fell after tripping over the bathroom rug. She was alert and oriented on admission but shaken by the experience. She takes alprazolam for anxiety "several times a week." She has no other medical history and takes no other prescribed medication. She does not exercise regularly and is inconsistent with her vitamin D and calcium intake. Postoperatively, Mrs. Oakley is conscious, follows directions, and responds to questions. She denies hip pain but is anxious and fidgety. She is pulling at the wound dressing and has removed it three times. The nurse is becoming frustrated and concerned. She questions Mrs. Oakley's pain level. Although Mrs. Oakley continues to deny pain, her behavior is consistent with a person having pain. The nurse wants to medicate her with morphine as ordered, but Mrs. Oakley keeps saying no.

Pain is expected after surgery. Surgery incites the physiologic and psychological stress, contributes to tissue damage, and generates hyperexcitable neural responses with increased sensitivity to noxious stimulation, resulting in heightened postoperative pain. Anesthesia further exacerbates these responses.

Up to 80% of adult patients report postoperative pain, with nearly 90% of these reporting moderate, severe, or extreme pain. More than 50% of adults over age 65 report having severe postoperative pain. In addition to surgically related pain, gerioperative patients experience pain due to aging, alterations in functional status, and comorbid diseases. Approximately 75% of community-dwelling older adults report having pain on a regular basis, with 25 to 50% reporting their pain as moderate to severe. Up to 80% of older adults living in nursing homes suffer from moderate to severe persistent pain. Musculoskeletal pain is the most common cause of pain in older adults.

Community-dwelling older adults and older adults in nursing homes may take one or more prescription medications to relieve persistent or acute pain. Over-the-counter medications and herbal remedies are also used to relieve pain. Many of these medications interfere or interact with preanesthetic medications, anesthesia, and postoperative analgesia.

Psychosocial/Health Factors
Age, gender, culture, cognition, comorbid
disease, functional status, mood state

Environmental Factors
Unit, equipment, noise/light,
room-unit activity

Preoperative Pain
Acute or persistent pain
present prior to surgery

Procedural Pain
Results from nursing or
medical procedure,
intervention, diagnostic test

Postoperative Pain
Results from surgical
invasion or operative
environment

Incident Pain
Occurs in response to activity such
as coughing, deep breathing,
moving, ambulating

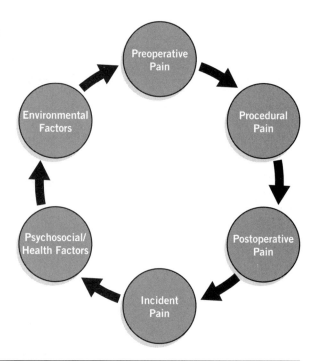

FIGURE 22.1
Context of Gerioperative Pain

Inadequate pain relief affects patient outcomes at every stage of the perioperative continuum.

Pain has a negative effect on all body systems. Inadequate perioperative pain relief can lead to poor gerioperative care outcomes. Hormonal response and physiologic sensitivity to the demands of surgical stress and trauma are increased in the presence of pain. Perioperative pain requires considerations of three key clinical concepts. First, inadequate relief of persistent preoperative pain predisposes the older adult to higher levels of postoperative pain. Second, pain is a postoperative complication that impedes surgical recovery. Finally, poor management of acute pain results in pathological changes in the aging nervous system that can lead to postsurgical persistent pain syndromes.

Recognizing the effect of age-related changes on pain perception, interpretation, behavior, and treatment creates a foundation for clinical judgment and collaborative decision-making needed to relieve pain in older adults. Pain is a complex phenomenon arising from multiple sources in the gerioperative patient and influenced by patient, environment, and provider interactions that contribute to each other and to the overall pain experience. Figure 22.1 shows the circular self-perpetuating nature of pain. This chapter examines the complex nature of gerioperative pain. Strategies are offered for enhancing pain assessment, identifying pain-related risk factors, preventing pain, and optimizing pain relief throughout the gerioperative continuum.

Gerioperative Pain Defined

McCaffery defined pain as "whatever the experiencing person says it is, existing whenever he [sic] says it does" (McCaffery & Paseo, 1999, p. 17). The International Association for the

Study of Pain uses the following terminology for classifying pain: "an unpleasant sensory and emotional experience associated with actual or potential tissue damage, or described in terms of such damage" (Merskey & Bogduk, 1994, p. 210).

The McCaffery and Pasero definition and International Association for the Study of Pain classification of pain address the subjective sensation and experience of pain, a critical perspective in optimizing pain relief with postoperative older adults. However, pain can also be considered an objective phenomenon in situations where the body, without the conscious awareness by the individual, responds physiologically to noxious stimuli. For example, a patient under anesthesia and not subjectively experiencing pain shows evidence of sympathetic responses consistent with a noxious stimuli. According to the subjective definition, the bodily response cannot be called "pain" because the person does not interpret the sensation as pain. Recognizing the potential for "objective pain" in patients without conscious interpretation of the sensation can help providers be more sensitive to the intraoperative and postoperative pain experience.

The definition of gerioperative pain reflects McCaffery and Paseo's definition and that of the International Association for the Study of Pain while keeping in mind the potential effects of noxious stimuli on physiologic responses. Gerioperative pain is defined as sensations that occur before, during, or after surgery that older adults characterize as painful or that occur in the absence of conscious interpretation. The personal and situational context in which the sensation occurs is part of the pain phenomenon.

Categories of Pain

Gerioperative pain is classified in terms of its temporal relationship to surgery, duration of pain, and type of pain. Timeframes for pain onset and duration are divided into acute or persistent, as well as according to perioperative timeline: preoperative, intraoperative, and postoperative. Pain experiences can be discrete, lasting only as long as the noxious stimuli or healing of tissue damage occurs. Type of pain is categorized by pain source: somatic, visceral, neuropathic, and nonphysical. Onset, duration, timeframe, and type of pain can overlap, creating complex patterns that challenge patients and care providers throughout the gerioperative continuum in finding ways of relieving the suffering and burden occasioned by pain.

ACUTE PAIN

Acute pain is a symptom of injury, inflammation, or disease with rapid onset or evolves over a short period of time. Preoperative surgically related acute pain is caused by the health condition requiring surgery (e.g., hip fracture or bowel obstruction). Postoperative acute pain is caused by direct tissue damage associated with the surgical procedure itself. Some evidence suggests that inflammatory reactions to general anesthesia can also cause acute postoperative pain. Medical treatments and procedures are common causes of acute gerioperative pain.

Pain from surgical procedures may be mild, moderate, or severe depending on the type of procedure and the response of the individual. Acute postoperative pain is usually of short or intermediate duration and improves as healing occurs over time. The pain is typically relieved through use of nonpharmacologic and pharmacologic interventions. Opioids are often used in the immediate postoperative period for relief of moderate to severe pain.

PERSISTENT PAIN

Persistent pain, also termed chronic pain, is defined as pain without apparent biological value that lasts beyond normal tissue healing time and is of sufficient duration or intensity to adversely affect the function or well-being of the patient. Persistent pain is considered a disease state resulting from pathophysiological changes in the peripheral and central nervous system. Exhibit 22.1 lists key points related to persistent pain in the gerioperative patient.

Continuous nerve cell activation can lead to pathophysiologic changes in pain pathways. Treatment of persistent pain often requires multimodal and interdisciplinary intervention. When assessing a patient with persistent pain, it is important to ask if the older adult has been on long-term opioid or adjuvant pain medications, such as antiepileptics and antidepressants. These medications can interact with preanesthetic medications, anesthetics, and postoperative analgesic medications. Careful monitoring is required to detect adverse drug effects and unexpected responses to dose.

PREEXISTING PAIN

Preexisting or preoperative pain is acute or persistent pain that occurs prior to surgery. The pain results from pathology related to the impending surgery, diagnostic procedures, comorbid disease, or age-related changes. When preexisting pain is inadequately relieved, pain pathways can be altered, causing increasing severity in postoperative pain. It is important for older adults with preexisting pain to receive optimal pain relief.

POSTOPERATIVE PAIN

Postoperative pain results from tissue damage and inflammation caused by surgical trauma. General anesthesia also stimulates inflammatory responses, contributing to postoperative pain severity. The experience of postoperative pain begins shortly after surgery as the patient recovers consciousness and anesthetic analgesia wanes. The patient's experience of

---

EXHIBIT 22.1 Key Points Regarding Persistent Pain in Gerioperative Patients

- Up to 72% of community-dwelling elders have moderate to severe persistent pain
- Between 50 and 83% of elders living in nursing homes report pain
- Preoperative persistent pain stems from multiple etiologies that may or may not be related to a surgical condition
- Persistent pain influences amount, type, and response to perioperative medications
- Persistent pain leads to:
  - Anxiety
  - Depression
  - Poor quality of life
  - Increased risk of falls
  - Impaired functional abilities
  - Increased health care costs
  - Higher levels of postoperative pain
  - Decrease in effectiveness of pain relief medications

postoperative pain is not limited to surgical injury. Other causes of postoperative pain are preoperative comorbid conditions, age-related changes in pain physiology, positioning during surgery, and postoperative therapeutic interventions and procedures, such as urinary catheters, nasogastric tubes, dressing changes, mobility, and deep breathing with coughing.

Over time as healing occurs, surgically related pain typically resolves. Unrelieved postoperative pain can alter pain physiology, leading to the development of persistent pain that can last weeks, months, or for an indefinite period of time after surgery.

Pain Origin

Physical pain often includes nociceptive pain and neuropathic pain. Nociceptive pain is further subdivided into somatic and visceral pain. Nonphysical pain describes suffering associated with intense or prolonged emotional, spiritual, or psychological pain. Different origins of pain necessitate different treatments. Knowing the origin of a patient's pain assists in determining effective pain assessment, prevention, and intervention choices.

SOMATIC PAIN

Somatic pain results from injury to the skin or musculoskeletal system and is usually well localized to the site of injury. Deep somatic pain that results from bone or muscle injury is perceived as "dull" or "aching." Surface somatic pain, also called cutaneous pain, is described as "sharp," "burning," or "prickling." Somatic pain can be mild, or it can be at a level of intensity to prevent the older adult from carrying out simple everyday activities. In the gerioperative patient, somatic pain may be associated with preexisting disease such as rheumatoid arthritis. Surgically related somatic pain usually occurs as a result of skin damage at the incision site or a result of direct injury or manipulation or positioning of joints, ligaments, muscle, or bone. The pain is usually well localized and often accompanied by inflammation, tenderness, and swelling. Additional sources of somatic pain in the postsurgical period are infection, coughing, excessive activity, or inactivity. Generally, nonpharmacologic interventions such as avoiding stimulation of the injured site, heat, cold, and pharmacologic interventions relieve somatic pain.

VISCERAL PAIN

Visceral pain originates in the organs of the thorax and abdomen. Stretching, distention, ischemia, smooth muscle spasm, or direct abdominal organ manipulation during surgery stimulate nociceptors. Visceral pain can be diffuse, radiating, or referred, making it difficult to determine the exact location. The pain is often felt at a site distant from the injury or damage, also known as referred pain. Jaw pain associated with a myocardial event or right scapular pain that can occur with gallbladder disease are examples of referred pain. Asking the older adult to "put a finger" on the location of visceral pain can lead to a vague waving of the hand toward a general area. Descriptors of visceral pain include "deep," "comes in waves," or a "feeling of weight or pressure." Visceral pain is often associated with a sense of distress with an overtone of threat or dread. Nausea and general malaise frequently occur with the onset of visceral pain. Intensity ranges from mild discomfort to severe, excruciating agony.

Older adults tend to be less sensitive to visceral pain, presenting a hazard when there is an acute pathology without adequate warning signals for early detection. A common example is the presence of appendicitis without complaints of the lower abdominal discomfort that are typically associated with the condition in a younger person.

Gerioperative patients with visceral pain require prompt attention and rapid diagnosis. Acute visceral pain can indicate postsurgical complications such as an ileus, urinary tract infection, a myocardial event, or a deep wound infection. The pathology may be well advanced before the older adult experiences pain.

Narcotics are frequently used to treat postoperative visceral pain. Oxycodone is more effective than morphine in treating visceral pain, particularly for patients who have had abdominal surgery. Spasmolytics are used to relieve pain originating from smooth muscle spasms.

NEUROPATHIC PAIN

Neuropathic pain is the result of injury to the spinal cord or peripheral nervous system. Compression of a spinal nerve, damage to nerves through disease such as diabetic neuropathy, nerve damage from chemotherapy and other medical treatments, or direct trauma such as limb amputation are common causes of neuropathic pain. Idiopathic neuropathic pain is caused when a dysfunction occurs in pain pathways without demonstrated physical evidence of tissue damage or injury. Age-related changes in vertebral structure or neurological function can cause idiopathic neuropathic pain. Neuropathic pain often lasts for long periods of time, leading to physical and emotional suffering. The pain is described as "burning," "sharp," "electric," or "deep and aching." Patients often complain of hyperesthesia or hyperanalgesia.

Treatment of neuropathic pain is difficult, often requiring multimodal and multidisciplinary interventions. In addition to analgesic medications, treatment can require the use of adjuvant medications such as antidepressants, anticonvulsants, anxiolytics, or antipsychotic medications. Onset and efficacy of adjuvant medications can be days to weeks, though use of these drugs is usually limited to patients with longstanding severe pain. Abrupt cessation of medications used to treat neuropathic pain, particularly antidepressant, anxiolytic, or narcotic medications, can lead to withdrawal symptoms. If neuropathic pain medications are discontinued, early detection of withdrawal symptoms and prevention of associated adverse effects depend on vigilant systematic monitoring. Medications for neuropathic pain should be restarted immediately after surgery to maintain continued pain relief. Nondrug interventions can be useful in combination with other pain relief methods, such as transcutaneous electrical nerve stimulation (TENS). Relaxation, hypnosis, physical therapy, and application of heat or ice are also effective.

NONPHYSICAL PAIN

Older adults experience pain without evidence of obvious tissue damage. Persistent physical pain, loss, grief, and social isolation can trigger pain sensations. Nonphysical pain is sometimes referred to as somatic psychological distress, emotional pain, suffering, mental anguish, or spiritual distress. Older adults experience high rates of change in health status, impaired ability to carry out activities of daily living, and loss of friends and loved ones that contribute to grief, emotional distress, and suffering that result in the sensation of pain. Nonphysical pain can be acute or persistent and can occur at any time during the perioperative care continuum.

Nonphysical pain is based on physiological changes and needs to be treated as seriously as physical pain.

Nonphysical pain is associated with changes in physiology. Responses in the limbic system and cingulate gyrus participate in the experience of nonphysical pain. Strong emotions trigger a neurochemical cascade inducing autonomic responses such as pallor, nausea, and changes in blood pressure and heart rate. The brain interprets the intense emotional sensation as pain. This autonomic response is similar to that evoked by physical pain.

Using language that infers pain is psychological or emotionally based without physical findings can evoke negative connotations, causing the patient's pain experience to be discounted. When an older adult describes a sensation as "pain," the pain is real to the person regardless of origin. Experiencing nonphysical pain escalates physical pain severity. Similarly, physical pain can escalate nonphysical pain. Being cognizant of the interaction between nonphysical and physical pain and the interaction on health outcomes is basic to effective gerioperative pain relief. Nonphysical pain should receive the same attention in assessment and treatment as that accorded to acute postoperative physical pain. Attending to nonphysical pain can be an intervention for physical pain.

Physiology of Pain

Pain is a safety mechanism alerting the organism to danger or injury from an external source or to harmful changes in internal body functions. The sensation of pain signals the need to take self-protective action to prevent further threat or damage to the system.

> *Pain is a self-protective physiologic mechanism essential for survival.*

Somatic pain involves nociceptors, which are specialized cells in the peripheral nervous system located in skin, bone, muscle, and some visceral organs. Nociceptors react to noxious stimuli such as direct mechanical or thermal injury. Injury triggers an inflammatory response that releases chemical mediators such as prostaglandins, histamines, and serotonin. The mediators further stimulate nociceptor response. Action potentials in nociceptors transmit signals to the dorsal horn of the spinal cord via peripheral sensory nerve fibers. Ascending spinal cord tracts transmit the sensation to the reticular activating system in the brainstem to the hypothalamus and thalamus. From the thalamus, the signal is transmitted simultaneously to other areas of the brain, particularly the somatosensory cortex, cingulate gyrus in the limbic system, and frontal cortex. It is in these areas that perception, interpretation, localization, and emotional-behavioral responses occur. It is at this point that the stimulus is translated as "pain." See Figure 22.2 for an overview of pain pathways.

Thus, pain is the result of the highly complex interactions that occur among motor, sensory, associative, autonomous, and limbic systems. The complex nature of acute pain and the even more complex neurophysiological changes associated with persistent pain challenge providers desiring to provide effective pain relief.

Pain modulation involves changing or inhibiting central nervous system transmission of pain impulses. As sensory information ascends the spinal cord and enters the cerebrum, neuromodulators in the spinal cord and brain are activated. Endogenous opioids (endorphins and enkephalins) and neurotransmitters (serotonin and norepinephrine) are activated by the brain to inhibit the transmission of pain signals. The endogenous opioids bind with opioid receptors in the brain and at the dorsal horn of the spinal cord to block pain impulses at both the presynaptic and postsynaptic junctions. These junctions are also the site of action of opioid medications. Endorphins are the major contributor to stress analgesia, the ability of an organism to continue to function under conditions of extreme pain.

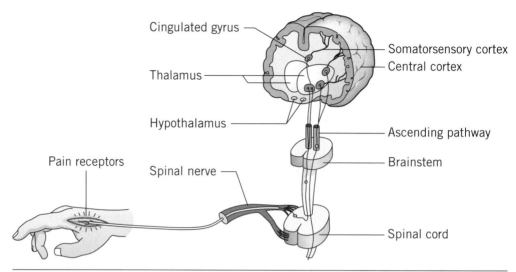

FIGURE 22.2
Pain Pathways

Facilitatory spinal fibers are descending pathways that increase sensory information and pain sensitivity. The increased sensitivity acts like an early alarm system to increase protective responses. Disruptions in the facilitatory process result in pain hypersensitivity and hyperalgesia. The altered function in the facilitatory modulating system that can occur as a result of surgical trauma or unrelieved pain is a potential factor in postoperative persistent pain syndromes. Adequate pain relief is central to maintaining normal pain mechanisms and preventing development of pathophysiological processes.

Surgical trauma damages tissues through direct stimulation of nociceptors in skin, musculoskeletal, or visceral tissues. Prostaglandins, histamine, and serotonin release bradykinin in response to the direct tissue damage. Bradykinin is a proinflammatory substance released in response to nocioceptor stimulation and a major chemical mediator enhancing nociceptor response. The presence of bradykinin may account for lingering pain sensations after the immediate pain cause is removed.

In addition to the direct trauma and inflammation caused by the surgical procedure, emerging evidence indicates that general anesthesia provokes neurogenic inflammatory processes. When added to the inflammatory response induced by surgical trauma, anesthesia-induced nociceptor stimulation further contributes to perioperative pain.

Pain threshold is the level of stimulus needed to trigger a pain response in an individual. Patients with higher thresholds have greater tolerance to noxious stimuli before perceiving the presence of pain. Lower thresholds mean there is less tolerance to noxious stimuli, and a pain sensation is elicited more readily. Patients with pain sensitization have lowered pain thresholds.

Pain sensitization occurs whenever injured tissue is subjected to intense, repeated, or prolonged pain stimuli. Peripheral sensitization lowers the level of pain stimulus necessary to activate nociceptors. Sensitization of peripheral nerve fibers results in a greater and more persistent barrage of nerve impulses firing to the central nervous system. Central sensitization is a long-term change in the nerve cells of the spinal cord and pain centers in the brain as a result of the continuing barrage of pain impulses from peripheral nerves. Once sensitization occurs, hyperalgesia results, when even a minor stimulation can elicit an intensified response. Sensitization can lead to onset of persistent pain from nerve cell dysfunction.

Pain interpretation is the meaning attached to a noxious stimulus. The same stimulus can be interpreted differently carrying different meanings. For example, pinching and tweaking the skin can be experienced as painful when caused by an irritating family member. Similar pinching and tweaking may be pleasurable when initiated by a significant other.

Beliefs about pain etiology influence pain perception. Patients who have a positive interpretation of their pain have a more positive affect regardless of pain severity. For example, many elder Chinese adults consider pain a positive sign of healing after surgery. Thus, pain assessment should involve information on pain affect, as well as pain intensity. Although patients establish a pain intensity level, the affect attached to the pain may not be at the same level of intensity. Intervention strategies are modified based on the interaction between pain intensity and pain affect. The context of the pain situation influences both pain intensity and the meaning the patient attaches to the stimulus.

AGE-RELATED CHANGES

Age-related changes result in an increase or decrease in pain sensation, perception, threshold, interpretation, and response. Changes in pain sensation and perception result from changes in number of nociceptors, alteration in nociception transmission, demyelinization of central and peripheral nerve fibers, decrease in the size and number of central nervous system neurons, and slowed response to neurotransmitters and neuromodulators. Although receptors may transmit pain signals more slowly, the response to pain may be more acute or severe due to reduced pain modulation in descending nerve pathways.

As age increases, the number of opioid receptors and the concentration of endogenous opioid-like substances in the spinal cord decrease. Changes in the efficacy of these endogenous analgesic systems reduce the ability of older adults to cope with severe pain. The reduced modulation reduces pain protective mechanisms such as muscle guarding and withdrawal. These age-related changes limit the reliability of behavioral cues. Changes in brain and spinal cord neurotransmitters and neuromodulators alter events in the facilitative and inhibitory pain pathways.

Older adults require higher levels of noxious stimulation to reach pain thresholds. Slowing of information processing time in the central nervous system increases the time needed to interpret the afferent sensation as pain, locate the pain site, and respond. The slowed response can increase the patient's exposure to harmful stimuli or disease progression, resulting in more extensive tissue damage. As tissue damage increases, inflammation increases, further intensifying pain.

A common myth among health care providers is that "age dulls the sense of pain," a misinterpretation of an increased pain threshold. An increased pain threshold does not mean less pain; it means pain, as an alert system signaling a problem, is not functioning effectively. By the time the pain threshold is triggered, the underlying pathology or damage can be extensive, increasing the risk of more serious consequences. In reality, older adults have more intense pain, but by the time they have pain, the damage resulting from the injury is more severe and the signal more intense. Understanding the relationship among higher pain thresholds, increased risk of damage to the organism, and sensitivity to pain is critical when caring for the gerioperative patient. Changes in pain transmission, transduction, and modulation demand that care providers be more alert and responsive when older adults complain of pain. Table 22.1 identifies provider and patient myths about pain and aging.

TABLE 22.1

Common Patient and Provider Pain Myths That Interfere With Effective Pain Relief

Myths	Facts
Older adults have less pain	Older adults are as sensitive to pain as younger age adults Condition may be more severe before pain indicated
Pain is a normal part of aging	Pain is due to pathophysiological changes
Older adults should not take opioids	Opioids are safe for use in older adults if carefully titrated and monitored
Morphine is addicting	Therapeutic use of morphine for acute pain is rarely addicting
You should wait until you really need pain medication before using it or it will not work	Early intervention is more effective and leads to better outcomes
Medication is the best form of pain relief	Nonpharmacologic pain relief methods are effective in relieving mild to moderate pain or as adjuncts for severe pain
Old people complain about everything	Old people complain when they have pain. Older people are at higher risk for pain due to age- and disease-related changes

Undertreated Pain Outcomes

Pain, regardless of severity or origin, leads to adverse affects and contributes to negative gerioperative outcomes, as shown in Table 22.2. Moderate to severe acute pain stimulates sympathetic response mechanisms increase heart rate, blood pressure, and myocardial oxygen consumption. Although age-related changes slow these autonomic responses, severe pain present in older adults at risk for a cardiac event can trigger myocardial ischemia. Unrelieved pain increases insulin resistance and interferes with glucose metabolism, increasing blood sugar.

Inadequate pain relief can affect all organ systems, increasing the older patient's vulnerability to postoperative complications. Pain delays wound healing, increases postsurgical infection, and contributes to constipation and paralytic ileus. Moderate to severe pain interferes with the patient's participation in postsurgical recovery activities, increasing the risk for atelectasis, pneumonia, deep vein thrombosis, and deconditioning. Pain increases energy expenditure and decreases appetite, interfering with hydration and caloric intake. Many older adults are in a catabolic state after surgery.

Uncontrolled pre- and postoperative pain in older adults results in loss of functional abilities, increased health care costs, and impaired quality of life.

Pain interrupts sleep patterns, increases anxiety, and contributes to depression. Uncontrolled or poorly controlled pain is identified as a risk factor for delirium, postoperative cognitive dysfunction, depression, and postsurgical persistent pain syndromes. Loss of functional ability, increased health care costs, and impaired quality of life have been associated with poor pain relief.

Poorly managed acute pain is associated with development of persistent pain that can cause long-term functional impairment. Attention to pain relief at all stages of the perioperative continuum can improve patient outcomes, decrease hospital length of stay, and lower health care costs. Systematic pain monitoring and an interdisciplinary integrated plan of

TABLE 22.2
Outcomes of Undertreated Pain

Organ System	Pain Effects	Consequences
Respiratory	Reduced cough Decreased lung excursion Sputum retention Hypoxemia	Pneumonia Atelectasis
Cardiovascular	Increased myocardial oxygen demand Cardiac ischemia	Myocardial infarction
Musculoskeletal	Impaired mobility Impaired activities of daily living	Pressure ulcers Depression Deep vein thrombosis Deconditioning
Genitourinary	Urinary retention	Urinary tract infection
Endocrine	Impaired glycemic control Protein catabolism Sodium retention	Increased insulin resistance Pressure ulcers Poor wound healing Increased risk of infection
Gastrointestinal	Decreased gastric emptying Reduced intestinal motility	Poor nutrition Constipation Partial ileus
Psychoemotional	Depression	Increased suffering, anxiety, Psychological distress
Neurological	Hypersensivity of nocireceptors Impaired sleep pattern	Persistent pain Fatigue Delirium
Immune system	Decreased immune response	Increased risk of infection
Overall system effects	Postoperative complications	Increased length of hospital stay Increased risk of hospital readmission

care that spans the perioperative continuum are needed to achieve continuous, effective pain relief and optimize patient outcomes.

Assessing Gerioperative Pain

QUANTIFYING THE SUBJECTIVE EXPERIENCE

Effective pain relief depends on accurate pain assessment. Accurate assessment depends on coordinating data from multiple sources. Data includes patient self-report, provider observation of patient behavior, recognition of individual variation in age-related changes in pain physiology, level of surgical trauma, and influence of comorbid diseases.

Assessing gerioperative pain can be difficult. Pain occurs within the patient, but the power to treat and relieve pain rests in the hands of providers. Patients often need to "sell" their pain to get attention and intervention. Providers and patients have differing levels of knowledge, attitudes, and beliefs regarding the experience and meaning of pain, and pain treatment. These differences create barriers to effective communication about pain and effective pain relief. Quality pain assessment rests on provider sensitivity to pain as a subjective experience and a perspective that the evaluation of pain by a third person is inherently incomplete and potentially harmful.

The presence of pain in older adults is more than a physical sensation. Pain raises concerns about being ill, fear of increasing dependency, and fear of becoming a burden. Fears about pain causation and its potential for progression, as well as concerns about medication effects, especially the possibility of addiction, lead older patients to ignore pain or minimize its severity.

Providers have inadequate preparation about aging effects on pain physiology or the effects of surgical trauma on aging pain physiology. A common myth among care providers is that older adults do not have pain as acute as that experienced by younger age groups. The extensive literature on adverse effects of medications leads many providers to limit analgesia for older adults.

The lack of knowledge and misconceptions about pain, pain relief interventions, and the effects of inadequate pain relief on surgical outcomes among providers and older adults create complex and multilayered barriers to accurate pain assessment and effective intervention. Common myths are listed in Table 22.1. Providers must evaluate the adequacy of their knowledge and the effect of personal beliefs about pain and aging before they are able to effectively manage the challenges in assessing pain and providing adequate pain relief to the gerioperative patient. Equally important, providers need to provide older adults and their families with accurate information and decisional support that facilitates pain assessment.

Patient self-reports are the gold standard in pain assessment. Family members and providers are poor predictors of a patient's pain level. Family members are more likely to overrate an older person's pain, while nurses and other health care providers tend to underestimate pain. Provider and family overrating or underestimating pain severity, intensity, and effect leads to poor pain relief.

Older adults often use vague verbal descriptors such as "pretty uncomfortable," "feeing sore," "aching," "being tired," or "not feeling well." When asked short or single sentence closed questions about pain, older adults respond with short, closed answers omitting critical details. Care provider–patient communication based on simple questions and short answers shuts down communication and limits the information sharing needed to make accurate pain assessment and intervention decisions. Eliciting a clear description of pain characteristics and severity from an older adult rests on the ability to establish rapport, listen carefully, and ask follow-up questions in response to verbal and nonverbal cues.

Older adults are reluctant to talk about pain. They do not want to be viewed as complainers or burdens. They want to be "good patients" and not bother nurses busy caring for patients "who are sicker." They want to protect their family members, who may be busy with their own lives, working or taking care of children. Admitting to pain or asking for assistance implies a need for help and the risk for becoming dependent on others. Beliefs that care providers do not care about or believe what they say about their pain create additional barriers to talking about their pain.

Patient self-report methods using standardized tools include descriptor, numeric, or illustrated ratings that are patient-directed or provider-directed. Patient-directed self-report asks older adults to describe their pain using their own words or a scale they devise. Provider-directed patient self-report asks patients to describe their pain using words, illustrations, or numbers provided by someone else or by a standard tool.

A drawback of single end-point tools is the limited information elicited about the patient's pain.

Patient-directed self-report begins with the patient's story. Listening to the patient demonstrates empathy, attentiveness, interest in the patient's experience, and commitment to helping the patient achieve pain relief. Attending to the patient's story of pain reinforces the dictum to treat the person not the pain.

The initial step in patient-directed self-reporting pain assessment is asking the older adult to describe the pain experience in their own words. Follow-up assessment of the patient's story is used to clarify elements of the patient's description and ensure that key elements of a pain assessment are reviewed: pain characteristics, intensity, location, duration, and alleviating or aggravating factors. For the gerioperative patient, it is important to ask how pain affects the patient's ability to complete postoperative pain activities and exercises.

Important to hearing the patient's pain description is attending to the words used by the patient to describe their pain. Asking patients what words they use to distinguish between mild, moderate, and severe pain further clarifies pain severity and intensity. Table 22.3 provides an example of a patient's response when asked how he would describe the differences between mild, moderate, and severe pain.

Health care providers can then continue using the patient's pain words and descriptors as a consistent framework for ongoing assessment and reassessment. Using the patient's words shows respect and avoids misinterpretations. The frames of reference created by different terminology and word usage can result in ineffective or inappropriate interventions.

The mnemonic WILDA (Fink, 2000) incorporates five elements of pain assessment: *w*ords, *i*ntensity, *l*ocation, *d*uration, and *a*lleviating or *a*ggravating factors. Including an "F" to represent function is an adaptation of the original WILDA that is important in assessing the gerioperative patient (Table 22.4). WILDA(F) is an easy tool for health care providers to use in the clinical setting and for families to use after the patient is discharged.

Provider-directed patient self-report uses standardized pain tools with predetermined provider language or methods. Standardized tools were established to provide consistency in pain care and to evaluate intervention effectiveness in relieving pain. Most standardized pain assessment tools are based on a visual analog, numeric rating, or similar Likert-type instruments that ask the patient to indicate pain intensity or severity on a scale ranging from no pain to severe pain.

Pain assessment tools used in acute care or ambulatory surgical centers for use with older adults are selected by a team of providers or a clinical committee as part of a pain protocol or standard of care. Protocols usually limit providers to using the tools identified in the protocol, rather than a tool selected by the gerioperative patient or one directed to the patient's needs and abilities.

The majority of tools are one-dimensional, scaled, and ask only about the patient's current pain severity, intensity, or a reassessment of changes in pain severity and intensity after intervention. A drawback to the single end-point tool is the limited information elicited about other important elements of the patient's pain experience. Unless care providers seek additional information about pain characteristics, onset, location, duration, and effect of pain on function, treatment decisions are based on incomplete, inaccurate, or misinterpretation of the data. The utility of single point systems for accurate pain assessment and effective pain relief in older adults remains in question.

No single pain tool is effective for use with all older adults across the perioperative continuum. Multiple factors influence the older adult's ability to use a pain assessment tool effectively: age-related cognitive changes, level of cognitive function, sensory functioning, clinical condition, health status, sociocultural influences, and personal preference. A major issue in perioperative care is the need to have a tool that can be used or adapted appropriately for

TABLE 22.3

Describing Pain Using Patient Descriptors

Mild	"Hurts some."
Moderate	"It hurts."
Severe	"Hurts like hell."

TABLE 22.4

WILDA(F) Mnemonic for Pain

Letters	Key Factors	Description
W	Words	Ask the patient to describe his/her pain or discomfort using words or qualifiers. Identifying the qualifiers enhances understanding of the patient's pain cause and should optimize pain treatment.
I	Intensity	Pain intensity should be evaluated at the present level, least, worst, at rest, or with movement. A personal comfort goal describing the level of pain that will allow functional and psychosocial comfort can also be elicited. A reassessment of pain experienced after analgesic or adjuvant drug administration, and/or use of nonpharmacologic approaches can also add information about the patient's level of pain after intervention. Pain intensity can be measured quantitatively with the use of a visual analog scale, numeric rating scale, or verbal descriptor scale.
L	Location	Ask where the pain(s) is located. Ask patient to identify all pain sources or location.
D	Duration	Understanding whether the pain is persistent, intermittent, or both will guide the intervention selection. Ask how long the patient had the pain. Ask if the pain is recent or longstanding.
A	Aggravating or alleviating factors	Ask the patient what makes the pain worse or better.
F	Function	How does the pain affect prehabilitation or post surgical activities.

Adapted with permission from Fink, R. (2000) Pain assessment: the cornerstone to optimal pain management. *Baylor University Medical Center Proceedings*, 13(3), 236-239.

use in preoperative assessment, and later, when the older adult is in a different clinical condition. The use of self-report scales rests on the functional ability of the person to use the scale. Before selecting a standardized assessment scale, a functional assessment is needed to evaluate the patient's ability to use the scale reliably and validly.

The McGill Pain Questionnaire and Brief Pain Inventory are multidimensional tools employing a comprehensive framework for pain assessment. A drawback to these multidimensional scales is the time required to complete the assessment, limiting their use in busy clinical settings.

Several pain assessment tools have been promoted as effective and useful for older adults. Studies are needed to explore the feasibility and benefit of using a single assessment tool across the care continuum. Using the same assessment scales across the perioperative continuum can facilitate continuity of care. The tool becomes familiar to the older adult, potentially making results more reliable.

Numerical rating scales, verbal descriptors, and FACES Pain Scales are easy for older adults to use. The Visual Analog Scale has been identified as difficult for many older adults because of the level of abstract thinking and cognitive processing required; its use is not recommended.

When using any pain scale, coaching the older adult is important in improving familiarity and ease of use. Providing time for practice sessions before using a pain scale in the clinical setting improves reliability in the individual patient. Verbal and visual cueing is important each time the older adult is asked to use a specific scale to rate pain severity. Older adults in pain or in unfamiliar environments may not retain information from one session to another.

Cueing allows for a gentle reminder that helps the older person recall the purpose of the pain assessment, the specific tool being used, and how to use the tool.

Older adults who rely on hearing aids or glasses need to have them clean and in place before being asked to use a pain scale that depends on adequate vision or hearing ability. Scales requiring adequate vision are the Visual Analog Scale, FACES Pain Scale, and the pain thermometer. The Visual Descriptor Scale requires the patient to be able to hear or read the words. Adapting visual scales is important. Enlarged font type, darkened print, illustrations and lines, and printing the assessment scales on no-glare paper can improve visibility and ease of use. Making these adaptations will benefit all older adults, not just those with moderate to severe visual impairment. Poor hospital lighting, fatigue, and medications can interfere with visual acuity, even in patients with minimal impairment.

Pain tool selection is based on the older person's functional abilities and comfort with the tool and should be consistent with the person's functional abilities. The selected tool should be documented so that all members of the health care team can be consistent in pain assessment throughout the perioperative process. However, a change in the patient's condition can necessitate reevaluation of the pain assessment process including the assessment tool. Any changes in the pain assessment process including the reason for the change should be documented and the information should be handed off to all members of the care team to ensure continuity of care. Table 22.5 identifies items to consider when selecting and using pain scales.

GERIOPERATIVE PAIN AND COGNITIVE IMPAIRMENT

An inability to communicate pain-related needs makes older adults more vulnerable to the consequences of under-treated or unrelieved pain. Yet, gerioperative patients with cognitive impairment or impaired communication have

Understanding sources of patient-provider pain miscommunication improves pain relief effectiveness.

TABLE 22.5

Pain Scale Considerations for Gerioperative Patients

Tool familiarity	• Use same tool across perioperative continuum unless changes in patient's clinical condition requires different tool
Adapting pain scales	• Large font • Dark print • Darkened illustrations • No-glare paper • Consider cognitive function • Consider clinical condition
Patient preference	• Pilot test variety of tools with patient • Collaborate with patient in selecting tool
Patient cueing	• Review tool purpose and instructions before each use
Provider pain assessment	• Location • Duration • Change in intensity • Characteristics
Document	• Name of tool • Initial findings • Changes in intensity • Patient comfort and ability using tool

Behavior change may be the only evidence of pain.

pain assessed less often and receive less medication than older adults without cognitive or communication changes.

Cognitive and communication impairment can be a preexisting condition or occur after anesthesia, surgical stress, or medical interventions. When assessing pain, impaired cognition and impaired communication require special considerations. Although self-report continues to be the gold standard when assessing pain in persons with limited verbal or cognitive skills, the pain assessment process must be matched to the needs and abilities of the patient. Asking older adults if they hurt and where they hurt remain critical questions that must be included as part of the pain assessment process. Self-report in older adults with cognition changes must be combined with observation and use of clinical judgment. When assessment findings are inconclusive, applying nonpharmacologic pain interventions provides a form of differential diagnosis. Occasionally, it may be necessary to use mild pharmacological interventions if observed behaviors continue. If behavioral symptoms continue after pharmacological intervention, an interdisciplinary consult should be considered.

Impaired cognition and communication are not barriers to pain assessment, but they do make accurate and comprehensive pain assessment more challenging. Cognitive impairment, depression, medication, and other factors can lead patients to have misconceptions about pain by either exaggerating or minimizing pain sensations. The older person with cognitive changes or impaired communication needs time to process and respond to questions. Assessment takes longer and requires a calm, focused communication process that relies heavily on nonverbal and behavioral cues. Exhibit 22.2 lists guidelines for assessing pain in older adults with cognitive or communication impairment.

Behavioral changes can be the first signs of pain in patients with impaired communication or cognition. Pain-related behavioral cues include facial grimacing, wincing, frowning,

---

EXHIBIT 22.2 Guidelines for Assessing Pain in Older Adults With Cognitive or Communication Impairment

- Establish and implement pain prevention strategies for known procedural, postoperative, and incident pain
- Appreciate that pain assessment will take longer
- Establish systematic pain assessment and reassessment plan
- Ask the older adult if he or she is in pain (Yes/No)
- Ask older adult to point to pain location: Where does it hurt?
- Observe patient behaviors to validate pain presence and pain location
- When necessary, ask companion-coach or family member about pain behaviors
- Implement nonpharmacologic interventions if cues suggest pain; conduct follow-up reassessment
- Conduct analgesia trial with reassessment if behaviors indicate continuing pain after nonpharmacologic intervention
- Continue to titrate nonpharmacologic and pharmacologic intervention until patient's verbal responses and observed behaviors indicate pain relief
- If patient behaviors continue to indicate distress, request immediate interdisciplinary team consult

muscle guarding, lack of movement, restlessness, rocking or fidgeting, moaning, changes in breathing pattern, or diaphoresis. Older adults with dementia demonstrating aggressive or fear-directed behaviors are often reflecting pain sensations. Behaviors include slapping at care providers, crying, withdrawal, or restlessness. Sudden onset of new behaviors requires immediate attention and follow-up investigation. Behavior change may be the only evidence of pain and an impending crisis. Often, family caregivers can help interpret behavioral cues and provide information indicating pain, illness, or other discomfort.

Pain assessment tools based on behavioral findings remain in development. Two tools have been tested for postoperative pain assessment in older adults with severe cognitive impairment: the Checklist of Nonverbal Pain Indicators and the Pain Assessment in Advanced Dementia. Both tools need further testing to determine reliability and validity with older adults in the perioperative clinical environment.

It is important for care providers to recognize that personal and professional attitudes, beliefs, and level of knowledge contribute to pain misconceptions. When making clinical judgments and decisions about pain assessment and treatment of older adults who have limited cognitive or communication ability, health care providers must collect data from multiple sources, including the observation of verbal and nonverbal cues, comparison of current findings with previous information, and coordination of current data with the patient's history.

VARIABLES IN PAIN ASSESSMENT

The combination of age and cultural norms compounds the difficulty of pain assessment and the use of standardized tools. It is important to remember that the population of older adults is composed of cohorts who are subcultures with their own cultural values and norms. Age, gender, religion, and geographical region constitute subcultures with norms and values that shape pain experiences.

> *Understanding the differences in verbal and nonverbal pain expressions across age cohorts and cultural backgrounds facilitates pain assessment.*

Age Cohorts

Age cohorts, the time period when a person was born, create subcultures. In the United States, people born in the 1920s and1930s, known as the Depression era, have significantly different attitudes about pain than those born after World War II, known as baby boomers. In the Depression era, pain due to trauma and childbirth was common. People did not visit physicians on a regular basis, had few medications for

> *Quality pain care can be achieved by working closely with the patient, family, professional interpreters, and members of the health care team.*

pain relief, and relied on home remedies for treatment of ailments. After World War II, health care became readily available, medication use increased, and there was less reliance on home remedies and more on medical intervention.

Historical events and the availability of health care have shaped pain beliefs and attitudes of older adults in other cultures and ethnic backgrounds. When asked if they are having pain or if their pain is relieved, older adults may nod "yes" because it is the "expected" or "good" response; the nod may not reflect the reality of the situation. In some cultures, for example with patients of eastern European descent, a head nod actually may mean "no." The older adult's willingness to discuss pain, the way pain is described, nonverbal behaviors, and affective responses are all shaped by cultural background and ethnicity. Providers must always validate behavioral cues.

Variations in pain sensitivity and tolerance are manifested differently across gender and cultural groups. Studies of pain severity reports in men and women show mixed results depending on study population age, setting, clinical situation, type of pain, and duration of pain experience. Differences in verbal and nonverbal language norms in peoples from different cultures, countries, races, and ethnicities create challenges to standardizing pain assessment in the hospitalized surgical older adult. When possible, it is helpful to ask the older adult or family member about pain beliefs, attitudes, and how pain is usually described.

Determining nonverbal behaviors associated with pain is important. African Americans or Asians traditionally indicate higher pain levels. Italian Americans express pain more readily and emotionally. Cultural expressions of pain may not be consistent with the level of pain experienced by the patient. In some cultures, stoicism is a way of coping with severe pain, while in other cultures, crying and wailing, even if pain is mild or moderate, is the accepted coping method. Exhibit 22.3 identifies strategies to facilitate culturally appropriate pain assessment.

Pain assessment tools that can be used with patients from diverse cultures are the 21-Point Numeric Rating Scale, FACES Pain Scale, Verbal Descriptor Scale, Brief Pain Inventory, and Iowa Pain Temperature scales. Several pain scales have been translated into multiple languages. Translation resources can be found at www.britishpainsociety.org and www.painknowledge.org.

While it is difficult to maintain expertise on cultural pain beliefs, attitudes, expressions, and treatments, it is important for health providers to bracket their beliefs and assumptions about what the patient believes or needs regarding pain relief. Demonstrating a willingness to listen and learn about pain attitudes and beliefs facilitates a more culturally congruent plan, which is important for achieving the patient's goal for pain relief.

Pain scales can be useful but should not be the sole dimension in assessing pain in older adults. The choice of instrument cannot be based solely on the provider or the institution. The selection of pain tools must be based on patient preference, ease of use, unique needs, and ability of the patient. Relying solely on assessment scales limits knowledge about type, quality, and location of the patient's pain. Pain scales cannot differentiate between new onset and

---

EXHIBIT 22.3 Strategies to Facilitate Culturally Appropriate Assessment

- Use assessment tools preferred by the individual
- Appreciate variations in affective response to pain
- Be sensitive to variations in communication styles
- Recognize that communication of pain may not be acceptable within a culture
- Appreciate that the meaning of pain varies between cultures
- Using knowledge of biological variations in pain sensation and pain relief
- Develop personal awareness of values and beliefs which may affect providers' interpretation and treatment
- Acknowledge the patient's perception, interpretation, and response to pain
- Arrange for professional interpreter for cultural pain norms as well as use of pain scales or verbal translation
- Incorporate patient-selected decision-makers per patient request

Adapted from Davidhizer and Giger (2004).

ongoing pain, between pain expected from surgical trauma and pain due to the development of complications, or between preexisting and surgical pain. Health providers must coordinate pain data from multiple sources and data from clinical judgment when making clinical decisions about pain prevention and treatment interventions. Findings and interventions must be documented and communicated to other care providers to ensure consistent, patient-centered pain care across the perioperative continuum.

Gerioperative Care

PREOPERATIVE CONSIDERATIONS

Optimal physical, emotional, and psychological pain relief is a major goal of gerioperative care. Uncontrolled pain or pain that interferes with a patient's functional ability should be carefully evaluated prior to surgery. Achieving high levels of pain relief before surgery decreases psychological distress, improves surgical outcomes, and decreases risk of postsurgical persistent pain.

A goal during the preoperative pain assessment is to identify pain-related risk factors and treatment regimens, determine needs for patient teaching, and establish a plan of care for assessing and relieving pain throughout the perioperative continuum. A comprehensive assessment analyzes the actual and potential effect of the patient's past and current pain history on postoperative pain. The preoperative interview is an opportunity to share information, review options, and initiate pain relief decisions.

HEALTH HISTORY AND PAIN ASSESSMENT

A history of current illnesses and health conditions is an essential element in preoperative pain assessment. Degenerative diseases such as diabetic neuropathy, osteoporosis, osteoarthritis, cancer, diverticulitis, peripheral vascular disease, angina, and degenerative spine disease are the most common causes of persistent somatic, visceral, or neuropathic pain in older adults. Exhibit 22.4 lists common sources of preoperative pain.

EXHIBIT 22.4 Sources of Preoperative and Persistent Pain

- Musculoskeletal pain
  - Osteoarthritis
  - Fibromyalgia
  - Gout
  - Postfracture
  - Vertebral collapse
  - Vertebral fracture
  - Osteoporosis
  - Rheumatoid arthritis
  - Polymyalgia rheumatica
  - Muscle spasms, leg cramps
- Cancer-related pain
- Cardiovascular disease
- Peripheral vascular disease
- Poststroke pain
- Soft-tissue damage
  - Skin ulcers
- Neuropathic pain
  - Diabetic neuropathy
  - Age-related neuropathy
  - Idiopathic neuropathy
  - Vascular neuropathy
  - Post herpes neuralgia

EXHIBIT 22.5 **Pain Risk Factors Assessed During Preoperative Screening**

- Cognition
- Mental status
- Vision and hearing
- Depression
- Anxiety

Pain caused by different etiologies results in a range of pain characteristics that require different interventions with varying levels of pain relief. The pain experienced from different etiologies creates differences in physiological, emotional, and psychological responses. Each pain source requires a comprehensive assessment.

Preoperative depression and cognitive impairment are risk factors for increased levels of postoperative pain. Changes in cognition can influence the ability of elders to effectively report pain using standardized pain assessment tools. Thus, preoperative screening with older adults at risk for depression or the presence of cognitive changes is important in achieving perioperative pain relief. Chapters 20 and 21 offer descriptions of screening tools for assessing depression and cognition. Findings from the screening assessment suggest if any adaptations are needed for conducting an effective pain assessment. Exhibit 22.5 lists items to be included in screening assessment.

Exhibit 22.6 lists topics to include in a comprehensive pain assessment. Using the human figures (Figure 22.3) allows the patient to point to the site(s) of acute or chronic pain. In a self-assessment, the patient can mark the site of acute pain with an "X" and chronic or persistent pain with a "Y." The pain assessment considers each pain site for pain type, characteristics, location, duration, triggers or aggravating factors, alleviating factors, impact on functional ability, cause of pain, and meaning of pain. Different types, sources of pain, or causation can have separate meanings. For example, pain in the abdomen may be linked with cancer-related pain while pain in the knee may be due to osteoarthritis. The meaning of pain is important in assessing patient anxiety about potential causes of pain related to the proposed surgery. Discussing pain causation and meaning of pain for the patient can decrease preoperative anxiety.

Pain assessment lays the foundation for a plan of care that will prevent unnecessary pain and effectively treat pain when it occurs. Preoperative pain assessment is multifaceted and includes a history of the older adult's past and current pain experiences, comprehensive health care history, and physical examination related to acute and persistent physical and nonphysical pain. Many preoperative pain checklists and self-assessment tools are designed to be completed by the patient. Examples of self-assessment tools are the Brief Pain Inventory and the Brief Impact Questionnaire. Both tools are multidimensional and assess for pain severity, functional interference, and impact of pain on psychosocial well-being.

During the preoperative interview, the nurse should evaluate the patient's ability to complete a self-administered questionnaire before giving the document to the patient. Barriers to self-administration include language, vision, cognition, functional capacity, pain, and fatigue. A family member or friend accompanying the patient or the interviewer can assist at the patient's request or if the patient is unable to complete the self-assessment independently. Reviewing the completed assessment tool with the older adult helps to ensure accuracy and completeness of the information.

Prescription and over-the-counter medications, herbal remedies, and all oral or topical preparations used to relieve pain must be carefully reviewed and documented. Documented

EXHIBIT 22.6 Guidelines for Preoperative Pain Assessment

Assessment Topic	Suggested Questions
Current or present pain	<ul><li>Ask if the patient is have any pain or discomfort at the present time or within the past week that is related to the planned surgery.</li><li>Ask if the patient has had any pain in the past week due to causes other than the reason for the planned surgery.</li><li>If no to both questions, reword using ache, hurts, or soreness.</li></ul>
Pain language	<ul><li>Discover the pain language/words the patient uses; use the same language/words unless the patient indicates otherwise.</li><li>Ask what words the patient uses most often to describe pain.</li><li>Prompts if the patient asks for explanation: sore, achy, uncomfortable, hurts, funny feeling.</li></ul>
Pain location	<ul><li>Show the patient the human figure diagram; ask the patient to mark or point to each pain area.</li><li>Indicate pain sites using the key.</li></ul>
Pain description	For each pain location, elicit the following information. Allow the patient to discuss each pain(s) location in his or her own words. If information does not include one of the following, use prompts to elicit information about: <ul><li>Onset</li><li>Duration</li><li>Location</li><li>Cause</li><li>Severity</li><li>Descriptors (sharp, dull, or other words used by the patient)</li><li>Continuous or intermittent</li></ul>
Pain causation	Ask the patient to describe the cause of the pain.
Pain triggers	Ask what makes the pain better or worse.
Pain effect on daily activities	Ask the patient what effect the pain has on the following daily activities: <ul><li>Appetite/eating</li><li>Sleeping</li><li>Moving about the home</li><li>Concentration</li><li>Hobbies or interests</li><li>Reading, watching television</li><li>Driving or shopping</li><li>Relationships with others</li><li>Other type of activities</li></ul>

(continued)

EXHIBIT 22.6 Guidelines for Preoperative Pain Assessment *(continued)*

Assessment Topic	Suggested Questions
Pain relief methods	Assess all forms of pain relief methods; ask for name, dose/amount, frequency of use of the following: • Over-the-counter medications (list name, dose, frequency) • Prescription pain medications (list medication, dose, frequency) • Prescription adjuvant medication: antidepressants, antianxiety, psychotropic, other (list medication, dose, frequency) • Herbal remedies (list type and frequency) • Nonpharmacologic (list method) • Alcohol or other drug use (list type, amount, frequency) • Roots, leaves for home remedies/teas • Other home remedies • Indicate sensitivities or allergies to any pain medication
Effectiveness of pain relief methods	• Identify the pain relief patient thinks most effective and how effectiveness is evaluated.
Response to pain	• How does the patient act or respond when having pain? • Allow patient to describe in own words. • Prompts may include irritation, anxiety, anger, fatigue, restlessness, inability to concentrate, stoicism, depression.
Meaning of pain	• What are some cultural implications or traditions that are important regarding pain? For example: "You aren't supposed to talk about your pain." or other norms that influence the patient's approach to pain. • How does the patient interpret the pain (e.g., annoying, debilitating, dying)?
Prior experience: surgery, postoperative pain, pain relief	• Has the patient ever had postoperative pain? If yes, go to next questions. • What was the previous surgery? • What was the experience with postoperative pain? Allow patient to describe the pain situation in his or her own words. • Use prompts to elicit information: pain severity, anxiety, interactions with care providers, pain relief methods, effectiveness of pain relief, side effects of analgesia.
Patient-controlled analgesia	• Has the patient ever used patient-controlled analgesia? • If so, did the patient have any difficulty or concerns about using it? • Does the patient want to self-administer medication. If not, why not? • Who does the patient prefer to act as authorized agent for patient-controlled analgesia (family member, friend (by name), nurse)?

(continued)

EXHIBIT 22.6 Guidelines for Preoperative Pain Assessment *(continued)*

Assessment Topic	Suggested Questions
Current surgery expectations and pain	• What are the patient's expectations about pain after the planned surgery? • What concerns does the patient have about the planned surgery?
Family or proxy knowledge of pain	• Who will be helping the patient with pain relief after surgery? • How well does the patient's family understand or interpret the patient's pain?
Pain assessment tool.	• Has the patient ever used a pain assessment tool? • If yes, what kind, how well did it work, and would it be a preferred tool for the patient to use?
Pain tolerance	• Using his or her own words, ask the patient to describe his or her pain tolerance. Confirm the level of tolerance by asking the patient to score pain tolerance as low tolerance, moderate tolerance, high tolerance. (This is important information for understanding the patient's rating of pain, limitations of participation in recovery activities, tolerance of painful procedures, and need for pain relief.)
Comfort level	• Explain it is not always possible to relieve pain 100% . • Ask the patient what comfort level of pain relief is needed to be able to move around in bed, cough, eat and drink, or walk. • Have the patient describe comfort/pain level using his or her own language. • If the patient is comfortable with a pain assessment scale, ask patient to indicate a pain level that best reflects needed comfort/pain level. • Assist the patient to set realistic levels based on the general rule that a level 4 or greater usually initiates intervention.

Documenting assessment	• Document data for use by providers across the perioperative period.
	• Use alerts for the following topics:
	  • Medication sensitivity and allergies
	  • Pain language used by patient
	  • Assessment tool reference
	  • Expected comfort level
	  • Pain tolerance level

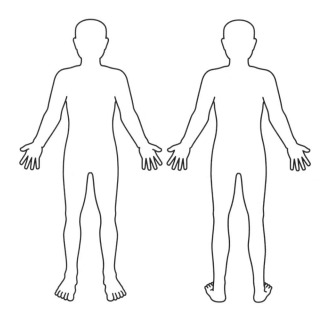

Point to where you have acute pain or mark with an X.
Point to where you have ongoing or persistent pain or
mark with a Y.

FIGURE 22.3
Human Figures for Indicating Pain Source

information includes medication or herbal name, dose, frequency, length of use, effective-ness, and if the patient experiences any side effects. The patient should be asked if a phar-macologic product was ever discontinued and why. Ask if the patient prefers to continue a specific pain relief method for a preexisting pain while in the hospital or after surgery. If the home remedy is contraindicated, discuss alternative modalities. Assessing patient beliefs and attitudes about the use of medication or type of medication is an important part of the medication history. Older adults often misunderstand or misinterpret informa-tion about medications, especially morphine, morphine derivatives, and pain relief. A com-mon misunderstanding is that old people can become addicted if they take morphine or morphine derivatives. Morphine is an important medication for postoperative pain relief. Clarifying misinformation and ensuring patient understanding about the benefits of mor-phine as a pain relief method contribute to achievement of successful postoperative pain relief outcomes.

Medication allergies and side effects must be labeled with a "medication alert," noting medication name, dose, and type of allergic reaction or side effect. Side effects should also be evaluated for onset and duration, noting if they are transient, episodic, or continuous. The information is used to evaluate medication risks and benefits, adjust dose, and identify the need for monitoring.

Older adults often use nonpharmacologic pain relief methods at home but may not think about continuing to use them in the hospital or after surgery. Patients often link the hospital with "medication." Older adults who may want to continue using nondrug interventions for pain relief after surgery should be encouraged to discuss the situation with their surgeon before surgery. Coaching the patient on how to communicate with providers about con-tinuing their nondrug interventions while in the perioperative setting can help initiate the discussion. Using pain relief methods that the older patient finds effective is important in relieving preexisting and postoperative pain.

No single tool has been documented to be effective in assessing pain in all older adults across the perioperative continuum. Multiple factors influence the older adult's ability to use a pain assessment tool effectively: age-related cognitive changes, cognitive processing, level of cognitive function, sensory function, clinical condition, health status, sociocultural influences, and personal preference. A major issue in perioperative care is the need to have a tool that can be used and adapted appropriately for use in preoperative assessment, and later, when the older adult's clinical condition has changed. The use of self-report scales rests on the functional ability of the person to use the scale. Before selecting a standardized assessment scale, a functional assessment is needed to evaluate the patient's ability to use the scale reliably and validly.

PHYSICAL ASSESSMENT

The patient's reported areas of pain should be carefully examined. Physical assessment includes observation and palpation of the painful site to assess for swelling, masses, or tenderness. Observing for circulatory changes and hypersensitivity to temperature and sensation provides information on peripheral circulation. Painful muscles and joints should be assessed for mobility, flexibility, and function. Congenital or acquired anatomical abnormalities of the spine or torso must be carefully evaluated to determine whether they create a risk for regional and local anesthesia, analgesia, and positioning.

Note the presence of topical pain preparations or devices. If the older adult is using a once-a-day analgesic patch, it should remain in place, its use should be documented on the preoperative database, and an anesthesia provider should be notified. The use of TENS units for chronic pain requires notification of the intraoperative and anesthesia team and documented in the medical record. Intraoperative equipment can interfere with the operation of the TENS unit.

DIAGNOSTIC TESTING

Reviewing laboratory values is important in considering vulnerability to adverse effects of perianesthesia and postoperative pain medications. Albumin levels and creatinine clearance are of particular relevance. Many analgesics bind to serum albumin, which causes the drug to be inactivated. Only the circulating drug is bioactive and available so the timing of the dose must be adjusted to prevent overmedicating. Patients with hypoalbuminemia must be monitored closely for early detection of adverse effects. Decreased blood flow to the liver and diminished renal function interferes with metabolism of analgesic medications.

Renal function studies, liver function panels, and serum albumin levels should be reviewed as they are available. Preoperative laboratory values should be compared with previous results to determine significant changes. Abnormal results should be reviewed with the surgeon and anesthesia provider.

INTERVENTION

A postoperative pain relief plan is developed and includes pain goals, pain assessment tools, and the use of preemptive analgesia. Exhibit 22.7 identifies topics and content to be included in information sharing and coaching with the older adult about postoperative pain and pain relief.

EXHIBIT 22.7 Preoperative Coaching About Postoperative Pain

- Pain is what the patient says it is
- Selection of patient preferred pain assessment scale
- Using patient-controlled analgesia: preference for self-administered or proxy-administered
- Communicating with care providers about surgical pain:
  - Need to report pain
  - How to report pain
  - To whom to report pain
  - Nonpharmacologic and pharmacologic pain relief methods
  - Reporting pain relief effectiveness
  - Establishing functional comfort level
- Informing care providers about causes and location of preoperative persistent pain
- Type of effective pain relief methods used by patient
- Identifying patient pain related goals and outcomes
- Postdischarge pain relief needs

Reinforcing the message that pain is unique to the individual and "pain is what the patient says it is" empowers older adults to talk about pain. Many older adults are hesitant to complain. Explaining the negative effects pain can have on surgical recovery and rehabilitation adds to the older person's knowledge, helping them feel more comfortable communicating to care providers that they have pain. Encourage the patient to select a family member or friend to serve as a companion-coach and to work with the health care team to ensure the patient has optimal pain relief. Older patients may be hesitant to ask someone to be a companion-coach out of concern that it will be a burden. Remind the patient that surgery is stressful, the postsurgical period can be overwhelming, and that both of these factors can limit a person's ability to be proactive. Older adults should discuss any concerns, attitudes, and goals regarding pain relief prior to surgery with the companion-coach to ensure effective advocacy after surgery.

Preoperative coaching on communicating with interdisciplinary team members promotes patient confidence about actively participating in pain care decisions across the perioperative continuum. Topics to include in preoperative coaching are pain expectations, establishing pain goals, using pain assessment tools, methods of pain relief, communicating with providers about pain, patient perceived levels of pain tolerance, use of patient-controlled analgesia (PCA), and attention to patient anxiety or depression.

Allow time for the older adult to raise questions and concerns about pain and pain relief after admission to the surgical setting and after surgery. Discussing concerns helps the patient to feel heard, a powerful psychological foundation for alleviating preoperative anxiety and stress. The older adult should be reassured that the health care team is committed to ensuring patient comfort and optimum pain relief.

The patient ultimately determines pain goals and interprets an acceptable level of pain during postoperative and recovery activities.

Older adults are familiar with different kinds of pain. Unless severely cognitively impaired, they have vast self-awareness of their response and coping strategies when they have pain and the methods they use to alleviate it. Care providers can use patient's self-knowledge to tailor pain relief methods and individualize the plan of care.

Consult the patient's goals for pain care. Emphasize that health care provider goals are to maximize patient comfort while minimizing adverse effects. Reassure the patient that health care providers are committed to the patient's comfort and ability to engage in recovery activities. It is equally important to help the patient recognize that his or her pain goal may not always be advisable. Pain is a protective mechanism designed to prevent the patient from activities that stress the body's resources too much, too soon after surgery. Pain relief should not override this protective mechanism or create adverse medication effects.

Older adults are highly vulnerable to side effects from analgesia. Balancing the benefits of pain relief with the risk of side effects is important in meeting realistic pain goals. Care providers and patients must work together to achieve pain relief at a level that maintains patient comfort and allows the patient to carry out recovery activities while avoiding adverse effects. Such cost-benefit decisions must be a joint evaluation between the older adult and the health care team.

PATIENT COACHING

The preoperative interview is an opportune time to coach the patient on how to use assessment scales, explain pain goals and comfort zones, discuss pain experiences with providers, and determine postoperative pain assessment. Older adults can use pain scales but find them difficult to use or prefer other methods. Coaching the older adult and providing time to practice with different types of scales improves patient ease and competence when the patient is having pain and may be asked to use a pain scale.

Coaching begins with asking if the patient has ever used a pain scale. If so, ask the patient to share the experience including the type of pain scale, ease of use, usefulness in explaining the pain experience to providers, and overall satisfaction with the assessment and follow-up activities. Use the patient's description to evaluate the patient's comfort and ability using pain scales and to select the type of pain scales to pilot test. Remind the patient that pain scales, unless stated otherwise, evaluate pain severity and that the patient needs to provide additional information about the pain including location, onset, duration, character, and whether the pain is of new onset or different from pain previously discussed.

Review the purpose of pain scales and how they assist in pain assessment and contribute to pain relief. Explain each of the tools commonly used in the surgical site. Have the patient use the scale to describe any preoperative pain.

Exhibit 22.8 presents an overview for helping gerioperative patients evaluate pain tools. Document the tools the patient identifies as easy to use and that accurately reflect the patient's pain severity.

If the patient is uncomfortable or unable to use a pain scale, attempt to identify the source of the discomfort and work with the older adult to resolve the discomfort. If the patient remains uncomfortable, engage the patient in selecting an alternate method. Caregivers providing intraoperative and postoperative care must be aware of the patient's preferred method for assessing pain. Document a "pain alert," noting the patient's difficulty using pain tools and explaining the patient's selected preferred method.

Pain Relief Interventions

The use of PCA for pain relief in older adults is effective. If PCA is a treatment option, preoperative coaching allows the older person to make an informed decision and to determine how and by whom the medication should be administered. Some older adults prefer to self-administer, while others prefer the nurse or a designated family member to activate the PCA.

EXHIBIT 22.8 Patient Evaluation of Pain Assessment Tools

- Ask the patient to pilot test three different types of assessment tools commonly used for postoperative pain assessment. The patient can use the tools to evaluate current pain level or a previous pain experience. Ask the patient to describe the situation as a context for tool selection.
- Review the different types of tools. Have the patient review each tool separately. Provide instructions before the use of each tool.
  - Visual analog
  - Verbal descriptor
  - Numeric rating
  - Pictures, illustrations (e.g., FACES Pain Scale)
- Have patient evaluate the usefulness of the human figure form for pain location.
- Assess comfort with three different type of assessment tools.
- First coach the patient on how to use each tool.
- Ask the patient to select a type of tool that is easiest for the patient to use.

The question of who administers PCA bolus is an important preoperative discussion. Families often want to administer medication or are asked to do so by the patient. The American Society for Pain Management Nursing published a position statement and clinical practice recommendations for caregiver authorized agents and controlled analgesia (Wuhrman et al., 2007). Authorized agent–controlled analgesia is the authorization of a person to assist in administration or to administer controlled analgesia in patients who are unable to self-administer. Most institutions allow patients to authorize someone other than the nurse to administer PCA medication on their behalf if the person receives training. Providers caring for the patient must monitor the process and the outcomes. Hospitals must have established protocols for caregiver authorized agents including the process for selecting, training, and monitoring of the agent.

PREEMPTIVE PAIN ANALGESIA

Preemptive analgesia administered before the start of surgery has mixed results. Several single studies and meta-analyses arrived at differing conclusions on the beneficial effects of preemptive analgesia on postoperative pain. The difference in conclusions results from differences in the type of preemptive analgesia administered and the definition of outcome variables. Decisions about preemptive analgesia should be considered in light of the needs of the individual patient, type of surgery, sensitivity to pain, and sensitivity to medication. The patient should be fully informed about the risks and benefits of preemptive analgesia before making a decision about its use.

EPIDURAL ANALGESIA

Epidural analgesia is used for anticipated moderate to severe postoperative pain and provides prolonged delivery of high-quality pain relief. Epidural analgesia offers immediate pain relief in patients who have had extensive surgical procedures or surgeries expected to cause severe postoperative pain such as thoracic or upper abdominal surgery. Epidural anesthesia decreases the amount of opioid medication required to achieve adequate pain relief.

The epidural catheter is usually placed preoperatively in the epidural space, and opioids are administered via the catheter. Opioids bind with opiate receptors in the dorsal horn of the spinal cord, blocking pain impulses to the cerebral cortex. Epidural opioids do not prevent, relieve, or treat the inflammation caused by injury at the pain site; they relieve the sensation or feeling of pain by interrupting of nerve pathways. Epidural analgesia allows the patient to be comfortable and participate in critical postoperative recovery and rehabilitation such as deep breathing, coughing, and early ambulation. Epidural analgesia is administered as continuous basal drip, continuous basal drip with an on-demand bolus, or on-demand bolus only. Narcotics commonly used for epidural anesthesia are preservative-free morphine sulfate and fentanyl. Hydromorphone can be used when patients have identified allergies.

Preoperative anxiety correlates strongly with higher levels and more prolonged postoperative pain, increased analgesia, and decreased participation in postoperative recovery activities. Attending to the patient's presurgery anxiety lowers postoperative anxiety and pain, as well as improves surgical recovery. Providing information and coaching the patient on prehabilitation self-care and postoperative recovery helps decrease anxiety. Coaching the older adult on how to communicate about pain has shown mixed results. However, coaching does improve competence and self-confidence, factors that contribute to decreasing anxiety.

INTRAOPERATIVE CONSIDERATIONS

Intraoperative interventions are directed to preventing intraoperative pain and decreasing postoperative pain. Chapter 8 discusses anesthesia and intraoperative medications.

Surgical positioning is a major source of postoperative pain. Attention to careful handling of joints and extremities during surgery can minimize postoperative musculoskeletal pain. Chapter 8 provides a more complete description of safe intraoperative positioning and prevention of postoperative pain. Environmental and physical nonpharmacologic interventions, initiated before and during surgery, are effective in decreasing patient stress and anxiety.

Listening to music immediately before surgery is effective in lowering anxiety in older adults. Having a nurse remain with the patient to provide a calm, supportive environment before and during induction of anesthesia and during emergence from anesthesia helps the patient feel safe and more secure. Physical methods focus on increasing patient comfort before and during surgery. Effective interventions include the use of warming blankets and physical touch, with permission, to reassure the patient.

POSTOPERATIVE CONSIDERATIONS

The major concern in the immediate postanesthesia period is ensuring recovery of an adequate airway, breathing, and circulation. Once stabilized, pain is the fourth element in the gerioperative patient evaluation. Depending on the extent of surgery and the surgical setting, postoperative pain is time-dependent, decreasing over time.

Pain severity in the immediate postoperative period can contribute to cardiovascular instability. Hypothermia, common in older adults during and after surgery, increases pain sensation. Anxiety, nausea, and disorientation further exacerbate the pain experience. In the postanesthesia care unit, vital signs with pain assessments are monitored frequently.

Pain assessment in the immediate postanesthesia period challenges older adults. Hearing and vision acuity, already diminished by age-related changes, are further distorted by resolving anesthetics. Stress, pain, anxiety, and anesthesia effects can be overwhelming and limit an older person's ability to focus on specific questions or provide detailed answers. Unless there is severe cognitive impairment or minimal consciousness, older adults can answer short, direct questions about pain. Questions in the immediate postanesthesia period may need to be limited to essential data: Are you in pain? Can you point to the pain? Do you need medication? Responses need to be confirmed for accuracy by correlating them with behavior, ability to function, and clinical condition. It is important to pinpoint pain location and severity to differentiate surgical pain from other discomforts such as nausea, pain caused by intraoperative positioning, catheters, or technological devices.

Pain interventions in the postanesthesia care unit focus on removing the pain source and initiating therapeutic interventions including medication and nonpharmacologic methods. Adjusting the patient's position, listening to music, and applying local warmth can be effective nonpharmacologic measures for relieving mild to moderate pain. Warming blankets are important not only in providing comfort but for relieving pain.

Reviewing preoperative assessment data and intraoperative activities allows the identification of patients at risk for severe pain levels. Predictors contributing to postoperative pain severity and analgesia use include level of preoperative anxiety and psychological distress and type of surgery: orthopedic, thoracic, abdominal, or emergency.

In the immediate postoperative period, if surgical pain is intense, fast-acting intravenous opioids are the first line of treatment: morphine, hydromorphone, and fentanyl. Some studies have suggested that oxycodone is a better choice for relieving visceral pain, although most drug choices depend on provider preference. Acetaminophen is effective as a solo medication for mild to moderate pain and as the foundation for multimodal analgesia for moderate to severe pain. Meperidine is contraindicated as an analgesic in older adults due to its association with onset of delirium and cognitive dysfunction. Intramuscular medications are not recommended.

Although pain relief in the postoperative period is a shared decision between provider and patient, the final determination of pain goals and setting an acceptable level of pain rests with the patient. If the patient is unable to make decisions about pain relief or if the decisions are counter to the patient's previous stated goals, family members or others may need to interpret or oversee the patient's decisions. Pain goals identified before surgery are reviewed with the patient, and changes are made as needed. The review is reassuring, signaling that care providers will remain attentive to the patient's perspectives and goals throughout the postoperative period. Pain goals and treatments are always individualized to the patient's clinical condition and in the context of patient preferences. The variation in types of pain, level of medication safety and interactions, individual response to medication effects, presence of comorbid health conditions, and the unique character of the patient's pain experience and response to treatment suggest that standard order sets for relieving pain in older adults must be carefully reviewed and revised based on the individual.

Review intervention decisions with the interdisciplinary team and the patient as soon after surgery as possible. Decisions are made available to all team members through careful documentation of the decisions, the basis for the decisions, and any areas remaining unresolved. Documentation should present the patient's level of involvement in developing the plan of care and the patient's understanding of the elements in the plan. Documentation prevents patient information and the plan of care from "falling through the cracks."

The World Health Organization's (WHO) three-step analgesia ladder for relieving cancer pain is adapted to postoperative pain relief in the geriatric patient. The step-up approach

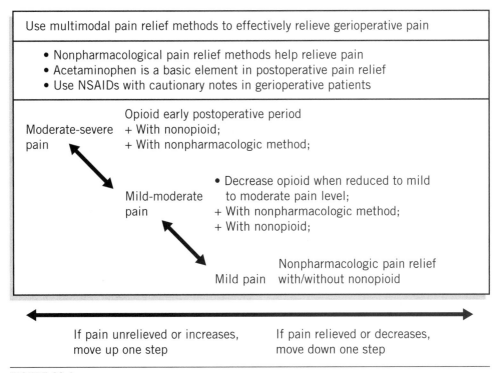

FIGURE 22.4
Gerioperative Pain Ladder

indicates that as pain increases, analgesia level increases. The ladder progresses from non-opioid intervention at the lowest step (one) to opioid plus the addition of one or more nonopioid medications and nonpharmacologic interventions at the highest step (three). Figure 22.4 is an adaptation of the WHO ladder to gerioperative care.

In the immediate postoperative period, when pain levels are highest, gerioperative patients are most likely to require analgesia at the top of the analgesia ladder, steps two or three, As pain decreases during postoperative recovery, analgesia intervention can transition to steps one and two based on patient assessment. Analgesia can return to higher steps if pain levels increase or pain relief methods at the lower level are not effective.

Multimodal analgesia is an important element of the WHO analgesic ladder. Nonopioid and nonpharmacologic pain relief methods are recommended at all steps. Multimodal analgesia can decrease the amount of opioid needed in older adults sensitive to the effects of opioids. Using a combination of drug and nondrug interventions can decrease the potential for adverse medication effects.

Nonpharmacologic pain methods are a basic component of effective pain relief. These methods are generally safe for older adults and result in few side effects. They can be used as a single intervention for mild to moderate pain or as part of a comprehensive pain relief program. The major side effect of nonpharmacologic intervention is inadequate pain relief. Nonpharmacologic pain relief methods can be classified as environmental, mind-body, and physical methods. Nonpharmacologic interventions can be highly effective as the sole intervention methods for mild or moderate pain or as part of a multimodal program for moderate to severe pain. Older adults, their caregivers, and their companion-coaches should be coached on how and when to use nonpharmacologic methods. Exhibit 22.9 list key points

> **EXHIBIT 22.9   Key Points of Nonpharmacologic Pain Relief**
>
> - Nonpharmacologic methods are effective in relieving pain with older adults
> - Teaching older adults about nonpharmacologic pain methods is best done in the preoperative period
> - Encourage older adults to practice different methods helps to:
>   - Identify modalities best suited to the individual
>   - Increase familiarity and comfort with how to use the method, facilitating its use when needed for pain relief
> - Older adults who use effective nonpharmacologic methods before surgery should be encouraged to continue their use after surgery if not contraindicated
> - Include family and companion-coach on how to help older adults use nonpharmacologic pain relief with patient agreement
> - Encourage older adults to share preferences with nonpharmacologic pain relief methods with providers, family, and companion-coach
> - Document patient preference preoperatively facilitates more effective postoperative pain relief planning

in considering patient use of nonpharmacologic pain relief. Table 22.6 lists commonly used nonpharmacologic interventions, indications, and cautions. Nonpharmacologic methods require documentation similar to analgesic medications. Documentation should include pain location, severity, nonpharmacologic intervention, and patient response to the intervention. Reassessment after nonpharmacologic intervention is as critical as reassessment after medication administration.

ENVIRONMENTAL STRATEGIES

Ambulatory and in-hospital postsurgical units are multisensory stimulating environments that are noisy, glaring, busy, and rapidly paced. The environment creates sensory overload for older adults. Loud noises, bright lights, and numerous unfamiliar providers entering and leaving the patient's room contribute to sleep deprivation, patient anxiety, disorientation, and confusion. Heightened sympathetic response systems, altered by age-related changes, increase the response to pain stimulation. Neural activity stimulated by sensory overload and pain increases demand for cerebral blood flow as the older adult struggles to assimilate environmental cues and the body attempts to maintain homeostasis. Providing "quiet time" for the older adult can release sensory tension. Decreasing sensory overload calms sympathetic responses that exacerbate pain sensation. Maintaining noninvasive monitoring and a patient observation system helps the older adult feel safe, cared for, and alleviates feelings of isolation.

MIND-BODY STRATEGIES

Decreasing cognitive, sensory, and physical stress helps to relieve pain. An often overlooked but effective intervention, reflective of the mind-body model, is the care provider therapeutic use of self. Therapeutic use of self is a planned intervention to alleviate the patient's fear or anxiety and provide reassurance. The use of self rests on a commitment to and the ability to

TABLE 22.6

Nonpharmacologic Pain Relief Methods in Older Adults

Category of Pain Relief	Action	Safety Considerations
Environmental	Minimize noise	Balance in room monitor alarm to achieve adequate volume within patient tolerance
	Decrease glare	Shut off overhead direct lighting
	Avoid interruptions	Limit interruptions; Schedule activities together
	Attend, observe, and monitor	Inform patient of observation and monitoring purpose and process
Mind-body	Music	Patient-selected music High-quality music player and earphones
	Guided imagery	Effective with chronic or persistent pain Coaching may be required Allow sufficient time Not recommended for older adults with moderate to severe cognitive impairment
	Relaxation	Coaching may be needed Decreases anxiety Relieves pain
Physical	Heat/cold	Protect the skin Warming blankets decrease anxiety Avoid cold in postanesthesia Avoid in patients with decreased peripheral sensation
	Massage	Avoid in older adults with fragile skin Ask for permission to use Apply at or near affected area Teach patient self-massage Use on shoulders, back, neck, hands, and feet for general relief Avoid with acute inflammation, risk of deep vein thrombosis, anticoagulant therapy

create patient-centered, relationship-oriented interactions. The ability to calm and focus the self on the patient and to extend that sense of calm and focus to the patient generates feelings of safety and security that relieves tension and contributes to pain relief.

Reducing pain triggers and minimizes pain signals, which in turn reduces pain sensation and perception. Mind-body integration relieves muscle strain that occurs with pain and escalates the pain cycle. Music, relaxation, guided imagery, and deep breathing help to reduce stress and anxiety that can exacerbate postoperative pain. When used alone, they are best used early in the pain cycle and limited to use with mild to moderate pain. In later stages of pain or in moderate to severe pain, mind-body modalities can be adjunct interventions in combination with other pain relief methods. The patient should learn about and practice mind-body pain relief methods before surgery or when the patient has minimal pain. Preoperative teaching provides the patient time to practice and consider how best to use the pain relief method based on the individual's needs. It is important to teach the companion-coach or family members who will be staying with the older person postoperatively how to facilitate the pain relief method.

Music is a well-established, nonpharmacologic therapy for postoperative pain relief. Studies on the most effective music indicate that patient preference is most likely to produce better pain relief. High-quality earphones or ear buds are needed to provide maximum clarity at low volumes. Older adults with hearing difficulties require quality equipment for maximum impact of the music intervention.

Guided imagery uses relaxation and mental visualization to reduce stress and promote emotional and physical well-being. The method has been used effectively in older adults with chronic or persistent pain from comorbid diseases as well as postoperative pain. Due to the need for concentration and attention, some older adults may find it difficult to use guided imagery in the immediate postoperative period. Others find focusing beneficial, as focusing shifts attention away from pain and discomfort. An experienced person familiar with the method should serve as a coach to help the patient use guided imagery effectively and safely in the immediate postoperative period. The use of guided imagery is not recommended for older adults who have a history of hallucinations or illusions.

Deep, conscious, and controlled breathing are important considerations in the relief of acute pain. Deep breathing releases muscle tension, a common response to heightened pain sensations and a risk factor for increased pain intensity. Focusing on deep breathing or muscle relaxation also serves as a distraction further contributing to pain relief.

PHYSICAL STRATEGIES

Physical pain relief strategies include cryotherapy, thermal therapy, massage, and physical activity. Cryotherapy is the use of cold modalities to decrease inflammation and muscle spasms and provide a local analgesic effect. Cold is particularly useful in relieving musculoskeletal pain and pain from surgical incisions.

Thermal therapy is the application of heat to relieve pain. Heat can relieve pain by increasing blood flow to the pain site. Increasing blood flow increases tissue oxygenation and provides nutrients and antibodies to the area. The removal of metabolites from the injured area by vasodilation further contributes to pain relief.

Heat can be soothing to superficial issues such as muscle or joint pain, soft-tissue discomfort, or when pain is more diffuse. Older adults are more likely to prefer heat to cold. Heat can be applied through warming blankets or moist compresses. Warming blankets provide a sense of comfort, reduce muscle tension, and decrease anxiety.

Temperature interventions must be used with caution. Superficial application of cold or heat can cause tissue injury secondary to age-related changes in skin sensitivity and age- or disease-related changes in peripheral nerves. Manufacturer recommendations for device parameters must be adhered to for patient comfort and safety.

Massage increases comfort and relieves stiffness and muscle spasm caused by positioning and immobility. Massage increases blood flow through an area, increases warmth, and reduces edema. It can be applied directly to or around a painful area. Caution is needed if the area is particularly sensitive or has diminished blood supply. Massage is also effective as a general comfort measure when applied to the back, neck, hands, feet, or shoulders. Massage should be used gently in older adults with fragile skin, as skin tearing or superficial blood vessel rupture can occur. It should not be used in patients with peripheral vascular disease or cellulitis.

Activity relieves pain. Joint stiffening and muscles cramping secondary to inactivity become additional sources of pain and exacerbate preexisting joint and bone pain. Repositioning, moving in bed, encouraging passive and active range of motion, and ambulating contribute to overall pain relief.

PHARMACOLOGIC STRATEGIES

Pharmacologic methods of pain control include nonopioid, opioid, and adjuvant analgesia. As with all medications administered to geriatric patients, care is needed to evaluate adequate doses consistent with patient's clinical status and prevention of adverse medication effects. Table 22.7 lists potential adverse effects of common medications used by older adults for persistent pain relief. Commonly used analgesics include acetaminophen, nonsteroidal anti-inflammatory drugs (NSAIDs), muscle relaxants, and opioids. Adjuvant therapy includes antidepressants, anticonvulsants, anxiolytics, psychotropics, and steroid-based anti-inflammatory medications.

Medicating the older adult for postoperative pain relief presents challenges. The therapeutic-risk ratio of analgesic medications is narrowed significantly after surgery. Hormonal stress response, anesthesia effects, extreme physiologic demands, fluid imbalance, and depletion of physiologic reserves alter drug metabolism, making older adults highly vulnerable to the small difference between therapeutic response and adverse effects of medications. Preexisting pulmonary, cardiac, or renal disease create additional physiologic threats. Postoperative vulnerability to adverse effects continues even after the immediate postanesthesia phase. Polypharmacy increases risk of drug-drug and drug-disease interactions. Acute pain intervention guidelines are available online (http://www.guideline.gov/content.aspx?id=10198).

Older adults are as vulnerable to undertreatment of pain due to provider fears of medication adverse effects as they are to overtreatment and overuse of medication. Concerns about adverse side effects need to be balanced with the need for adequate pain relief. Pharmacologic analgesia is based on pain severity, type of pain, and type of medication, medication dose, administration route, and reassessment.

"Start low and go slow" is the universal recommendation for medication use in older adults. Analgesic medications must never be administered based solely on the results of a pain scale rating. The goal is to balance the dose of medication required to achieve pain relief

TABLE 22.7
Common Analgesia Medications With Selected Concerns

Analgesic	Preexisting Concerns	Postoperative Concerns
Opioids	Cardiac disease Respiratory disease Low albumin Decreased renal clearance Decreased liver function Polypharmacy Preexisting persistent pain	Dehydration Respiratory rate Free opioid in blood stream Nonexcreted opioid Nonmetabolized opioid Drug interactions Loss of medication effectiveness
Acetaminophen	Decreased renal clearance Decreased liver function	Increased renal toxicity Increased liver toxicity
Nonsteroidal anti-inflammatory drugs	Decreased liver function Heart failure Anticoagulants	Increased blood pressure Fluid retention Increased bleeding times
Antidepressants		Anticholinergic effects Drowsiness Exacerbate hypertension

goals with the need to avoid adverse medication effects. Diligent pain assessment with systematic monitoring of patient response before and after an intervention, and ongoing observation must be implemented if health care providers are to meet the goals of patient comfort, adequate pain relief, and prevention of adverse events.

NONOPIOID ANALGESIA

Nonopioid analgesics can be effective adjuncts to opioids when opioids alone are ineffective. Synergistically, they can reduce the level of opioid needed to relieve pain. Nonopioids can replace opioids when pain levels decrease in response to healing and recovery.

NSAIDs are useful for pain associated with inflammation. Doses should be kept at the minimum level needed to achieve therapeutic goals. Depending on severity, NSAIDs can be contraindicated in gerioperative patients who have impaired hepatic or renal function, dehydration, use diuretic medications, or have heart failure. A major concern with NSAID administration is gastrointestinal bleeding. Patients on anticoagulants should not be receiving NSAID medications. NSAIDs should be for short-term use and administered with caution in older adults. Acetaminophen is a preferred analgesic in older adults, especially in the absence of inflammation.

Acetaminophen has a weaker analgesic effect than a comparable dose of NSAIDs and has no anti-inflammatory action. It offers relief for mild to moderate postoperative pain and is an integral component of multimodal regimens in the relief of severe pain. Acetaminophen is metabolized in the liver. Age- and disease-related changes in hepatic function can alter acetaminophen metabolism. The potential for acetaminophen toxicity is increased in older adults with reduced hepatic function, decreased hepatic blood flow, or a history of excessive alcohol use. Toxicity is of special concern in older adults who take acetaminophen for long-term persistent pain. Patients taking acetaminophen long-term require careful counseling about the effects of alcohol on the liver and the potential for acetaminophen toxicity.

OPIOID ANALGESIA

Older adults are highly sensitive to the therapeutic and adverse effects of opioids, requiring careful titration and close monitoring. Response to opioids is based on the individual's physical, physiological, and psychoemotional characteristics. Initial doses in older adults should begin 25 to 50% below the recommended dose for adults. If pain is unrelieved, dosage can be increased slowly in 25% increments until the patient's comfort and functional pain goal has been achieved. Adding nonopioid analgesia and nonpharmacologic interventions minimizes the amount of drug needed for effective analgesia and decreases adverse side effects. Meperidine, codeine, and methadone are not recommended for older adults due to their potential for causing delirium and cognitive dysfunction. Exhibit 22.10 lists guidelines for use of opioids in older adults.

Opioids affect almost all organ systems. Common side effects are sedation, respiratory depression, constipation, orthostatic hypotension, and cognitive changes. Signs of sedation precede respiratory depression. Sedation can also indicate the onset of hypoactive delirium. Whenever an older adult shows any changes in cognition, level of alertness, or affect, a full assessment, including current drug regimen, is needed. Opioids are withheld and alternative analgesia is administered until the cause is determined.

Providers are likely to limit opioid administration due to concerns about delirium. However, unrelieved pain can also cause delirium. It is important to balance the risk of delirium due to medication with the risk of delirium caused by unrelieved pain. Limiting

EXHIBIT 22.10 **Guidelines for Opioid Use in Older Adults**

- Schedule opioid medication around the clock for acute moderate to severe pain
- Use opioids with short half-lives (morphine, hydromorphone, oxymorphone, oxycodone)
- Avoid use of meperidine and codeine
- Avoid intramuscular administration (painful, unpredictable absorption due to less muscle, more fat)
- Treat opioid side effects prophylactically
- Establish bowel regimen and sleep protocols at first dose of opioid
- If side effects, decrease dose if analgesia sufficient for patient comfort
- Establish patient monitoring system for sedation and respiratory depression
- Use around-the-clock dosing for early, severe postoperative pain
- Start with low dose (25 to 50% of usual adult dose), titrate up slowly
- Use adjuncts (acetaminophen or nonsteroidal anti-inflammatory) for opioid-sparing effect
- Consider use of nonpharmacologic or nonopioid medication to decrease amount of opioid needed
- Monitor for drug-drug interactions (sedatives, antiemetics, antihypertensive medications with sedative side effects, drugs with anticholinergic effects)

medication can lead to severe, unrelieved pain, contributing to the onset of delirium; unrelieved pain is more likely to cause delirium than therapeutic levels of opioids.

A major concern with opioid administration is poor quality sleep, specifically a disruption in rapid eye movement and slow wave sleep. Poor sleep quality contributes to increased pain sensation, resulting in the need for more analgesia. The cycle of opioid-impaired sleep may contribute to cognitive changes often seen after surgery. Sleep disturbance also is linked with impaired cognition. A sleep protocol should be initiated with the first dose of opioid. Key to the success of a protocol is remaining within patient preference and previous habits. Ask patients what they do to get to sleep at home and replicate those practices as much as possible. When patient practices cannot be replicated, suggesting methods in a sleep protocol can be useful. Suggested sleep protocols include decreasing environmental stimuli, ensuring patient comfort including warmth or coolness depending on patient preference, positioning, a warm drink, and soothing music.

Constipation is the most common side effect from opioid medication, occurring in almost 100% of patients. Older adults have slowed intestinal motility due to age-related changes. The added effect of slowed intestinal motility resulting from opioids heightens the risk of constipation and paralytic ileus. A preemptive bowel regimen should be initiated in any older adult receiving opioid therapy as soon as the first dose is given. Prevention of constipation using a combined regimen of stool softener and stimulant laxative is most effective. Maintaining a high-fiber diet, ambulation, and hydration are basic elements in preventing constipation and are integral to preventing opioid-induced constipation.

Pruritis is a distressing side effect occurring in up to 50% of patients receiving opioid therapy. Pruritis is less common in older adults. However, it is common in older patients receiving epidural opioids. Pruritis should not be considered a minor side effect due to its potential for causing infection in the older adult. Aging skin is friable. Cracks in the skin can result in infections, and opioids reduce immunity. The postoperative older adult is further suppressed immunologically from age-related changes and surgical stress. Ondansetron and naloxone are suggested medications for treating pruritis, though their effectiveness is not well established and highly variable. Adding medications to treat medication side effects can result in a prescribing cascade. Changing the route of administration, altering dose levels, or changing to another analgesic is an alternate to adding more medications. There is little published data on effectiveness of nonpharmacologic interventions for older adults with opioid-induced pruritis.

Intravenous or Epidural Strategies

Intravenous or epidural-controlled anesthesia can be highly effective in relieving postoperative pain in older adults. Patient-controlled epidural or intravenous administration routes are easy titrated to meet individual patient needs. When continuous infusions are used, conservative basal rates are administered in older adults, especially those who have not used opioids previously or who have preexisting pulmonary or renal disease.

Major side effects associated with epidural opioid administration are respiratory depression, nausea and vomiting, pruritis, and urinary retention. Naloxone is the drug of choice to reverse respiratory depression. Antiemetics can be used to prevent or treat nausea and vomiting, with naloxone indicated for relief of severe nausea. Urinary retention can be treated with intermitted bladder catheterization or naloxone administration.

Older adults receiving epidural analgesia are vulnerable to adverse effects and should be assessed regularly for bladder distention, lower extremity motor function, respiratory depression, placement of epidural tubing, and intact dressing. Vital signs, intake, and output should be monitored on a regular basis and compared with previous results. Assessment results and comparison data should be documented and the information included in every care provider handoff.

Opioids continue to be used in older adults even with the high potential for adverse effects in vulnerable older adults. Consistent monitoring for early detection of impending side effects, awareness of atypical signs and symptoms, and critical analysis of information during handoffs are needed to protect the older adult from adverse opioid events, balanced with achievement of optimal pain relief goals.

Intramuscular Administration

Intramuscular administration routes are not used in older adults. Decreased muscle mass and diminished circulation alter drug absorption at intramuscular sites. Delayed medication onset or prolonged medication effects can result, making it difficult to titrate drug dose and increasing the risk of adverse effects.

Oral Administration

Oral analgesic medications are recommended for patients with mild to moderate pain. Oral administration of medication is least invasive and a safer route for opioid administration. Gerioperative patients should be given oral analgesia as soon as they can tolerate taking fluids by mouth. A full glass of water or liquids assists in passing the oral medications to the stomach.

Changing from parenteral to oral pain medication administration can result in too much or too little medication, causing oversedation or inadequate pain relief. Patients must be monitored at regular intervals for evidence of sedation or unrelieved pain until a stable level of comfort is achieved without adverse effects. It is more difficult to achieve initial pain relief with oral opioids than to maintain ongoing pain relief. Regaining an adequate level of comfort is difficult once it is lost. It is especially difficult after a change in administration routes.

Equianalgesic Dosing

An equianalgesic dosing table guides the transition from one route of administration to another for the initial dose selection. Close monitoring is required to determine medication effectiveness or early detection of adverse effects. Before converting to a new opioid or administration route, evaluate the effectiveness of the current regimen and presence of any side effects. Maintaining effectiveness can be achieved by selecting an initial dose comparable to current use. Pain relief that is inadequate at the time of transition may require an increase in initial dose during conversion to a different route until effectiveness is determined. Careful and attentive monitoring is needed when converting from one opioid to another or from one administration route to another.

DOCUMENTATION

Pain relief prevention and intervention are not well documented. Major gaps in pain documentation include limited or absent assessment data, lack of reassessment, and lack of information on follow-up when reassessment indicates inadequate pain relief. Nonpharmacologic pain relief methods are rarely documented either as an intervention or in terms of effectiveness. Poor documentation results in poor communication across units of care and among members of the health care team. Poor communication contributes to inadequate pain relief, impedes patient recovery, imperils patient safety, and increases risk of patient care errors and suboptimal outcomes.

Transferring accurate, timely information is crucial for providing safe, quality care. Documentation provides information about the patient's pain severity and frequency, progress toward pain relief goals, onset of new pain, and effectiveness of prevention and intervention methods.

DISCHARGE CONSIDERATIONS

Providing clear, basic, easily understandable information about pain assessment and pain medication is critical in maintaining adequate pain relief for older adults discharged to home care or assisted living. Older adults are reluctant to "bother the doctor" unless their pain level is severe. They also are reluctant to bother busy family members.

Before an older adult is discharged, review preoperative coaching about the importance of adequate pain relief in promoting recovery. The reinforcement provides support for the patient or family member who may be hesitant to contact a physician or designated care provider about pain issues after discharge. Remind the family to ask the patient about pain and reinforce the importance of "being honest" with the patient. Education and coaching can facilitate pain-related communication between caregivers and the older adult. Ask the patient about the type and effectiveness of nonpharmacologic methods used at home. If methods are effective and not contraindicated, encourage the patient to continue using them.

Pain relief promotes recovery.

Medication prescriptions should be reviewed carefully with the older adult before discharge, emphasizing how the medication is to be used and safely administered. An important area for discussion is the older person's ability to obtain medications in a timely manner. Inform patients when the next dose of pain medication can be administered and ensure that medications will be available for the next dose.

Patients with analgesic medication prescriptions should be informed about adverse medication effects. An explanation of what the patient should do and who should be notified if side effects occur is important to ensure postdischarge safety. Balancing the need to decrease dosing and type of analgesia as recovery continues with the need to maintain comfort of the older adult requires discussion. Older adults will be discharged with pain relief medications related to surgical pain while needing to maintain medication use for persistent pain. The analgesia needs can be very different, calling for different medications. An analgesia medication reconciliation should be done at the first follow-up visit with the surgeon or primary care provider.

All information should be written out in language easily understood by the patient and caregivers. Encouraging the patient or family to write down the information in addition to receiving written information can be useful for retaining important details. Having the patient and caregivers explain their understanding of analgesic medication, expectations for pain relief, and potential side effects back to the provider can reinforce patient understanding and allow for follow-up clarification.

Older adults who enter a nursing home or rehabilitation center after discharge require medications to be reconciled at the time of hospital discharge and as soon as admitted to the new facility. Medication reconciliation is important to ensure that preadmission medications for persistent pain are continued after hospitalization. Hospital-initiated pain relief should be continued until the older person is fully recovered from surgery.

PATIENT REPORT DISCUSSION: Mrs. Oakley

The nurse initially assumes Mrs. Oakley is confused possibly due to dementia. Mrs. Oakley's nonverbal behaviors are consistent with the behavior of someone who is in pain and has cognitive impairment. Discovering Mrs. Oakley has no preadmission history of dementia, the nurse redefines the problem as delirium. However, Mrs. Oakley does not show evidence of fluctuating mental changes, and she is oriented. The nurse decides to talk with Mrs. Oakley more closely about her behavior. When questioned, Mrs. Oakley admits she is uncomfortable but not at a level she would call pain. Her incision site is sore and bothers her. She also reports feeling "antsy" and tense. She keeps rubbing her stomach because it helps relieve the discomfort and also helps relieve the tension. The nurse reviews the medication record, notes the aprazolam was not restarted after surgery, and contacts the physician to restart it. At the same time, the nurse suggests that acetaminophen be added to increase her general comfort and decrease the opioid dose. The nurse explains the situation to Mrs. Oakley who feels reassured. With the new medication regimen, Mrs. Oakley is more comfortable, stops removing her dressing, recovers well, and returns home.

Mrs. Oakley has been a healthy older adult. Prior to surgery she was active, socially engaged, and showed no evidence of cognitive decline. The benzodiazepine she was on before surgery poses a slight risk for postoperative delirium and postoperative cognitive dysfunction. The timeline, signs, and symptoms do not support either diagnosis. The stress of surgery increased her anxiety, making it difficult for her to attend completely to her surroundings and to articulate her discomfort. Further, the use of the pain scale focused on pain severity, and she didn't have pain. She had sufficient discomfort that, when combined with aftereffects of surgery and anesthesia, the effects of her anxiety, and aftereffects of benzodiazepine withdrawal, interfered with her ability to articulate that pain was not the problem but that she was anxious and uncomfortable. Pain assessment involves asking about discomfort as well as asking about pain. Patients and providers often use different language or use similar language that has different meanings. The nurse caring for Mrs. Oakley used clinical judgment and a problem-solving process to redefine the problem and arrive at a successful solution.

SUMMARY

Pain is a complex phenomenon. No two persons or even the same person at different points in time experience pain the same. The uniqueness of the pain experience is the basis for the belief that "pain is whatever the person says it is and occurs whenever the person says it occurs." Objective surgical pain can result in severe postoperative pain even though the older adult may have no conscious memory of the pain experience.

Age-related changes in pain physiology, psychology, and coping mechanisms combined with comorbid disease and medication sensitivity make older adults highly vulnerable to the negative outcomes of poor pain relief. The highly individualized nature of pain and pain response changes with age, reinforcing the dictum to treat the person in pain, not the pain.

Health providers who care for gerioperative patients must apply an understanding of the physiology, etiology, and effects of preoperative and postoperative pain on gerioperative outcomes. Current evidence indicates that providers remain inattentive to pain in older adults even though pain is a well-established risk factor for intraoperative and postoperative complications. Such evidence suggests there continues to be a serious lack of geriatric and gerontological knowledge among members of the health care team. Pain protocols and guidelines established by the International Society for Pain Management, the American Geriatrics Society, and the Anesthesia Society of America dictate that providers and institution leadership attend to system-based causes of inadequate pain relief.

KEY POINTS

- Age- and disease-related changes have significant effects on pain physiology in older adults.
- Pain as a safety factor for body systems diminishes with aging. Therefore, more damage occurs in body systems before the pain alarm signal is triggered.
- Older adults have highly individualized responses to acute pain requiring diligent assessment and monitoring.
- Unrelieved preoperative and postoperative pain negatively affects every body system, delays prehabilitation and recovery, and triggers postoperative persistent pain. Staying ahead of the pain curve prevents suffering, lost rehabilitation time, and decreased quality of life.
- Many providers are inadequately prepared about aging effects on pain physiology and the subsequent implications for achieving adequate pain relief.
- Gerioperative patients benefit from coaching in use of pain assessment tools, nonpharmacologic pain relief, and communicating with providers about pain and pain relief.
- Pain is a major cause of postoperative complications in the gerioperative patient.
- Pain prevention is more cost-effective than pain intervention.

TWENTY-THREE

Promoting Discharge Wellness

Raelene V. Shippee-Rice, Susan J. Fetzer, and Jennifer V. Long

PATIENT REPORT: Ms. Carter

Ms. Carter had a hemicolectomy for diverticulitis. During the surgery, there was an injury to her ureter, and she had a subsequent percutaneous nephrostomy. Prior to admission she considered herself to be healthy "for an old gal" and able to take care of herself. She is 83 years old and lives alone in her own house half a mile from the center of the small town where she has lived for 50 years. She has been a widow for 20 years and works part-time at a local office doing filing work and helping with billing. Her income is very limited but she manages as long as she is careful. Her two daughters live 30 minutes and 3 hours away, respectively. They are close and visit on the telephone regularly and occasionally help financially. She sees the daughter who lives nearby quite regularly. However, they are unable to provide daily or regular help due to their own families and work.

Her preoperative medical history indicates hypertension, heart failure, and moderately severe osteoarthritis. Her preoperative medications include furosemide 20 mgm a day, potassium 20 mEq daily, metoprolol 25 mg twice a day, aspirin 81 mg, and acetaminophen 500 mg every 6 hours. She is getting ready for discharge and will be returning home on self-care.

Patient-centered, relationship-oriented transitional care starts with the patient. The transitional care process first responds to patient questions and concerns, and then moves to information sharing and coaching on continuing postoperative recovery, and finally to promoting a long-term wellness program. Gerioperative care follows the older adult from the hospital or ambulatory surgical center until the first postdischarge visit with the surgeon or primary care provider. Transitional care support is a keystone to achieving optimal patient outcomes and preventing unnecessary hospital readmissions.

Planning for discharge begins at the time the patient agrees to surgery with the question: Given the older adults' clinical condition, functional status, available resources, type of surgery, and risk factors, what will this person need to maintain and continue surgical recovery after being discharged? The preadmission interview provides the data and determines the initial plan at time of admission. The plan is revised and adapted in response to changes in the patient's clinical condition or functional status during the perioperative period.

Transitional care is challenging when there are multiple providers involved in multiple discharge order sets. Older adults with multiple comorbidities requiring multiple medications are highly vulnerable to drug-drug and drug-disease interactions and adverse medication events (see Chapter 5).

Discharge after surgery with transition to a new care setting is a vulnerable period for the older adult. The shift from perioperative health care providers to elder self-care, informal care providers, or alternative health care providers in long-term care or the community requires critical coordination.This chapter reviews issues and concerns associated with transitional care of the gerioperative patient and provides strategies for improving patient-centered discharge that will promote surgical recovery, best care outcomes, and optimal wellness.

Background

Discharge planning and continuity of care have been sources of frustration for providers, patients, families, and payers for over 30 years. Community health nurses and nurses in long-term care institutions have long lamented the poor communication between hospital providers and those caring for the older adult as they transition out of the hospital. Patients and families have long complained about not knowing what they were supposed to do when the patient arrived home. Gerontological and geriatric nurses and other health care leaders have argued that professional providers and assistive personnel should have knowledge about the special care needs of older adults, yet families have been expected to provide complex care with little to no training and minimal information. The consequences of inadequate patient preparation for self-care and family preparation for care giving include lack of follow-up care after discharge, high rates of hospital readmission, diminished quality of life, and poor patient outcomes.

Up to 16% of older adults who have had surgery return to the hospital within 30 days with 27% readmitted within 90 days (Jencks, Williams, & Coleman, 2009). Up to 70% of patients with hospital readmission after surgery are readmitted for a medical problem related to surgery with pneumonia and medication adverse events as the primary cause of readmission. As many as two-thirds of the cited medication errors are preventable. Readmission costs up to $15 billion annually.

More than 40% of older adults cannot state the purpose of their medications. Fewer than half of older adults discharged from the hospital know their diagnosis. Of older adults needing assistance with activities of daily living, slightly over 80% did not have a home care referral. Almost two-thirds stated that no one at the hospital talked with them about how they would manage care at home (Makaryus & Friedman, 2005).

Current discharge teaching is accomplished in less than 10 minutes on average. Patients are highly passive, asking few questions. Due to fatigue, the fast pace of information transfer, pain, discomfort, or medication effects, most adults nod "Yes" to "Do you understand?" or "No" to "Do you have any questions?" Of eight recommended elements that should be included in discharge preparation (see Exhibit 23.1), less than four are covered 50% of the time, and six or less are covered in 30% of discharges (Makaryus & Friedman, 2005). Until recently, discharge planning and implementation was important on paper but received little attention in practice.

The paradigm is changing. Transitional care is becoming a central focus for improving patient outcomes after surgery. Medicare, the Joint Commission, the Institute of Medicine, and the Institute for Health Care Improvement along with professional organizations and health policy advocates are advocating for models that prevent readmission and promote

long-term health in older adults. Most postsurgical readmissions are preventable when there is effective discharge
planning and preparation of the patient and caregiver for
home-based care.

Nurses are key players in the effort to improve discharge planning and transitional care.

Nurses are key players in the effort to improve discharge
planning and transitional care processes. Gerioperative facil-
itated care uses a transitional care model across the perioperative continuum, incorporating a
discharge process that begins as soon as surgery is planned. The plan is continuously adapted
and redesigned as the patient's clinical conditions warrants, focused on self-care for immediate
surgical recovery and extended to ongoing wellness. Nurses are in direct contact with patients,
caregivers, and companion-coaches on a daily basis, allowing for the continuous information
sharing and coaching essential to preparation for home discharge. Medicare's changing reimbursement mechanisms support the older adult's return to home and reinforce discharge and
transitional care behaviors shown to improve patient outcomes.

Transitional Care Goals

Transitional care does not occur at a point in time during the discharge of the patient from
one setting to another. Rather, transitional care is a process concerned with the older adult's
preparedness for leaving one care setting, the adequacy of resources to continue the recovery
process, and the achievement of best patient outcomes and the patient's health care goals.
Resource availability refers to the knowledge, skills, and ability of the older adult for self-care
or of care providers at the new care site. Resources also include access to health care and
social support services.

The goals of transitional care involve the elder, caregiver, and new providers or care
(Exhibit 23.1). The goals are met by coordinating a care team that includes the patient, informal

---

EXHIBIT 23.1 Gerioperative Transitional Care Goals

- Establish specific outcomes in collaboration with gerioperative patient related to
  surgical recovery, general health
- Determine recovery outcomes pertinent to specific type of surgery
- Maximize the older adult's competence, confidence and ability for self-care consistent with the patient's level of physical and cognitive functional status
- Prepare patient and family for the psychosocial reactions and needs associated
  with transition to a new care setting and address concerns about long-term outcomes (e.g., partial recovery, palliation, functional status changes, death)
- Ensure caregiver understanding of care needs of the older adult, safety of home
  care environment, or adequacy of institutional support services
- Evaluate caregiver readiness, competence, confidence, and ability to assist older
  adult with surgical recovery
- Provide health coaching with patient and caregivers targeted to long-term health
  goals and well-being
- Conduct follow-up visits and ongoing contact to ensure resources are in place and
  the older adult is safe, comfortable, healing, and working toward agreed upon goals

caregivers, companion-coach, and providers from health and social support services and agencies. Coaching, a primary provider role during transitional care (see Chapter 6), targets short- and long-term health goals and well-being. Interactions to meet transitional care goals include follow-up visits by the geriatric care facilitator (GCF) and ongoing contact. Visits confirm that resources are in place and that the older adult is safe, comfortable, health, and working toward the agreed upon health goals.

The GCF or gerioperative nurse collaborates with the patient, family, companion-coach, and health care team to meet the transitional care goals specific to gerioperative care and to the patient. Sharing information and coaching with the patient and caregiver improves knowledge and skills needed for continuing postoperative recovery activities. Helping older adults and caregivers feel comfortable with contacting and communicating with providers, service agencies, and health care organizations increases feelings of safety and security after discharge. Although older adults who are discharged home receive most of the information on provider contact, older adults in any care setting must have access to outside providers who can be called upon to attend to their needs. Access is highly relevant to institutionalized elders.

Gerioperative Considerations

Gerioperative transitional care is divided into four stages: transition planning, comprehensive geriatric assessment, health coaching, and transition support.

TRANSITION PLANNING

Transition planning begins as soon as the patient agrees to surgery and continues throughout the perioperative continuum (Exhibit 23.2). Included in the preoperative information is an explanation of the multiple transitions the patient will experience during perioperative care: preadmission, admission, preoperative care, intraoperative care, postanesthesia care, postoperative care, and posthospital care. Guiding the older adult through these multiple transitions and helping them navigate the process promotes feelings of safety and security. Transition to home, rehabilitation setting, or long-term care facility is a vulnerable period for older adults as care shifts from one group of providers to another. Inadequate coordination and poor communication increase the risk for poor outcomes and adverse events. The GCF or gerioperative nurse follows the patient across the perioperative continuum linking preoperative information to anticipated care needs, intended outcomes, and plans for care after leaving the surgical center or hospital.

Preoperative planning sets a foundation for subsequent transitions and allows providers to plan ahead to what is needed to optimize patient outcomes. Changes that occur in the patient's clinical situation, as the perioperative journey progresses, will require reevaluating decisions for postoperative and posthospital care.

Plans for discharge and transitional care derive from the preoperative assessment. The goal is to return the older adult to a level equal to or better than the patient's preoperative level of function, health, and well-being. Knowledge of the older adult's preoperative health and functional ability establishes beginning patient goals for use after discharge.

Providing and supporting transitional care of the gerioperative patient is particularly challenging. Many older adults have medical comorbidities in addition to surgical needs and general self-care concerns. The complex self-care often needed for surgical recovery involves pain relief, medication management, wound care and healing, nutrition, mobility, activity,

EXHIBIT 23.2 Gerioperative Transitional Care Flow Chart

Stage I: Initial contact
- Introduce gerioperative care facilitator
- Outline facilitator role, responsibilities in relation to gerioperative patient
- Identify companion-coach
- Outline perioperative continuum
- Respond to patient questions, concerns

Stage II: Preoperative assessment
- Comprehensive geriatric assessment and screening with a written plan of care
- Prehabilitation based on comprehensive geriatric assessment and screening priorities
- Interdisciplinary action plan
- Postdischarge recovery plan considers comprehensive geriatric assessment priorities plus surgically related priorities
- Home modifications recommended and a plan for completing developed
- Preplanning regarding community resource availability and access information

Stage III: Perioperative continuum
- Monitor high-risk, potentially inappropriate, and anticholinergic medications with interdisciplinary team
- Attention to patient/caregiver questions, concerns
- Ongoing patient, companion-coach, caregiver coaching regarding progress, diagnoses, complications, prevention, therapeutic interventions, action plan
- Interdisciplinary action plan
- Written information to patient, caregiver, companion-coach
- Ongoing reflect back by patient, caregiver, companion-coach to ensure understanding, need for clarification, coaching, support
- Discharge plan revised/adapted as patient's clinical condition, functional status, care needs change

Stage IV: Preparing for transition to self-care
- Attention to patient concerns, questions, fear, expectations, outcomes
- Medication reconciliation
- Prescription, over-the-counter, herbal remedy review, and health coaching
- Demonstration and self-care coaching for care specific to surgical procedure
- Attention to basic postoperative care needs: pain relief, analgesia use, activity, rest/activity balance, mobility, stairs, driving, incision care, bathing, oral hygiene, nutrition/diet, symptom management
- Review of self-care goals, action plans related to comprehensive geriatric assessment priorities, patient readiness
- Resource provider to contact with questions, concerns: name and contact information of resource individual(s)
- Discussion of situations requiring contact with resource person
- Discussion of possible complications requiring intervention, early symptoms, early patient response to contact resource person, primary care provider, surgeon, emergency services
- Follow-up appointments: physical therapy, occupational therapy, primary care provider, surgeon, other members of interdisciplinary team

(continued)

EXHIBIT 23.2 Gerioperative Transitional Care Flow Chart *(continued)*

- Schedule for obtaining medications
- Start schedule of health, social support services
- Written plan of care with pictures, diagrams, websites, resource sites targeted to patient education, literacy, language, sensory changes, cognitive status
- Review, clarify, and validate patient, caregiver, companion-coach written notes
- Patient, caregiver, companion-coach reflect back to ensure congruity of understanding
- Follow-up appointment/telephone contact gerioperative care facilitator, gerioperative nurse, other resource persons

Stage IV (Alternative): Preparing for transition to nursing home
- Written plan of care including statement of patient concerns
- Results of medication reconciliation: anticholinergic risk, potentially inappropriate medications, dose, schedule, reasons for continuing, reason for discontinuing, plans for tapering if appropriate
- Care needs: pain relief, diet, elimination, incision care, activity, mobility, sleep, balance rest/activity, hygiene, hydration, follow-up schedule with surgeon and primary care provider, therapies
- Discharge summary detailing diagnoses, surgical procedure, progress and complications, comprehensive geriatric assessment and screening results, test results, therapies
- Name of resource person to contact with questions, concerns
- Referral to local aging and disability resource center for follow-up

Stage V: Follow-up contact
- Telephone call within 48 hours of discharge to assess progress, clarify information, questions, concerns
- In-home contact within 1 week of discharge or earlier depending on results of telephone call
- In-home, email, telephone contact as needed until first primary care provider and surgeon visits completed.
- Plan for termination

Stage VI: Transition to continuing self-care and support services
- Transition to full self-care, caregiver, home care nurse, other support services
- Written documentation regarding perioperative care history, patient concerns, care expectations, patient goals, patient care preferences, plans for long-term or ongoing care

and function. Care of comorbid conditions increase concerns about self-care when added to the demands of surgical recovery even in patients who have been managing chronic illness conditions for many years and become highly competent.

Transition to a long-term care facility, rehabilitation setting, or assisted living facility is difficult if it occurs in response to changes in health conditions that occurred due to surgery. The move is often unplanned. Providers, families, and friends are important support resources. It is important to send explicit and patient-sensitive discharge information to the new care setting before the older adult is discharged so the transitional care goals are better realized. Having information in advance encourages new providers and provides time to ensure that special care needs are in place prior to the patient's arrival.

COMPREHENSIVE GERIATRIC ASSESSMENT

Surgical stress, trauma, and anesthesia impact every body system at varying degrees of intensity dependent on the purpose, type, and extent of the surgical procedure. Results of the discharge assessment are compared with preadmission data to evaluate the extent of the changes in the patient's clinical and functional status that influence self-care abilities and the potential need for follow-up services. The gerioperative discharge screening assessment combines the standard discharge criteria associated with a specific surgical procedure with the screening comprehensive geriatric assessment elements used during preadmission (see Chapter 7). Table 23.1 reviews the elements of the comprehensive geriatric discharge assessment along with recommendations for patient and caregiver coaching.

Areas of special concern for the gerioperative patient include cognition and depression, medications, pain, mobility, nutrition, and wound care. Alterations in any of these elements increase the vulnerability for hospital readmission and poor discharge outcomes. Interventions must be developed in context of the patient's postdischarge environment, available resources, and ability of the older adult or caregiver to carry out the care intervention. Helping older adults understand that many self-care activities are interconnected to achieve a common outcome and are not discrete tasks that must be accomplished linearly is helpful. Focusing on the interaction and outcomes shifts attention from the number of self-care behaviors to the desired outcomes of behaviors that will promote recovery. Patients who see self-care behaviors as individual actions can be overwhelmed by the number of things they have to do. Coordinating overlapping behaviors that target a solution or outcome to a specific care need helps make the information less overwhelming.

COGNITION AND DEPRESSION

Cognitive changes are highly distressing to older adults and family caregivers. Assessing cognition before discharge, comparing results with preoperative baseline data, and sharing results with caregivers and the older adult is important for avoiding unnecessary distress and maintaining patient safety. The stress of surgery often triggers cognitive impairment in older adults with undetected mild cognitive impairment. Older adults functioning in day-to-day activities in a familiar environment can be tipped into demonstrable impairment secondary to the stress of surgery and hospitalization, pain, and medication effects. Changes in cognition may not be noticed until after the older adult returns to the preoperative environment and caregivers become aware of the change. Hospital-based changes are often overlooked as a normal response to the hospital environment. Upon return home, the behaviors take on a new significance that can be alarming to caregivers and to the patient.

Behavioral or cognitive changes after discharge can be alarming to caregivers and to the patient.

The onset of postoperative cognitive dysfunction (POCD) or depression frequently occurs after the patient is discharged. Caregivers and the older adult often assume cognitive changes and depression are a normal consequence of aging, surgery, and hospitalization. Coaching caregivers to understand that depression and cognitive changes are not normal and the importance of reporting changes in cognition or mood will assist in acting quickly to prevent and treat POCD. These actions can be critical to preserving cognition, well-being, and quality of life of the older adult. Ignoring the onset of cognitive impairment or changes in mood increases the older adult's vulnerability to poor health outcomes. Although prevention interventions of POCD are not well established, older adults are encouraged to be as physically active as possible, engage in regular physical and cognitive exercises, and have adequate

TABLE 23.1

Discharge Comprehensive Geriatric Assessment and Screening Elements, Information Sharing, Health Coaching

Element	Discharge Assessment	Information Sharing, Health Coaching, and Patient Talk Back
Surgical condition	Evaluate clinical condition in comparison with discharge criteria: wound, temperature, nutrition, bowel function, voiding, mobility, vital sign stability Evaluate criteria related to type of anesthesia Evaluate criteria related to type of surgery and surgery-specific discharge needs	Self-care regimen Surgery-specific self-care needs Schedule follow-up telephone call, home visit Schedule follow-up surgeon visit Schedule follow-up primary care clinic visit Provide patient written summary of surgery and recovery to date including postdischarge instructions Conduct reflect-back to ensure patient or caregiver understanding
Wound	Wound condition Patient understanding of wound care	Wound care management Surgery-specific wound care (e.g., ostomy care, cast care, staple removal) Ability to do wound care: self or others Type of equipment needed and where to obtain Return demonstration, description of wound care
Comorbid disease	Changes in self-care regimen Changes in clinical status Attend to patient concerns, questions	Coaching on self-care regimen Review any changes between postoperative regimen and preoperative regimen Clear written instructions Schedule postdischarge visits with PCP, IDT Ensure companion-coach, family member, gerioperative care facilitator attends first postoperative visits Patient review of self-care regimen
Functional status	ADLs, IADLs, advanced ADLs Self-care ability and limitations Review expected return of function if impaired since surgery	Need for assistive devices Demonstration correct use of assistive devices
Mobility	Ambulatory assistance needed Distance walking Gait, balance evaluation Fall risk assessment Exercise limitations Need for assistive devices	Ambulation safety Activity restrictions Exercise Avoid extended periods in reclining chairs Balance rest and activity Driving restrictions Need for assistive devices Demonstration correct use of assistive devices

(continued)

TABLE 23.1

Discharge Comprehensive Geriatric Assessment and Screening Elements, Information Sharing, Health Coaching *(continued)*

Element	Discharge Assessment	Information Sharing, Health Coaching, and Patient Talk Back
Cognition	Conduct Mini-Cog or institution-specific cognitive assessment Identify changes in cognitive function Evaluate recovery from hospital-based delirium	Safety precautions Cognitive exercises Physical exercise Social interaction Balance rest and activity Sleep support Medication review for potentially inappropriate and anticholinergic medications Discuss potential for postoperative cognitive dysfunction especially in patients discharged in less than 7 days after surgery. Explain condition, review signs and symptoms, when to notify provider, discuss interventions Follow-up visits with PCP, IDT Caregiver and patient brief intervention counseling
Depression/mood	Conduct GDS-SF Assess mood Evaluate appetite and sleep pattern	Address patient concerns about surgery, diagnosis, home care, potential for recovery Review signs and symptoms depressed mood When to contact care provider Establish exercise regimen Support social interaction Explain sleep protocol Review risks and benefits of sleep aids
Pain	Pain level related to surgically caused pain Pain level due to preexisting pain Pain level due to iatrogenic events	Conduct pain medication reconciliation Pain relief prescriptions for postoperative pain and preexisting pain Evaluate for drug interactions Tapering postoperative pain medication Use of nonpharmacologic pain relief methods Integration of postoperative medication regimen with preoperative pain relief regimen for preexisting pain Provider review of instruction notes prepared by patients, caregivers, or companion coach Review potential side effects of pain relief medications Discuss patient actions if medication side effects occur When to notify providers Give contact information of provider, gerioperative care facilitator, gerioperative care nurse Reinforce importance of contacting provider Ask patient, caregiver, or companion-coach for a "reflect back" to ensure understanding

(continued)

TABLE 23.1

Discharge Comprehensive Geriatric Assessment and Screening Elements, Information Sharing, Health Coaching *(continued)*

Element	Discharge Assessment	Information Sharing, Health Coaching, and Patient Talk Back
Nutrition and hydration	Appetite at time of discharge Weight Hydration	Dietary restrictions and recommendations specific to surgical procedure Discuss target goal for weight if underweight or overweight Hydration needs Nutritional consult as needed
Polypharmacy	Conduct medication reconciliation Identify high-risk medications, potentially inappropriate medications, anticholinergic medications Patient talk back regarding medication regimen	Review discharge medication list with preoperative medication list—explain changes and reasons for change Provide written copy of prescribed medications with drug name, dose, schedule, brief side effects, toxic effects, when to contact provider Review herbal medication safety Review restrictions on alcohol use Ask patient to explain medication self-administration
Sleep	Current sleep patterns Changes in sleep patterns after surgery	Review importance of sleep Review sleep protocol Provide written sleep protocol
Smoking	Patient intent to smoke	Reward nonsmoking during surgical recovery Provide smoking cessation health coaching Refer to smoking cessation clinic, PCP
Social support	Availability of caregiver Ability of caregiver to provide needed care Ongoing support of companion coach Assess caregiver knowledge, skills, support needs Availability of support system for shopping, obtaining medications Availability of community health, social service resources	Referral to Aging and Disability Resource Center options counselor Referral to community support services Transportation from hospital Obtaining support for instrumental activity needs (e.g., transportation, bill paying, shopping, laundry) Determining wait time for initiation of support services Follow-up phone calls from gerioperative care facilitator, companion-coach to ask, What do you need?
Home environment Patient safety	Safety issues: home access, bedroom access, bathroom access, stair railings, bathroom handrails, shower/bathtub safety, raised toilet seat, throw rugs, cooking facilities, refrigerator, hot water, distance to pharmacy Environmental safety Lifeline or other emergency call system Home modifications completed since preoperative review	Referral to volunteer home rehabilitation-modification organization Schedule IDT home visit Navigating the environment

(continued)

TABLE 23.1

Discharge Comprehensive Geriatric Assessment and Screening Elements, Information Sharing, Health Coaching *(continued)*

Element	Discharge Assessment	Information Sharing, Health Coaching, and Patient Talk Back
Spiritual support	Identify patient's sources of strength Evaluate feelings of security and readiness to move forward with challenges of recovery Assess patient concerns and feelings of uncertainty about the future especially if surgery related to diagnosis of cancer	Referral for home visit from minister, pastor, or other spiritual support person Explore patient's concerns about the future Attend to feelings of uncertainty
Patient's strengths	Feelings of competence to manage self-care activities Areas of insecurity regarding self-care Concerns about caregiver readiness Willingness to reach out to providers with questions and concerns	Review patient progress on self-care Reinforce self-care ability Refer to follow up support from gerioperative care facilitator, companion-coach, and IDT Provide information on caregiver support services Reinforce importance of reaching out to providers

ADLs, activities of daily living; GDS-SF, Geriatric Depression Scale-Short Form; IADLs, instrumental activities of daily living; IDT, interdisciplinary team; PCP, primary care provider.

nutrition and hydration, and rest and sleep. These POCD interventions have been shown to be of benefit in maintaining cognitive function and decreasing depressive symptoms.

POLYPHARMACY

Polypharmacy is a major cause of cognitive change in older adults. Over 50% of postdischarge hospital readmissions are due to medication errors at the time of discharge or inability or unwillingness of the older adult or caregiver to understand and follow through with the medication regimen. Medication safety improves with discharge medication reconciliation. Discharge medication reconciliation compares discharge prescriptions with the patient's admission medication list and all medications prescribed throughout the preoperative and postoperative stay. Disposition of prescribed medications are noted. Disposition includes discontinued on admission, continued on admission, discontinued before surgery, continued after surgery, discontinued on discharge, or continued on discharge. New prescriptions written at time of discharge are compared with previously prescribed medications to determine duplication. Comparison includes drug name, dose, administration schedule, and route. Prescriptions are reviewed for potentially inappropriate medications, anticholinergic burden, drug-drug interactions, and nonprescription-prescription drug interactions. Questions, concerns, and discrepancies are referred to the interdisciplinary care team.

Older adults taking multiple medications on a routine schedule find changes in medication dosing and scheduling challenging. Discharge medication regimens that differ from preoperative regimens can be disrupting for older adults. Particularly disrupting are changes in drug dose, schedule, or when drugs that have a similar effect have different names. For example, at the time of discharge, a patient may receive a new prescription for a drug to treat a preexisting medical condition. The newly prescribed drug has similar action but a different name from the drug previously taken. The patient may fill the new prescription and then resume the older prescription at home, not understanding that they are duplicate prescriptions. It should be explained to the older adult that the only medications to be taken are those written on the discharge instruction form. Telling the patient that old medications are not to be restarted on return home unless told to do so helps to eliminate the problem. It is important for patients to know they should take all containers of all the medications they took preoperatively plus the medications they are taking postoperatively to the first follow-up visit with the surgeon or primary care provider. Explaining the importance of asking the provider to clarify which medications should be continued and at what dosing schedule makes it easier for the patient to talk with the provider about medication use. If the patient has questions before the professional visit, the contact person should be notified. Reinforcing the message to the patient that the contact resource person or the provider must be called whenever there is a treatment question helps to prevent complications and adverse events as well as provides support to the older adult.

Over time, the new regimen becomes the norm but during transition, medication changes can be particularly troublesome and prone to error. Complex directions involving how medications are to be taken, such as with meals or without meals, before, with, or after other medications, morning dose or evening dose, and alternating days or several times a week, easily lead to adverse drug events. Directions that state a drug is to be discontinued but does not provide a specific date for discontinuing the drug creates uncertainty. For example, a pain medication that is to be discontinued "when no longer needed" raises patient concerns about stopping the medication too early or too late.

Instructions that seem obvious to providers can seem incomprehensible to older adults. The role of the gerioperative care nurse is to ensure the older adult, companion-coach, and caregivers have sufficient clarity about the medication regimen for patient safety. Safety centers on correct medication, correct dose, correct information about side effects and adverse effects, and correct action to take should either occur. For patients with multiple medications, the task seems daunting.

Several barriers interfere with effective medication teaching during the discharge process. Time is a major barrier for providers, while physical and psychological energy is a major patient barrier. Discharge coaching must be scheduled in advance. Scheduling sets aside time for providers to focus on the patient and for the patient to focus on the material. Scheduling also establishes a message that discharge teaching is important and takes time to accomplish. Medication information should be written out in advance in easy-to-read font and print size. There should be room on the information sheet for the patient or caregiver to make notes about the medication or to write questions after returning home.

Instructions that seem obvious to providers may be incomprehensible to elders.

A general approach begins with medications that retain the same schedule as preoperative regimen followed by medications that are the same but have a new dose or new schedule. New medications are discussed last. This approach moves from easy to more difficult information. If the patient is easily fatigued, starting with new content while the patient is not yet fatigued may be reasonable. A third approach is to ask the patient the method he or she prefers. There is no right answer that fits all situations. The answer rests on clinical judgment and sensitivity to the patient's fatigue, concerns, attention span, and presence and attitude of companion-coach or family member.

It is a decision the nurse makes in context of the individual patient and situation. Coaching must be explicit, concrete, in step with the patient's ability to absorb, and responsive to the patient's questions, concerns, knowledge level, and feelings of competence and confidence.

Older adults often do not consider smoking and alcohol use to be medication-related. However, nicotine and alcohol are substances that alter the body's physiology and affect the neurological system similar to medications. Helping the older adult realize that cigarette smoking and alcohol use have side effects and negative effects similar to that caused by medications provides a different lens for observing their behavior. Older adults, if asked, would not continue taking a medication that had negative side effects. Encouraging them to discontinue overuse of alcohol or the use of cigarettes using the example of discontinuing medications with negative side effects provides a different source of motivation. Chapter 6 outlines the 5As, a brief intervention health coaching process for smoking cessation and management of alcohol intake.

PAIN

Effective pain relief at home is based on principles of prevention, early detection, and immediate intervention. Caregivers express concerns about overmedicating and harming the older adult especially when using opioid medications. Informal caregivers overestimate the older person's discomfort, while older adults hesitate to express pain due to burden worry and concerns about dependence. Facilitating communication between older adults and informal caregivers remains a high priority for improving home-based care of the older adult.

Assessing patient and caregiver beliefs about pain and medication is essential in coaching patient and caregiver decisions about pain relief methods in the home. Differences in beliefs, about how pain should be treated and how much pain a person should experience before having medication or other interventions, interfere with effective pain relief. Explaining to caregivers that "pain is what the patient says it is," is an important aspect of health coaching. Encouraging use of medication around the clock to promote a low level of pain is often counter to many patient and caregiver beliefs. The common approach to pain is to "take something when it hurts." Coping with postoperative pain requires a different approach. Maintenance doses of acetaminophen around the clock can be highly effective in treatment of mild to moderate pain especially when combined with nonpharmacologic interventions. Moderate to severe pain is managed with low dose-opioids at a level to keep pain at a comfortable level. Persistent, severe postoperative pain requires evaluation by a provider. Reassure caregivers and older adults that providers prefer to be called with questions and concerns rather than to have pain, or the condition causing pain, to escalate to a point where emergency care or readmission is needed. Convincing older adults and caregivers that prevention is better for the provider and for the patient is an important message to reinforce. Providing a 24/7 contact information number and contact name minimizes patient and caregiver hesitancy about calling.

MOBILITY, ACTIVITY, AND FUNCTIONAL STATUS

Assess the amount of assistance the patient needs to carry out recovery activities, basic and instrumental activities of daily living, and to ambulate or move around within the environment. The assessment provides a baseline for immediate and longer-term exercise and activity goals. Comparing discharge assessment data with preoperative assessment provides target goals for recovery as well as establishes a baseline for measuring recovery after discharge.

Returning to the preoperative environment can set back the older adult's in-hospital activity level and mobility. Relief at being out of the hospital and being in one's own surroundings and one's own bed predisposes patients to being resistant to activity. Older adults who have had day surgery may not consider exercise important to their postoperative recovery.

With discharge after day surgery and short in-hospital stays, the risk for postoperative complications extends after discharge. Patients often assume that once home, the danger is past. Reinforcing the information that postoperative complications remain a risk until further recovery and that mobility is a primary prevention mode can serve as a motivation. Effective methods for increasing activity and exercise include chair yoga and walking.

Chair yoga, involving upper and lower extremity and torso exercises, is excellent for improving muscle strength and flexibility. Incorporating deep breathing and muscle relaxation as part of the chair yoga exercises also helps with relaxation to decrease discomfort, anxiety, and improve depressive symptoms. Walking as much as possible remains the gold standard for exercise. Walking can be done in any environment, around the house, outdoors, or in stores. Establishing a chair yoga and walking exercise program as part of postoperative recovery can easily be extended into a longer-term health behavior change to improve overall health and well-being. Many shopping malls have walking clubs, and chair yoga is offered in many health centers and clinics. However, walking and chair yoga can easily be done at home.

Safety is always a concern, and balancing the needs for rest and activity must be used to guide the amount of exercise during early stages of recovery. Activity is increased as the patient gains strength. Monitoring the interaction of pain and discomfort with activity is important. Pain and activity are bidirectional. Pain can increase or decrease activity, and activity can increase or decrease pain. Clinical judgment and knowledge of the patient are key variables in considering coaching for mobility and activity goals and action plans. Decisions must be made in context of what the patient was doing prior to surgery, at time of discharge, short- and long-term limitations caused by surgery, and the short- and long-term goals.

The companion-coach and caregivers are essential in providing support, encouragement, and cheerleading the older adult to continue moving. Older adults are more likely to participate in exercise and activity if others join them in the effort. Having the companion-coach and caregivers do the exercises and walking with the older adult makes the "work" more fun and improves the overall health and well-being for all participants.

WOUND HEALING AND NUTRITION

Wound care and healing are immediate concerns and high anxiety factors in the gerioperative patient. Concerns center on how to care for the wound, prevent injury, possible complications particularly bleeding or infection, showering and bathing, and removal of staples or stitches. The older adult has an increased level of risk for infection and slowed healing due to age-related changes in the immune system, changes in the skin, effects of comorbid disease on healing, and ability to perform self-care due to vision changes and flexibility. Assessing functional ability, flexibility, and vision to see the wound, and availability of someone to assist with wound care are important discharge assessment considerations.

Wound care is highly specific to the type of surgery; wound site; extent of wound; type of dressings; presence of ostomy, drains, or other tubes; and if there are staples or stitches. If the wound is large or complicated, demonstration of wound care with talk back by the patient is critical to improving the patient's feelings of competence managing wound care. Providing information on activities to avoid, whether the patient can shower or bathe, and how to protect the wound during activity decreases patient anxiety. Discussion regarding the amount of bleeding from the wound that is expected for the type of wound, signs and symptoms of infection, how to prevent wound problems, alert signals that indicate the beginning of a complication, when to call a provider, and the name and telephone number of a resource person to contact if there are any questions are basic to quality discharge coaching about wounds.

Patients do not routinely understand the importance of nutrition when thinking about how to take care of surgical wounds. Explaining the role of nutrition in wound care serves to improve wound healing and overall nutrition, important in energy production and restoring nutritional reverses depleted by surgery.

Inadequate nutrition is a continuing health problem in older adults especially for those with comorbid disease, living alone, or facing difficulty with transportation. In the gerioperative patient, nutrition is essential to recovery as it impacts wound healing, energy levels, and the body's ability to replenish protein and fat stores used in managing the stress of surgery.

Patients do not consider nutrition when thinking about wound care.

Conducting the discharge nutrition assessment focuses on factors that will influence postdischarge nutrition. Support factors such as meal preparation, shopping transportation, and financial resources to purchase quality foods such as fruits, vegetables, and protein sources are just as important in assessing the patient's ability to attain adequate nutrition as is the type of foods he or she eats.

Appetite often improves in older adults after discharge with the return to a familiar environment with access to familiar "comfort" foods. The concern is the quality of the comfort foods. Comparing preoperative diets with postoperative nutritional needs establishes priority areas for nutrition coaching. Age-related changes in taste and smell, together with activity, comfort, and sleep patterns altered by surgery interfere with postoperative nutrition. Recommendations to improve home nutrition must be adapted to the care setting and resource availability. Frequent high-nutrition meals or between meal high-nutrition snacks and drinks is often more effective than increasing meal size to improve nutrition. Vitamin supplements, particularly vitamin C and a multivitamin, contribute to wound healing and should be encouraged. Older adults at risk for poor nutrition should have an interdisciplinary team consult or, at a minimum, a nutritionist and social worker referral.

SOCIAL SUPPORT

Older adults rely to a large extent on family caregivers after surgery. Incorporating family caregivers as part of the overall health care team throughout the perioperative continuum is critical. Incorporating family in the transitional care process with the permission of the older adult cannot be overlooked. Discharge planning and health coaching must be done in the presence of the companion-coach or the person who is going to serve as an informal caregiver.

The caregiver is often an older adult who also has age-related and disease-related changes. Caregiving is physically, psychologically, and emotionally stressful. Concern and uncertainty about the future health and well-being of the patient, worry about patient safety, feelings of inability to provide the care needed or fear of harming the older adult contribute to heightened caregiver stress. Patients not wanting to overburden family members often make caregiving more difficult by denying their needs with "don't worry" or "don't bother" when caregivers attempt to provide needed care.

Caregiving is emotionally stressful and exhausting.

Assessing social support includes attention to the care needs of the caregiver as well as an assessment of the knowledge, abilities, and capabilities of the caregiver to meet the patient's care needs. Facilitating the older adult, caregiver, and the companion-coach as a team working together for common goals is a message throughout the perioperative continuum and a message that needs to continue as part of the transitional care process. Although coaching centers on self-care of the older adult, caregivers often contribute to that self-care. Coaching caregivers on not doing too much for the older adult while also not doing too little and how to tell the difference is helpful to both the older adult and caregivers.

Coaching the patient and caregiver on contacting community health and social agencies and resources to meet short- or long-term care goals contributes to improving patient recovery. Aging and disability resource centers provider caregiver support services and counseling on long-term care needs of older adults and family caregivers. One of the goals of aging and disability resource centers is to help patients and caregivers coordinate community resources. Older adults who are discharged to a long-term care or rehabilitation facility should be referred to the local aging and disability resource center for follow-up counseling on community supports and resources.

Plans for follow-up care are part of the discharge care responsibilities. Patients should have follow-up appointments with primary care providers, specialists, and surgeons prior to leaving the surgical care site. Patients are also provided with a discharge summary that includes their diagnosis, surgery, medications, and discharge action plan. Explain that the patient is to take the discharge summary to all postoperative follow-up appointments and review the document with the provider.

HEALTH COACHING

A major component of the discharge wellness promotion is health coaching. Health coaching begins with the patient's concerns, questions, fears, expectations, and goals. What does the patient want to know? Although older adults and their caregivers have questions, they often

TABLE 23.2

Barriers to Effective Transitional Discharge Care

Gerioperative Patient or Caregiver Characteristics	Provider Characteristics	System Characteristics

• Age-related changes
  • Cognition
  • Psychomotor processing
  • Sensoriperceptual
• Disease-related changes
  • Functional capacity
  • Depression
  • Diminished reserve
• Literacy
• Health literacy
• Hesitancy to ask questions
• Unfamiliar with questions to ask
• Inadequate resources
• Complex care needs
	• Poor communication
	• Inadequate time
	• Lack of written instructions
	• Written instructions not sensitive to patient characteristics
	• Prescription medications
	  • High alert medications
	  • Potentially inappropriate medications
	  • Anticholinergic medications
	• Poor communication
	• Inadequate information transfer
	• Overestimation of patient knowledge
	• Inattention to talk back process
		• Inadequate medication reconciliation process
		• Inattention to discharge planning as element of care
		• Single practice settings (e.g., primary care, hospitalist)
		• Lack of care integration by gerioperative care facilitator or gerioperative care nurse
		• Inadequate transfer of discharge summary to interdisciplinary team, primary care provider, clinic

do not ask them. Patient, provider, and system characteristics, as identified in Table 23.2, create barriers to effective information exchange and active participation by the patient.

Older adults are overwhelmed before and during the transition to home or discharge care setting. Getting prepared to move to a different location and concerns about the future interfere with attention and decrease retention. Fatigue, stress, and concerns about managing care needs contribute to feelings of incompetence and inability to cope. Managing the discharge information needs of the patient requires clinical judgment, artful communication, and sensitivity to the unique context of the patient's clinical condition, self-competence and -confidence, new location of care, and goals for the future.

Older adults rate pain, activity, wound care symptom management, and management of complications as high concern topics. Table 23.3 lists discharge informational needs identified by older adults or provider groups. Patient who have had abdominal surgery suggest elimination as an additional important issue.

TABLE 23.3

Discharge Informational Needs Identified by Patients, Nurses, and Physicians

Patient Concerns[1] (Postoperative)	Gerioperative Facilitated Care	Nurse-Identified Concerns (Postoperative)	Society of Hospital Medicine[2] (Elderly Patient)	Transitional Care Pillars[3] (Medical-Surgical)
Pain	Polypharmacy	Medication	Medication education	Medication
Wound care, bathing	Wound healing, nutrition	Wound care	Patient instructions	Patient self-care record
Activity	Mobility, activity, functional status	Psychosocial	Cognition	Red flags (monitoring complications)
Monitoring complications	Surgical condition Comorbid disease	Patient-identified concerns	Discharge summary	Follow-up with primary care and specialist providers
Symptom management	Health coaching		Provider-provider contact	
Contact person	Cognition Depression		Hazardous medication Follow-up	
Elimination	Pain		Follow-up	
Quality of life	Spiritual support Sleep Social support Home environment Patient strengths Follow-up care			

[1]Pieper et al., 2006.
[2]Society of Hospital Medicine, 2005.
[3]The Care Transitions Program, 2007.

Nurses identify psychosocial concerns, medication, wound care, and patient-identified concerns as core discharge information. Other provider groups suggest that medication, patient instructions, ensuring outside providers have information about the patient's condition and progress, monitoring complications, and establishing follow-up plans improve patient outcomes after discharge.

The gerioperative facilitated care model relies on the geriatric comprehensive assessment, the specific care needs associated with the type of surgery, and patient concerns as the foundation for determining and attending to discharge information needs. Priorities are decided by collaboration: with the older adult, informal caregivers or formal care providers, and the gerioperative nurse or GCF.

Attending to the patient's concerns demonstrates respect for the individual and acceptance of the gerioperative patient's immediate fears. Connecting self-care information with the older adult's strengths and previous experience as patient or caregiver with information gained throughout the perioperative experience helps decrease information overload and increase feelings of competence and confidence. Checking in with the patient using the "talk back" or "reflect back" process indicates whether information is being assimilated or more clarification is needed. The responsibility of the discharge health coach is to begin within the patient's frame of reference and then gently guide the patient to new areas of self-care.

DISCHARGE INFORMATION

Written information serves as a reference point for information sharing. Taking the written information home or to the next care setting also contributes to feelings of competence and confidence. The patient has information on hand to turn to for self-care recommendations and as validation for contacting providers with questions. However, how providers' present written information and how patient's read, think about, or interpret the information often lacks congruency. Reviewing the written document, encouraging the patient to ask questions, and then adapting the information and writing it to the patient's own language use and style make it easier for the patient to understand the information at a later date. The patient or caregiver(s) is encouraged to include additional notes if needed to make the information clearer. However, it is important for the gerioperative care provider to review the notes for accuracy.

The amount of information patients must absorb can be overwhelming. Determining how to make the quantity of information manageable presents a challenge. The information must be relevant, succinct, focused, accurate, and easy for a layperson to understand at the fifth- or sixth-grade level, regardless of the patient's level of education. Stress reduces the ability to absorb new data.

Discharge information can be divided into several classifications. One approach to classifying discharge information is on the basis of urgent, need, or nice to know. Urgent refers to information the patient must have and be able to use in order to provide safe self-care. Examples include knowledge of high-risk medications and prevention of infection. High-risk medication coaching includes learning the name, dose, administration schedule, side effects, response, and treatment of side effects. The needed discharge information refers to information that promotes the patient's immediate recovery needs. Nice to know information is that which is important for promoting ongoing health and well-being but can be reviewed at a later date when immediate safety and recovery needs have been met.

How information is classified into the three categories varies from individual to individual. Classification depends on patient variables such as level of frailty or wellness, clinical condition, status of comorbid condition, ability to provide self-care, and risk factors pertinent to the individual discharge situation. Surgical variables include type of surgery, presence of postoperative complications, and surgery-specific self-care needs.

There is a consistent theme across provider groups that medication instruction is a major challenge. The priority reflects the high number of discharge-associated medication errors and the number of older adults readmitted to the hospital as a result of medication error or misinformation. Medication information can be classified as urgent, needed, or nice to know. For example, discharge medication regimens that are consistent with the regimen the patient was taking at time of admission and at same dose and schedule create a less urgent situation than a regimen that involves one or more high-alert medications such as anticoagulant, hypoglycemic, opioid, antibiotic, or corticosteroid medications. Older adults transitioning to a long-term care or a rehabilitation facility will have a less immediate need for information on medication safety and administration than older adults transitioning to home, where the patient is responsible for self-medication or an informal caregiver administers the medication.

Information can be classified during the discharge coaching process in response to patient need, knowledge base, questions, and concerns. Questions for the provider to consider when determining information needs include: How much information and at what level does this older adult need or want to safely carry out self-care in relations to a specific self-care variable? The ability to organize and simplify information while retaining its critical elements is a communication art sorely needed by providers responsible for discharge information and health coaching.

The success of information sharing and health coaching rests on the clinical judgment and expert knowledge of the gerioperative care nurse or GCF. Clinical judgment and expert knowledge guide decisions about what must be included at an information exchange meeting as well as how to present the discharge information in a way that remains patient-centered, supports patient safety, promotes continuing recovery, and stimulates patient commitment. Thus, decisions on discharge informational needs and sharing do not rest on a checklist of items; the decisions rest on recognizing and respecting the unique character of the individual and the situation, the ability to adapt information to the goals and needs of the individual, and maintaining a focus on patient safety, progress toward recovery, and achieving patient-centered short- and long-term health goals.

TRANSITION SUPPORT

Transition to another care setting is anxiety provoking even when the care setting is familiar. The patient has been through a stressful experience with new short-term care needs and the potential for long-term care needs. The first few days or week after discharge can be highly challenging to older adults living alone or when caregiving is limited to a single family member. The following example illustrates this point.

Mrs. Jameson was caring for her husband after his discharge from the hospital for total knee replacement. She was highly concerned about his safety and feared he would try to get around by himself. He complained of being unable to move easily and had difficulty getting from the house to the car and in and out of the car. He refused to go shopping. Mrs. Jameson did not want to leave him but had no one to help with getting groceries and medications or going to the post office or laundromat. The nurses had been very helpful in explaining what she needed to do to take care of her husband and to encourage him to take care of himself, but no one had anticipated the difficulty with managing the day-to-day activities. "It was very different when we got home; very different from it was when we talked about it in the hospital."

"It was very different when we got home."

The stress of surgery and hospitalization plus the stress and anticipation of going home or to another care setting inhibits the older patient's ability to think ahead to what the instrumental care needs will be. Questions from the GCF or gerioperative care nurse prompt patients and caregivers to identify concerns and potential barriers to meeting their own needs. Caregivers are often elderly and experience age- or disease-related changes, stress, and anxiety related to their own health and function as well as the perioperative patient's situation. Once home, problems that were not considered in the abstract discussion become clear. Knowing that someone will be doing a follow-up telephone call or home visit within 24 or 48 hours of discharge decreases stress and helps to contain feelings of security and well-being. Having the name of a contact person or telephone number adds to feelings of comfort and control. Older adults living in rural communities with limited access to support services are particularly vulnerable and require special care.

Home support services may take several weeks to initiate. Lack of transportation interferes with securing dressing supplies and medications. The presence of a companion-coach provides an immediate support system able to run errands and shop or remain with the gerioperative patient while the family caregiver does the shopping. Asking the patient about instrumental activities of daily living support prompts consideration of constraints to re-entering the home environment and getting the environment well stocked with the needed resources. Exploring availability of formal and informal supports helps ensure the readiness of the home environment.

Older adults hesitate to call providers. However, if providers call older adults, the older adult is more likely to ask questions, express concerns, and ask for advice or help. Follow-up telephone calls allow providers to assess patient safety, needs, progress toward identified goals, and adherence to recommended treatment and action plans. Phone calls focus on the individual patient as well as general surgical and geriatric assessment guidelines. A review of each element enables the gerioperative care nurse or GCF to assess status of current concerns as well as the emergence of new problems. The telephone appointment is best scheduled before the older adult leaves the hospital. A follow-up reminder mailed to the older adult with sample questions from the GCF or nurse helps the older adult prepare for the call. Sample questions asked by the GCF may include: How have you been feeling since you have been home? What has concerned you since you left the surgical care unit? How have you been managing your pain? Have you had any concerns about your medications? What does the wound look like? and Tell me what a typical day is like for you.

Schedule follow-up appointments before discharge.

Often, patients do not see that the home is unsafe, creating a hazard, or interfering with recovery. A provider looks at the home environment with a different lens. Although the older adult is not always willing or able to make recommended changes to the environment that facilitate self-care or safety, the nurse or GCF will have a better context for understanding environmental supports and barriers.

A follow-up visit to the home or care facility after discharge is the most comprehensive mechanism for ensuring a safe, effective transitional care process. Assessing the patient in the context of the care facility guides the questions that need to be asked and the ongoing coaching of older adult and the caregivers. The home visit includes an assessment of the patient's recovery progress, identifies any barriers that have disrupted progress, and data for continued coaching on recovery or longer-term health goals. Conducting a review of elements including the screening comprehensive geriatric assessment guides the evaluation of the patient's recovery progress. Continue contact with the perioperative patient until the patient has the first follow-up visit with the surgeon and primary care providers. Attending the first visit with the patient provides data for the complete transition of the patient to self health care management with assistance from family members or significant others.

Generally, older adults will be in late-stage recovery and able to maintain progress. In the event that the older adult continues to need care after the follow-up visit, the GCF works with the patient and family to develop an action plan that will provide ongoing care and ensure the older adult's continued progress toward health and well-being.

Evaluating Transitional Care

There is mixed evidence on the effectiveness of the traditional discharge planning model in improving patient outcomes, decreasing hospital readmissions, or promoting long-term health behavior change and wellness. Most reviews indicate little benefit. Evaluation of transitional care programs with integrated health coaching and follow-up contacts demonstrates improved patient outcomes and better long-term health gains. Evaluating the effects of transitional care throughout the perioperative continuum on patient outcomes at each stage has yet to be completed. Table 23.4 identifies evaluation criteria for current transitional care models. Providing financial incentives as well as establishing standards of care that support a transitional care model through the patient's surgical care process will improve short-term goals related to patient satisfaction, quality patient care, and immediate patient outcomes, as well as contribute to overall health and well-being and quality of life.

TABLE 23.4
General Criteria to Evaluate Transitional Care

- Patient satisfaction
- Self-care competence and confidence
- Ability to state self-care goals
- Established action plan to achieve self-care goals
- Patient-identified goals
- Patient clinical status
- Patient functional status
- Hospital readmission rates
- Surgery-related complication rates after discharge
- Morbidity rate
- Mortality rate
- Medication error
- Hospital costs
- Provider satisfaction

PATIENT REPORT: Ms. Carter

The GCF meets with Ms. Carter and her daughter at 10:00 a.m. the day before her discharge. During the comprehensive discharge assessment, the GCF learns that Ms. Carter is doing well. She is recovering quickly and feels ready to go home. Ms. Carter says she is used to taking care of herself and has "it all worked out." However, there are several areas that concern Ms. Carter. Ms. Carter has received no information on how to care for her nephrostomy. Ms. Carter states she has none of "those bags or anything else" to take home with her.

Ms. Carter has no close friends in town, though she has friends in town who are going to help her with shopping. Her daughter will stay with her for a few days after she gets home, but then she will be alone. Ms. Carter is able to take care of her hygiene, although very slowly.

Ms. Carter is alert, oriented, and carries a conversation well, but complains about "feeling fuzzy" in her head. She pats the top of her head and says, "It just doesn't feel right up here. I am fine but just doesn't feel right."

She reports her pain is okay. The nurses give her something when she complains, which is not often. When asked how she will manage her pain at home, Ms. Carter says it will not be a problem: "If it hurts too much, I will take something and go lie down until it feels better. I know how to take care of myself." The GCF asks her what she will take. Ms. Carter is not sure but whatever they tell her to take will be fine. They will probably tell her to just take some aspirin or an extra acetaminophen or something.

Ms. Carter does her own cooking. "I make a lot of sandwiches. You know with bologna and ham. It's easy and pretty nutritious too. I cook a chicken now and then. That is easy too. I don't drink very much water. Makes me go to the bathroom all the time. Just a cup of coffee in the morning."

She reports sleeping well: "Like a log as a matter of fact. Go to bed around 10 or 11 and up around 7. Got a full day ahead of me. Have to keep ahead of my housework so I can be ready to go to the office. Working is really good for me. Keeps me out of trouble. And I don't have time to get down in the dumps." She does not anticipate any problems with sleeping when she gets home.

Social support is primarily her daughters and her neighbors. One of her daughters will stay with her the first three or four days. If she needs help after that, the daughter who lives half an hour away can drive up and help her. The neighbors will take care of her immediate needs. "Everything will be fine. Don't you worry," is her summation to the GCF.

The GCF summarizes the issues and suggests they start with working on the issues that concern Ms. Carter. The laundry and shopping turn out to be easily solved. The daughter who will be staying with Ms. Carter will see that everything is caught up while she is there. The laundry will be done and food, medicine, supplies, and anything else that she needs will be stocked and available. The house will be cleaned and everything in order before she leaves. The daughter who lives closer will take Ms. Carter shopping and do the laundry once a week. The neighbors will fill in as needed in between times. Ms. Carter feels a bit guilty about making her daughter drive over an hour every week to do her laundry. When reassured that it would not be a problem and not to worry, she finally accepts the plan.

The GCF also decided to check with the staff nurses about the nephrostomy and abdominal wound care and make sure Ms. Carter had the information and supplies she would need before going home. She asked if Ms. Carter was up to meeting a while longer to go over some of the GCF's concerns. Ms. Carter states she was getting a bit uncomfortable and would like to rest for a bit. The GCF makes an appointment to come back after lunch.

On returning to see Ms. Carter, the staff nurse reports he met with Ms. Carter and reviewed nephrostomy care, abdominal wound care, and that supplies would be ready for her to take home. Ms. Carter was relieved and feeling much better. The daughter was with her during the teaching session and would pass the information along to the other daughter who would be staying with Ms. Carter for the first few days.

The GCF meets with Ms. Carter and asks about the teaching session. When Ms. Carter confirms that she feels fine, the GCF explains they need to review Ms. Carter's diet and medications. Ms. Carter is quite surprised. She thought she was doing just fine. She didn't see anything wrong with her diet, and she had been managing her medications for years. The GCF reassures her that she has been managing her medications well. Her discharge prescriptions remain the same with no change in medication, dose, or schedule. However, with the surgery and the abdominal and nephrostomy wounds, attention to her diet becomes even more important for both wound healing and maintenance of her low sodium intake. The GCF suggests that Ms. Carter meet with one of the dieticians and go over her meal plans to look at the sodium and nutritional quality in relation to wound healing. The dietician will review comfort foods that will be easy to prepare but are lower in sodium and higher in nutrition to help her wounds to heal. Ms. Carter agreed to listen to what the dietician had to say and see if it made sense.

The GCF then addressed pain relief and medication. Ms. Carter said she never takes anything but sometimes increases the aspirin or acetaminophen when her knee begins bothering her too much. She does not like to take pills. The GCF reminds her it is important to keep pain at a minimum so she can do the walking she needs to do to keep up her recovery, keep her knee in shape, get stronger, and continue sleeping well. Ms. Carter will be discharged with a prescription for combination acetaminophen and oxycodone. The GCF reviews safety issues related to sedation and fall risk. With her osteoarthritis, her age, and her postsurgical status, she is at risk for falls unless she is very careful to take preventative measures.

As the prescribed pain medication has acetaminophen as an ingredient, the GCF explains that Ms. Carter will not need to take her acetaminophen when she takes the prescription pain medication. It will be helpful if she keeps a record of when she takes her acetaminophen for pain and when she takes her prescription pain medication. Also, she should take aspirin only as prescribed by the provider and not increase the dose for her knee pain. The GCF asks if there is anything else Ms. Carter does when she has pain to make her feel better. Ms. Carter mentions she sometimes uses a heating pad on her knee when it bothers her and that sometimes calling one of her friends helps. The GCF encourages her to continue these pain relief methods for her knee and adds that they can also be used for minor abdominal or nephrostomy discomfort. The facilitator reminds her that if pain at either of the surgical sites increases more than it has been in the hospital or if the pain does not improve after she goes home, she should call the GCF or the surgeon immediately.

A final discussion focuses on Ms. Carter's "fuzzy feeling" in her head. The GCF explains that sometimes surgery or being in the hospital can cause this to happen but often it goes away after a while. It may take quite some time for the feeling to disappear, perhaps as long as 6 months or a year. The GCF explains there is no treatment to cure the fuzzy feeling; it should improve over time. However, getting enough sleep, keeping up with her exercising, maintaining her diet, and socializing with her friends and family on a regular basis may help decrease the fuzziness.

The GCF encourages Ms. Carter to discuss the fuzzy feeling with the surgeon before she goes home. The GCF will notify the surgeon to discuss the issue with Ms. Carter. Also, the GCF will see Ms. Carter before she goes home the next day. The GCF gives Ms. Carter a telephone number where the GCF can be reached at any time. The GCF reinforces that calling is very important if Ms. Carter or her daughters have any questions about her care. "It is much better to call and get your questions answered than not call and have a problem become more serious. " The GCF asks for the telephone number of the daughter who will be staying with Ms. Carter so they can talk about the action plan.

The dietician is contacted to meet with Ms. Carter and her daughter that evening. A visiting nurse service is contacted for a home visit to help Ms. Carter with dressing changes and reviewing medications, diet, exercise, and activity.

The GCF schedules a follow-up telephone call and a home visit with Ms. Carter with plans for additional telephone calls and home visits. The GCF makes arrangements to attend Ms. Carter's follow-up visit with the surgeon. Ms. Carter states she is a bit overwhelmed by all the planning and feels like she's being told a lot of "you need to do this and don't do that."

The GCF agrees there is a lot to think about and reviews the action plan step by step to help Ms. Carter and her daughter clarify their notes. They make a schedule for the first few days at home. Although the visiting nurse will receive a copy of the action plan, Ms. Carter can discuss the action plan with the nurse at the first home visit.

The facilitator asks Ms. Carter to explain the self-care notes. Ms. Carter explains her medication schedule and the importance of taking her pain medication and to balance it with the acetaminophen for her knee. She knows she needs to take it easy but also to exercise and do her self-care with help as needed. Her daughter agrees and says they will learn more from the dietician about her diet. Ms. Carter and the GCF will review the action plan and her progress during follow-up contacts. Longer-term health goals will be established when Ms. Carter is ready. Ms. Carter states she feels better and is confident that with the help of her daughters, the visiting nurse, neighbors, and the GCF, everything "will work out just fine."

SUMMARY

Helping the older adult to continue the recovery trajectory after the transition from hospital or outpatient surgery is critical to optimizing the patient outcomes. Full recovery occurs after the patient leaves the care center. The predischarge meeting is focused on the patient's questions and concerns, the care environment, availability of supports, and the care needs specific to the surgery. Coaching the patient on wound care, pain relief, activity, exercise, and managing medications is a challenge to the older adult and to the provider. Elder-sensitive care based on findings from the discharge comprehensive geriatric assessment guide the discharge process. The goal is to ensure the safety and well-being of the older adult and promote feelings of confidence and competence in managing immediate and longer-term self-care needs with support and assistance from available resources.

KEY POINTS

- Most postsurgical readmissions are preventable when there is effective discharge planning and preparation of the patient and caregiver for home-based care.
- On a daily basis, nurses are in the ideal position through daily contact to prepare and educate patients, caregivers, and companion-coaches about discharge preparations and arrangements.
- Helping older adults and caregivers feel comfortable contacting and communicating with providers, service agencies, and health care organizations increases feelings of safety and security.
- Medications that have different names can be confusing to patients and families, and must be carefully reviewed to avoid duplication.
- Coaching must be clear, concise, concrete, and responsive to patient questions and concerns.
- Managing discharge information requires clinical judgment, artful communication, and sensitivity to the uniqueness of patients' condition, self-competence, self-confidence, new location of care, and goals for the future.
- A follow-up visit to the home or care site after discharge is the most comprehensive mechanism for ensuring a safe, effective transitional care process.

TWENTY-FOUR

Summary

Susan J. Fetzer, Raelene V. Shippee-Rice, and Jennifer V. Long

An individual's chronological age, the number of whole years since birth, is a poor representation of health. Aging, the accumulation of changes over time, depends on genetic composition, environmental exposures, and lifestyle. Healthy aging reflects an ability to resist environmental exposures and adopt a healthy lifestyle. Genetic predisposition, inflammatory processes, and general wear and tear decrease the functional capacity of cells, organs, and the entire organism. With aging, elements in the body begin to lose functional capacity beginning in some systems around age 30. Changes in body function are highly individualized within and across individuals. All body systems do not age at the same rate, and some have minimal age-related changes. However, the aging process does inhibit the ability and effectiveness of cells and organs to protect the individual from internal and external stressors.

Normal aging is not disease. It is critical to differentiate the aging process from age-related diseases. Normal aging predisposes the elder to disease onset, the result of age-related changes, genetics, and lifestyle effects. Age-related changes make older adults more vulnerable to diseases that younger adults more easily resist.

Age is not a contraindication to surgery. Centenarians undergo surgery and anesthesia with optimum outcomes. Achieving optimum outcomes depends on the efforts of the patient, caregivers, coaches, and health care providers, particularly nurses, to consider the impact of aging on an elder's ability to maintain or regain homeostasis. Surgery and anesthesia generate physiological, psychological, social, and emotional stress. Managing the stress imposed by surgery requires recognizing the demands placed on reserve capacity that may be limited in the older adult.

Gerioperative care aims to promote adaptation to the stress of surgery and anesthesia. Nursing is fundamental in the implementation of gerioperative care and achieving positive care outcomes. The nurse must understand the potential impact of age-related changes while implementing evidence-based interventions to minimize their effects. Balancing the competing needs and demands of gerioperative care is a complex process requiring conscious application of clinical judgment, critical thinking, and reasoning. Identifying elder's physiological and psychological reserve is challenging. Mobilizing reserve requires a delicate approach. The margin between doing good and doing harm narrows with the progression of age-related changes. This margin narrows even further with preexisting disease, surgical stress, and deconditioning.

Throughout the perioperative period, the older adult is bombarded with physiological and psychological stimuli. Gerioperative care minimizes adverse stimuli while promoting positive, adaptive responses. Preoperative considerations identify baseline function and encourages development of reserves. Interventions focus on minimizing risk factors and maximizing function. Intraoperative considerations maintain function and prevent adverse responses to noxious stimuli. Postoperative considerations focus on returning the elder to optimum function and promoting wellness.

The emergence of gerioperative care as a focus of study has illuminated the dearth of direct evidence available to guide gerioperative nurses. While guidelines and protocols have been developed, additional research to support and improve prevention and interventions is needed. Additional attention to the population of older adults undergoing surgery and anesthesia is sorely needed.

Communication among the interdisciplinary care team that includes the patient, companion-coach, family, and health care providers within and across transitions is a best practice mandate to promote prevention and early intervention that will optimize care outcomes. A major factor in the proactive approach is clear and concise communication among care providers and throughout care transitions.

Education on age-related changes as a foundation for providing quality elder care begins with basic nursing education and continues as a lifelong pursuit. Academic programs must include gerioperative care across the curricula. Clinical educators conducting educational needs assessments with nursing staff providing surgical care must assess knowledge and skills needed to provide quality gerioperative care. Administrators must specify gerioperative competencies in performance evaluation tools. Providers caring for gerioperative patients have a professional responsibility for maintaining education and practice standards in the care of older adults. Journal publications, geriatric reference texts, professional conferences, and professional websites are excellent resources for advancing education and evidence based practice.

Gerioperative care is patient-focused. Gerioperative facilitated care allows the nurse to join older adults throughout the perioperative journey. Providers must focus on listening to the elders' stories and appreciating their journey. The elder is the best teacher.

APPENDIX I

Protocol for Prevention, Early Detection, and Treatment of Postoperative Delirium in the Older Adult

Outcome: Reduce the incidence of delirium in older adults who have had surgery

- Preadmission protocol
  - Conduct cognitive assessment using standardized screen (e.g., Mini-Cog)
  - Conduct depression assessment using Geriatric Depression Scale-Short Form
  - Refer patient with positive results to interdisciplinary team or primary provider
  - Attach an alert notice to patient's medical record

- Postoperative protocol
  - Review preoperative record to determine cognitive status or depression
  - Refer patients with history of cognitive impairment or depression or with other high-risk profile to interdisciplinary team
  - Evaluate risk factors
    - Review preoperative risk assessment
    - Baseline or preoperative cognitive assessment
    - Medication review
    - Pain assessment
    - Metabolic changes
    - Hydration status
    - Infection
    - Environment
    - Mobility, activity, function level
    - Changes in medical or surgical parameters

- Institute prevention protocol immediately postsurgery
  - Review preoperative and postoperative medication list
    - Determine anticholinergic burden
    - Evaluate use of benzodiazepines, phenothiazines
    - Evaluate necessity for continuing high-risk medications
    - Discontinue high-risk medications if possible

- Implement hydration protocol
- Implement sleep protocol
- Implement pneumonia protocol, catheter care protocol, wound care protocol to minimize postoperative infection
- Implement mobility protocol
  - Range of motion, ambulation, activity protocols immediately after surgery within surgical limitations and patient functional capacity every 1 to 2 hours
  - Alternate activity with rest periods
  - Avoid prolonged bed rest, chair rest
- Implement pain protocol
  - Conduct pain assessment every 2 hours or at request of patient or family member.
  - Maintain nonopioid baseline and nonpharmacologic pain relief
  - Administer additional analgesia to achieve effective pain relief if needed
  - Monitor side effects of pain and pain relief methods at regular intervals
- Administer supplemental oxygen as needed
- Ensure sensory aids are in place, clean, and functioning properly
- Initiate bowel regimen
- Establish routine toileting
- Maintain familiar environment
  - Maintain regular care provider
  - Minimize number of people entering room
  - Eliminate room changes.
- Communicate effectively
  - Calm presence
  - Quiet clear voice at patient's hearing level
- Family, companion-coach engagement
  - Provide family/companion-coach information and support
  - Encourage family/companion-coach interaction; demonstrate or coach as needed
  - Engage patient in preferred activities, puzzles, games that prompt cognition
- Manage environment
  - Keep noise at comfort level for patient
  - Keep lights at soft level, prevent shadows
  - Provide low-level music with patient's permission
  - Use white board information: name, room number, day/date/daily action plan, schedule
  - Provide clocks, calendars, family photographs
  - Avoid clutter

- Institute early detection protocol
  - Frequency of assessment:
    - At least once every shift
    - Whenever patient demonstrates behavioral or cognitive changes
    - Whenever family member or companion-coach reports a change in patient behavior
  - Assessment elements
    - Evaluation of cute onset of behavior change
    - Fluctuations in behavior, symptoms
    - Level of alertness: fluctuates from stuporous to hypervigilant
    - Attention span: inattentive, easily distractible, may have difficulty shifting attention from one focus to another; has difficulty keeping track of what is being said

- Orientation: disoriented to time and place; should not be disoriented to person
- Memory: inability to recall events of hospitalization and current illness; unable to remember instructions; forgetful of names, events, activities, current news, etc.
- Thinking: disorganized thinking; rambling, irrelevant, incoherent conversation; unclear or illogical flow of ideas; unpredictable switching from topic to topic; difficulty in expressing needs and concerns; speech may be garbled
- Perception: perceptual disturbances such as illusions and visual or auditory hallucinations, misperceptions such as calling a stranger by a relative's name
- Psychomotor activity: may fluctuate between hypoactive, hyperactive, mixed subtypes
- Document assessment results

- Establish rapid intervention plan
  - Evaluate potential precipitating factors
    - Changes in medical/surgical parameters
    - Medications
    - Pain relief effectiveness
    - Dehydration, infection, bowel, urinary, metabolic impairment
    - Sensory stability
    - Evaluate sleep patterns
    - Family, companion-coach interaction with patient
    - Staff interaction, familiarity
  - Immediate treatment of precipitating factors

Adapted from Tullman, Mion, Fletcher, & Foreman (2008).

Reprinted with permission from Springer Publishing Company.

Medication Reconciliation Protocol

Outcome: Reduce incidence of gerioperative medication errors

Admission Reconciliation Process
1. The medication reconciliation process begins when the gerioperative patient is admitted to the hospital or surgical center.
2. The patient is asked to bring a list of medications to the hospital including prescription, over-the-counter, and herbal medications or remedies. Additional sources of medication information include preoperative admission notes, family members, companion-coach, gerioperative care facilitator, primary care office, or pharmacy.
3. Ask if patients have stopped a medication prior to surgery. If so, is the medication included on the patient's list.
4. A member of the interdisciplinary care team, usually a nurse or pharmacist, compares the complied list of admitting medications to the admitting physician orders. Any medication not on the physician's prescribing list is noted in the patient medical record for follow-up review or on the institution's medication reconciliation form. A medication reconciliation form specific to gerioperative patients should include the following information:
    a. Patient's height, weight and allergies
    b. Medication list with dose, schedule, route, and time of day the patient usually takes the medication
    c. Patient statement of adherence with prescribed medications; use always, usually, generally, sometimes, never
    d. Each medication has a statement of intent to continue in the hospital, hold in the hospital, discontinue permanently, change the dose, change the dosing schedule, change the route of each medication listed
5. Medications ordered on admission are reviewed for:
    a. Potentially inappropriate medication designation
    b. Analysis of contribution to anticholinergic burden
    c. Analysis of dose adjustment for gerioperative patients
    d. Determination of medication-anesthesia interaction
    e. Alert notice indicating to be used with cautionary note with note included
    f. Analysis of drug-drug interaction
6. Questions about any aspect of the patient's admission medication list or prescribed medications must be referred to the pharmacist, physician, and/or interdisciplinary team for review and action.

7. Unreconciled medications must be reviewed by a pharmacist or nurse and physician within 24 hours of admission.
8. Once complete, the medication reconciliation document is maintained in the medical record.

Inpatient Transfer Reconciliation Process

1. Patients transferred to or from the surgical services area, intensive care unit, or from one unit to another must have a review of current medications at the time of transfer.
   a. Medications currently ordered on the transfer out unit are compared to the level of medications ordered on the transfer in unit
   b. New orders on the transfer in unit are reviewed for: potentially inappropriate medications; anticholinergic burden; and documentation of adjusted dose and scheduling for administration to gerioperative patients

Inpatient Discharge Reconciliation Process

1. Upon discharge, medications ordered at time of discharge for patient to take at home or at next care setting will be compared with the current in-hospital medication administration record and with the patient's home medication list.
2. Medications on the original home medication list will be noted as discontinued in hospital, discontinued at time of discharge, restarted for home use, continued for home use. Reasons for discontinuing drugs will be noted. Changes in dose, schedule, or route of administration will be documented. Discrepancies between the home medication and discharge lists must be brought to the attention of a pharmacist or provider.
3. Timeline for duration of drug should be noted.
4. The patient is given a written description of the medication list and disposition of each medication. Patients are to be informed on how to destroy old medications safely without danger to self, others, or the environment.
5. Discharge medications are reviewed for potentially inappropriate drugs, anticholinergic burden, and adjusted dose for older adult and context of patient's clinical condition.
6. A complete list of the patient's medication is provided to the gerioperative care facilitator, transferred to the next provider of service when a patient is referred or transferred to another setting, and communicated to primary care or service practitioner.
7. No older adult will be discharged until the medication reconciliation is documented, signed, and attached to the medical record.

APPENDIX II

Hendrich II Fall Risk Model©		
Risk Factor	**Risk Points**	
Confusion disorientation impulsivity	4	
Symptomatic depression	2	
Altered elimination	1	
Dizziness certigo	1	
Male gender	1	
Any administered antiepileptics (anticonvulsants)[1]: Carbamazepine, divalproex sodium, ethotoin, ethosuximide, felbamate, fosphenytoin, gabapentin, lamotrigine, mephenytoin, methsuximide, phenobarbital, phenytoin, primidone, topiramate, trimethadione, valproic acid	2	
Any administered benzodiazepines[2]: Alprazolam, chlordiazepoxide, clonazepam, clorazepate dipotassium, diazepam, flurazepam, halazepam,[3] lorazepam, midazolam, oxazepam, temazepam, triazolam	1	
Get-up-and-go test If unable to assess, monitor for change in activity level, assess other risk factors, document both on patient chart with date and time.		
Ability to rise in a single movement—no loss of balance with steps	0	
Pushes up, successful in one attempt	1	
Multiple attempts, but successful	3	
Unable to rise without assistance during test (*or* if a medical order states the same and/or complete bed rest is ordered) *If unable to assess, document this on the patient chart with the date and time	4	
A score of 5 or greater = high risk	**Total Score**	
2011 AHI of Indiana, Inc. All Rights Reserved. United States Patent #7,282,031 and U.S. Patent No. 7,682,308. Federal Laws prohibits the replication, distribution or use without written permission from AHI of Indiana, Inc.		

Ongoing Medication Review Updates:

[1]Levetiracetam (Keppra) was not assessed during the original research conducted to create the Hendrich Fall Risk Model. As an antieptileptic, levetiracetam does have a side effect of somnolence and dizziness, which contributes to its fall risk and should be scored (effective June 2010).

[2]The study did not include the effect of benzodiazepine-like drugs since they were not on the market at the time. However, due to their similarity in drug structure, mechanism of action and drug effects, they should also be scored (effective January 2010).

[3]Halazepam was included in the study but is no longer available in the United States (effective June 2010).

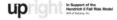

Geriatric Depression Scale–Short Form

Instructions:	Give the answer that best describes how you felt over the past week.

1. Are you basically satisfied with your life?   yes   no

2. Have you dropped many of your activities and interests?   yes   no

3. Do you feel that your life is empty?   yes   no

4. Do you often get bored?   yes   no

5. Are you in good spirits most of the time?   yes   no

6. Are you afraid that something bad is going to happen
   to you?   yes   no

7. Do you feel happy most of the time?   yes   no

8. Do you often fell helpless?   yes   no

9. Do you prefer to stay at home, rather than going out
   and doing things?   yes   no

10. Do you feel that you have more problems with memory
    than most?   yes   no

11. Do you think it is wonderful to be alive now?   yes   no

12. Do you feel worthless the way you are now?   yes   no

13. Do you feel full of energy?   yes   no

14. Do you feel that your situation is hopeless?   yes   no

15. Do you think that most people are better off than
    you are?   yes   no

Total Score _____

Geriatric Depression Scale Scoring Instructions

Instructions:	Score 1 point for each bolded answer. A score of 5 or more suggest depression

1. Are you basically satisfied with your life?	yes	**no**
2. Have you dropped many of your activities and interests?	**yes**	no
3. Do you feel that your life is empty?	**yes**	no
4. Do you often get bored?	**yes**	no
5. Are you in good spirits most of the time?	yes	**no**
6. Are you afraid that something bad is going to happen to you?	**yes**	no
7. Do you feel happy most of the time?	yes	**no**
8. Do you often fell helpless?	**yes**	no
9. Do you prefer to stay at home, rather than going out and doing things?	**yes**	no
10. Do you feel that you have more problems with memory than most?	**yes**	no
11. Do you think it is wonderful to be alive now?	yes	**no**
12. Do you feel worthless the way you are now?	**yes**	no
13. Do you feel full of energy?	yes	**no**
14. Do you feel that your situation is hopeless?	**yes**	no
15. Do you think that most people are better off than you are?	**yes**	no

A score of ≥ 5 suggests depression   ***Total Score*** _____

Ref. Yes average: The use of Rating Depression Series in the elderly, in Poon (ed.): Clinical Memory Assessment of Older Adults, American Psychological Association, 1986

Patient Health Questionnaire (PHQ-9)

NAME: _____   **DATE:** _____

Over the *last 2 weeks*, how often have you been bothered by any of the following problems? *(use "✓" to indicate your answer)*	Not at all	Several days	More than half the days	Nearly every day
1. Little interest or pleasure in doing things	0	1	2	3
2. Feeling down, depressed, or hopeless	0	1	2	3
3. Trouble falling or staying asleep, or sleeping too much	0	1	2	3
4. Feeling tired or having little energy	0	1	2	3
5. Poor appetite or overeating	0	1	2	3
6. Feeling bad about yourself—or that you are a failure or have let yourself or your family down	0	1	2	3
7. Trouble concentrating on things, such as reading the newspaper or watching television	0	1	2	3
8. Moving or speaking so slowly that other people could have noticed. Or the opposite—being so fidgety or restless that you have been moving around a lot more than usual	0	1	2	3
9. Thoughts that you would be better off dead, or of hurting yourself in some way	0	1	2	3

add columns: _____ + _____ + _____

(Healthcare professional: For interpretation of TOTAL, please refer to accompanying scoring card.)   **TOTAL:** _____

10. If you checked off *any* problems, how *difficult* have these problems made it for you to do your work, take care of things at home, or get along with other people?	**Not difficult at all** _____
	Somewhat difficult _____
	Very difficult _____
	Extremely difficult _____

Fold back this page before administering this questionnaire

INSTRUCTIONS FOR USE

for doctor or healthcare professional use only

PHQ-9 QUICK DEPRESSION ASSESSMENT

For initial diagnosis:

1. Patient completes PHQ-9 Quick Depression Assessment on accompanying tear-off pad.

2. If there are at least 4 ✓s in the blue highlighted section (including Questions #1 and #2), consider a depressive disorder. Add score to determine severity.

3. ***Consider Major Depressive Disorder***
   —if there are at least 5 ✓s in the blue highlighted section (one of which corresponds to Question #1 or #2)

   Consider Other Depressive Disorder
   —if there are 2 to 4 ✓s in the blue highlighted section (one of which corresponds to Question #1 or #2)

   Note: Since the questionnaire relies on patient self-report, all responses should be verified by the clinician and a definitive diagnosis made on clinical grounds, taking into account how well the patient understood the questionnaire, as well as other relevant information from the patient. Diagnoses of Major Depressive Disorder or Other Depressive Disorder also require impairment of social, occupational, or other important areas of functioning (Question #10) and ruling out normal bereavement, a history of a Manic Episode (Bipolar Disorder), and a physical disorder, medication, or other drug as the biological cause of the depressive symptoms.

To monitor severity over time for newly diagnosed patients or patients in current treatment for depression:

1. Patients may complete questionnaires at baseline and at regular intervals (eg, every 2 weeks) at home and bring them in at their next appointment for scoring or they may complete the questionnaire during each scheduled appointment.

2. Add up ✓s by column. For every ✓: Several days = 1   More than half the days = 2   Nearly every day = 3

3. Add together column scores to get a TOTAL score.

4. Refer to the accompanying PHQ-9 Scoring Card to interpret the TOTAL score.

5. Results may be included in patients' files to assist you in setting up a treatment goal, determining degree of response, as well as guiding treatment intervention.

PHQ-9 SCORING CARD FOR SEVERITY DETERMINATION

for healthcare professional use only

Scoring—add up all checked boxes on PHQ-9
For every ✓: Not at all = 0; Several days = 1;
More than half the days = 2; Nearly every day = 3

Interpretation of Total Score

Total Score	Depression Severity
1-4	Minimal depression
5-9	Mild depression
10-14	Moderate depression
15-19	Moderately severe depression
20-27	Severe depression

The NEECHAM Confusion Scale*

The Neelon and Champagne Confusion (NEECHAM) scale was developed as an instrument for rapid and nonintrusive assessment of normal information processing, early changes in information processing, and for documentation of confusional behavior, including delirium. It can be scored by the nurse "at the bedside" in a manner similar to other vital function measurements during routine or required nursing assessments. It makes maximum use of already collected data. Because the NEECHAM places a minimal response burden on the patient, NEECHAM ratings can be repeated at frequent intervals to monitor changes in the patient's status and the response to treatment.

SUMMARY OF PSYCHOMETRIC DATA

The validity and reliability of the NEECHAM scale has been evaluated in elderly patients hospitalized for acute medical illness.[1,2] Inter-rater and retest reliability were also tested in a sample of stable elderly nursing home residents.[3]

Inter-rater (Pearson $r = 0.96$) and test-retest reliability (Pearson $r = 0.98$) in stable elderly subjects were strong. Internal consistency for the total score was high (Cronbach's alpha = 0.91, Study 1; 0.90, Study 2). There were high correlations with Mini-Mental State Examination (MMSE) ($r = 0.87$, Study 1) and with the sum of *Diagnostic and Statistical Manual of Mental Disorders, Third Edition, Revised (DSM-IIIR)* positive items (Pearson $r = -0.91$). Correlation was good with the *DSM-IIIR* criteria positive score ($r = -0.70$). All items except vital function and oxygen stability showed a good corrected item-total correlation, loading on one factor, explaining 60% of the variance.

The NEECHAM total score range runs from 0 (minimal responsiveness) to 30 (normal function). The NEECHAM has nine scaled items divided into three domains (subscales) of assessment: cognitive processing, behavior, and physiological control. Subscale One measures key cognitive functions and is given the greatest weight (0–14). Subscale Two (0–10) measures behavioral manifestations. Subscale Three (0–6) is given the least weight because hospitalized patients in general are likely to have abnormal values on one or more of these items. A NEECHAM score below 25 predicts confusion as measure by two of three other clinical indicators (*DSM-III* criteria, MMSE, report of mental status change) with a sensitivity of 0.95 and specificity of 0.78.

---

*Neelon/Champagne/McConnell (c'85,87)

INSTRUCTIONS FOR SCORING THE NEECHAM CONFUSION SCALE

Points are assigned for the item level description that represents the patient's response or behavior during the rater's interaction. Accurate scoring of the NEECHAM requires sensitivity to cultural differences and awareness of physical disabilities (visual, hearing, motor, etc.) that may affect the subject's response. The patient need not exhibit every behavior in the item description level to score at that point level, but behavior(s) should be representative. Although some training is required, inter-rater reliability of professional nurses is good. Data needed to score the NEECHAM can be collected during 10 minutes of routine patient observations and vital sign assessment.

Cognitive-Information Processing

Note patient's level of responsiveness on entering the room—eye contact, recognition, etc.

Note whether patient can maintain attentiveness and understand both verbal and visual information. Does the patient require repeated contact to stay focused or aroused? Do verbal or facial cues suggest understanding of interaction (e.g., patient anticipates required action by visual cues [opens mouth to visual thermometer cue]).

Observe for complex or cued command responses. Is patient able to initiate/complete a telephone call or nurse "call" procedure? Depending on the type of system and after initial orientation to procedure, the subject's ability to "call" the nurse can be used as a measure of complex command processing. Observe how he/she would "find and activate call system" (a "complex" system requires locating the "call instrument," picking it up from bedside table, activating nurse signal amongst several possible choices, and responding to call-back). Is the task completed with normal speed and without prompting? Can the patient only respond to "cued" commands (visual or touch cues)?

Orientation and short-term memory can be tapped without typical "do you know what day/date this is" question. What part of the day, what meal he/she has eaten, what place this is are all examples of information obtained in routine care interaction.

Behavior and Performance

Score patient's awareness and actions in managing appearance, posture, and position (do not rate routine nursing hygiene care, only patient function).

Are there "hyperactive" movements or purposeless movements?

Does the subject show abnormal hand/finger movements—"picking" at sheets?

Differentiate between culturally grounded slow speech and difficulty in speaking, initiating speech, appropriate speech, etc.

Physiologic Control

The vital signs are scored as defined in scale. Observe patient's response and awareness. Does he/she anticipate procedure and assist or require repeated prompting or cueing?

Oxygen stability is scored by a noninvasive measure of oxygen saturation (pulse oximetry). Note subject's position and whether oxygen is being administered (flow-rate). In place of oximeter measurements, scoring can be done by scoring 1 point loss for required oxygen therapy and 1 point loss for the presence of apnea (greater than 15-second period during a 1-minute observation and more than one observation).

Scoring continence is confounded by clinical care factors as well as by interactive effects of deteriorating cognitive and physical function in those who develop acute confusion. Score as defined in item but note whether subject needs assistance to toilet, requested help, and whether help was delayed.

SCORING:		POINTS
Items 1–3	Processing—Attention = 0–4	
	Processing—Command = 0–5	
	Orientation—Memory = 0–5	
		0–14
Items 4–6	Behavior—Appearance = 0–2	
	Behavior—Motor = 0–4	
	Behavior—Verbal = 0–4	
		0–10
Items 7–9	Vital Function = 0–2	
	Oxygen Stability = 0–2	
	Continence = 0–2	
		0–6
Total		0–30

Scores of:
27–30: "Not confused," or normal processing
25–26: "Not confused," but at risk for confusion
20–24: Mild or early developing confusional state
0–19: Moderate to severe confusion

Scores for subjects with severe chronic cognitive impairment may differ from the above ranges (with or without superimpose acute confusional state).

Helpful Hints for Scoring the NEECHAM Confusing Scale

- Score the NEECHAM at the completion of the interaction. Read all scoring options for each item before selecting item score.
- In scoring a patient, it is not uncommon for a 1- or 2-point difference to occur between ratings—a change of more than 2 points is considered clinically significant and warrants a more complete assessment.
- Be creative and develop an approach that is comfortable and gets the necessary information. The key is to be consistent in assessment and scoring.
- Cognitive ability may fluctuate even in a short 15-minute period. Should this occur, score the lowest level observed during the entire interaction.
- Pay attention to the patient's awareness or reaction to surroundings as well as what occurs in your interaction.
- Avoid asking yes and no questions as the basis for scoring.
- Record only what you observe during the present interaction, not what was seen previously.
- Score patient as observed regardless of possible cause (recent sedation or narcotic medication, etc.). Make a note of circumstances that might affect scoring.

NEECHAM Confusion Scale

NAME/IDENTIFICATION: _____   DATE: _____ TIME:_____
                                                SCORED BY: _____

LEVEL I—PROCESSING

PROCESSING—ATTENTION: (Attention-Alertness-Responsiveness)

4   **Full attentiveness/alertness:** responds immediately and appropriately to calling of name or touch—eyes, head turn, fully aware of surroundings, attends to environmental events appropriately.

3   **Short or hyper attention/alertness:** either shortened attention to calling, touch, or environmental events or hyperalert, overattentive to cues/objects in environment.

2   **Attention/alertness inconsistent or inappropriate:** slow in responding, repeated calling or touch required to elicit/maintain eye contact/attention; able to recognize objects/stimuli, though may drop into sleep between stimuli.

1   **Attention/alertness disturbed:** eyes open to sound or touch; may appear fearful, unable to attend/recognize contact, or may show withdrawal/combative behavior.

0   **Arousal/responsiveness depressed:** eyes may/may not open; only minimal arousal possible with repeated stimuli; unable to recognize contact.

PROCESSING—COMMAND: (Recognition-Interpretation-Action)

5   **Able to follow a complex command:** "Turn on nurse's call light." (Must search for object, recognize object, perform command.)

4   **Slowed complex command response:** requires prompting or repeated directions to follow/complete command. Performs complex command in "slow"/overattending manner.

3   **Able to follow a simple command:** "Lift your hand or foot Mr. . . .." (Only use one object.)

2   **Unable to follow direct command:** follows commands prompted by touch or visual cue—drinks from glass placed near mouth. Responds with calming affect to nurse contact and reassurance or handholding.

1   **Unable to follow visual guided command:** responds with dazed or frightened facial features, and/or withdrawal-resistive response to stimuli, hyper-/hypoactive behavior; does not respond to nurse gripping hand lightly.

0   **Hypoactive, lethargic:** minimal motor/responses to environmental stimuli.

PROCESSING—ORIENTATION: (Orientation-Short-term Memory-Thought/Speech Content)

5   **Oriented to time, place, and person:** thought processes, content of conversation or questions appropriate. Short-term memory intact.

4   **Oriented to person to place:** minimal memory/recall disturbance, content and response to questions generally appropriate; may be repetitive, requires prompting to continue contact. Generally cooperates with requests.

3   **Orientation inconsistent:** oriented to self, recognizes family but time and place orientation fluctuates. Uses visual cues to orient. Thought/memory disturbance common, may have hallucinations or illusions. Passive cooperation with requests (cooperative cognitive protecting behaviors).

(continued)

NEECHAM Confusion Scale *(Continued)*

2	**Disoriented and memory/recall disturbed:** oriented to self/recognizes family. May question actions of nurse or refuse requests, procedures (resistive cognitive protecting behaviors). Conversation content/thought disturbed. Illusions and/or hallucinations common.
1	**Disoriented, disturbed recognition:** inconsistently recognizes familiar people, family, objects. Inappropriate speech/sounds.
0	**Processing of stimuli depressed:** minimal responses to verbal stimuli.

LEVEL 2—BEHAVIOR

BEHAVIOR—APPEARANCE:

2	**Controls posture, maintains appearance, hygiene:** appropriately gowned or dressed, personally tidy, clean. Posture in bed/chair normal.
1	**Either posture or appearance disturbed:** some disarray of clothing/bed or personal appearance, or some loss of control of posture, position.
0	**Both posture and appearance abnormal:** disarrayed, poor hygiene, unable to maintain posture in bed.

BEHAVIOR—MOTOR:

4	**Normal motor behavior:** appropriate movement, coordination and activity, able to rest quietly in bed. Normal hand movement.
3	**Motor behavior slowed or hyperactive:** overly quiet or little spontaneous movement (hands/arms across chest or at sides) or hyperactive (up/down, "jumpy"). May show hand tremor.
2	**Motor movement disturbed:** restless or quick movement. Hand movements appear abnormal—picking at bed objects or bed covers, etc. May require assistance with purposeful movements.
1	**Inappropriate, disruptive movements:** pulling at tubes, trying to climb over rails, frequent purposeless actions.
0	**Motor movement depressed:** limited movements unless stimulated; resistive movements.

BEHAVIOR—VERBAL:

4	**Initiates speech appropriately:** able to converse, can initiate and maintain conversation. Normal speech for diagnostic condition, normal tone.
3	**Limited speech initiation:** responses to verbal stimuli are brief and un-complex. Speech clear for diagnostic condition, tone may be abnormal rate may be slow.
2	**Inappropriate speech:** may talk to self or not make sense. Speech not clear for diagnostic condition.
1	**Speech/sound disturbed:** altered sound/tone. Mumbles, yells, swears, or is inappropriately silent.
0	**Abnormal sounds:** groaning or other disturbed sounds. No clear speech.

© 1985/89 Neelon/Champagne/McConnell

(continued)

NEECHAM Confusion Scale *(Continued)*

LEVEL 3—PHYSIOLOGIC CONTROL

PHYSIOLOGICAL MEASUREMENTS:

Recorded Values:	Normal:		
_____ Temperature	$(36°–37°)$	_____ Periods of apnea/hypopnea present?	
		1 = yes, 0 = no	
_____ Systolic blood pressure	(100–160)	_____ Oxygen therapy prescribed?	
		0 = no, 1 = yes, but not on,	
		2 = yes on now	
_____ Diastolic blood pressure	(50–90)		
_____ Heart rate	(60–100)		
Regular/irregular	(circle one)		
_____ Respirations	(14–22) (Count for 1 full minute)		
_____ Oxygen saturation	(93 or above)		

VITAL FUNCTION STABILITY: (Count abnormal systolic blood pressure and/or diastolic blood pressure as one value; count abnormal and/or irregular heart rate as one; count apnea and/or abnormal respiration as one; and abnormal temperature as one)

2   Blood pressure, heart rate, temperature, respiration within normal range with regular pulse

1   Any one of the above in abnormal range

0   Two or more in abnormal range

OXYGEN SATURATION STABILITY:

2   Oxygen saturation in normal range (93 or above)

1   Oxygen saturation 90 to 92 or is receiving oxygen

0   Oxygen saturation below 90

URINARY CONTINENCE CONTROL:

2   Maintains bladder control

1   Incontinent of urine in last 24 hours or has condom catheter

0   Incontinent now or has indwelling or intermittent catheter or is anuric

_____ **LEVEL 1 Score:** Processing (0–14 points)	Total Score of:	Indicates:	
	0–19	Moderate to severe confusion	
	20–24	Mild or early development of confusion	
_____ **LEVEL 2 Score:** Behavior (0–10 points)	25–26	"Not Confused," but at high risk of confusion	
	27–30	"Not Confused," or normal function	
_____ **LEVEL 3 Score:** Integrative Physiological Control (0–6 points)			
_____ **TOTAL NEECHAM** (0–30 points)			

References

Agency for Healthcare Research and Quality. (2010, October 25). Hospitalizations for medication and illicit drug-related conditions on the rise among Americans ages 45 and older. Retrieved March 17, 2011, from www.ahrq.gov/news/press/pr2010/hospmedpr.htm

Alano, G., Pekmezaris, R., Wolf-Klein, G., Tai, J., Hussain, M., Jeune, J., . . . Wolf-Klien, G. P. (2010). Factors influencing older adults to complete advance directives. *Palliative and Supportive Care, 8*(3), 267–275.

Amador, L., & Loera, J. (2007). Preventing postoperative falls in the older adult. *Journal of the American College of Surgeons, 204*(3), 447–453.

American Geriatrics Society. (n.d.). Geriatrics for specialists. Retrieved October 20, 2008, from www.americangeriatrics.org/specialists/involved.shtm

American Nurses Association. (2001). *Code of ethics for nurses with interpretive statements.* Silver Spring, MD: American Nurses Association.

American Nurses Association. (2004). *Nursing: Scope and standards of practice.* Washington, D.C.: American Nurses Association.

American Nurses Association. (2010). *Nursing: Scope and standards of practice* (2nd ed.). Silver Spring, MD: American Nurses Association.

American Psychiatric Association. (2000). *Diagnostic and statistical manual of mental disorders, 4th edition, Text Revision.* Arlington, VA: American Psychiatric Association.

Ansaloni, L., Catena, F., Chattat, R., Fortuna, D., Franceschi, C., Mascitti, P., & Melotti, R. M. (2010). Risk factors and incidence of postoperative delirium in elderly patients after elective and emergency surgery. *British Journal of Surgery, 97*(2), 273–280.

Appelbaum, P. S. (2007). Assessment of patients' competence to consent to treatment. *New England Journal of Medicine, 357*(18), 1834–1840.

Arias, E. (2007). United States life tables 2004. *National Vital Statistics Report, 56,* (9). Hyattsville, MD: National Center for Health Statistics.

Arora, V., McGory, M., & Fung, C. (2007). Quality indicators for hospitalization and surgery in vulnerable elders. *Journal of the American Geriatrics Society, 55*(Supplement 2), s347–s358.

Artnak, K. (1997). Informed consent in the elderly: assessing decisional capacity. *Seminar in Perioperative Nursing, 6,* 59–64.

Avidan, M., Searleman, A., Storandt, M., Barnett, K., Vannucci, A., Saager, L., . . . Evers, A. S. (2009). Long-term cognitive decline in older subjects was not attributable to non-cardiac surgery or major illness. *Anesthesiology, 111*(5), 964–970.

Baecker, N., Tomic, A., Mika, C., Gotzmann, A., Platen, P., Gerzer, R., & Heer, M. (2003). Bone resorption is induced on the second day of bed rest: results of a controlled crossover trial. *Journal of Applied Physiology, 95*(3), 977–982.

Balas, M. (2005). The course of delirium in older surgical intensive care unit patients. *Scholarly commons: Repository*. Retrieved March 23, 2011, from repository.upenn.edu/dissertations/AAI3179703/

Bass, D., Attix, D., Phillips-Bute, B., & Monk, T. (2008). An efficient screening tool for preoperative depression: The Geriatric Depression Scale-Short Form. *Anesthesia and Analgesia, 106*(3), 805–809.

Baumhover, L., & McNicoll, L. (2007). Providing a geriatric-friendly environment for the older surgical patient. *Perioperative Nursing Clinics, 2*(4), 309–316.

Becker, P. M. & Jamieson, A. O. (1992). Common sleep disorders in the elderly: Diagnosis and treatment. *Geriatrics, 47*, 41–52.

Bedford, P. (1955). Adverse cerebral effects of anaesthesia on old people. *Lancet, 269*(6884), 259–263.

Beers, M. H. (1992). Inappropriate medication prescribing in skilled-nursing facilities. *Annals Internal Medicine, 117*(8), 684–689.

Beers, M. (1997). Explicit criteria for determining potentially inappropriate medication use by the elderly. An update. *Archives of Internal Medicine, 157*(14), 1531–1536.

Berg, J., Appelbaum, P., Lidz, C., & Parker, L. (2001). *Informed consent: Legal theory and clinical practice* (2nd ed.). New York, NY: Oxford University Press.

Berwick, D. (2002). A user's manual for the IOM's "Quality Chasm" report. *Health Affairs, 21*(3), 80–90.

Billimoria, K., Bentrem, D., Ko, D., Stewart, A., Winchester, D., & Talamonti, M. (2007). National failure to operate on early stage pancreatic cancer. *Annals of Surgery, 246*(2), 173–180.

Birkmeyer, J., Dimick, J., & Birkmeyer, N. (2004). Measuring the quality of surgical care: structure, process, or outcomes? *Journal of the American College of Surgeons, 198*(4), 626–632.

Bonk, M., Krown, H., Matuszewski, K., & Oinonen, M. (2006). Potentially inappropriate medications in hospitalized senior patients. *American Journal of Health-System Pharmacy, 63*(12), 1161–1165.

Borson, Scanlan, Brush, Vitallano, & Dokmak. (2000). The mini-cog: a cognitive 'vital signs' measure for dementia screening in multi-lingual elderly. *International Journal of Geriatric Psychiatry, 15*(11), 101–107.

Borson, S., Scanlan, J. M, Chen, P. & Ganguli, M. (2003). The Mini-Cog as a screen for dementia: validation in a population-based sample. *Journal of the American Geriatrics Society, 51*(10), 1451–1454.

Boult, C., Giddens, J., Frey, K., Reider, L., & Novak, T. (2009). *Guided care: A new nurse-physician partnership in chronic care*. New York, NY: Springer Publishing Company.

Brown, C., Friedkin, R., & Inouye, S. (2004). Prevalence and outcomes of low mobility in hospitalized older patients. *Journal of the American Geriatrics Society, 52*(8), 1263–1270.

Brown, C., Redden, D., Flood, K., & Allman, R. (2009). The underrecognized epidemic of low mobility during hospitalization of older adults. *Journal of the American Geriatrics Society, 57*(9), 1660–1665.

Browning, L., Denehy, L., & Scholes, R. (2007). The quantity of early upright mobilization performed following upper abdominal surgery is low: An observational study. *The Australian Journal of Physiotherapy, 53*(1), 47–52.

Buchner, D., & Wagner, E. (1992). Preventing frail health. *Clinics in Geriatric Medicine, 8*(1), 1–17.

Butler, R. (1969). Ageism: another form of bigotry. *Gerontologist, 9*, 243–246.

Butler, R. (1975) *Why survive? Being old in America*. New York, NY: Harper & Row.

Butterworth, S., Linden, A., & McClay, W. (2007). Health coaching as an intervention in health management programs. *Disease Management and Health Outcomes, 15*, 299–307.

Capezuti, E., Zwicker, D., Mezey, M., & Fulmer, T. (2008). *Evidence-based geriatric nursing protocols for best practice* (3rd ed.). New York, NY: Springer Publishing Company.

The Care Transitions Program. (2007). The Care Transitions Intervention: Improving transitions across sites of care. Retrieved March 11, 2011, from www.caretransitions.org/documents/manual.pdf

Carli, F., Charlebois, P., Stein, B., Feldman, L., Zavorsky, G., Kim, D., . . . Mayo, N. E. (2010). Randomized clinical trial of prehabilitation in colorectal surgery. *The British Journal of Surgery, 97*(8), 1187–1197.

Carli, F., & Zavorsky, G. (2005). Optimizing functional exercise capacity in the elderly surgical population. *Current Opinion in Clinical Nutrition and Metabolic Care, 8*(1), 23–32.

Carreon, L., Puno, R., Dimar, J., Glassman, S., & Johnson, J. (2003). Perioperative complications of posterior lumbar decompression and arthrodesis in older adults. *The Journal of Bone and Joint Surgery, 85,* 2089–2092.

Cassell, E. (2005). Consent or obedience? Power and authority in medicine. *New England Journal of Medicine, 352,* 328–330.

Centers for Disease Control and Prevention. (2010, September 17). QuickStats: Life expectancy at birth, by race and sex—United States, 1970–2007. Retrieved April 7, 2011, from www.cdc.gov/mmwr/preview/mmwrhtml/mm5936a9.htm?s_cid=mm5936a9_w

Centers for Disease Control and Prevention. (2011). National diabetes fact sheet. Retrieved April 10, 2011, from www.cdc.gov/diabetes/pubs/factsheet11.htm

Champagne, M. T., Neelon, V. J., McConnell, E. S., & Funk, S. G. (1987). The NEECHAM scale: assessment of acute confusion in the hospitalized elderly. *The Gerontologist, 27*(October Special), 4A.

Chang, Y., Tsai, Y., Lin, P., Chen, M., & Liu, C. (2008). Prevalence and risk factors for postoperative delirium in a cardiovascular intensive care unit. *American Journal of Critical Care, 17*(6), 567–575.

Chen, T., Anderson, D., Chopra, T., Choi, Y., Schmader, K., & Kaye, K. (2010). Poor functional status is an independent predictor of surgical site infections due to methicillin-resistant Staphylococcus aureus in older adults. *Journal of the American Geriatrics Society, 58*(3), 527–532.

Cherniack, E. (2002). Increasing use of DNR orders in the elderly worldwide. Whose choice is it? *Journal of Medical Ethics, 28*(5), 303–307.

Cherry, D. K., Burt, C. W., & Woodwell, D. A. (2001). Ambulatory Medical Care Survey: 1999 Summary. Advance data from ambulatory and health statistics.

Clancy, C. (2008). SCIP: Making complications of surgery the exception rather than the rule. *AORN Journal, 87*(3), 621–624.

Clancy, C. (2009, September/October). AHRQ: One decade after *To Err is Human. Patient Safety and Quality Health Care.* Retrieved December 1, 2010, from www.psqh.com/septemberoctober-2009/234-september-october-2009-ahrq

Clarke, L., & Griffin, M. (2008). Failing bodies: Body image and multiple chronic conditions in later life. *Qualitative Health Research, 18*(8), 1084–1095.

Coleman, E. (2003). Falling through the cracks: Challenges and opportunities for improving transitional care for persons with continuous complex care needs. *Journal of the American Geriatrics Society, 51*(4), 549–555.

Coleman, E., Parry, C., Chalmers, S., & Min, S. (2006). The care transitions intervention: Results of a randomized controlled trial. *Archives of Internal Medicine, 166*(17), 1822–1828.

Committee on Identifying and Preventing Medication Errors. (2006). Preventing medication errors: Quality chasm series. National Academies Press.

Cook, J., Marshall, R., Masci, C., & Coyne, J. (2007). Physicians' perspectives on prescribing benzodiazepines for older adults: A qualitative study. *Journal of General Internal Medicine, 22*(3), 303–307.

Cuddy, A., Norton, M., & Fiske, S. (2005). This old stereotype: The pervasiveness and persistence of the elderly stereotype. *Journal of Social Issues, 61*(2), 267–285.

Currie, L. (2008). Fall and injury prevention. In R. G. Hughes (Ed.), *Patient safety and quality: An evidence-based handbook for nurses* (pp. 1-195–1-250). Rockville, MD: Agency for Healthcare Research and Quality.

Dasgupta, M. & Dumbrell, A. C. (2006). Preoperative risk assessment for delirium after noncardiac surgery: A systematic review. *Journal of the American Geriatrics Society, 54,* 1578–1589.

Dasgupta, M., Rolfson, D., Stolee, P., Borrie, M., & Speechley, M. (2009). Frailty is associated with postoperative complications in older adults with medical problems. *Archives of Gerontology and Geriatrics, 48*(1), 78–83.

Davidhizer, R., & Giger, J. N. (2004). A review of the literature on care of clients in pain who are culturally diverse. *International Nursing Review, 51*(1), 47–55.

del Carmen, M., & Joffe, S. (2005). Informed consent for medical treatment and research: A review. *The Oncologist, 10*(8), 636–641.

dePender, W., & Ikeda-Chandler, W. (1990). *Clinical ethics: An invitation to healing professionals* (1st ed.). New York, NY: Praeger.

Detroyer, E., Dobbels, F., Verfaillie, E., Meyfroidt, G., Sergeant, P., & Milisen, K. (2008). Is preoperative anxiety and depression associated with onset of delirium after cardiac surgery in older patients? A prospective cohort study. *Journal of the American Geriatrics Society, 56*(12), 2278–2284.

Ditmyer, M., Topp, R., & Pifer, M. (2002). Prehabilitation in preparation for orthopaedic surgery. *Orthopaedic Nursing, 21*(5), 52–54.

Dykes, P., Carroll, D., Hurley, A., Lipsitz, S., Benoit, A., Chang, F., . . . Middleton, B. (2010). Fall prevention in acute care hospitals: A randomized trial. *Journal of the American Medical Association, 304*(17), 1912–1918.

Engel, G., & Romano, J. (2004). Delirium, a syndrome of cerebral insufficiency. *The Journal of Neuropsychiatry and Clinical Neurosciences, 16,* 526–538.

Ershler, W. (2007). A gripping reality: Oxidative stress, inflammation, and the pathway to frailty. *Journal of Applied Physiology, 103*(1), 3–5.

Etzioni, D., Liu, J., Maggard, M., O'Connell, J., & Ko, C. (2003). Workload projections of surgical oncology: Will we need more surgeons? *Annals of Surgical Oncology, 10,* 1112–1117.

Fearing, M., & Inouye, S. (2009). Delirium. *Focus, 7*(1), 53–63.

Federal Interagency Forum on Aging-Related Statistics. (2008). Older Americans 2008: Key indicators of well-being. Retrieved October 28, 2008, from www.agingstats.gov/Agingstatsdotnet/Main_Site/Data/Data_2008.aspx

Fick, D., Cooper, J., Wade, W., Waller, J., Maclean, J., & Beers, M. (2003). Updating the Beers criteria for potentially inappropriate medication use in older adults: Results of a US consensus panel of experts. *Archives of Internal Medicine, 163*(22), 2716–2724.

Fink, A. S., Prochazka, A. V., Henderson, W.G., Bartenfeld, D., Nirenda, C., Webb, A., . . . Parmelee, P. (2010) Enhancement of surgical informed consent by addition of repeat back: A multicenter, randomized controlled clinical trial. *Annals of Surgery, 252*(1), 27–36.

Fink, R. (2000). Pain assessment: the cornerstone to optimal pain management. *Baylor University Medical Proceedings, 13,* 236–239.

Finucane, M., Slovic, P., Hibbard, J., Peters, E., Mertz, C., & McGregor, D. (2002). Aging and decision making competence: An analysis of comprehension and consistency skills in older versus younger adults considering health plan options. *Journal of Behavioral Decision-Making, 15*(2), 141–164.

Fiore, M. C., Bailey, W.C., & Cohen, S. J. (2000). *Treating tobacco use and dependence: Quick reference guide for clinicians.* Rockville, MD: U.S. Department of Health and Human Services.

Fiscella, K., Franks, P., Meldrum, S., & Barnett, S. (2005). Racial disparity in surgical complications in New York State. *Annals of Surgery, 242*(2), 151–155.

Fiske, A., Wetherell, J., & Gatz, M. (2009). Depression in older adults. *Annual Review of Clinical Psychology, 5*, 363–389.

Foley, D. J., Monjan, A. A., Brown, S. L., Simonsick, E. M., Wallace, R. B., & Blazer, D. G. (1995). Sleep complaints among elderly persons: an epidemiologic study of three communities. *Sleep, 18*, 425–432.

Folstein, M., Folstein, S., & McHugh, P. (1975). "Mini-mental state," a practical method for grading the cognitive state of patients for the clinician. *Journal of Psychiatric Research, 12*, 189–198.

Fong, H., Sands, L., & Leung, J. (2006). The role of postoperative analgesia in delirium and cognitive decline in elderly patients: a systematic review. *Anesthesia and Analgesia, 102*, 1255–1266.

Foust, J., Naylor, M., Boling, P., & Cappuzzo, K. (2005). Opportunities for improving post-hospital home medication management among older adults. *Home Health Care Services Quarterly, 24*(1-2), 101–122.

Fox, W., & Wold, J. (1996). Baccalaureate student gerontological nursing experiences: raising consciousness levels and affecting attitudes. *Journal of Nursing Education, 35*, 348–155.

Freter, S., Dunbar, M., MacLeod, H., Morrison, M., MacKnight, C., & Rockwood, K. (2005). Predicting post-operative delirium in elective orthopaedic patients: the Delirium Elderly At-Risk (DEAR) instrument. *Age & Aging, 34*(2), 169–171.

Fried, L., Hadley, E., Walston, J., Newman, A., Guralnik, J., Studenski, S., . . . Ferrucci, L. (2005). From bedside to bench: Research agenda for frailty. *Science of Aging Knowledge Environment, 31*, 24.

Fried, L., Tangen, C., Walston, J., Newman, A., Hirsch, C., Gottdiener, J., . . . McBurnie, M. (2001). Frailty in older adults: evidence for a phenotype. *Journals of Gerontology. Series A Biological Sciences and Medical Sciences, 56*(3), M134–M135.

Gatt, M., Anderson, A., Reddy, B., Hayward-Sampson, P., Tring, I., & MacFie, J. (2005). Randomized clinical trial of multimodal optimization of surgical care in patients undergoing major colonic resection. *The British Journal of Surgery, 92*(11), 1354–1362.

Geriatrics Interdisciplinary Advisory Group. (2006). Interdisciplinary care of older adults with complex needs: American Geriatrics Society Position Statement. *Journal of the American Geriatrics Society, 54*(5), 849–852.

Gillis, A., & MacDonald, B. (2005). Decondition in the hospitalized elderly. *The Canadian Nurse, 101*(6), 16–20.

Girish, M., Trayner Jr., E., Damman, O., Pinto-Plata, V., & Bartolome, C. (2001). Symptom-limited stair climbing as a predictor of postoperative cardiopulmonary complications after high-risk surgery. *Chest, 120*(4), 1147–1151.

Gittell, J., Fairfield, K., Bierbaum, B., Head, W., Jackson, R., Kelly, M., . . . Zuckerman, J. (2000). Impact of relational coordination on quality of care, postoperative pain and functioning, and length of stay: A non-hospital study of surgical patients. *Medical Care, 38*(8), 807–819.

Givens, J., Jones, R., & Inouye, S. (2009). The overlap syndrome of depression and delirium in older hospitalized patients. *Journal of the American Geriatrics Association, 57*, 1347–1353.

Goldmann, A., Hoehne, C., Fritz, G., Unger, J., Ahlers, O., Nachtigall, I., & Boemke, W. (2008). Combined vs. isoflurane/fentanyl anesthesia for major abdominal surgery: Effects on hormones and hemodynamics. *Medical Science Monitor: International Medical Journal of Experimental and Clinical Research, 14*(9), 445–452.

Glover, J., Edwards, F., & Hitchcock, K. (2007). What steps can reduce morbidity and mortality caused by hip fractures? *Journal of Family Practice, 56*(11), 44–46.

Greene, N., Attix, D., Weldon, B., Smith, P., McDonagh, D., & Monk, T. (2009). Measures of executive function and depression identify patients at risk for postoperative delirium. *Anesthesiology, 110*(4), 788–795.

Gyomber, D., Lawrentschuk, N., Wong, P., Parker, F., & Bolton, D. (2010). Improving informed consent for patients undergoing radical prostatectomy using multimedia techniques: A prospective randomized cross over study. *BJU International, 106*, 1152–1156.

Hale, L., Griffin, A., Cartwright, O., Moulin, J., Alford, S., & Fleming, R. (2008). Potentially inappropriate medication use in hospitalized older adults: a DUE using the full Beers criteria. *Formulary, 43*, 326–339.

Hamman, C., & Minaker, K. (2009). Approach to frailty in older adults. In A. H. Goroll & A. G. Mulley (Eds.), *Primary care medicine: Office evaluation and management of the adult patient* (6th ed.) (pp. 1550–1554). Philadelphia, PA: Lippincott Williams & Wilkins.

Hamel, M., Toth, M., Legedza, A., & Rosen, M. (2008). Joint replacement surgery in elderly patients with severe osteoarthritis of the hip or knee: Decision making post operative recovery and clinical outcomes. *Archives of Internal Medicine, 168*(13), 1430–1440.

Hartford Institute for Geriatric Nursing, New York University College of Nursing. (2011, January 5). Specialty nursing association global vision statement on care of older adults. Retrieved February 22, 2011, from http://consultgerin.org/uploads/File/REASN_Global_Vision_Statement.pdf

Hendrich, A., Bender, P., & Nyhuis, A. (2003). Validation of the Hendrich II Fall Risk model: A large concurrent case/control study of hospitalized patients. *Applied Nursing Research, 16*(1), 9–21.

Herrera, A., Snipes, S., King, D., Torress-Vigil, I., Goldgerg, D., & Weinberg, A. (2010). Disparate inclusion of older adults in clinical trials: Priorities and opportunities for policy and practice change. *American Journal of Public Health, 100*(s1), s105–s112.

Hicks, R. W., Becker, S. C., Krenzischeck, D., & Beyea, S. C. (2004). Medication errors in the PACU: A secondary analysis of MEDMARX. *Journal of PeriAnesthesia Nursing, 19*(1), 18–28.

Hines, S., Moss, A., & Badzek, L. (1997). Being involved or just being informed: Communication preferences of seriously ill, older adults. *Communication Quarterly, 45*(3), 268–281.

Hubbard, R., O'Mahoney, M. S., & Woodhouse, K. (2009). Characterising frailty in the clinical setting—a comparison of different approaches. *Age and Ageing, 38*(1), 115–119.

Huffman, M. H. (2009). Health coaching: a fresh, new approach to improve quality outcomes and compliance for patients with chronic conditions. *Home Healthcare Nurse, 27*(8), 490–496.

Huffman, M., Bello, T., & Bissontz, K. (2008). *Health coaching made easy for healthcare providers.* Winchester, TN: The National Society of Health Coaches.

Hughes, R., & Clancy, C. (2007). Improving the complex nature of care transitions. *Journal of Nursing Care Quality, 22*(4), 289–292.

Institute for Healthcare Improvement. (n.d.) Reconcile Medications at all Transition Points. Available at http://www.ihi.org/knowledge/Pages/Changes/ReconcileMedicationsatAll TransitionPoints.aspx

Institute for Healthcare Improvement. (2007, April 19). Institute for Healthcare Improvement: High-alert medications require heightened vigilance. Retrieved January 9, 2011, from www.ihi.org/IHI/Topics/PatientSafety/MedicationSystems/ImprovementStories/FS HighAlertMedsHeightenedVigilance.htm

Institute for Safe Medication Practices. (2008). ISMP's list of high-alert medications. Retrieved April 3, 2011, from www.ismp.org/tools/highalertmedications.pdf

Institute of Medicine. (2000). *To err is human: Building a safer health system*. Washington, DC: National Academies Press.

Institute of Medicine. (2004). *Improving medical education: Enhancing the behavioral and social science content of medical school curricula*. Washington, DC: National Academies Press.

Institute of Medicine. (2008). *Retooling for an aging America*. Washington, DC: National Academies Press.

Institute of Medicine Committee on Quality of Health Care in America. (2001). *Crossing the quality chasm: A new health system for the 21st century*. Washington, DC: National Academies Press.

Inouye, S., Bogardus, S., Baker, D., Leo-Summers, L., & Cooney Jr., L. (2000). The Hospital Elder Life program: A model of care to prevent cognitive and functional decline in older hospitalized patients. *Journal of the American Geriatrics Society, 48*(12), 1697–1706.

Inouye, S., & Charpentier, P. (1996). Precipitating factors for delirium in hospitalized elderly persons. Predictive model and interrelationship with baseline vulnerability. *Journal of the American Medical Association, 275*(11), 852–857.

Inouye, S., Wagner, D., Acampora, D., Horwitz, R., Cooney, L. J., Hurst, L., & Tinetti, M. E. (1993). A predictive index for functional decline in hospitalized elderly medical patients. *Journal of General Internal Medicine, 8*(12), 645–652.

Iorio, R., Robb, W., Healy, W., Berry, D., Hozack, W., Kyle, R., . . . Parslet, B. S. (2008). Orthopaedic surgeon workforce and volume assessment for total hip and new replacement in the United States: Preparing for an epidemic. *The Journal of Bone and Joint Surgery, 90*, 1598–1605.

Kaestli, L., Wasilewski-Rasca, A., Bonnabry, P., & Vogt-Ferrier, N. (2008). Use of transdermal drug formulations in the elderly. *Drugs & Aging, 25*(4), 269–280.

Katz, J. (1984) *The silent world of doctor and patient*. New York, NY: Free Press.

Katz, S., Down, T. D., Cash, H. R., & Grotz, R. C. (1970). Progress in the development of the index of ADL. *The Gerontologist, 10*(1), 20–30.

Katznelson, R., Djaiani, G., Borger, M., Friedman, Z., Abbey, S., Fedorko, L., . . . Beattie, W. S. (2009). Preoperative use of statins is associated with reduced early delirium rates after cardiac surgery. *Anesthesiology, 110*(1), 67–73.

Kennedy. (2003).

Kingsnorth, A. N., & Majid, A. A. (2006). *Fundamentals of surgical practice* (2nd ed.). Leiden, Netherlands: Cambridge University Press.

Kite, M., Stockdale Jr., G., Whitley, B. E., & Johnson, B. (2005). Attitudes toward younger and older adults: An updated meta-analytic review. *Journal of Social Issues, 61*(2), 241–266.

Kojodjojo, P., Gohil, N., Barker, D., Youssefi, P., Salukhe, T., & Choong, A. (2008). Outcomes of elderly patients aged 80 and over with symptomatic, severe aortic stenosis: Impact of patient's choice of refusing aortic valve replacement on survival. *QJM, 101*(7), 567–573.

Kolcaba, K. (2001). Evolution of the mid-range theory of comfort for outcomes research. *Nursing Outlook, 49*(2), 86–92.

Kolcaba, K., Tilton, C., & Drouin, C. (2006). Comfort theory: A unifying framework to enhance the practice environment. *Journal of Nursing Administration, 36*(11), 538–544.

Kortebein, P., Symons, T., Ferrando, A., Paddon-Jones, D., Ronsen, O., Protas, E., . . . Evans, W. J. (2008). Functional impact of 10 days of bed rest in healthy older adults. *The Journals of Gerontology Series A, Biological Sciences and Medical Sciences, 63*(10), 1076–1081.

Kovner, C., Mezey, M., & Harrington, C. (2002). Who cares for older adults? Workforce implications of an aging society. *Health Affairs, 21*(5), 78–90.

Kraus, L., Stoddard, S., & Gilmartin, D. (1996). *Chartbook on disability in the United States.* Washington, DC: National Institute on Disability and Rehabilitation Research, U.S. Department of Education Publication.

Kristjansson, S., Nesbakken, A., Jordhøy, M., Skovlund, E., Audisio, R., Johannessen, H., . . . Wyller, T. B. (2010). Comprehensive geriatric assessment can predict complications in elderly patients after elective surgery for colorectal cancer: A prospective observational cohort study. *Clinical Reviews in Oncology/Hematology, 76,* 208–217.

Kurtz, S., Ong, K., Lau, E., Mowat, F., & Halpern, M. (2007). Projections of primary and revision hip and knee arthroplasty in the United States from 2005 to 2030. *The Journal of Bone and Joint Surgery, 89*(4), 780–785.

Kuzawa, C., & Sweet, E. (2008). Epigenetics and the embodiment of race: Developmental origins of US racial disparities in cardiovascular health. *American Journal of Human Biology, 21*(1), 2–15.

Landefeld, C., Palmeer, R., Kresevic, D., Fortinsky, R., & Kowal, J. (1995). A randomized control trial of care in a hospital medical unit especially designed to improve the functional outcomes of acutely ill older patients. *New England Journal of Medicine, 332,* 1338–1344.

Lapid, M., Rummans, T., Pankratz, V., & Appelbaum, P. (2004). Decisional capacity of depressed elderly to consent to electroconvulsive therapy. *Journal of Geriatric Psychiatry, 17*(1), 42–46.

Lauerman, C. (2008). Surgical patient education related to smoking. *AORN Journal, 87*(3), 599–609.

Lawton, M. P. & Brody, E. M. (1969). Assessment of older people: Self-maintaining and instrumental activities of daily living. *The Gerontologist, 9*(3), 179–186.

Leung, J., Sands, L., Mullen, E., Wang, Y., & Vaurio, L. (2005). Are preoperative depressive symptoms associated with postoperative delirium in geriatric surgical patients? *Journals of Gerontology Series A Biological Sciences and Medical Sciences, 60*(12), 1563–1568.

Lien, C. A. (2011). Thermoregulation in the elderly. Syllabus on Geriatric Anesthesiology. American Society of Anesthesiologists. Available at: http://asatest.asahq.org/clinical/geriatrics/thermo.htm

Litaker, D., Locala, J., Franco, K., Bronson, D., & Tannous, Z. (2001). Preoperative risk factors for postoperative delirium. *General Hospital Psychiatry, 23*(2), 84–89.

Liu, J., Etzioni, D., O'Connell, J., Maggard, M., & Ko, C. (2004). The increasing workload of general surgery. *Archives of Surgery, 139,* 423–428.

Lubin, M., Smith, R., Dodson, T., Spell, N., & Walker, H. (2006). *Medical management of the surgical patient: A textbook of perioperative medicine.* Cambridge, UK: Cambridge University Press.

Lyder, C., & Ayello, E. (2008). Pressure ulcers: A patient safety issue. In R. G. Hughes (Ed.), *Patient safety and quality: An evidence-based handbook for nurses* (pp. 1-267–1-340). Rockville, MD: Agency for Healthcare Research and Quality. Retrieved March 11, 2011, from www.ahrq.gov/qual/nurseshdbk/docs/lyderc_pupsi.pdf

Mahoney, F. I. & Barthel, D. W. (1965). Functional evaluation: The Barthel index. *Maryland State Medical Journal, 14,* 61–65.

Mainz, J. (2003). Defining and classifying quality indicators for quality improvement. *International Journal for Quality in Health Care, 15*(6), 523–530.

Majumdar, S., Kim, N., Colman, I., Chahal, A., Raymond, G., Jen, H., . . . Rowe, B. H. (2005). Incidental vertebral fractures discovered with chest radiography in the emergency department: Prevalence, recognition, and osteoporosis management in a cohort of elderly patients. *Archives of Internal Medicine, 165*(8), 905–909.

Makary, M., Segev, D., Pronovost, P., Syin, D., Bandeen-Roche, K., Patel, P., . . . Fried, L. (2010). Frailty as a predictor of surgical outcomes in older patients. *Journal of the American College of Surgeons, 210*(6), 901–908.

Makaryus, A., & Friedman, E. (2005). Patients' understanding of their treatment plans and diagnosis at discharge. *Mayo Clinic Proceedings, 80*(8), 991–994.

Maldonado, J. (2008). Delirium in the acute care setting: Characteristics, diagnosis and treatment. *Critical Care Clinics, 24*(4), 657–722.

Marcantonio, E., Juarez, G., Goldman, L., Mangione, C., Ludwig, L., Lind, L., . . . Lee, T. H. (1994). The relationship of postoperative delirium with psychoactive medications. *Journal of the American Medical Association, 272*(19), 1518–1522.

Marcucci, C., Seagull, F., Loreck, D., Bourke, D., & Sandson, N. (2010). Capacity to give surgical consent does not imply capacity to give anesthesia consent: Implications for anesthesiologists. *Anesthesia & Analgesia, 110*(2), 596–600.

Martens, A., Goldenberg, J., & Greenberg, J. (2005). A terror management perspective. *Journal of Social Issues, 63*(2), 223–239.

McCaffery, M., & Paseo, C. (1999) *PAIN clinical manual* (2nd ed.). Philadelphia, PA: Mosby.

McCarthy, E., Pencina, M., Kelly-Hayes, M., Evans, J., Oberacker, E., D'Agostino, R. B., Sr., . . . Murabito, J. M. (2008). Advance care planning and health care preferences of community-dwelling elders: The Framingham Heart Study. *Journal of Gerontology, 63*(9), 951–959.

McCleskey, C. (1997). *Geriatric anesthesiology*. Baltimore, MD: Williams & Wilkins.

McGory, M., Kao, K., Shekelle, P., Rubenstein, L., Leonardi, M., & Parikh, J. (2009). Developing quality indicators for elderly surgical patients. *Annals of Surgery, 250*(2), 338–347.

McGory, M., Shekelle, P., Rubenstein, L., Fink, A., & Ko, C. (2005). Developing quality indicators for elderly patients undergoing abdominal operations. *Journal of the American College of Surgeons, 201*, 870–873.

McKinlay, J. B. (1986). A case for refocusing upstream: the political economy of illness. In P. Conrad & R. Kern (Eds.), *The Sociology of Health and Illness: Critical Perspectives* (2nd ed.) (pp. 502–517). New York: St. Martin's Press.

McKneally, M., & Martin, D. (2000). An entrustment model of consent for surgical treatment of life-threatening illness: Perspective of patients requiring esophagectomy. *Journal of Thoracic and Cardiovascular Surgery, 120*(2), 264–269.

McNicoll, L., & Besdine, R. (2007). The future of delirium research: Promising but still room for improvement. *Aging Clinical and Experimental Research, 19*(3), 169–171.

Meiner, S., & Lueckenotte, A. (2006). *Gerontological nursing* (3rd ed.). St. Louis, MO: Mosby.

Merskey, H., & Bogduk, N. (1994). Part III: Pain terms, a current list with definition and notes on usage. In H. Merskey & N. Bogduk (Eds.). *Classification of chronic pain* (2nd ed.) (pp. 209–214). Seattle, WA: International Association for the Study of Pain Press.

Mezey, M., Boltz, M., Esterson, J., & Mitty, E. (2005). Evolving models of geriatric nursing. *Geriatric Nursing, 26*(1), 11–15.

Mezey, M., & Fulmer, T. (2002). The future history of gerontological nursing. *Journal of Gerontology Series A: Biological Sciences and Medical Sciences, 57A*, M438–M441.

Miller, N. (2010). Motivational interviewing as a prelude to coaching in healthcare settings. *Journal of Cardiovascular Nursing, 25*(3), 247–251.

Mitchell, P. (2008). Defining patient safety and quality care. In R. G. Hughes (Ed.), *Patient safety and quality: An evidence-based handbook for nurses* (pp. 1–5). Rockville, MD: Agency for Healthcare Research and Quality.

Mitty, E., & Post, L. (2008). Health care decision making. *Evidence-based geriatric nursing protocols for best practice* (3rd ed.). New York, NY: Springer Publishing Company.

Moss, F. & Halmandaris, V. J. (1977). *Too old, too sick, too bad. Nursing homes in America.* Germantown, MD: Aspen Systems.

National Center for Health Statistics. (2003). Health, Unites States 2003: Special excerpt: Trend tables on 65 and older population. Hyattsville, Maryland.

National Center for Health Statistics. (2011). Health, United States, 2010: With special feature on death and dying. Hyattsville, Maryland.

National Guideline Clearinghouse. (n.d.). Home page. Retrieved March 10, 2011, from www.guideline.gov/

National Institutes of Health. (1987). *Geriatric assessment methods for clinical decision making.* Bethesda, MD: National Institutes of Health, Office for Medical Applications of Research.

National Quality Forum. (2004). National voluntary consensus standards for nursing-sensitive care: An initial performance measure set. Retrieved April 10, 2011, from www.nursing center.com/library/JournalArticle.asp?Article_ID=798122

National Quality Forum. (2005). Implementing a national voluntary standard for informed consent for health care professionals. Retrieved from www.qualityforum.org/Publications/2005/09/Implementing_a_National_Voluntary_Consensus_Standard_for_Informed_Consent__A_User%E2%80%99s_Guide_for_Healthcare_Professionals.aspx

Naylor, M., Brooten, D., Campbell, R., Jacobsen, B., Mezey, M., Pauly, M., & Schwartz, J. S. (1999). Comprehensive discharge planning and home follow-up of hospitalized elders: A randomized controlled trial. *Journal of the National Medical Association, 281,* 613–620.

Naylor, M., Brooten, D., Campbell, R., Maislin, G., McCauley, K., & Schwartz, J. (2004). Transitional care of older adults hospitalized with heart failure: A randomized, controlled trial. *Journal of the American Geriatrics Society, 52,* 675–684.

Neelon, V. J., Champagne, M. T., Carlson, J. R., & Funk, S. G. (1996). The NEECHAM confusion scale: construction, validation and clinical testing. *Nurs Research, 45,* 324–330.

Neelon, V. J., Champagne, M. T., McConnell, E., Carlson, J., & Funk, S. G. (1992). Use of the NEECHAM Confusion Scale to assess acute confusional states of hospitalized older patients. In S. G. Funk & E. M. Tornquist (Eds.), *Key aspects of elder care: managing falls, incontinence and cognitive impairment* (278–289). New York, NY: Springer Publishing Company.

Nelson, T. (2005). Ageism: Prejudice against our feared future self. *Journal of Social Issues, 61*(2), 207–221.

Neuman, M., Speck, R., Karlawish, J., Schwartz, J., & Shea, J. (2010). Hospital protocols for the inpatient care of older adults: Results from a statewide survey. *Journal of the American Geriatrics Society, 58,* 1959–1964.

Nielsen, P., Jorgensen, L., Dahl, B., Pedersen, T., & Tonnesen, H. (2010). Prehabilitation and early rehabilitation after spinal surgery: Randomized clinical trial. *Clinical Rehabilitation, 24*(2), 137–148.

Nitz, J., Hourigan, S., & Steer, M. (2007). A study of two sitting positions in frail, older, non-mobile and totally dependent residents of aged care facilities. *Australian Journal on Ageing, 26*(2), 77–80.

Noimark, D. (2009). Predicting the onset of delirium in the post-operative patient. *Age and Ageing, 38*(4), 368–373.

Nussbaum, J., Pitts, J., Huber, F., Krierger, J. R., & Ohs, J. (2005). Ageism and ageist language across the life span: Intimate relationship and non-intimate interactions. *Journal of Social Issues, 61*(2), 287–305.

Office of Minority Health. (n.d.). Health information resource database. Retrieved February 24, 2011, from www.health.gov/nhic/nhicscripts/Entry.cfm?HRCode=HR2339

Office of Minority Health Resource Center. (2006). Retrieved from Diabetes Data/Statistics. http://minorityhealth.hhs.gov/templates/browse.aspx?lvl=3&lvlid=5

Olver, I., Whitford, H., Denson, L., Peterson, M., & Olver, S. (2009). Improving informed consent to chemotherapy: A randomized controlled trial of written information versus an interactive multimedia CD-ROM. *Patient and Counseling, 74*(2), 197–204.

Ory, M., Hoffman, M., Hawkins, M., Sanner, B., & Mockenhaupt, R. (2003). Challenging aging stereotypes: Strategies for creating a more active society. *American Journal of Preventive Medicine, 25*(3), s164–s171.

Ottenbacher, K., Graham, J., Al Snih, S., Raji, M., Samper-Ternent, R., Ostir, G., & Markides, K. S. (2009). Mexican Americans and frailty: Findings from the Hispanic established populations epidemiologic studies of the elderly. *American Journal of Public Health, 99*(4), 673–679.

Palmer, S., Tubbs, I., & Whybrow, A. (2003). Health coaching to facilitate the promotion of health behavior and achievement of health-related goals. *International Journal of Health Promotion and Education, 41*(3), 91–93.

Panno, J., Kolcaba, K., & Holder, C. (2000). Acute care for elders (ACE): A holistic model for geriatric orthopaedic nursing care. *Orthopaedic Nursing, 19*(6), 53–60.

Penrod, J., Litke, A., Hawkes, W., Magaziner, J., Doucette, J., Koval, K., . . . Siu, A. L. (2008). The association of race, gender, and comorbidity with mortality and function after hip fracture. *Journals of Gerontology Series A, Biological Sciences and Medical Sciences, 63*(8), 867–872.

Pew-Fetzer Task Force. (1994). *Health professions education and relationship-centered care.* San Francisco, CA: Pew Health Professions Commission.

Picone, D., Titler, M., Dochterman, J., Shever, L., Kim, T., Abramowitz, P., . . . Qin, R. (2008). Predictors of medication errors among elderly hospitalized patients. *American Journal of Medical Quality, 23*(2), 115–127.

Pieper, B., Sieggreen, M., Freeland, B., Kulwicki, P., Frattaroli, M., Sidor, D., . . . Garretson, B. (2006). Discharge information needs of patients after surgery. *Journal of Wound, Ostomy and Continence Nursing, 33*(3), 281–289.

Pippins, J. R., Gandhi, T. K., Hamann, C., Ndumele, C. D., Labonville, S. A., Diedrichsen, E. K., . . . Schnipper, J. L. (2008). Classifying and predicting errors of inpatient medication reconciliation. *Journal of General Internal Medicine, 23*(9),1414–1422.

Pleis, J. R., Ward, B. W., & Lucas, J. W. (2009). Summary health statistics for U.S. adults. National Health Interview Survey 2009. National Center for Health Statistics. *Vital Health Statistics, 10*(249), 2010.

Podsiadlo, D., & Richardson, S. (1991). The timed "Up & Go": A test of basic functional mobility for frail elderly persons. *Journal of the American Geriatrics Society, 39*(2), 142–148.

Prochaska, J., & DiClemente, C. (1983). Stages and processes of self-change of smoking: Toward an integrative model of change. *Journal of Consulting and Clinical Psychology, 51*(3), 390–395.

Prochaska, J., & Velicer, W. (1997). The transtheoretical model of health behavior change. *American Journal of Health Promotion, 12*(1), 38–48.

Qaseem, A., Snow, V., Fitterman, N., Hornbake, E., Lawrence, V., Smetana, G., . . . Weiss, K. B. (2006). Risk assessment for and strategies to reduce perioperative pulmonary complications for patients undergoing noncardiothoracic surgery: A guideline from the American College of Physicians. *Annals of Internal Medicine, 144*(8), 575–80.

Quartin, A., Schein, R., Kett, D., & Peduzzi, P. (1997). Magnitude and duration of the effect of sepsis on survival. *Journal of the American Medical Association, 277*(13), 1058–1063.

Ricker, J. H. & Axelrod, B. N. (1994). Analysis of an oral paradigm for the trail making test. *Assessment, 1*, 47–52.

Rockwood, K., Fox, R., Stolee, P., Robertson, D., & Beattie, B. (1994). Frailty in elderly people: An evolving concept. *Canadian Medical Association Journal, 150*(4), 489–495.

Rolfson, D., Majumdar, S., Tsuyuki, R., Tahir, A., & Rockwood, K. (2006). Validity and reliability of the Edmonton Frail Scale. *Age and Ageing, 35*(5), 526–529.

Rollnick, S., Miller, W. R., & Butler, C. C. (2008). *Motivational interviewing in health care: Helping patients change behavior.* New York, NY: Guilford Press.

Rooks, D., Huang, J., Bierbaum, B., Bolus, S., Rubano, J., Connolly, C., . . . Katz, J. N. (2006). Effect of preoperative exercise on measures of functional status in men and women undergoing total hip and knee arthroplasty. *Arthritis and Rheumatism, 55*(5), 700–708.

Rothman, M., van Ness, P., O'Leary, J., & Fried, T. (2007). Refusal of medical and surgical interventions by older persons with advanced chronic disease. *Journal of General Internal Medicine, 22*(7), 982–987.

Royall, D., Cordes, J., & Polk, M. (1998). CLOX: An executive clock drawing task. *Journal of Neurology, Neurosurgery, & Psychiatry with Practical Neurology, 64*(5), 588–594.

Rubenstein, L., Josephson, K., Wieland, G., English, P., Sayre, J., & Kane, R. (1984). Effectiveness of a geriatric evaluation unit: A randomized clinical trial. *New England Journal of Medicine, 311*, 1664–1670.

Rudolph, J., Salow, M., Angelini, M., & McGlinchey, R. (2008). The anticholinergic risk scale and anticholineric adverse effects in older persons. *Archives of Internal Medicine, 168*(5), 508–513.

Ryan, C. (2011, January 24). Care transitions: What do these programs look like? And how can the aging network play a role? *Affordable Care Act Webinar.* Lecture conducted from Administration on Aging.

Sackett, D., Rosenbery, W. M. C., Gray, J. A. M., Haynes, R. B., & Richardson, W. S. (1996). Evidence based medicine: what it is and what it isn't. *British Medical Journal, 312*, 71–72.

Saczynski, J., Beiser, A., Seshadri, S., Auerbach, S., Wolf, P., & Au, R. (2010). Depressive symptoms and risk of dementia: The Framingham Heart Study. *Neurology, 75*(1), 35–41.

Schoonhoven, L., Defloor, T., van der Tweel, I., Buskens, E., & Grypdonck, M. (2002). Risk indicators for pressure ulcers during surgery. *Applied Nursing Research, 16*(2), 163–173.

Schouchoff, B. (2002). Pressure ulcer development in the operating room. *Critical Care Nursing Quarterly, 25*(1), 76–82.

Shue, C., McNeley, K., & Arnold, L. (2005). Changing medical students' attitudes about older adults and future older patients. *Academic Medicine, 80*(Supplement 10), s6–s9.

Shumway-Cook, A., Baldwin, M., Polissar, N. L., & Gruber, W. (1997). Predicting the probability for falls in community-dwelling older adults. *Physical Therapy, 77*(8), 812–819.

Shumway-Cook, A., Brauer, S., & Woollacott, M. (2000). Predicting the probability for falls in community-dwelling older adults using the Timed Up & Go Test. *Physical Therapy, 80*(9), 896–903.

Sieber, F. E. (2007). *Geriatric anesthesia.* New York, NY: McGraw-Hill Professional.

Silverstein, J., Rooke, G., Reves, J., & McLeskey, C. (2008). *Geriatric anesthesiology* (2nd ed.). New York, NY: Springer Publishing Company.

Smetana, G., Lawrence, V., & Cornell, J. (2005). Preoperative pulmonary risk stratification for noncardiothoracic surgery: Systematic review for the American College of Physicians. *Annals of Internal Medicine, 144*, 581–595.

Society of Hospital Medicine. (2008). BOOSTing care transitions. Retrieved March 11, 2011, from www.hospitalmedicine.org/ResourceRoomRedesign/RR_CareTransitions/CT_Home.cfm

Sorensen, E., & Wang, F. (2009). Social support depression, functional status, and gender differences in older adults undergoing first-time coronary artery bypass graft surgery. *Heart and Lung, 38*(4), 306–317.

Stenvall, M., Olofsson, B., Lundström, M., Englund, U., Borssén, B., Svensson, O., . . . Gustafson, Y. (2007). A multidisciplinary, multifactorial intervention program reduces postoperative falls and injuries after femoral neck fracture. *Osteoporosis International, 18*(2), 167–175.

Stern, C., & Jayasekara, R. (2009). Interventions to reduce the incidence of falls in older adult patients in acute-care hospitals: A systematic review. *International Journal of Evidence-based Healthcare, 7*(4), 243–249.

Stulberg, J., Delaney, C., Neuhauser, D., Aron, D., Fu, P., & Koroukian, S. (2010). Adherence to surgical care improvement project measures and the association with postoperative infections. *Journal of the American Medical Association, 303*(24), 2479–2485.

Suchman, A. (2006). A new theoretical foundation for relationship-centered care. Complex responsive processes of relating. *Journal of General Internal Medicine, 21*(Supplement 1), S40–S44.

Sündermann, S., Dademasch, A., Praetorius, J., Kempfert, J., Dewey, T., Falk, V., . . . Walther, T. (2011). Comprehensive assessment of frailty for elderly high-risk patients undergoing cardiac surgery. *European Journal of Cardiothoracic Surgery, 39*, 33–37.

Tanner, C. (2006). Thinking like a nurse: A research-based model of clinical judgment in nursing. *Journal of Nursing Education, 45*(6), 204–211.

Tauber, A. (2005). *Patient autonomy and the ethics of responsibility.* Cambridge, MA: The MIT Press.

Teno, J., Gruneir, A., Schwartz, Z., Nanda, A., & Wetle, T. (2007). Association between advance directives and quality of end-of-life care: A national study. *Journal of the American Geriatrics Society, 55*, 189–194.

Thorpe Jr., R., Brandon, D., & LaVeist, T. (2008). Social context as an explanation for race disparities in hypertension: Findings from the Exploring Health Disparities in Integrated Communities (EHDIC) Study. *Social Science & Medicine, 67*(10), 1604–1611.

Tinetti, M., Doucette, J., & Claus, E. (1995). The contribution of predisposing and situational risk factors to serious fall injuries. *Journal of American Geriatrics Society, 43*(11), 1207–1213.

Tomlin, K., Walker, R., & Grover, J. (2005). *Trainer's guide to motivational interviewing: Enhancing motivation for change—A learner's manual for the American Indian/Alaskan Native Counselor.* Portland, OR: One Sky National Resource Center and Oregon Health & Sciences University.

Topp, R., Ditmyer, M., King, K., Doherty, K., & Hornyak 3rd, J. (2002). The effect of bed rest and potential of prehabilitation on patients in the intensive care unit. *AACN Clinical Issues, 13*(2), 263–276.

Tullman, D. F., Mion, L. C., Fletcher, K., & Foreman, M. D. (2008). Delirium: Prevention, early recognition, and treatment. In E. Capezuti, D. Zwicker, M. Mezey, & T. Fulmer (Eds.). *Evidence-based geriatric nursing protocols for best practice* (3rd ed.). (pp. 111–125). New York, NY: Springer Publishing Company.

Tunzi, M. (2001). Can the patient decide? Evaluating patient capacity in practice. *American Family Physician, 64*(2), 299–308.

U.S. Census Bureau. (2011). Births, deaths, marriages, & divorces: Life expectancy. *The 2011 Statistical Abstract: The National Data Book.* Retrieved January 28, 2011, from www.census.gov/compendia/statab/cats/births_deaths_marriages_divorces/life_expectancy.html

U.S. Census Bureau. (2011). Statistical Abstracts of the United States, 2011. Resident population by sex and age. Retrieved from http://www.census.gov/compendia/statab/2011/tables/11s0008.pdf

U.S. Department for Health and Human Services. (2010, May 20). Deaths: Final data for 2007. *National Vital Statistics Reports, 58*. Retrieved January 20, 2011, from www.cdc.gov/NCHS/data/nvsr/nvsr58/nvsr58_19.pdf

Van Norman, G. (1998). Informed consent in the operating room: Ethical topic in medicine. *University of Washington School of Medicine.* Retrieved January 21, 2011, from http://depts.washington.edu/bioethx/topics/infc.html

Velanovich, V., Gabel, M., Walker, E., Doyle, T., O'Bryan, R., Szymanski, W., ... Lewis Jr., F. R. (2002). Causes for the undertreatment of elderly breast cancer patients: Tailoring treatments to individual patients. *Journal of the American College of Surgeons, 194*(1), 8–13.

Vollmer, K. (2010). Introduction to progressive mobility. *Critical Care Nurse, 30*(2), S3–S5.

Wadlund, D. (2006). Prevention, recognition, and management of nursing complications in the intraoperative and postoperative surgical patient. *Nursing Clinics of North America, 41*, 151–171.

Wagner, Byrne, & Kolcaba. (2006). Effects of comfort warming on preoperative patients. *AORN Journal, 84*(3), 427–428.

Walston, J., McBurnie, M., Newman, A., Tracy, R., Kop, W., Hirsch, C., ... Fried, L. P. (2002). Frailty and activation of the inflammation and coagulation systems with and without clinical comorbidities. *Archives of Internal Medicine, 162*, 2333–2341.

Warner, D. (2005). Preoperative smoking cessation: The role of the primary care provider. *Mayo Clinic Proceedings, 80*(2), 252–258.

Warner, D. (2009). Feasibility of tobacco interventions in anesthesiology practices: A pilot study. *Anesthesioloy, 110*(6), 1223–1228.

Webster's New World Dictionary of the American Language. (1970). Second College Edition. New York: The World Publishing Company.

Weed, H., Lutman, C., Young, D., & Schuller, D. (1995). Preoperative identification of patients at risk for delirium after major head and neck cancer surgery. *Laryngoscope, 105*(10), 1066–1068.

Wertheimer, A., & Miller, F. (2008). Payment for research participation: A coercive offer? *Journal of Medical Ethics, 34*(5), 389–392. Retrieved October 19, 2010, from http://jme.bmj.com/content/34/5/389.full

Whitbourne, S. (2002). *The aging individual: Physical and psychological perspectives* (2nd ed.). New York, NY: Springer Publishing Company.

Williams, S. L., Jones, P. B., & Pofahl, W. E. Preoperative management of the older patient-A surgeon's perspective: Part I. Clinical Geriatrics, January 17, 2008, 24-28. Downloaded March 24 2008. Available at http://www.clinicalgeriatrics.com/articles/Preoperative-Management-Older-Patient-Surgeon's-Perspective-Part-I

Wilson, L. & Kolcaba, K. (2004) Practical application of comfort theory in the perianesthesia setting. *Journal of PeriAnesthesia Nursing, 19*(3), 164–173.

Wolf, Z. (1989). Medication errors and nursing responsibility. *Holistic Nursing Practice, 4*(1), 8–17.

Wong, J. D., Bajcar, J. M., Wong, G. G., Alibhai, S. M., Huh, J. H., Cesta, A., ... Fernandes, O. A. (2008). Medication reconciliation at hospital discharge: Evaluating discrepancies. *The Annals of Pharmacotherapy, 42*(10), 1373–1379.

World Health Organization. (1996). *Cancer pain relief and palliative care (technical report series)* (2nd ed.). Geneva, Switzerland: World Health Organization. Retrieved May 17, 2010, from www.who.int/cancer/palliative/painladder/en/

Wren, S., Martin, M., Yoon, J., & Bech, F. (2010). Postoperative pneumonia—prevention program for the inpatient surgical ward. *Journal of the American College of Surgeons, 210*(4), 491–495.

Wuhrman, E., Cooney, M. F., Dunwoody, C. J., Eksterowicz, N., Merkel, S., & Oakes, L. L. (2007). Authorized and unauthorized ("PCA by Proxy") dosing of analgesic infusion pumps: Position statement with clinical practice recommendations. *Pain Management Nursing, 8*(1), 4–11.

Zheng, W., & Chodobski, A. (2005). *The blood-cerebrospinal fluid barrier.* Boca Raton, FL: Taylor & Francis.

Bibliography

A Place for Mom. (n.d.). Elderly dehydration. Retrieved June 16, 2010, from http://nursing-homes.aplaceformom.com/articles/elderly-dehydration

Academy of Medical-Surgical Nurses. (n.d.). *Care of the older adult*. Pitman, NJ: Academy of Medical-Surgical Nurses.

Academy of Medical-Surgical Nurses. (2007). *Scope and standards of medical-surgical nursing practice* (4th ed.). Pitman, NJ: Academy of Medical-Surgical Nurses.

Adelman, R., Capello, C., LoFaso, V., Greene, M., Konopasek, L., & Marzuk, P. (2007). Introduction to the older patient: A "first exposure" to geriatrics for medical students. *Journal of the American Geriatrics Society, 55*, 1445–1450.

Afilalo, J., Eisenberg, M., Morin, J., Bergman, H., Monette, J., Noiseux, N., . . . Boivin, J. (2010). Gait speed as an incremental predictor of mortality and major morbidity in elderly patients undergoing cardiac surgery. *Journal of the American College of Cardiology, 56*(20), 1668–1676.

Aging and Wellness Module. (n.d.). Development states and theories of aging. Retrieved February 17, 2011, from http://itde.vccs.edu/uploads/nur/114/agingandwellnesslecture/agingandwellnesslecture4.html

Agostini, J., Concato, J., & Inouye, S. (2007). Improving sedative-hypnotic prescribing in older hospitalized patients: Provider-perceived benefits and barriers of a computer-based reminder. *Journal of General Internal Medicine, 23*(Supplement 1), 32–36.

Ahmed, N., Mandel, R., & Fain, M. (2007). Frailty: An emerging geriatric syndrome. *The American Journal of Medicine, 120*, 748–753.

Alagiakrishnan, K., Marrie, T., Rolfson, D., Coke, W., Comicioli, R., Duggan, D., . . . Magee, B. (2007). Simple cognitive testing (Mini-Cog) predicts in-hospital delirium in the elderly. *Journal of the American Geriatrics Society, 55*(2), 314–316.

Alfieri, W., & Borgogni, T. (2010). Through the looking glass and what frailty found there: Looking for resilience in older adults. *Journal of the American Geriatrics Society, 58*(3), 602–603.

Alt-White, A. (1995). Obtaining "informed" consent from the elderly. *Western Journal of Nursing Research, 17*(6), 700–705.

American College of Surgeons. Statement on advance directives by patients: "Do Not Resuscitate" in the operating room. Retrieved November 27, 2010, from www.facs.org/fellows_info/statements/st-19.html

The American Federation for Aging Research. (n.d.). Theories of aging based on predetermined or programmed events. Retrieved February 18, 2011, from www.healthandage.com/html/min/afar/content/other2_3.htm

American Geriatrics Society Panel of Pharmacological Management of Persistent Pain in Older Persons. (2009). Pharmacological management of persistent pain in older persons. *Journal of the American Geriatrics Society, 57,* 1331–1346.

American Medical Directors Association. (2003). Pain assessment in advanced dementia (PAINAD) scale. Retrieved March 10, 2011, from www.amda.com/publications/caring/may2004/painad.cfm

American Nurses Association. (2010). *Nursing: Scope and standards of practice* (2nd ed.). Silver Spring, MD: American Nurses Association.

American Society of Anesthesiologists. (2001; reaffirmed 2008). *Ethical guidelines for the anesthesia care of patients with do-not-resuscitate orders or other directives that limit treatment.* Park Ridge, IL: American Society of Anesthesiologists. Retrieved November 27, 2010, from www.asahq.org/

American Society for Anesthesiologists. (2009, October 21). *Standards, guidelines, and statements.* Retrieved March 10, 2011, from http://www.asahq.org/For-Healthcare-Professionals/Standards-Guidelines-and-Statements.aspx

American Society of Anesthesiologists Task Force on Acute Pain Management. (2004). Practice guidelines for acute pain management in the perioperative setting. *Anesthesiology, 100*(6), 1573–1581.

American Society of PeriAnesthesia Nurses. (n.d.). A position statement on the geriatric patient. Retrieved December 2, 2010, from http://www.aspan.org/Portals/6/docs/ClinicalPractice/PositionStatement/1012/Pos_Stmt_11_Geriatric_Pt.pdf

Association of periOperative Registered Nurses. (2010). AORN position statement on care of the older adult in perioperative settings. Retrieved December 2, 2010, from www.aorn.org/PracticeResources/AORNPositionStatements/OlderAdult

Arola, H., Nicholls, E., Mallen, C., & Thomas, E. (2010). Self-reported pain interference and symptoms of anxiety and depression in community-dwelling olderadults: Can a temporal relationship be determined? *European Journal of Pain, 14*(9), 966–971.

Arntz, A., & Claassens, L. (2004). The meaning of pain influences its experienced intensity. *Pain, 109*(1–2), 20–25.

Ashcroft, G., Mills, S., & Ashworth, J. (2002). Ageing and wound healing. *Biogerontology, 3,* 337–45.

Asher, M. (2004). Surgical considerations in the elderly. *Journal of Perianesthesia Nursing, 19*(6), 406–414.

Assess the person, not just the pain. (1993, September). *Pain clinical updates: Assess the person, not just the pain.* Retrieved February 5, 2011, from www.iasp-pain.org/AM/AMTemplate.cfm?Section=HOME,HOME&TEMPLATE=/CM/ContentDisplay.cfm&SECTION=HOME,HOME&CONTENTID=7627

Aubrun, F., & Marmion, F. (2007). The elderly patient and postoperative pain treatment. *Best Practice & Research Clinical Anesthesiology, 21*(1), 109–127.

Bass, D., Atix, D. K., Phillips-Bute, B., & Monk, T. G. (2008). An efficient screening tool for preoperative depression: The geriatric depression scale-short form. *Ambulatory Anesthesiology, 106,* 805–809.

Barrowclough, F., & Pinel, C. (1981). The process of ageing. Journal of Advanced Nursing, 6, 319–325.

Bapoje, S., Whitaker, J., Schulz, T., Chu, E., & Albert, R. (2007). Preoperative evaluation of the patient with pulmonary disease. *Chest, 132*(5), 1637–1645.

Barnett, S. (2009). Polypharmacy and perioperative medications in the elderly. *Anesthesiology Clinics, 27*(3), 377–389.

Barnes, D. E. Alexopoulos, G. S., Lopez, O. L. Williamson, J. D., & Yaffe, K. (2006). Depressive symptoms, vascular, disease, and mild cognitive impairment. Findings from the cardio-vascular health study. *Archives General Psychiatry, 63,* 273–280.

Barrera, R., Shi, W., Amar, D., Thaler, H., Gabovich, N., Bains, M., & White, D. (2005). Smoking and timing of cessation. Impact on pulmonary complications after thoracotomy. *Chest, 127*(6), 1977–1983.

Baumgartner, R. (1997). Three dimensions of ethics. *Vocational Education and Work Adjustment Bulletin, 39*(Winter), 94–98.

Beliveau, M., & Multach, M. (2003). Perioperative care for the elderly patient. *Medical Clinics of North America, 87*, 273–289.

Bell, C., Bajcar, J., Bierman, A., Li, P., Mandani, M., & Urbach, D. (2006). Potentially unintended discontinuation of long-term medication use after elective surgical procedures. *Archives of Internal Medicine, 166*, 2525–2531.

Bell, M. (1999). Postoperative pain management in the non-Hispanic white and Mexican American older adult. *Seminars in Perioperative Nursing, 8*(1), 7–11.

Belmaker, R. H., & Agam, G. (2008). Major depressive disorder. *New England Journal of Medicine, 358*, 55–68.

Bennett, J. (2000). Dehydration: Hazards and benefits. *Geriatric Nursing, 21*(2), 84–88.

Bennett, J., Thomas, V., & Riegel, B. (2004). Unrecognized chronic dehydration in older adults: examining prevalence rate and risk factors. *Journal of Gerontologic Nursing, 30*(11), 22–28.

Benson, J., & Forman, W. (2002). Comprehension of written health care information in an affluent geriatric retirement community: Use of the test of functional health literacy. *Gerontology, 48*, 93–97.

Bergman, H., Ferrucci, L., Guralnik, J., Hogan, D., Hummel, S., Karunananthan, S., & Wolfson C.. (2007). Frailty: An emerging research and clinical paradigm—issues and controversies. *Journal of Gerontology Series A Biological Sciences and Medical Sciences, 62A*(7), 731–737.

Bergman, S., & Coletti, D. (2006). Perioperative management of the geriatric patient. Part 1: Respiratory system. *Oral Surgery, Oral Medicine, Oral Pathology, Oral Radiology and Endodontics, 102*(3), e1–6.

Bhat, R., & Rockwood, K. (2007). Delirium as a disorder of consciousness. *Journal of Neurology, Neurosurgery, and Psychiatry, 78*(11), 1167–1170.

Bhattacharya, S. (2008). Falls and mobility problems in older adults. *POGOe Portal of Geriatric Online Education*. Retrieved April 24, 2011, from www.pogoe.org/productid/20273

Bianchi, J., & Cameron, J. (2008). Assessment of skin integrity in the elderly 1. *British Journal of Community Nursing, 13*(3), S26, S28, S30–S32.

Bjoro, K., & Herr, K. (2008). Tools for pain assessment in older adults with end-stage dementia. *AAHPM Bulletin, 9*(3), 1–4.

Bodolea, C., Hagau, N., Coman, I., Pintea, S., Cristea, I.A., Cristea, T., & Negrutiu, S. (2008). Postoperative cognitive dysfunction in elderly patients. An integrated psychological and medical approach. *Journal of Cognitive and Behavioral Psychotherapies, 8*(1), 117–132.

Boldt, J. (2000). Volume replacement in the surgical patient—Does the type of solution make a difference? *British Journal of Anaesthesia, 84*(6), 783–793.

Boldt, J., Ducke, M., Kumie, B., Papsdorf, M., & Zurmeyer, E. (2004). Influence of different volume replacement strategies on inflammation and endothelial activation in the elderly undergoing major abdominal surgery. *Intensive Care Medicine, 30*(3), 416–422.

Bonk, M., Krown, H., Matuszewski, K., & Oinonen, M. (2006). Potentially inappropriate medications in hospitalized senior patients. *American Journal of Health-System Pharmacy, 63*, 1161–1165.

Borson, S. Scanlan, J. M., Watanabe, J., Tu, S.-P., & Lessig, M. (2005) Simplifying detection of cognitive impairment: Comparison of the Mini-Cog and Mini-Mental State Examination in a multiethnic sample. *Journal of the American Geriatrics Society, 53*, 871–874.

Bortz, W. (2002). A conceptual framework of frailty: A review. *Journal of Gerontology Series A. Biological Sciences and Medical Sciences, 57A*(5), M283–M288.

Bortz, W. (2010). Understanding frailty. *Journal of Gerontology Series A. Biological Sciences and Medical Sciences, 65A*(3), 255–256.

Boult, C., Giddens, J., Frey, K., Reider, L., & Novak, T. (2009). *Guided care. A new nurse physician partnership in chronic care.* New York, NY: Springer Publishing Company.

Brandes, R., Fleming, I., & Busse, R. (2005). Endothelial aging. *Cardiovascular Research, 66*(2), 286–294.

Brandstrup, B. (2006). Fluid therapy for the surgical patient. *Best Practice & Research Clinical Anaesthesiology, 20*(2), 265–283.

Brett, M. (1998). Informed consent—Ethics and the elderly. *British Journal of Theatre Nursing, 8*(7), 21–27.

Brown, C., Holcomb, L., Maloney, J., Naranjo, J., Gibson, C., & Russell, P. (2005). Caring in action: The patient care facilitator role. *International Journal for Human Caring, 9*(3), 51–58.

Brown, C., Roth, D., Allman, R., Sawyer, P., Ritchie, C., & Roseman, J. (2009). Trajectories of life-space mobility after hospitalization. *Annals of Internal Medicine, 150*(6), 372–328.

Brown, D. (2004). A literature review exploring how healthcare professionals contribute to the assessment and control of postoperative pain in older people. *Journal of Clinical Nursing, 13*(6B), 74–90.

Bruce, A., Ritchie, C., Blizard, R., Lai, R., & Raven, P. (2007). The incidence of delirium associated with orthopedic surgery: A meta-analytic review. *International Psychogeriatrics, 19*(2), 197–214.

Bruce, D. (2009). Medication errors: Another important surgical problem. *ANZ Journal of Surgery, 79*(9), 583–584.

Brunicardi, F., Anderson, D., Billiar, T., Dunn, D., Hunter, J., & Pollock, R. (2006). *Schwartz's manual of surgery.* New York. NY: McGraw-Hill Professional.

Buchner, D. (1992). Preventing frail health. *Clinics in Geriatric Medicine, 8*(1), 1–17.

Bundgaard-Nielsen, M., Secher, N., & Kehlet, H. (2009). "Liberal" vs. "restrictive" perioperative fluid therapy—a critical assessment of the evidence. *ACTA Anaesthesiologica Scandanavia, 53*(7), 843–851.

Burda, S., Hobson, D., & Pronovost, P. (2005). What is the patient really taking? Discrepancies between surgery and anesthesiology perspective. *Quality & Safety in Health Care, 14*, 414–416.

Buss, M., Vanderwerker, L., Inouye, S., Zhang, B., Block, S., & Prigerson, H. (2007). Associations between caregiver-perceived delirium in patients with cancer and generalized anxiety in their caregivers. *Journal of Palliative Medicine, 10*(5), 1083–1092.

Butler, R. (1969). Ageism: another form of bigotry. *Gerontologist, 9*, 243–246.

Butler, R. (1975) *Why survive? Being old in America.* New York, NY: Harper & Row.

Butterworth, A. (2004). Advance directives. Vital to quality care for elderly patients. *ADVANCE for Nurse Practitioners, 12*(3), 69–75.

Calkins, E., Boult, C., Wagner, E., & Pacala, J. (1999). *New ways to care for older people: Building systems based on evidence.* New York, NY: Springer Publishing Company.

Callen, B., Mahoney, J., Wells, T., Enloe, M., & Hughes, S. (2004). Admission and discharge mobility of frail hospitalized older adults. *MEDSURG Nursing, 13*(3), 156–163.

Callen, J., McIntosh, J., & Li, J. (2010). Accuracy of medication documentation in hospital discharge summaries: a retrospective analysis of medication transcription errors in manual and electronic discharge summaries. *International Journal of Medical Informatics, 79*(1), 58–65.

Calvin, R., & Lane, P. (1999). Perioperative uncertainty and state anxiety of orthopaedic surgical patients. *Orthopaedic Nursing, 18*(6), 61–66.

Campbell, C. (n.d.). Deconditioning: The consequence of bed rest. *Institute of Aging.* Lecture conducted from University of Florida. Retrieved February 15, 2011, from www.aging.ufl .edu/files/lectures/reconditioning_campbell.pdf

The Care Transitions Program. (2007). The Care Transitions Intervention: Improving transitions across sites of care. Retrieved March 11, 2011, from www.caretransitions.org/ documents/manual.pdf

Carli, F., & Zavorsky, G. (2005). Optimizing functional exercise capacity in the elderly surgical population. *Current Opinion in Clinical Nutrition and Metabolic Care, 8*(1), 23–32.

Cassel, C. (n.d.). Geriatrics: A vital core of hospital medicine. *Caring for the Hospitalized Elderly: Current Best Practice and New Horizons.* Retrieved March 26, 2011, from http:// www.hospitalmedicine.org/AM/Template.cfm?Section=The_Hospitalist&Template=/ CM/ContentDisplay.cfm&ContentFileID=1447

Chaboyer, W., McMurray, A., & Wallis, M. (2008). *Standard operating protocol for implementing bedside handover in nursing.* Sydney, Australia: Australian Commission on Safety and Quality in Healthcare.

Chang, J., & Ganz, D. (2007). Quality indicators for falls and mobility problems in vulnerable elders. *Journal of the American Geriatrics Society, 55*(Supplement 2), S327–S334.

Chibnall, J., & Tait, R. (2001). Pain assessment in cognitively impaired and unimpaired older adults: a comparison of four scales. *Pain, 92,* 173–186.

Chunta, K. (2009). Expectations, anxiety, depression, and physical health status as predictors of recovery in open-heart surgery patients. *Journal of Cardiovascular Nursing, 24*(6), 454–464.

Cigolle, C., Ofstedal, M., Tian, Z., & Blaum, C. (2009). Comparing models of frailty: The health and retirement study. *Journal of the American Geriatrics Society, 57,* 830–839.

Clark, G., Lucas, K., & Stephens, L. (1994). Ethical dilemmas and decisions concerning the do-not-resuscitate patient undergoing anesthesia. *AANA Journal, 62*(3), 253–256.

Clark, J. (2004). An aging population with chronic disease compels new delivery systems focused on new structures and practices. *Nursing Administration Quarterly, 28*(2), 105–115.

Clarke, M., Kennedy, K., & Macdonagh, R. (2008). Discussing life expectancy with surgical patients: Do patients want to know and how should this information be delivered? *BMC Medical Informatics and Decision Making, 8*(24). Retrieved March 11, 2011, from www .biomedcentral.com/1472-6947/8/24

Classen, D., Jaser, L., & Budnitz, D. (2010). Adverse drug events among hospitalized Medicare patients: Epidemiology and national estimates from a new approach to surveillance. *The Joint Commission Journal on Quality and Patient Safety, 36*(1), 12–21.

Clavet, H., Hebert, P., Fergusson, D., Doucette, S., & Trudel, G. (2008). Joint contracture following prolonged stay in the intensive care unit. *Canadian Medical Association Journal, 178*(6), 691–697.

Clayton, J. (2008). Special needs of older adults undergoing surgery. *AORN Journal, 87*(3), 557–570.

Collier, E. (2005). Latent age discrimination in mental health care. *Mental Health Practice, 8*(6), 42–45.

Congdon, N., Vingerling, J., Klein, B., West, S., Friedman, D. S., Kempen, J., . . . Taylor, H. R. (2004). Prevalence of cataract and pseudophakia/aphakia among adults in the United States. *Archives of Ophthalmology, 122,* 487–494.

Cook, D., & Rooke, G. (2003). Priorities in perioperative geriatrics. *Anesthesia and Analgesia, 96*(6), 1823–1836.

Counsell, S., Callahan, C., Buttar, A., Clark, D., & Frank, K. (2006). Geriatric resources for assessment and care of elders (GRACE): A new model of primary care for low-income seniors. *Journal of the American Geriatrics Society, 54*, 1136–1141.

Cox, K. (n.d.). Care of older adults. *Academy of Medical-Surgical Nurses.* Retrieved December 2, 2010, from www.amsn.org/cgi-bin/WebObjects/AMSNMain.woa/1/wa/viewSection?s_id=1073744079&ss_id=536873598&wosid=8SKq6AAWb5QE2OL6Ufl4vC

Crawford, R. (1980). Healthism and the medicalization of everyday life. *International Journal of Health Services: Planning, Administration, Evaluation, 10*(3), 365–388.

Cyr, N. (2007). Depression and older adults. *AORN Journal, 85*(2), 397–401.

D'Ambrosia, R. (2005). Epidemiology of osteoarthritis. *Orthopedics, 28*(2 Supplement), s201–s205.

Dahl, J., & Moiniche, S. (2004). Pre-emptive analgesia. *British Medical Bulletin, 71*, 13–27.

Dahlke, S., & Phinney, A. (2008). Caring for hospitalized older adults at risk for delirium: The silent, unspoken piece of nursing practice. *Journal of Gerontological Nursing, 34*(6), 41–47.

Das, S., Forrest, K., & Howell, S. (2010). General anaesthesia in elderly patients with cardiovascular disorders: Choice of anaesthetic agent. *Drugs & Aging, 27*(4), 265–282.

Dasgupta, M., Rolfson, D., Stolee, P., Borrie, M., & Speechley, M. (2009). Frailty is associated with postoperative complications in older adults with medical problems. *Archives of Gerontology and Geriatrics, 48*, 78–83.

Davidson, J., Griffin, R., & Higgs, S. (2007). Introducing a clinical pathway in fluid management. *Journal of Pharmacy and Pharmacology, 17*(6), 248–256.

Davidhizer, R., & Giger, J. N. (2004). A review of the literature on care of clients in pain who are culturally diverse. *International Nursing Review, 51*(1), 47–55.

Decker, S. (2009). Behavioral indicators of postoperative pain in older adults with delirium. *Clinical Nursing Research, 18*(4), 33–347.

de Jonghe, J., Kalisvaart, K., Dijkstra, M., van Dis, H., Vreeswijk, R., Kat, M., . . . van Gool, W. A. (2007). Early symptoms in the prodromal phase of delirium: A prospective cohort study in elderly patients undergoing hip surgery. *The American Journal of Geriatric Psychiatry, 15*(2), 112–121.

Delaney, C., Senagore, A., Gerkin, T., Beard, T., Zingaro, W., Tomaszewski, K., . . . Poston, S. A. (2010). Association of surgical care practices with length of stay and use of clinical protocols after elective bowel resection: Results of a national survey. *The American Journal of Surgery, 199*, 299–304.

Devlin, J. W., Fong, J. J., Howard, E. P., Skrobik, Y., McCoy, N., Yasuda, C., Marshall, J. (2008) Assessment of delirium in the intensive care unit: Nursing practices and perceptions. *American Journal of Critical Care, 17*, 555–565.

DeVries, E., Ramrattan, M., Smorenburg, S., Gouma, D., & Boermeester, M. (2008). The incidence and nature on in-hospital adverse events: A systematic review. *Quality & Safety in Health Care, 17*(3), 216–223.

DeWaters, T., Faut-Callahan, M., McCann, J., Paice, J., Fogg, L., Hollinger-Smith, L., . . . Stanaitis, H. (2008). Comparison of self-reported pain and the PAINAD Scale in hospitalized, cognitively impaired and intact older adults after hip fracture surgery. *Orthopedic Nursing, 27*(1), 21–28.

Dewing, J. (2002). Older people with confusion: Capacity to consent and the administration of medicines. *Nursing Older People, 14*(8), 23–28.

Dindo, D., Demartines, N., & Clavien, P. (2004). Classification of surgical complications: A new proposal with evaluation in a cohort of 6336 patients and results of a survey. *Annals of Surgery, 240*(2), 205–213.

Doerflinger, D. C. (2009). Older adult surgical patients: presentation and challenges. *AORN Journal, 90*(2), 223–240.

Donahue, J. L., Lowenthal, D. T., & Ouslander, J. (1997). Clinical physiology-pharmacology: The old, old bladder. *Geriatric Nephrology and Urology*, 6, 181–188.

Dotson, V., Beydoun, M. A., & Zonderman, A. B. (2010) .Recurrent depressive symptoms and the incidence of dementia and mild cognitive impairment. *Neurology*, 75, 27–34.

Duppils, G., & Wikblad, K. (2007). Patients' experiences of being delirious. *Journal of Clinical Nursing*, 16, 810–818.

DuVal, G., Sartorius, L., Clarridge, B., Gensler, G., & Danis, M. (2001). What triggers requests for ethics consultations. *Journal of Medical Ethics*, 27, i24–i29.

Dybec, R. (2004). Intraoperative positioning and care of the obese patient. *Plastic Surgical Nursing*, 24(3), 118–122.

Ead, H. (2004). Post-anesthesia tracheal extubation. *Dynamics*, 15(3), 20–25.

Ebell, M. (2007). Predicting delirium in hospitalized older patients. *American Family Physician*, 76(10), 1527–1529.

Ebersole, P. (1996). A little knowledge can be dangerous. *Geriatric Nursing*, 17(5), 197–198.

Eid, T. (2008). Documenting and implementing evidence-based post-operative pain management in older patients with hip fractures. *Journal of Orthopedic Nursing*, 12(2), 90.

Eilers, H., & Niemann, C. (2003). Clinically important drug interactions with intravenous anaesthetics in older patients. *Drugs & Aging*, 20(13), 969–980.

Ekstein, M., Gavish, D., Ezri, T., & Weinbroum, A. (2008). Monitored anaesthesia care in the elderly: guidelines and recommendations. *Drugs & Aging*, 25(6), 477–500.

Ene, K., Nordberg, G., Sjostrom, B., & Bergh, I. (2003). Prediction of postoperative pain after radical prostatectomy. *BMC Nursing*, 7(14), 1–9.

Engel, C., Oxman, T., Yamamoto, M., Gould, D., Barry, S., Stewart, P., . . . Dietrich, A. J. (2008). RESPECT-Mil: Feasibility of a systems-level collaborative care approach to depression and post-traumatic stress disorder in military primary care. *Military Medicine*, 173(10), 935–940.

Erikson, K. I., Raji, C. A., Lopez, O. I., Becker, J. T., Rosano, C., Newman, A. B., . . . Kuller, L. H. (2010). Physical activity predicts gray mater volume n late adulthood: The Cardiovascular Health Study. *Neurology*, 75, 1415–1422.

Ertel, K., Glymour, M., Glass, T., & Berkman, L. (2007). Frailty modifies effectiveness of psychosocial intervention in recovery from stroke. *Clinical Rehabilitation*, 21, 511–522.

Eskicioglu, C., Forbes, S., Aarts, M., Okrainec, A., & McLeod, R. (2009). Enhanced recovery after surgery (ERAS) programs for patients having colorectal surgery: A meta-analysis of randomized trials. *Journal of Gastrointestinal Surgery*, 13(12), 2321–2329.

Espinoza, S., & Walston, J. (2005). Frailty in older adults: Insights and interventions. *Cleveland Clinic Journal of Medicine*, 72(12), 1105–1112.

Espiritu, J. (2008). Aging-related sleep changes. *Clinics in Geriatric Medicine*, 24, 1–14.

Evans, W. (2010). Skeletal muscle loss: Cachexia, sarcopenia, and inactivity. *American Journal of Clinical Nutrition*, 91(4), 1123–1127.

Fagerlin, A., & Schneider, C. E. (2004). Enough: The failure of the living will. *The Hastings Center Report*, 34(March–April), 30–42.

Fairhall, N., Aggar, C., Kurrle, S., Sherrington, C., Lord, S., Lockwood, K., . . . Cameron, I. D. (2008). Frailty Intervention Trial (FIT). *BMC Geriatrics*, 8(27). Retrieved February 18, 2011, from www.biomedcentral.com/1471-2318/8/27

Farage, M. A., Miller, K. W., Berardesca, E., & Maibach, H. I. (2009). Clinical implications of aging skin. *American Journal of Clinical Dermatology*, 10(2), 73–86.

Farrell, T., & Dosa, D. (2007). The assessment and management of hypoactive delirium. *Medicine Health Rhode Island*, 90(12), 393–395.

Fay, V. (n.d.). Theories of aging. Retrieved February 17, 2011 from www.scribd.com/doc/44680788/Age-Theories-1

Fedarko, N. S. (2011). The biology of aging and frailty. *Clinics in Geriatric Medicine, 27,* 27–37.

Feldt, K. S. (2000). The checklist of non verbal pain indicators (CNPI). *Pain Management Nursing, 1*(1), 13–21.

Felley, C., Perneger, T. V., Goulet, I., Rouillard, C., Azar-Pey, N., Dorta, G., . . . Frossard, J. L. (2008). Combined written and oral information prior to gastrointestinal endoscopy compared with oral information alone: A randomized trial. *BMC Gastroenterology, 8*(22). Retrieved March 10, 2011, from www.biomedcentral.com/1471-230X/8/22

Ferrari, A., Radaelli, A., & Centola, M. (2003). Aging and the cardiovascular system. *Journal of Applied Physiology, 95*(6), 2591–2597.

Fick, D., Hodo, D., Lawrence, F., & Inouye, S. (2007). Recognizing delirium superimposed on dementia. *Journal of Gerontological Nursing, 33*(2), 40–48.

Fick, D., Mion, L., Beers, M., & Walker, J. (2008). Health outcomes associated with potentially inappropriate medication use in older adults. *Research in Nursing & Health, 31,* 42–51.

Fillit, H., & Butler, R. (2009). The frailty identity crisis. *Journal of the American Geriatrics Society, 57*(2), 348–352.

Fine, P. (2004). Difficulties and challenges in the treatment of chronic pain in the older adult. *American Journal of Pain Management, 14*(2 Supplement), 2S–8S.

Finfgeld-Connett, D. (2005). Clarification of social support. *Journal of Nursing Scholarship, 37*(1), 4–9.

Fiske, A., Wetherell, J. L., & Gatz, M. (2009) Depression in older adults. *Annual Review of Clinical Psychology,* 5, 363–389.

Flaherty, J., Rudolph, J., Shay, K., Kamholz, B., Boockvar, K., Shaughnessy, M., . . . Edes, T. (2007). Delirium is a serious and under-recognized problem: Why assessment of mental status should be the sixth vital sign. *Journal of the American Medical Directors Association, 8*(5), 273–275.

Forster, A., Murff, H., Peterson, J., Ganchi, T., & Bates, D. (2005). Adverse drug events occurring following hospital discharge. *Journal of General Internal Medicine, 30,* 317–323.

Fortinsky, R., Covinsky, K., Palmer, R., & Landefeld, C. (1999). Effects of functional status changes before and during hospitalization on nursing home admission of older adults. *Journal of Gerontology Series A Biological Sciences and Medical Sciences, 54*(10), M521–526.

Foust, J., Naylor, M., Boling, P., & Cappuzzo, K. (2005). Opportunities for improving post-hospital home medication management among older adults. *Home Health Care Services Quarterly, 24*(1–2), 101–122.

Frank, C., Heland, D. K., Chen, B., Farquhar, D., Myers, K., & Iwaasa, K. (2003). Determining resuscitation preferences of elderly inpatients: A review of the literature. *Canadian Medical Association Journal, 169*(8), 795–799.

Fried, L., Ferrucci, L., Darer, J., Williamson, J., & Anderson, G. (2004). Untangling the concepts of disability, frailty, and comorbidity: Implications for improved targeting and healthcare. *Journal of Gerontology, 59*(3), 255–263.

Friedman, S., Mendelson, D., Kates, S., & McCann, R. (2008). Geriatric co-management of proximal femur fractures: Total quality management and protocol-driven care result in better outcomes for a frail patient population. *Journal of the American Geriatrics Society, 56,* 1349–1356.

Fukuse, T., Satoda, N., Hijiya, K., & Fujinaga, T. (2005). Importance of a comprehensive geriatric assessment in prediction of complications following thoracic surgery in elderly patients. *Chest, 127*(3), 886–891.

Ganai, S., Lee, K., Merrill, A., Lee, M., Bellantonio, S., Brennan, M., & Lindenauer, P. (2007). Adverse outcomes of geriatric patients undergoing abdominal surgery who are at high risk for delirium. *Archives of Surgery, 142*(11), 1072–1078.

Garcia, A. (2008). The effect of chronic disorders on sleep in the elderly. *Clinics in Geriatric Medicine, 24,* 27–38.

Gary, C., & Peter, C. (2008). The use of the pain assessment checklist for seniors with limited ability to communicate (PACSLAC) by caregivers in dementia care facilities. *The New Zealand Medical Journal, 121*(1286), 21–30.

Gekoski, W., & Knox, V. (1990). Ageism or healthism? Perceptions based on age or health status. *Journal of Aging and Health, 2,* 15–27.

Gibson, S., & Helme, R. (2001). Age-related differences in pain perception and report. *Clinics in Geriatric Medicine, 17*(3), 433–456.

Gelinas, C., & Arbour, C. (2009). Behavioral and physiologic indicators during a nociceptive procedure in conscious and unconscious mechanically ventilated adults: similar or different? *Journal of Critical Care, 24,* 7–17.

Gibson, S., & Farrell, M. (2004). A review of age differences in the neurophysiology of nociception and the perceptual experience of pain. *The Clinical Journal of Pain, 2*(4), 227–239.

Gill, T., Baker, D., Gottschalk, M., Peduzzi, P., Allore, H., & Byers, A. (2002). A program to prevent functional decline in physically frail, elderly persons who live at home. *New England Journal of Medicine, 347*(14), 1068–1074.

Gillon, R. (1994). Medical ethics: Four principles plus attention to scope. *British Medical Journal, 309,* 184.

Ginaldi, L., Benedetto, M. D., & Martinis, M. D. (2005). Osteoporosis, inflammation and ageing. *Immunity and Ageing, 4*(2), 14.

Gloth III, F. M., (2001) Principles of perioperative pain management in older adults. *Clinics in Geriatric Medicine, 17*(3), 553–573.

Gobbens, R., Assen, M. V., Luijkx, K., Wijnen-Sponselee, M., & Schols, J. (2010). Determinants of frailty. *Journal of the American Medical Directors Association, 11*(5), 356–364.

Gordon, S. (2004, June 16). Geriatric otolaryngology. *Grand Rounds Presentation.* Lecture conducted from University of Texas Medical Branch Department of Otolaryngology, Galveston, Texas.

Goroll, A. H., and Mulley, A. G. (Eds.). (2009). *Primary care medicine: Office evaluation and management of the adult patient* (6th ed.). Philadelphia, PA: Lippincott Williams & Wilkins.

Gore, D. (2007). Preoperative maneuvers to avert postoperative respiratory failure in elderly patients. *Gerontology, 53,* 438–444.

Gorski, L. (2008). Implementing home health standards in clinical practice. *Home Healthcare Nurse, 26*(5), 308–316.

Green, C., Anderson, K., Baker, T., Campbell, L., Decker, S., Fillingim, E., . . . Vallerand, A. H. et al. (2003). The unequal burden of pain: Confronting racial and ethnic disparities in pain. *Pain Medicine, 4*(3), 277–294.

Griffith, J., Brosnan, M., Lacey, K., Keeling, S., & Wilkinson, T. J. (2004). Family meetings— a qualitative exploration of improving care planning with older people and their families. *Age and Ageing, 33*(6), 577–581.

Griffiths, R., & Jones, C. (2007). Delirium, cognitive dysfunction and posttraumatic stress disorder. *Current Opinion in Anaesthesiology, 20*(2), 124–129.

Groban, L. (2005). Diastolic dysfunction in the older heart. *Journal of Cardiothoracic and Vascular Anesthesia, 19*(2), 228–236.

Grossman, S., & Lange, J. (2006). Theories of aging as basis for assessment. *MEDSURG Nursing, 15*(2), 77–83.

Gruber, R., Koch, H., Doll, B., Tegtmeier, F., Einhorn, T., & Hollinger, J. (2006). Fracture healing in the elderly patient. *Experimental Gerontology, 41*(11), 1080–1093.

Gyomber, D., Lawrentschuk, N., Wong, P., Parker, F., & Bolton, D. (2010). Improving informed consent for patients undergoing radical prostatectomy using multimedia techniques: A prospective randomized crossover study. *BJU International, 106*(8), 1152–1156.

Hagert, E. (2010). Proprioception of the wrist joint: A review of current concepts and possible implications on the rehabilitation of the wrist. *Journal of Hand Therapy, 23*(1), 2–16.

Halaszynski, T. (2009). Pain management in the elderly and cognitively impaired patient: The role of regional anesthesia and analgesia. *Current Opinion in Anaesthesiology, 22*(5), 594–599.

Halverson, J. L., & Walaszek, A. (2010, February 3). Late-onset depression. *eMedicine Psychiatry*. Retrieved January 19, 2011, from http://emedicine.medscape.com/article/286759-overview

Hamilton, H., Gallagher, P., & O'Mahony, D. (2009). Inappropriate prescribing and adverse drug events in older people. *BMC Geriatrics, 9*(5). Retrieved April 11, 2011, from www.biomedcentral.com/1471-2318/9/5

Hardin, R., & Zenilman, M. (2006). Surgical considerations in older adults. In F. Brunicardi, D. Anderson, T. Billiar & D. Dunn (Eds.), *Schwartz's manual of surgery* (8th ed.) (pp. 1188–1200). New York, NY: McGraw-Hill Professional.

Hardy, S., & Gill, T. (2004). Recovery from disability among community-dwelling older persons. *Journal of the American Medical Association, 291*(13), 1596–1602.

Harrison, N., & Nau, C. (2008). Sensitization of nociceptive ion channels by inhaled anesthetics—A pain in the gas? *Molecular Pharmacology, 74*, 1180–1182.

Hashizume, K., Suzuki, S., Takeda, T., Shigematsu, S., Ichikawa, K., & Koizumi, Y. (2006). Endocrinologoical aspects of aging: Adaptation to and acceleration of aging by the endocrine system. *Geriatrics & Gerontology, 6*(1), 1–6.

Hedenstierna, G. (1997). Atelectasis during anesthesia: can it be prevented? *Journal of Anesthesia, 11*, 219–224.

Helms, J., & Barone, C. (2008). Physiology and treatment of pain. *Critical Care Nurse, 28*(6), 38–49.

Hendrich, A. (2007). Predicting patient falls. *American Journal of Nursing, 107*(11), 50–58.

Henrickson, S., Wadhera, R., ElBardissi, A., Wiegmann, D., & Sundt, T. (2009). Development and pilot evaluation of a preoperative briefing protocol for cardiovascular surgery. *Journal of the American College of Surgeons, 208*, 1115–1123.

Herr, K., Bjoro, K., & Decker, S. (2006). Tools for assessment of pain in nonverbal older adults with dementia: A state-of-the-science review. *Journal of Pain and Symptom Management, 31*(2), 170–192.

Herr, K., Coyne, P., Key, T., Manworren, R., McCaffery, M., Merkel, S., . . . Wild, L. (2006). Pain assessment in the nonverbal patient: Position statement with clinical practice recommendations. *Pain Management Nursing, 7*(2), 44–52.

Herr, K., & Decker, S. (2004). Older adults with severe cognitive impairment: Assessment of pain. *Annals of Long-Term Care: Clinical Care and Aging, 12*(4), 46–52.

Herr, K., Spratt, K., Mobily, P., & Richardson, G. (2004). Pain intensity assessment in older adults: Use of experimental pain to compare psychometric properties and usability of selected pain scales with younger adults. *Clinical Journal of Pain, 20*(4), 207–219.

Herrick, C., Steger-May, K., Sinacore, D., Brown, M., Schechtman, K., & Binder, E. (2004). Persistent pain in frail older adults after hip fracture repair. *Journal of the American Geriatrics Society, 52*, 2062–2068.

Hofmann, J. C., Wenger, N. S., Davis, R., Teno, J., Connors Jr., A., Desbiens, N., . . . Phillips, R. S. (1997). Patient preferences for communication with physicians about end-of-life decisions. *Annals of Internal Medicine, 127*(1), 1–12.

Hommersom, A., Groot, P., Lucas, P., Marcos, M., & Martinez-Salvador, B. (2008). A constraint-based approach to medical guidelines and protocols. *Studies in Health Technology and Informatics, 139*, 213–222.

Hoogerduijn, J., Schuurmans, M., Duijnstee, M., Rooij, S. D., & Grypdonck, M. (2007). A systematic review of predictors and screening instruments to identify older hospitalized patients at risk for functional decline. *Journal of Clinical Nursing, 16*(1), 46–57.

Horgas, A. L., & Yoon, S. L. (2008). Pain management. In E. Capezuti, D. Zwicker, M. Mezey, & T. Fulmer (Eds.), *Evidence-based geriatric nursing protocols for best practice* (3rd ed.) (pp. 199–222). New York, NY: Springer Publishing.

Houston, D., Schwartz, A., Cauley, J., Tylavsky, F., Simonsick, E., Harris, T., . . . Kritchevsky, S. (2008). Serum parathyroid hormone levels predict falls in older adults with diabetes mellitus. *Journal of the American Geriatrics Society, 56*(11), 2027–2032.

Hubbard, R., O'Mahony, M., & Woodhouse, K. (2009). Characterizing frailty in the clinical setting—a comparison of different approaches. *Age & Ageing, 38*(1), 115–119.

Ille, R., Lahousen, T., Schweiger, S., Hofmann, P., & Kapfhammer, H. (2007). Influence of patient-related and surgery-related risk factors on cognitive performance, emotional state, and convalescence after cardiac surgery. *Cardiovascular Revascularization Medicine, 8*, 166–169.

Inouye, S., Bogardus Jr., S., Charentier, P., Leo-Summers, L., Acompara, D., Holford, T., & Cooner Jr., L. (1999). A multicomponent intervention to prevent delirium in hospitalized older adults. *New England Journal of Medicine, 340*, 669–767.

Insel, K.C., & Badger, T.A. (2002). Deciphering th 4D's: Cognitive decline, delirium, depression and dementia – a review. *Journal of Advanced Nursing, 38*(4), 360–368.

Institute of Medicine, Committee on Quality of Health Care in America. (2001). *Crossing the quality chasm: a new health system for the 21st century.* Washington, DC: National Academies Press.

International Association for the Study of Pain. (n.d.). Visceral pain. *Pain clinical updates.* Retrieved March 17, 2011, from www.iasp-pain.org/AM/AMTemplate.cfm?Section=HOME&SECTION=HOME&CONTENTID=7583&TEMPLATE=/CM/ContentDisplay.cfm

Ip, H., Abrishami, A., Peng, P., Wong, J., & Chung, F. (2009). Predictors of postoperative pain and analgesic consumption: A qualitative systematic review. *Anesthesiology, 111*, 657–677.

Jackson, E., & Warner, J. (2002). How much do doctors know about consent and capacity? *Journal of The Royal Society of Medicine, 95*, 601–603.

Jacobson, T. (2006). Overcoming "ageism" bias in treatment of hypercholesteremia. *Drug Safety, 29*(5), 421–448.

Jacoby, R. (2002). Old age psychiatry and the law. *British Journal of Psychiatry, 180*, 116–119.

Jencks, S., Williams, M., & Coleman, E. (2009). Rehospitalizations among patients in the Medicare fee-for-service program. *New England Journal of Medicine, 360*(14), 1418–1428.

John, A., & Sieber, F. (2004). Age associated issues: Geriatrics. *Anesthesiology Clinics of North America, 22*, 48–58.

The Joint Commission. (2011, January 7). Universal protocol for preventing wrong site, wrong procedure, wrong person surgery. Retrieved from http://www.jointcommission.org/assets/1/18/Universal%20Protocol%201%204%20111.PDF

Jones, D., Song, X., & Rockwood, K. (2004). Operationalizing a frailty index from a standardized comprehensive geriatric assessment. *Journal of the American Geriatrics Society, 52*, 1929–1933.

Journal Watch General Medicine: Medical Articles and Commentary. (n.d.). Do not resuscitate: Patients want a say. Retrieved March 19, 2011, from http://general-medicine.jwatch.org/cgi/content/full/1988/726/1

Juneja, R. (2006). Anaesthesia for the elderly cardiac patient. *Annals of Cardiac Anaesthesia, 9*(1), 67–77.

Kaasalainen, S. (2007). Pain assessment in older adults with dementia: Using behavioral observation methods in clinical practice. *Journal of Gerontological Nursing, 33*(6), 6–10.

Kagan, S. (2004). Gero-Oncology Nursing Research. *Oncology Nursing Forum, 21*(2), 293–297.

Kallenbach, L. (2007, January 1). Geriatric pharmacotherapy: ACOVE indicators. Retrieved March 27, 2010, from http://www2.kumc.edu/coa/education/FacDevPowerPoint/MedicationUse_ACOVE.ppt

Kamel, N., & Gammack, J. (2006). Insomnia in the elderly: Cause, approach, and treatment. *American Journal of Medicine, 119*(6), 463–469.

Kane, R., Flood, S., Keckhafer, G., Bershadsky, B., & Lum, Y. (2002). Nursing home residents covered by Medicare risk contracts: Early findings from the EverCare Evaluation Project. *Journal of the American Geriatrics Society, 50,* 719–727.

Kane, R., Keckhafer, G., Flood, S., Bershadsky, B., & Siadaty, M. (2003). The effect of Evercare on hospital use. *Journal of the American Geriatrics Society, 51,* 1427–1434.

Karp, J. F., Shega, J. W., Morone, N. E., & Weiner, D. K. (2008). Understanding the mechanisms and management of persistent pain in older adults. *British Journal of Anesthesia, 101*(1), 111–120.

Katz, S. (1992). Growing number of elderly patients will mean more ethical issues for MDs, conference told. *Canadian Medical Association Journal, 147*(8), 1239–1241.

Kaye, K., Anderson, D., Sloane, R., Chen, L., Choi, Y., Link, K., . . . Schmader, K. E. (2009). The effect of surgical site infection on older operative patients. *Journal of the American Geriatrics Society, 57,* 46–54.

Kemper, R., Steiner, V., Hicks, B., Pierce, L., & Iwuagwu, C. (2007). Anticholinergic medications: Use among older adults with memory problems. *Journal of Gerontological Nursing, 33*(1), 21–29.

Kennedy, G. (2008). Brief evaluation of executive dysfunction: An essential refinement in the assessment of cognitive impairment. *Annals of Long Term Care.* Retrieved March 16, 2011, from www.annalsoflongtermcare.com/article/7048

Kenney, W., & Munce, T. (2003). Invited review: Aging and human temperature regulation. *Journal of Applied Physiology, 95*(6), 2598–2603.

Kerr, P., Shever, L., Titler, M., Qin, R., Kim, T., & Picone, D. (2010). The unique contribution of the nursing intervention pain management on length of stay in older patients undergoing hip procedures. *Applied Nursing Research, 23,* 36–44.

Khosla, S., Atkinson, E., Melton, L., & Riggs, B. (1997). Effects of age and estrogen status on serum parathyroid hormone levels and biochemical markers of bone turnover in women: A population-based study. *Journal of Clinical Endocrinology and Metabolism, 82*(5), 1522–1527.

Kiely, D., Cupples, L., & Lipsitz, L. (2009). Validation and comparison of two frailty indexes: The MOBILIZE Boston Study. *Journal of the American Geriatrics Society, 57,* 1532–1539.

Kim, E., Mordiffi, S., Bee, W., Devi, K., & Evans, D. (2007). Evaluation of three fall-risk assessment tools in an acute care setting. *Journal of Advanced Nursing, 60*(4), 427–435.

Kim, G., Chiriboga, D., & Jang, Y. (2009). Cultural equivalence in depressive symptoms in older white, black, and Mexican-American adults. *Journal of the American Geriatrics Society, 57*(5), 790–796.

Kim, S., & Zenilman, M. (2008). The elderly surgical patient. In *ACS surgery principles and practice* (pp. 1–15). New York, NY: WebMD Professional Publishing. DOI 10.2310/7800.2008.S09C01. Available at http://www.acssurgery.com/acs/pdf/acs0901.pdf

Kingsnorth, A., & Majid, A. A. (2006). *Fundamentals of surgical practice* (2nd ed.). Cambridge, UK: Cambridge University Press.

Kirshner, H. (2007). Delirium: A focused review. *Current Neurology and Neuroscience Reports, 7*, 479–482.

Kleinpell, R., Fletcher, K., & Jennings, B. (2008). Reducing functional decline in hospitalized elderly. In R. G. Hughes (Ed.), *Patient safety and quality: An evidence-based handbook for nurses* (pp. 251–265). Rockville, MD: Agency for Healthcare Research and Quality.

Ko, F. (2011). The clinical care of frail, older adults. *Clinics in Geriatric Medicine, 27*(1), 89–100.

Kolcaba, K., & Kolcaba, R. (1991). An analysis of the concept of comfort. *Journal of Advanced Nursing, 16*, 1301–1310.

Kopf, A., Banzhaf, A., & Stein, C. (2005). Perioperative management of the chronic pain patient. *Best Practice & Research Clinical Anaesthesiology, 19*(1), 59–76.

Kortebein, P. (2009). Rehabilitation for hospital-associated deconditioning. *American Journal of Physical Medicine and Rehabilitation, 88*(1), 66–77.

Krenk, L., Rasmussen, L. S., & Kehlet, H. (2010). New insights into the pathophyiology of postoperative cognitive dysfunction. *Acta Anesthesiological Scandanavia, 54*, 951–956.

Kronenberg, R. S., & Drage, C. W. (1973). Attenuation of the ventilatory and heart rate response to hypxia and hypercapnia with aging in normal men. *Journal of Clinical Investigations, 52*(8), 1812–1819.

Kuh, D. (2007). A life course approach to healthy aging, frailty, and capability. *Journal of Gerontology, 62A*(7), 717–721.

Kurtz, S., Ong, K., Lau, E., Mowat, F., & Halpern, M. (2007). Projections of primary and revision hip and knee arthroplasty in the United States from 2005 to 2030. *The Journal of Bone and Joint Surgery, 89*(4), 780–785.

Lakatta, E. (2003). Arterial and cardiac aging: major shareholders in cardiovascular disease enterprises: Part III: Cellular and molecular clues to heart and arterial aging. *Circulation, 107*(3), 490–497.

Lakatta, E. (2008). Arterial aging is risky. *Journal of Applied Physiology, 105*(4), 1321–1322.

Landis, J. (2008, March). Make a move. Take steps to keep elderly patients. *The Hospitalist.* Retrieved February 22, 2010, from www.the-hospitalist.org/details/article/187763/Make_a_Move.html

Lassen, K., Soop, M., Nygren, J., Cox, P., Hendry, P., Spies, C., . . . Dejong, C. (2009). Consensus review of optimal perioperative care in colorectal surgery: Enhanced Recovery After Surgery (ERAS) Group recommendations. *Archives of Surgery, 144*(10), 961–969.

Lavretsky, H., & Irwin, M. (2007). Resilience and aging. *Aging Health, 3*(3), 309–323.

Lawrence, V., Cornell, J., & Smetana, G. (2005). Strategies to reduce postoperative pulmonary complications after noncardiothoracic surgery: Systematic review for the American College of Physicians. *Annals of Internal Medicine, 144*, 596–608.

Lawrence, V., Hazuda, H., Cornell, J., Pederson, T., Bradshaw, P., Mulrow, C., & Page, C. (2004). Functional independence after major abdominal surgery in the elderly. *Journal of the American College of Surgeons, 199*(5), 762–772.

Lawton, S. (2007). Addressing the skin-care needs of the older person. *British Journal of Community Nursing, 12*(5), 203–210.

Lee, J., Singletary, R., Schmader, K., Anderson, D., Bolognesi, M., & Kaye, K. (2006). Surgical site infection in the elderly following orthopaedic surgery. Risk factors and outcomes. *The Journal of Bone and Joint Surgery (American Volume), 88*(8), 1705–1712.

Lehmann, M., Monte, K., Barach, P., & Kindler, C. (2010). Postoperative patient complaints: a prospective interview study of 12,276 patients. *Journal of Clinical Anesthesia, 22*, 13–21.

Leino-Kilpi, H., Välimäki, M., Dassen, T., Gasull, M., Lemonidou, C., Scott, P. A., . . . Kalijonen, A. (2003). Perceptions of autonomy, privacy and informed consent in the care of elderly people in five European countries: Comparison and implications for the future. *Nursing Ethics, 10*(1), 58–66.

Lekan, D. (2009). Frailty and other emerging concepts in care of the aged. *Southern Online Journal of Nursing Research, 9*(3). Retrieved March 11, 2011, from http://snrs.org/publications/SOJNR_articles2/Vol09Num03Art04.html

Lenze, E., Munin, M., Skidmore, E., Dew, M., Rogers, J., Whyte, E., . . . Reynolds 3rf, C. (2007). Onset of depression in elderly persons after hip fracture: Implications for prevention and early intervention of late-life depression. *Journal of the American Geriatrics Society, 55,* 81–86.

Lesser, J. M., Hughes, S. V., Jemelka, J. R., & Griffith, J. (2005). Sexually inappropriate behaviors. Assessment necessitates careful medical and psychological evaluation and sensitivity. *Geriatrics, 60*(1), 34–37.

Leung, J. (2010). Postoperative delirium: Are there modifiable risk factors? *European Journal of Anaesthesiology, 27*(5), 403–405.

Leung, J., & Dzankic, S. (2004). Relative importance of preoperative health status versus intraoperative factors in predicting postoperative adverse outcomes in geriatric surgical patterns. *Journal of the American Geriatrics Society, 49,* 1080–1085.

Leung, J., & Sands, L. (2009). Long-term cognitive decline. Is there a link to surgery and anesthesia? *Anesthesiology, 111,* 931–932.

Levers, M., Estabrooks, C., & Ross Kerr, J. (2006). Factors contributing to frailty: Literature review. *Journal of Advanced Nursing, 56*(3), 282–291.

Levine, W., Mehta, V., & Landesberg, G. (2006). Anesthesia for the elderly: Selected topics. *Current Opinion in Anaesthesiology, 19,* 320–324.

Lindgren, M., Unosson, M., Krantz, A., & Ek, A. (2002). A risk assessment scale for the prediction of pressure sore development: Reliability and validity. *Journal of Advanced Nursing, 38*(2), 190–199.

Lindgren, M., Unosson, M., Krantz, A., & Ek, A. (2005). Pressure ulcer risk factors in patients undergoing surgery. *Journal of Advanced Nursing, 50*(6), 605–612.

Litwack, K. (2006). Adjusting postsurgical care for older patients. *Nursing, 36*(1), 66–67.

Litwack, K. (2009). *Clinical coach for effective perioperative nursing care.* Philadelphia: F. A. Davis.

Liu, C. (2011). Exercise as an intervention for frailty. *Clinics in Geriatric Medicine, 27*(1), 101–110.

Liu, S., & Kehlet, H. (2009). Postoperative pain. In *ACS surgery: Principles and practice.* New York, NY: WebMD Publishing. Available at: http://www.acssurgery.com/acs/pdf/ACS0106.pdf

Ljubuncic, P., & Reznick, A. (2009). The evolutionary theories of aging revisited—a minireview. *Gerontology, 55,* 205–126.

Loeser, R. (2010). Age-related changes in the musculoskeletal system and the development of osteoarthritis. *Clinics in Geriatric Medicine, 26*(3), 371–386.

Loran, D., Hyde, B., & Zwischenberger, J. (2005). Perioperative management of special populations: the geriatric patient. *Surgical Clinics of North America, 85,* 1259–1266.

Mackensen, G., & Geth, A. (2004). Postoperative cognitive deficits: More questions than answers. *European Journal of Anaesthesiology, 21,* 85–88.

Madsen, J., & Graff, J. (2004). Effects of ageing on gastrointestinal motor function. *Age and Ageing, 33*(2), 154–159.

Mahoney, J. (1998). Immobility and falls. *Clinics in Geriatric Medicine, 14*(4), 699–726.

Makaryus, A., & Friedman, E. (2005). Patients' understanding of their treatment plans and diagnosis at discharge. *Mayo Clinic Proceedings, 80*(8), 991–994.

Malani, P. (2009). Functional status assessment in the preoperative evaluation of older adults. *Journal of the American Medical Association, 302*(14), 1582–1583.

Malloy, D., Williams, J., Hadjistavropoulos, T., Krishnan, B., & Jeyaraj, M. (2008). Ethical decision-making about older adults and moral intensity: an international study of physicians. *Journal of Medical Ethics, 34*(4), 285–296.

Mamaril, M. (2006). Nursing considerations in the geriatric surgical patient: The perioperative continuum of care. *Nursing Clinics of North America, 41*(2), 313–328.

Mancuso, C., Sculco, T., Wickiewicz, T., Jones, E., Robbins, L., Warren, R., & Williams-Russo, P. (2001). Patients' expectations of knee surgery. *The Journal of Bone and Joint Surgery (American Volume), 83-A*(7), 1005–1012.

Manno, M., & Hayes, D. (2006). How medication reconciliation saves lives. *Nursing, 36*(3), 63–64.

Markle-Reid, M., & Browne, G. (2003). Conceptualizations of frailty in relation to older adults. *Journal of Advanced Nursing, 44*(1), 58–68.

Markowitz, A., & Pantilat, S. (2006). Palliative care for frail older adults: "There are things I can't do anymore that I wish I could." *Journal of the American Medical Association, 296*(24), 2967.

Martin, F. (2006). Recognizing depression after a coronary artery bypass graft. *British Journal of Nursing, 15*(13), 703–706.

Martin, T. A., & Bush, S. (2008). Ethical considerations in geriatric neuropsychology. *NeuroRehabilitation, 23*, 447–454.

Matta, J., Cornett, P., Miyares, R., Abe, K., Sahibzada, N., & Ahern, G. (2008). General anesthetics activate a nociceptive ion channel to enhance pain and inflammation. *Proceedings of the National Academy of Sciences, 105*(25), 8784–8789.

McAvay, G., Van Ness, P., Bogardus Jr., S., Zhang, Y., Leslie, D., Leo-Summers, L., & Inouye, S. (2007). Depressive symptoms and the risk of incident delirium in older hospitalized adults. *Journal of the American Geriatrics Society, 55*(5), 684–691.

McBride-Henry, K., & Foureur, M. (2006). Medication administration errors: Understanding the issues. *The Australian Journal of Advanced Nursing, 23*(3), 33–41.

McCarthy, M. (2003). Situated clinical reasoning: Distinguishing acute confusion from dementia in hospitalized older adults. *Research in Nursing & Health, 21*, 90–101.

McCarthy, E., Pencina, M., Kelly-Hayes, M., Evans, J., Oberacker, E., D'Agostino, R., . . . Murabito, J. (2008). Advance care planning and health care preferences of community-dwelling elders: The Framingham Heart Study. *Journal of Gerontology A Biological Sciences and Medical Sciences, 63A*(9), 951–959.

McCorkle, R., Strumpf, N., Naumah, N., Adler, D., Cooley, M., Jepson, C., . . . Torosian, M. (2000). A specialized home care intervention improves survival among older post surgical care patients. *Journal American Geriatrics Society, 48*(12), 1732–1733.

McDougall, G., & Balyer, J. (1998). Decreasing mental frailty in at-risk elders. *Geriatric Nursing, 19*(4), 220–224.

McKenzie, L. H., Simpson, J., and Stewart, M. (2010). A systematic review of pre-operative predictors of post-operative depression and anxiety in individuals who have undergone coronary artery bypass graft surgery. *Psychology, Health & Medicine, 15*(1), 74–93.

McKinlay, J. (1979). A case for refocusing upstream: The political economy of illness. In E. G. Jaco (Ed.), *Patients, physicians and illness: A sourcebook in behavioral science and health* (3rd ed.) (pp. 9–25). New York, NY: The Free Press.

McLaughlin, M. (2001). The aging heart. State-of-the-art prevention and management of cardiac disease. *Geriatrics, 56*(6), 45–49.

McLaughlin, M., Orosz, G., Magaziner, J., Hannan, E., McGinn, T., Morrison, R., . . . Siu A. (2006). Preoperative status and risk of complications in patients with hip fracture. *Journal of General Internal Medicine, 21*(3), 219–225.

McMain, L. (2010). Pain management in recovery. *Journal of Perioperative Practice, 20*(2), 59–65.

Meagher, D., Moran, M., Raju, B., Gibbons, D., Donnelly, S., Saunders, J., & Trzepacz, P. (2007). Phenomenology of delirium: Assessment of 100 adult cases using standardised measures. *British Journal of Psychiatry, 190*, 135–141.

Mercado, D., & Petty, B. (2003). Perioperative medication management. *Medical Clinics of North America, 87*, 41–57.

Michaels, A., Spinler, S., Leeper, B., Ohman, E., Alexander, K., Newby, L., . . . Gibler, W. (2010). Medication errors in acute cardiovascular and stroke patients. A scientific statement from the American Heart Association. *Circulation, 121*, 1–19.

Michaud, L., Büla, C., Berney, A., Camus, V., Voellinger, R., Stiefel, F., & Burnand, B. (2007). Delirium: Guidelines for general hospitals. *Journal of Psychosomatic Research, 62*, 371–383.

Michota, F., & Frost, S. (2002). Perioperative management of the hospitalized patient. *Medical Clinics of North America, 86*, 731–748.

Mick, D., & Ackerman, M. (2004). Critical care nursing for older adults: Pathophysiological and functional considerations. *Nursing Clinics of North America, 39*(3), 473–493.

Miller, C. (2003). Safe medication practices: Nursing assessment of medications in older adults. *Geriatric Nursing, 24*(5), 314–317.

Miller, D. (2010, October 29). Frailty, strength, and the promise of vitamin D. *ACP-Indiana and IMDA Annual Scientific Meeting.* Lecture conducted from Indiana University School of Medicine.

Miller, W. (1983). Motivational interviewing with problem drinkers. *Behavioral Psychotherapy, 11*, 147–172.

Miller, W., & Rollnick, S. (2002). *Motivational interviewing: Preparing people for change.* New York, NY: Guilford Press.

Mintzer, J., & Burns, A. (2000). Anticholinergic side-effects of drugs in elderly people. *Journal of the Royal Society of Medicine, 93*, 457–462.

Minville, V., Lubrano, V., Bounes, V., Pianezza, A., Rabinowitz, A., Gris, C., . . . Fourcade, O. (2008). Postoperative analgesia after total hip arthroplasty: Patient-controlled analgesia versus transdermal fentanyl patch. *Journal of Clinical Anesthesia, 20*(4), 280–283.

Mitty, E., & Flores, S. (2009). Sleepiness or excessive daytime somnolence. *Geriatric Nursing, 30*(1), 53–60.

Modrego, P. J., & Ferrandez, J. (2004) Depression in patients with mild cognitive impairment increases the risk of developing dementia of Azheimer type: A prospective cohort study. *Archives of Neurology, 61*, 1290–1293.

Mok, E., & Wong, K. (2003). Effects of music on patient anxiety. *AORN Journal, 77*(2), 396–410.

Mold, J., Vesely, S., Keyl, B., Schenk, J., & Roberts, M. (2004). The prevalence, predictors, and consequences of peripheral sensory neuropathy in older patients. *Journal of the American Board of Family Medicine, 17*(5), 309–318.

Moody, H. R. (1998). Cross-cultural geriatric ethics: Negotiating our differences. *Generations, 22*(3), 32–39.

Morley, J. (2003). Hormones and the aging process. *Journal of the American Geriatric Society, 51*(7 Supplemental), S333–S337.

Morrison, R., Flanagan, S., Fischberg, D., Cintron, A., & Siu, A. (2009). A novel interdisciplinary analgesic program reduces pain and improves function in older adults after orthopedic surgery. *Journal of the American Geriatrics, 57*, 1–10.

Mundy, G. (2007). Osteoporosis and inflammation. *Nutrition Reviews, 65*(12), S147–S151.

Muscular system - skeletal muscles. (n.d.). In *Science Encyclopedia.* Retrieved March 19, 2011, from http://science.jrank.org/pages/4503/Muscular-System-Skeletal-muscles.html

Myer, A. (2000). The effects of aging on wound healing. *Topics in Geriatric Rehabilitation, 16*(2), 1–10.

Naylor, M. (2004). Transitional care for older adults: A cost-effective model. *LDI Issue Brief, 9*(6), 1–4.

Naylor, M., Brooten, D., Campbell, R., Jacobsen, B., Mezey, M., Pauly, M., Schwartz, J. S. (1999). Comprehensive discharge planning and home follow-up of hospitalized elders: A randomized controlled trial. *Journal of the National Medical Association, 281*, 613–620.

Naylor, M., & Keating, S. (2008). Transitional care. *American Journal of Nursing, 108*(9), 58–68.

Need, A., O'Loughlin, P., Morris, H., Horowitz, M., & Nordin, B. (2004). The effects of age and other variables on serum parathyroid hormone in postmenopausal women attending an osteoporosis center. *Journal of Clinical Endocrinology and Metabolism, 89*(4), 1646–1649.

Nemeroff, C. B. (2008). Recent findings in the pathophysiology of depression. *Focus, 6*, 3–14. Retrieved from http://focus.psychiatryonline.org/cgi/content/full/6/1/3

Never been the same since: Delirium in older people might have permanent effects on the brain. *Harvard Health Letter, 32*(6), 4.

New York State Department of Health. Task Force on Life and the Law. (1994, May). When death is sought. Albany, NY: New York State Department of Health. Retrieved November 13, 2008, from www.health.ny.gov/regulations/task_force/reports_publications/death.htm

New York University College of Nursing. (n.d.-a). Certification. Retrieved January 21, 2011, from www.consultgerirn.org/certification

New York University College of Nursing. (n.d.-b). Evidence-based geriatric topics. Retrieved January 21, 2011, from http://consultgerirn.org

New York University College of Nursing. (2010, January 5). Specialty Nursing Association endorse global vision statement on care of older adults. Retrieved January 15, 2011, from http://consultgerirn.org/specialty_practice/Global_Vision_Statement/

Niedert, K. C., & Dorner, B. (2004). *Nutrition care of the older adult: A handbook for dietetics professionals working throughout the continuum of care* (2nd ed.). Chicago, IL: American Dietetic Association.

Nilsson, U., Rawal, N., Enqvist, B., & Unosson, M. (2003). Analgesia following music and therapeutic suggestions in the PACU in ambulatory surgery; a randomized controlled trial. *ACTA Anaesthesiologica Scandanavia, 47*, 278–283.

Nilsson, U., Unosson, M., & Rawal, N. (2005). Stress reduction and analgesia in patients exposed to calming music postoperatively: A randomized controlled trial. *European Journal of Anaesthesiology, 22*, 96–102.

Nilsson, U. (2008). The anxiety- and pain-reducing effects of music interventions: A systematic review. *AORN Journal, 87*(4), 780–807.

Nimalasuylya, K., Compton, M. T., & Guillory, V.J. (2009). Screening adults for depression in primary care: A position statement of the American College of Preventive Medicine. *The Journal of Family Practice, 58*(10), 535–538.

O'Connell, M. (2006). Positioning impact on the surgical patient. *Nursing Clinics of North America, 41*(2), 173–192.

O'Mahony, D., & Gallagher, P. (2008). Inappropriate prescribing in the older population: Need for new criteria. *Age and Ageing, 37*, 138–141.

Ollivere, B., Ellahee, N., Logan, K., Miller-Jones, J., & Allen, P. (2008). Asymptomatic urinary tract colonisation predisposes to superficial wound infection in elective orthopaedic surgery. *International Orthaepedics, 33*(2), 847–850.

Olorunto, W., & Galandiuk, S. (2006). Managing the spectrum of surgical pain: Acute management of the chronic pain patient. *Journal of the American College of Surgeons, 202*(1), 169–175.

Olver, I., Whitford, H., Denson, L., Peterson, M., & Olver, S. (2009). Improving informed consent to chemotherapy: A randomized controlled trial of written information versus an interactive multimedia CD-ROM. *Patient Education and Counseling, 74,* 197–204.

Ottenbacher, K., Graham, J., Al Snih, S., Raji, M., Samper-Ternent, R., Ostir, G., & Markides, K. (2009). Mexican Americans and frailty: Findings from the Hispanic established populations epidemiologic studies of the elderly. *American Journal of Public Health, 99*(4), 673–679.

Ouldred, E., & Bryant, C. (2008). Dementia care. Part 1: Guidance and the assessment process. *British Journal of Nursing, 17*(3), 138–145.

Ozay, F. (2007). Social support and resilience to stress: From neurobiology to clinical practice. *Psychiatry, 4*(5), 35–40.

Paciaroni, E., Fraticelli, A., & Antonicelli, R. (1996). Arterial hypertension in the elderly: A review. *Archives of Gerontology and Geriatrics, 23*(3), 257–264.

Page, R., & Ruscin, J. (2006). The risk of adverse drug events and hospital-related morbidity and mortality among older adults with potentially inappropriate medication use. *The American Journal of Geriatric Pharmacotherapy, 4*(4), 297–305.

Paillaud, E., Ferrand, E., Lejonc, J., Henry, O., Bouillanne, O., & Montagne, O. (2007). Medical information and surrogate designation: Results of a prospective study in elderly hospitalised patients. *Age and Ageing, 36,* 274–279.

Palmer, M. (2004). Physiologic and psychologic age-related changes that affect urologic clients. *Urologic Nursing, 24*(4), 247–252.

Palmisano-Mills, C. (2007). Common problems in hospitalized older adults: Four programs to improve care. *Journal of Gerontological Nursing, 33*(1), 48–54.

Pandharipande, P., & Ely, E. (2006). Sedative and analgesic medications: Risk factors for delirium and sleep disturbances in the critically ill. *Critical Care Clinics, 22*(2), 313–327.

Pandi-Perumal, S., Srinivasan, V., Spence, D., & Cardinali, D. (2007). Role of the melatonin system in the control of sleep: Therapeutic implications. *CNS Drugs, 21*(12), 995–1018.

Parker, S., Peet, S., McPherson, A., Cannaby, A., Abrams, K., Baker, R., . . . Jones, D. (2002). A systematic review of discharge arrangements for older people. *Health Technology Assessment, 6*(4), 1–183.

Pass, S., & Simpson, R. (2004). Discontinuation and reinstitution of medications during the perioperative period. *American Journal of Health-System Pharmacy, 61*(9), 899–912.

Passarino, G., Montesanto, A., DeRango, F., Garasto, S., Berardelli, M., Domma, F., . . . De Benedictis, G. (2007). A cluster analysis to define human aging phenotypes. *Biogerontology, 8,* 283–290.

Pathy, M. (2006). *Principles and practice of geriatric medicine* (4th ed.). Chichester, UK: John Wiley & Sons.

Pel-Littel, R., Schuurmans, M., Emmelot-Vonk, M., & Verhaar, H. (2009). Frailty: Defining and measuring of a concept. *The Journal of Nutrition, Health & Aging, 13*(4), 390–394.

Penrod, J., Litke, A., Hawkes, W., Magaziner, J., Doucette, J., Koval, K., . . . Siu, A. (2008). The association of race, gender, and comorbidity with mortality and function after hip fracture. *Journals of Gerontology Series A, Biological Sciences and Medical Sciences, 63*(8), 867–872.

Penson, R., Daniels, K., & Lynch Jr., T. (2004). Too old to care? *The Oncologist, 9*(3), 343–352.

Perell, K., Nelson, A., Goldman, R., Luther, S., Prieto-Lewis, N., & Rubenstein, L. (2001). Fall risk assessment measures: An analytic review. *Journals of Gerontology Series A, Biological Sciences and Medical Sciences, 56*(12), M761–M766.

Pergolizzi, J., Böger, R., Budd, K., Dahan, A., Erdine, S., Hans, G., . . . Sacerdote, P. (2008). Opioids and the management of chronic severe pain in the elderly: consensus statement of an International Expert Panel with focus on the six clinically most often used World Health Organization Step III opioids (buprenorphine, fentanyl, hydromorphone, methadone, morphine, oxycodone). *Pain Practice, 8*(4), 287–313.

Peterson, J. F., Pun, B. T., Dittus, R. S., Thomason, J. W. W., Jackson, J. C., Shintani, A. K., et al (2006) Delirium and its motoric subtypes: A study of 614 critically ill patients. *Journal of the American Geriatrics Society, 54*, 479–484.

Peterson, R. C. (2004). Mild cognitive impairment as a diagnostic entity. *Journal of Internal Medicine, 256*, 183–194.

Phillips, P., Johnston, C., & Gray, L. (1993). Distrubed fluid and electrolyte homoeostatsis following dehydration in elderly people. *Age and Ageing, 22*(1), S26–S33.

Picone, D., Titler, M., Dochterman, J., Shever, L., Kim, T., Abramowitz, P., . . . Qin, R. (2008). Predictors of medication errors among elderly hospitalized patients. *American Journal of Medical Quality, 23*(2), 115–127.

Pieper, B., Sieggreen, M., Freeland, B., Kulwicki, P., Frattaroli, M., Sidor, D., . . . Garretson, B. (2006). Discharge information needs of patients after surgery. *Journal of Wound, Ostomy and Continence Nursing, 33*(3), 281–289.

Pippins, J., Gandhi, T., Hamann, C., Ndumele, C., Labonville, S., Diedrichsen, E., . . . Schnipper, J. (2008). Classifying and predicting errors of inpatient medication reconciliation. *Journal of General Internal Medicine, 23*(9), 1414–1422.

Podrazik, P. (2009). CHAMP (Curriculum for the Hospitalized Aging Medical Patient) the hospitalized frail elder: Teaching strategies for identification and assessment. *POGOe - Portal of Geriatric Online Education*. Retrieved April 24, 2011, from www.pogoe.org/productid/20106

Poldermans, D., Hocks, S., & Feringa, H. (2008). Pre-operative risk assessment and risk reduction before surgery. *Journal of the American College of Cardiology, 51*(20), 1913–1924.

Porth, C. (1998). *Pathophysiology: Concepts of altered health states* (7th ed.). Philadelphia, PA: Lippincott Williams & Wilkins.

Powell, C. (1997). Frailty: Help or hindrance? *Journal of the Royal Society of Medicine, 32*, 23–26.

Pratt, W., Callery, M., & Vollmer Jr., C. (2008). Optimal surgical performance attenuated physiologic risk in high-acuity operations. *Journal of American College of Surgeons, 207*, 717–730.

Prestwood, K., & Kenny, A. (1998). Osteoporosis: Pathogenesis, diagnosis, and treatment in older adults. *Clinics in Geriatric Medicine, 14*(3), 577–599.

Price, J., Sear, J., & Venn, R. (2002). Perioperative fluid volume optimization following proximal femoral fracture. *Cochrane Database System Reviews, 1*. Retrieved March 11, 2011, from www2.cochrane.org/reviews/en/ab003004.html

Prowse, M. (2007). Postoperative pain in older people: A review of the literature. *Journal of Clinical Nursing, 16*, 84–97.

Pugh, K., & Wei, J. (2001). Clinical implications of physiological changes in the aging heart. *Drugs & Aging, 18*(4), 263–276.

Puts, M., Visser, M., Twisk, J., Deeg, D., & Lips, P. (2005). Endocrine and inflammatory markers as predictors of frailty. *Clinical Endocrinology, 63*(4), 403–411.

Quintana, J., Escobar, A., Aguirre, U., Lafuente, I., & Arenaza, J. (2009). Predictors of health-related quality-of-life change after total hip arthroplasty. *Clinical Orthopaedics and Related Research, 467*(11), 2886–2894.

Rahman, M., & Beattie, J. (2005). Managing post-operative pain through giving patients control. *The Pharmaceutical Journal, 275*, 145–148.

Rakel, B., & Herr, K. (2004). Assessment and treatment of postoperative pain in older adults. *Journal of Perianesthesia Nursing, 19*(3), 194–208.

Ramer, L., Richardson, J., Cohen, M., Bedney, C., Danley, K., & Judge, E. (1999). Multimeasure pain assessment in an ethnically diverse group of patients with cancer. *Journal of Transcultural Nursing, 10*, 94.

Rattan, S. (2006). Theories of biological aging: Genes, proteins, and free radicals. *Free Radical Research, 40*(12), 1230–1238.

Ray, W., Griffin, M., & Shorr, R. (1990). Adverse drug reactions and the elderly. *Health Affairs, 9*(3), 114–122.

Raymond, D., Pelletier, S., Crabtree, T., Schulman, A., Pruett, T., & Sawyer, R. (2001). Surgical infection and the aging population. *Journal of the American College of Surgeons, 67*(9), 827–832.

Redelmeier, D., McAlister, F., Kandel, C., Lu, H., & Daneman, N. (2010). Postoperative pneumonia in elderly patients receiving acid suppressants: A retrospective chart analysis. *British Medical Journal, 340*, c2608.

Reed, A. E., Mikels, J. A., & Simon, K. I. (2008). Older adults prefer less choice than young adults. *Psychology and Aging, 23*(3), 671–675.

Rengo, F., Acanfora, D., Trojano, L., Furgi, G., Picone, C., Iannuzzi, G., . . . Ferrara, N. (1996). Congestive heart failure in the elderly. *Archives of Gerontology and Geriatrics, 23*(3), 201–223.

Riall, T., & Lillemore, K. (2007). Underutilization of surgical resection in patients with localized pancreatic cancer. *Annals of Surgery, 246*(2), 181–182.

Ritz, P. (2000). Physiology of aging with respect to gastrointestinal, circulatory and immune system changes and their significance for energy and protein metabolism. *European Journal of Clinical Nutrition, 54*(Supplement 3), S21–S25.

Robinson, T., Eiseman, B., Wallace, J., Church, S., McFann, K., Pfister, S., . . . Moss, M. (2009). Redefining geriatric preoperative assessment using frailty, disability and co-morbidity. *Annals of Surgery, 250*(3), 449–455.

Rocchi, A., Chung, F., & Forte, L. (2002). Canadian survey of postsurgical pain and pain medication experiences. *Canadian Journal of Anesthesia, 49*(10), 1053–1056.

Rockwood, K., Fox, R., Stolee, P., Robertson, D., & Beattle, B. (1994). Frailty in elderly people: An evolving concept. *Canadian Medical Association Journal, 150*(4), 489–495.

Rockwood, K., Song, X., MacKnight, C., Bergman, H., Hogan, D., McDowell, I., & Mitmitski, A. (2005). A global clinical measure of fitness and frailty in elderly people. *Canadian Medical Association Journal, 173*(5), 489–495.

Rockwood, K., & Mitnitski, A. (2007). Frailty in relation to the accumulation of deficits. *Journal of Gerontology, 62A*(7), 723–727.

Rolfson, D. (2006, March 31). Bringing frailty into sharp clinical focus. *Medical Grand Rounds*. Lecture conducted from University of Alberta, Canada.

Rolfson, D. (2007, December 4). Is frailty a meaningful construct? Lecture conducted from Edmonton Senior's Coordinating Council, Edmonton, Alberta, Canada.

Rollnick, S., Miller, W., & Butler, C. (2008). *Motivational interview in health care: Helping patients change behavior*. New York, NY: Guilford Press.

Ronda, L., & Falce, C. (2002). Skin care principles in treating older people. *Primary Health Care, 12*(7), 51–57.

Rønning, B., Wyller, T., Seljeflot, I., Jordhøy, M., Skovlund, E., Nesbakken, A., & Kristjansson, S. (2010). Frailty measures, inflammatory biomarkers and post-operative complications in older surgical patients. *Age & Ageing, 39*(6), 758–761.

Rooke, G. (2003). Cardiovascular aging and anesthetic implications. *Journal of Cardiothoracic and Vascular Anesthesia, 17*(4), 512–523.

Rooks, D., Huang, J., Bierbaum, B., Bolus, S., Rubano, J., Connolly, C., . . . Katz, J. (2006). Effect of preoperative exercise on measures of functional status in men and women undergoing total hip and knee arthroplasty. *Arthritis and Rheumatism, 55*(5), 700–708.

Rosenthal, R., Zenilman, M., & Katlic, M. (2001). *Principles and practice of geriatric surgery.* New York, NY: Springer-Verlag.

Rubin, F., Williams, J., Lescisin, M., Mook, W., Hassan, S., & Inouye, S. (2006). Replicating the Hospital Elder Life program in a community based hospital and demonstrating effectiveness using quality improvement methodology. *Journal of the American Geriatrics Society, 54*(6), 969–974.

Rudolph, J., Jones, R., Rasmussen, L., Silverstein, J., Inouye, S., & Marcantonio, E. (2007). Independent vascular and cognitive risk factors for postoperative delirium. *The American Journal of Medicine, 120,* 807–813.

Russell, R. (1992). Changes in gastrointestinal function attributed to aging. *American Journal of Clinical Nutrition, 55*(6 Supplemental), S1203–S1207.

Russell, R. (2000). The aging process as a modifier of metabolism. *American Journal of Clinical Nutrition, 72*(2 Supplemental), S529–S532.

Saczynski, J. S., Beiser, A., Seshadri, S., Auerbach, S., Wolf, P. A., & Au, R. (2010). Depressive symptoms and risk of dementia. The Framingham heart study. *Neurology, 75,* 35–41.

Safar, M. (2006). Systolic hypertension in elderly patients. *Seminars in Cardiothoracic and Vascular Anesthesia, 10*(3), 203–205.

Sahni, M., Lowenthal, D., & Meuleman, J. (2005). A clinical, physiology and pharmacology evaluation of orthostatic hypotension in the elderly. *International Urology and Nephrology, 37*(3), 669–674.

Salzman, C. (2008). Pharmacologic treatment of disturbed sleep in the elderly. *Harvard Review of Psychiatry, 16*(5), 271–278.

Samuels, J., & Fetzer, S. (2009). Pain management documentation quality as a reflection of nurses' clinical judgement. *Journal of Nursing Care Quality, 24*(3), 223–231.

Sauaia, A., Min, S., Leber, C., Erbacher, K., Abrams, F., & Fink, R. (2005). Postoperative pain management in elderly patients: Correlation between adherence to treatment guidelines and patient satisfaction. *Journal of the American Geriatrics Society, 53,* 274–782.

Saufl, N. (2004). Preparing the older adult for surgery and anesthesia. *Journal of Perianesthesia Nursing, 19*(6), 372–378.

Schmader, K., Hanlon, J., Pieper, C., Sloane, R., Ruby, C., Twersky, J., . . . Cohen, H. (2004). Effects of geriatric evaluation and management on adverse drug reactions and suboptimal prescribing in the frail elderly. *American Journal of Medicine, 116,* 394–401.

Schopp, A., Valimaki, M., Leino-Kilpi, H., Dassen, T., Gasull, M., Lemonidou, C., . . . Kalijonen, A. (2003). Perceptions of informed consent in the care of elderly people in five European countries. *Nursing Ethics, 10*(1), 48–57.

Schouchoff, B. (2002). Pressure ulcer development in the operating room. *Critical Care Nursing Quarterly, 25*(1), 76–82.

Schuurmans, M. J., Shortridge-Baggett, L. M., & Duursma, S. A. (2003). The delirium observation screening scale: Screening Instrument for delirium. *Research and Theory for Nursing Practice: An International Journal, 17*(1), 31–50.

Scott, P., Välimäki, M., Leino-Kilpi, H., Dassen, T., Gasull, M., Lemonidou, C., & Arndt, M. (2003). Autonomy, privacy and informed consent 3: elderly care perspective. *British Journal of Nursing, 12*(3), 158–168.

Scott-Williams, S. (n.d.). Perioperative pressure ulcer prevention program (PPUPP): An innovative effort to prevent pressure ulcers in surgical patients. *American Academy of Nursing.* Retrieved March 11, 2011, from www.aannet.org/files/public/PPUPP_template.pdf

Severn, A. (2007). Anaesthesia and the preparation and management of elderly patients undergoing surgery. *European Journal of Cancer, 43*, 2231–2234.

Shardell, M., Hicks, G., Miller, R., Kritchevsky, S., Andersen, D., Bandinelli, S., . . . Ferrucci, L. (2009). Association of low vitamin D levels with the frailty syndrome in men and women. *Journal of Gerontology, 64A*(1), 69–75.

Sheahan, S., & Musialowski, R. (2001). Clinical implications of respiratory system changes in aging. *Journal of Gerontological Nursing, 27*(5), 26–34.

Sheehy, C., Perry, P., & Cromwell, S. (1999). Dehydration: Biological considerations, age-related changes, and risk factors in older adults. *Biological Research for Nursing, 1*(1), 30–37.

Shega, J., Emanuel, L., Vargish, L., Levine, S., Bursch, H., Herr, K., . . . Weiner, D. (2007). Pain in persons with dementia: Complex, common, and challenging. *The Journal of Pain, 8*(5), 373–378.

Shepard, S. (2009, August 21). Hospital discharge planning: Best practices to reduce preventable readmission. Lecture conducted by The Doctors Company. Available at http://www.gha.org/telnet/2422Hospital.pdf

Shields, G. (2004, June 16). Geriatric otolaryngology. *Grand Rounds Presentation*. Lecture conducted from University of Texas Medical Branch Department of Otolaryngology, Galveston, TX.

Shillerstrom, J. E., Horton, M. S., & Royall, D. R. (2005). The impact of medical illness on executive function. *Psychosomatics, 46*(6), 508–516.

Shippee-Rice, R. & Long, J. (2007, March 30). A new look at an old problem Part II: Gerioperative Care. *Annual Meeting*. Lecture conducted from New England Assembly of Nurse Anesthetists, Burlington, MA.

Shipton, E. A. (2008). Pain assessment in dementia. *The New Zealand Medical Journal, 121*(1286), 9–11.

Siebens, H., Aronow, H., Edwards, D., & Ghasemi, Z. (2000). A randomized controlled trial of exercise to improve outcomes of acute hospitalization in older adults. *Journal of the American Geriatrics Society, 48*(12), 1545–1552.

Sieber, F. E. (2007). *Geriatric anesthesia*. New York, NY: McGraw-Hill Professional.

Sigworth, S. (2008). Preoperative evaluation of hospitalized patients. *Mt. Sinai Journal of Medicine, 75*(5), 442–448.

Silverman, D., & Rosenbaum, S. (2009). Integrated assessment and consultation for the preoperative patient. *Medical Clinics of North America, 93*, 963–977.

Smetana, G., Lawrence, V., & Cornell, J. (2005). Preoperative pulmonary risk stratification for noncardiothoracic surgery: Systematic review for the American College of Physicians. *Annals of Internal Medicine, 144*, 581–595.

Society of Hospital Medicine. (2005). Ideal discharge for the elderly patient: a hospital checklist. (2005). Retrieved April 5, 2011, from http://www.hospitalmedicine.org/AM/Template.cfm?Section=QI_Clinical_Tools&Template=/CM/ContentDisplay.cfm&ContentID=10303

Society of Hospital Medicine. (2008). BOOSTing care transitions. Retrieved March 11, 2011, from www.hospitalmedicine.org/ResourceRoomRedesign/RR_CareTransitions/Boost

Solomonow, M. (2006). Sensory-motor control of ligaments and associated neuromuscular disorders. *Journal of Electromyography and Kinesiology, 16*(6), 549–567.

Spiller, J. (2006) Hypoactive delirium: Assessing the extent of the problem for inpatient specialist palliative care. *Palliative Care, 20*, 17–23.

Sprung, J., Gajic, O., & Warner, D. (2006). Review article: Age related alterations in respiratory function—anesthetic considerations. *Canadian Journal Anaesthesia, 53*(12), 1244–1257.

St-Arnaud, D., & Paquin, M. (2000). Safe positioning for neurosurgical patients. *AORN Journal*, *87*(6), 1156–1172.

Steinman, M., Landefeld, C., Rosenthal, G., Berthenthal, D., Sen, S., & Kaboli, P. (2006). Polypharmacy and prescribing quality in older people. *Journal of the American Geriatrics Society*, *54*, 1516–1523.

Steinmetz, J., & Rasmussen, L. (2010). The elderly and general anesthesia. *Minerva Anestesiologica*, *76*(9), 745–752.

STERIS Corporation. (2003). *Intraoperative patient positioning: It's more than just comfort.* Mentor, OH: STERIS Corporation.

Stibich, M. (2009, January 24). Why we age—theories and effects of aging. *Understanding Aging.* Retrieved February 17, 2011, from http://longevity.about.com/od/longevity101/a/why_we_age.htm

Stotts, N., & Wu, H. (2007). Hospital recovery is facilitated by prevention of pressure ulcers in older adults. *Critical Care Nursing Clinics of North America*, *19*(3), 269–275.

Stovring, H., Gyrd-Hansen, D., Kristiansen, I. S., Nexoe, J., & Nielsen, J. (2008). Communicating effectiveness of intervention for chronic diseases: What single format can replace comprehensive information? *BMC Medical Informatics and Decision Making*, *8*(25). Retrieved March 11, 2011, from http://www.biomedcentral.com/1472-6947/8/25

Studenski, S., Perera, S., Patel, K., Rosano, C., Faulkner, K., Inzitari, M., . . .Guralnik, J. (2011). Gait speed and survival in older adults. *Journal of the American Medical Association*, *305*(1), 50–58.

Sullivan, E. (2004). Issues of informed consent in the geriatric population. *Journal of Perianesthesia Nursing*, *19*(6), 430–432.

Suter, P. Depression revealed: The need for screening, treatment and nursing. *Home Healthcare Nurse*, *26*(9), 543–550.

Swaminathan, A., & Naderi, S. (2010, March 15). Pneumonia, aspiration. *eMedicine.* Retrieved October 14, 2010, from emedicine.medscape.com/article/807600-print

Tan, T., Ding, Y., & Lee, A. (2001). Impaired mobility in older persons attending a geriatric assessment clinic: Causes and management. *Singapore Medical Journal*, *42*(2), 68–72.

Theadon, A., & Cropley, M. (2006). Effects of preoperative smoking cessation on the incidence and risk of intraoperative and postoperative complications in adult smokers: a systematic review. *Tobacco Control*, *15*(5), 352–358.

Theou, O., & Kloseck, M. (2008). Tools to identify community-dwelling older adults in different stages of frailty. *Physical & Occupational Therapy in Geriatrics*, *26*(3), 1–21.

Thomas, D. (2001). Age-related changes in wound healing. *Drugs & Aging*, *18*(8), 607–620.

Thomas, E., Peat, G., Harris, L., Wilkie, R., & Croft, P. (2004). The prevalence of pain and pain interference in a general population of older adults: Cross-sectional findings from the North Staffordshire Osteoarthritis Project (NorStOP). *Pain*, *110*, 361–368.

Titler, M., & Herr, K. (2004). Evidence-based assessment of acute pain in older adults: Current nursing practices and perceived barriers. *Clinical Journal of Pain*, *20*(5), 331–340.

Topinkova, E. (2008). Aging, disability and frailty. *Annals of Nutrition and Metabolism*, *52*(Supplement 1), 6–11.

Topp, R., Swank, A., Quesada, P., Nyland, J., & Malkani, A. (2009). The effect of prehabilitation exercise on strength and functioning after total knee arthroplasty. *Physical Medicine & Rehabilitation*, *1*(8), 729–735.

Torpy, J. (2006). Frailty in older adults. *The Journal of the American Medical Association*, *296*(18), 2280.

Torres, M., & Moayedi, S. (2007). Evaluation of the acutely dyspneic elderly patient. *Clinics in Geriatric Medicine*, *23*, 307–325.

Tulsky, J. A. (2005). Interventions to enhance communication among patients, providers, and families. *Journal of Palliative Medicine, 8*(s1), S95–S102.

Turnheim, K. (2003). When drug therapy gets old: Pharmacokinetics and pharmacodynamics in the elderly. *Experimental Gerontology, 38*, 843–853.

Twiss, E., Seaver, J., & McCaffrey, R. (2006). The effect of music listening on older adults undergoing cardiovascular surgery. *Nursing in Critical Care, 11*(5), 224–231.

U.S. Census Bureau. (2008). U.S. interim projections by age, sex, race, and Hispanic origin: 2000–2050. *Population projections.* Retrieved March 11, 2011, from www.census.gov/population/www/projections/usinterimproj/

Vadivelu, N., Whitney, C., & Sinatra, R. (2009). Pain pathways and acute pain processing. In R. S. Sinatra, O. A. de Leon-Cassasola, B. Ginsberg, & E. R. Viscusi (Eds.), *Acute pain management* (pp. 3–11). Cambridge: Cambridge University Press.

Variand, H., & Gopal, Y. V. (2008). Late-onset depression: Issues affecting clinical care. *Advances in Psychiatric Treatment, 14*, 152–158.

Van Norman, G. (1998). Informed consent in the operating room. *Ethics in medicine.* Available at: http://depts.washington.edu./bioethx/topics/infc.html

Van Rompaey, B., Elseviers, M. M., Schuurmans, M. J., Shortbridge-Baggett, L. M., Truijen, S., & Bossaert, L. (2009). Risk factors for delirium in intensive care patients: A prospective cohort study. *Critical Care,13*(3). Retrieved from http://ccforum.com/content/13/3/R77 doi:10.1186/cc7892

Veterans' Administration Center for Medication Safety. (2006). *Adverse drug events, adverse drug reactions and mediation errors: frequently asked question.* Washington, DC: Veterans Administration Center for Medication Safety.

Vicky, R. N. (2009, August 2). *Theories of aging (part 3) - sociological theories.* Retrieved Retrieved Feburary 18, 2011, from http://allnurses-central.com/showthread.php?t=412760

Voyer, P. Cole, M. G., McCusker, J., & Belzile, E. (2006). Signs and symptoms of delirium superimposed on dementia. *Clinical Nursing Research,15*, 46–66.

Voyer, P., Cole, M. G., Mccusker, J., St-Jacques, S., & Laplante, J. (2008) Accuracy of nurse documentaion of delirium symptoms in medical charts. *International Journal of Nursing Practice, 14*, 165–177.

Wade, P. (2002). Aging and neural control of the GI tract. Age-related changes in the enteric nervous system. *American Journal of Physiology Gastrointestinal and liver physiology, 283*(3), G489–G495.

Wadensten, B. (2006). An analysis of psychosocial theories of ageing and their relevance to practical gerontological nursing in Sweden. *Scandinavian Journal of Caring Sciences, 20*(3), 347–354.

Walston, J. (2006). Frailty as a model of aging. In P. M. Conn (Ed.), *Handbook of models for human aging* (pp. 697–702). Amsterdam, Netherlands: Elsevier Academic Press.

Waltson, J., McBurnie, M., Newman, A., Tracy, R., Kop, W., Hirsch, C., . . . Fried, L. (2002). Frailty and activation of the inflammation and coagulation systems with and without clinical comorbidities. *Archives of Internal Medicine, 162*, 2333–2341.

Wanzer, L. (2005). Perioperative initiatives for medication safety. *Patient Safety First, 82*(4), 663–666.

Warden, V., Hurley, A., & Volicer, L. (2003). Development and psychometric evaluation of the pain assessment in advanced dementia (PAINAD) scale. *Journal of the American Medical Directors Association, 4*(1), 9–15.

Waszynski, C., & Petrovic, K. (2008). Nurses' evaluation of the Confusion Assessment Method. *Journal of Gerontological Nursing, 34*(4), 49–56.

Watson, R. (1994). Practical ethical issues related to the care of elderly people with dementia. *Nursing Ethics, 1*(3), 151–162.

Weinberger, M. I., Raue, P. J., Meyers, B. S., & Bruce, M. L. (2009). Predictors of new onset depression in medically ill, disables older adults at 1 year follow-up. *American Journal of Geriatric Psychiatry, 17*(9), 802–809.

Weiner, D., Herr, K., & Rudy, T. (2002). *Persistent pain in older adults: An interdisciplinary guide for treatment.* New York, NY: Springer Publishing Company.

Weinert, B., & Timiras, P. (2003). Invited review: Theories of aging. *Journal of Applied Physiology, 95*(4), 1706–1716.

Weisbein, J. (n.d.). Introduction to IV therapy. Lecture conducted from Westchester General Hospital, Miami, FL.

Westerdahl, E., & Moller, M. (2010). Physiotherapy-supervised mobilization and exercise following cardiac surgery: A national questionnaire survey in Sweden. *Journal of Cardiothoracic Surgery, 25*(5), 67.

Wetsch, W., Pircher, I., Lederer, W., Kinzi, J., Traweger, C., Heinz-Erian, P., & Benzer, A. (2009). Preoperative stress and anxiety in daycare patients and in patients undergoing fast-track surgery. *British Journal of Anaesthesia, 103*(2), 199–205.

Whinney, C. (2009). Perioperative medication management: General principles and practical applications. *Cleveland Clinic Journal of Medicine, 76*(Supplement 4), S126–S132.

Whiting, N. (2009). Skin assessment of patients at risk of pressure ulcers. *Nursing Standard, 24*(10), 40–44.

Whitson, H., Purser, J., & Cohen, H. (2007). Frailty thy name is . . . phrailty? *Journal of Gerontology Series A Biological Sciences and Medical Sciences, 62A*(7), 728–730.

Williams, A. (2008). Post-operative pain. *Nursing Standard, 23*, 59.

Williams, A., Sloan, F., & Lee, P. (2006). Longitudinal rates of cataract surgery. *Archives of Ophthalmology, 124*, 1308–1314.

Williams, B., Anderson, M., & Day, R. (2007). Undergraduate nursing student knowledge of and attitudes toward aging: A comparison of context-based learning and a traditional program. *Journal of Nursing Education, 46*(3), 115–120.

Williams, C. (2002). Using medications appropriately in older adults. *American Family Physician, 66*(10), 1917–1924.

Williams Jr., T., & Ellison, E. (2008). Population analysis predicts a future critical shortage of surgeons. *Surgery, 144*, 548–556.

Willson, H. (2000). Factors affecting the administration of analgesia to patients following repair of a fractured hip. *Journal of Advanced Nursing, 31*(5), 1145–1154.

Wilson, R. S., Hoganson, G. M., Rajan, K. B., Barnes, L. L. Mendes de Leon, C. F., & Evans, D. A. (2010). Temporal course of depressive symptoms during the development of Alzheimer disease. *Neurology, 75*, 21–26.

Wilson-Barnett, J. (1986). Ethical dilemmas in nursing. *Journal of Medical Ethics, 12*(3), 123–126, 135.

Windsor, J., & Hill, G. (1988). Risk factors for postoperative pneumonia: The importance of protein depletion. *Annals of Surgery, 208*(2), 209–214.

Witherington, E., Pirzada, O., & Avery, A. (2008). Communication gaps and readmissions to hospital for patients aged 75 years and older: Observational study. *Quality & Safety in Health Care, 17*(1), 71–75.

Wong, C., Holroyd-Leduc, J., Simel, D. L., & Straus, S. E. (2010). Does this patient have delirium?: Value of bedside instruments. *Journal of the American Medical Association, 304*(7), 779–786.

Wong, J., Bajcar, J., Wong, G., Alibhai, S., Huh, J., Cesta, A., . . . Fernandes, O. (2008). Medication reconciliation at hospital discharge: Evaluating discrepancies. *Annals Of Pharmacotherapy, 42*(10), 1373–1379.

Woolcott, J., Richardson, K., Wiens, M., Patel, B., Marin, J., Khan, K., & Marra, C. (2009). Meta-analysis of the impact of 9 medication classes on falls in elderly persons. *Archives of Internal Medicine, 169*(21), 1952–1960.

Woolger, J. (2008). Preoperative testing and medication management. *Clinics in Geriatric Medicine, 24*, 573–583.

World Health Organization India. (n.d.). Principles of geriatric surgery. Retrieved March 16, 2011, from www.whoindia.org/LinkFiles/Health_Care_for_the_Elderly_Guidelines_com_surg_interventaion_3.pdf

World Union of Wound Healing Societies. (2004). Minimizing pain at wound dressing-related procedures: a consensus document. *Principles of best practice: A World Union of Wound Healing Societies' Initiative.* Retrieved March 16, 2011 from www.wuwhs.org/datas/2_1/2/A_consensus_document_-_Minimising_pain_at_wound_dressing_related_procedures.pdf

Wren, S., Martin, M., Yoon, J., & Bech, F. (2010). Postoperative pneumonia—prevention program for the inpatient surgical ward. *Journal of the American College of Surgeons, 210*(4), 491–495.

Wrenn, H. (2006) Perioperative nursing. Retrieved from http://cfcc.edu/adn/documents/PerioperativeNursing.pdf

Wuhrman, E., Cooney, M., Dunwoody, C., Eksterowicz, N., Merkel, S., & Oakes, L. (2007). Authorized and unauthorized ("PCA by Proxy") dosing of analgesic infusion pumps: Position statement with clinical practice recommendations. *Pain Management Nursing, 8*(1), 4–11.

Yeager, M., & Spence, B. (2006). Perioperative fluid management: Current consensus and controversies. *Seminars in Dialysis, 19*(6), 472–479.

Young, J. (2007) Red flags in geriatrics: Diagnoses not to be missed in acute units. *Clinical Medicine, 7*(5) 512–514.

Young, J., & Inouye, S. (2007). Delirium in older people. *British Medical Journal, 334*, 842–846.

Zeeh, J. (2001). The aging liver: Consequences for drug treatment in old age. *Archives of Gerontology and Geriatrics, 32*(3), 255–263.

Zegerman, A., Ezri, T., & Weinbroum, A. (2008). Postoperative discomfort (other than pain)—a neglected feature of postanesthesia patient care. *Journal of Clinical Monitoring and Computing, 22*, 279–284.

Index